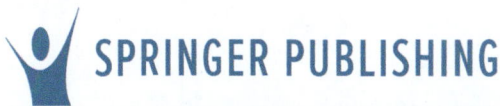 

GET THE MOST FROM YOUR BOOK

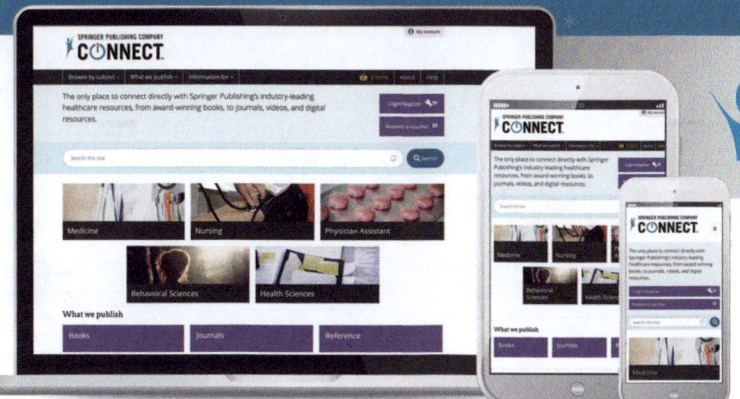

VOUCHER CODE:

PF4EU5V8

Online Access

Your print purchase of *DNP Role Development for Doctoral Advanced Nursing Practice,* Third Edition, includes **online access via Springer Publishing Connect**™ to increase accessibility, portability, and searchability.

Insert the code at http://connect.springerpub.com/content/book/978-0-8261-8137-4 or scan the QR code and insert the voucher code today!

Having trouble? Contact our customer service department at **cs@springerpub.com**

Instructor Resource Access for Adopters

Let us do some of the heavy lifting to create an engaging classroom experience with a variety of instructor resources included in most textbooks SUCH AS:

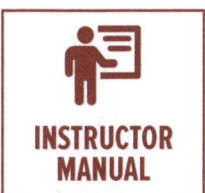  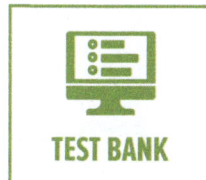

Visit **https://connect.springerpub.com/** and look for the **"Show Supplementary"** button on your **book homepage** to see what is available to instructors! First time using Springer Publishing Connect?

Email **textbook@springerpub.com** to create an account and start unlocking valuable resources.

DNP Role Development for Doctoral Advanced Nursing Practice

H. MICHAEL DREHER, PhD, RN, FAAN, ANEF, has long been an innovator in nursing and healthcare professions, both nationally and internationally. He is currently Professor of Nursing and Interim Dean of Health Sciences at the College of Staten Island, City University of New York (CUNY). He was also recently the Acting Chair of the Department of Nursing, overseeing the DNP program. Previously, he was Assistant Vice President and Associate Provost at Medgar Evers College, CUNY, in Brooklyn. At Medgar, he launched a BS in Financial Economics, the first fully online undergraduate degree program at CUNY. He served as Associate Vice President for Healthcare Innovation and Special Projects at The College of New Rochelle from 2017 to 2019 and Dean of the School of Nursing and Healthcare Professions from 2014 to 2017. At Drexel, he co-created a 5-year Co-op BS in Nursing, which became the largest provider of baccalaureate-prepared nurses in Pennsylvania, and developed an MS in Nursing Innovation. As the founding Chair of the Doctoral Nursing Department, he also launched one of the first Doctor of Nursing Practice programs in the United States, which included the first mandatory study abroad program for doctoral students. He has served as Associate Editor of *Holistic Nursing Practice*, writing a column on "Innovation, Health, and Healing," Associate Editor of *Clinical Scholars Review: The Journal of Doctoral Nursing Practice*, and Column Editor for "Practice Evidence." He is recognized as a national and international scholar on the professional/ practice doctorate. In 2010, he was appointed as the only non-UK citizen to the UK Council on Graduate Education's *2011 Report on Professional Doctorates* Review Panel. He is the co-author of six books, three of which have won the *American Journal of Nursing* Book-of-the-Year Award. His most recent book was by ME Smith Glasgow, HM Dreher, MD Dahnke, and J. Gyllenhammer (JD), *Legal and Ethical Issues in Nursing Education: An Essential Guide, 2e* (2021). He has been funded by the John A. Hartford Foundation, the Center for American Nurses, HRSA, and various other agencies. He was inducted as a Fellow in the American Academy of Nursing in 2012 and an Academy of Nursing Education Fellow in 2017. He is a graduate of the University of South Carolina, Widener University, and the University of Pennsylvania.

MARY ELLEN SMITH GLASGOW, PhD, RN, ACNS-BC, ANEF, FNAP, FAAN, serves as Dean and Professor of Duquesne University School of Nursing. She has also served as Vice-Provost of Research during part of her current tenure at Duquesne. Dr. Glasgow previously served as Associate Dean for Nursing, Undergraduate Health Professions, and Continuing Education and Chair of Undergraduate Programs at Drexel University. Dr. Glasgow was selected as a 2009 Robert Wood Johnson Foundation Executive Nurse Fellow. As dean, under her leadership, enrollment and NCLEX-RN scores increased, and research and scholarship significantly expanded. Duquesne University School of Nursing is recognized as a national leader in nursing education, emphasizing social justice, digital technologies, and graduates with strong ethical reasoning skills. In 2015, she led the development of the first dual undergraduate Biomedical Engineering and Nursing Program in the country, and in 2017, a PhD in Nursing Ethics. Dr. Glasgow is an innovator in nursing and health professions, both nationally and internationally. At Drexel, she created a BSN Co-op Program, a BSN Accelerated Career Entry Program, Pathway to Health Professions Program, and other forward-thinking educational programs. She also advanced online pedagogy, developing one of the largest online nursing programs in the country. She previously served as Associate Editor for *Oncology Nursing Forum*, responsible for the Leadership and Professional Development feature column. She is the co-author of four books, two of which have won first place in the *American Journal of Nursing* Book-of-the-Year Award. Dr. Glasgow has authored over 100 articles and book chapters and has presented nationally and internationally. She was inducted as a Fellow in the American Academy of Nursing, NLN Academy of Nursing Education Fellow, and as a Distinguished Fellow in the National Academies of Practice. She has been honored with the Villanova University College of Nursing Alumni Medallion for Distinguished Contribution to Nursing Education and received the Distinguished Alumni Award from Gwynedd-Mercy University. Recently, she served on the Health Service Executive and National Nursing and Midwifery Quality-Care Metrics Project Team to develop quality metrics for the country of Ireland.

MICHAEL D. DAHNKE, PhD, is a philosopher and bioethicist. He received his PhD in philosophy from Temple University and a BA in liberal studies from Bowling Green State University. In his career, he has worked across many interdisciplinary fields: Healthcare Ethics, Nursing Ethics, Medical Humanities, Healthcare Administration, Philosophy of Science in Nursing Practice, and Cultural Issues in Healthcare. His early work was in Aesthetics. He is the author and coauthor of four books: *Film, Art, and Filmart: An Introduction to Aesthetics Through Film* (2007); first author on *Philosophy of Nursing Science for Nursing Practice: Concepts* (2011), which received a five-star review from *Doody's* (less than 2% of all health profession books reviewed earn this distinction). The second edition of this book (2016) received second place in the *American Journal of Nursing's* Book-of-the-Year Awards in the Research Category. He was also coauthor of ME Smith Glasgow, HM Dreher, MD Dahnke, and J. Gyllenhammer's (2020) *Legal and Ethical Issues in Nursing Education: An Essential Guide*. He has taught students in healthcare fields including nursing (bachelor's, master's, and doctoral), physician assistant, behavioral health science, and healthcare administration, as well as undergraduates from all types of majors in his Introduction to Philosophy, Ethics, Logic, and Business Ethics courses. He has published (and sometimes mentored undergraduate students as first author) in *Critical Care Nurse, Journal of Bioethical Enquiry, Emergency Nursing, Advances in Health Sciences Education, International Journal of Healthcare Management, Journal of Neonatal Nursing, Holistic Nursing Practice, Auslegung: A Journal of Philosophy, MedSurg Nursing,* and *Philosophy Now.* Dr. Dahnke's most influential work has been examining some fewer known aspects of the Terri Schiavo case, publishing "What we learn (and don't learn) from the Terri Schiavo autopsy" in *Functional Neurology, Rehabilitation, and Ergonomics* and "Levinas and the face of Terri Schiavo: Bioethical and phenomenological reflections on a public spectacle and private tragedy" in *Theoretical Medicine and Bioethics*. He was previously Clinical Associate Professor in the Department of Health Administration and Division of Graduate Nursing at Drexel University and Clinical Associate Professor in the School of Nursing and Health Professions at The College of New Rochelle. He is currently Adjunct Assistant Professor at the College of Staten Island, City University of New York (CUNY) and teaches at Seton Hall University.

VALERIE T. COTTER, DrNP, AGPCNP-BC, FAANP, FAAN is Associate Professor, Johns Hopkins University, with a joint appointment in the School of Nursing and School of Medicine, Department of Psychiatry and Behavioral Sciences. She received academic degrees from Drexel University (DrNP), University of Pennsylvania (MSN), and University of Massachusetts (BSN). Dr. Cotter leads with four decades of sustained experience in nursing education, research, and specialty care of persons with dementia and their care partners. She has extensive teaching experience in academic nursing and interprofessional programs, as Director of the University of Pennsylvania's Gerontological Nurse Practitioner Program and Educational Director of the Alzheimer's Disease and Research Center as well as core faculty of Cognitive Impairment Programs at the Delaware Valley Mid-Atlantic Geriatric Education Center. She is a Fellow of the American Association of Nurse Practitioners and American Academy of Nursing, Cambia Health Foundation Sojourns Scholar, and coeditor/author of two books, over 50 publications and numerous national and international presentations.

DNP Role Development for Doctoral Advanced Nursing Practice

THIRD EDITION

H. Michael Dreher, PhD, RN, FAAN, ANEF

Mary Ellen Smith Glasgow, PhD, RN, ACNS-BC, ANEF, FNAP, FAAN

Michael D. Dahnke, PhD

Valerie T. Cotter, DrNP, AGPCNP-BC, FAANP, FAAN

EDITORS

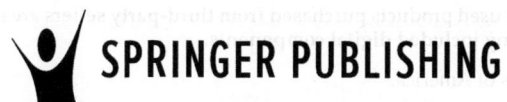

Copyright © 2025 Springer Publishing Company, LLC

All rights reserved.

First Springer Publishing edition 978-08261-0556-1 (2010); subsequent editions 2016

No part of this publication may be reproduced, stored in a retrieval system, or transmitted in any form or by any means, electronic, mechanical, photocopying, recording, or otherwise, without the prior permission of Springer Publishing Company, LLC, or authorization through payment of the appropriate fees to the Copyright Clearance Center, Inc., 222 Rosewood Drive, Danvers, MA 01923, 978-750-8400, fax 978-646-8600, info@copyright.com or at www.copyright.com.

Springer Publishing Company, LLC
902 Carnegie Center, Suite 140, Princeton, NJ 08540
www.springerpub.com
connect.springerpub.com

Acquisitions Editor: Joseph Morita
Production Editor: Dennis Troutman
Compositor: Exeter Premedia Services Pvt Ltd.

ISBN: 978-0-8261-8136-7
ebook ISBN: 978-0-8261-8137-4
DOI: 10.1891/9780826181374

SUPPLEMENTS:

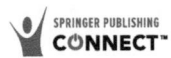 A robust set of instructor resources designed to supplement this text is located at http://connect.springerpub.com/content/book/978-0-8261-8137-4. Qualifying instructors may request access by emailing textbook@springerpub.com.

Instructor Materials:
PowerPoints 978-0-8261-8138-1
Transition Guide 978-0-8261-8162-6
Course Cartridge 978-0-8261-8161-9
AACN Mapping Grid 978-0-8261-8139-8

24 25 26 27 / 5 4 3 2 1

The author and the publisher of this Work have made every effort to use sources believed to be reliable to provide information that is accurate and compatible with the standards generally accepted at the time of publication. Because medical science is continually advancing, our knowledge base continues to expand. Therefore, as new information becomes available, changes in procedures become necessary. We recommend that the reader always consult current research and specific institutional policies before performing any clinical procedure or delivering any medication. The author and publisher shall not be liable for any special, consequential, or exemplary damages resulting, in whole or in part, from the readers' use of, or reliance on, the information contained in this book. The publisher has no responsibility for the persistence or accuracy of URLs for external or third-party Internet websites referred to in this publication and does not guarantee that any content on such websites is, or will remain, accurate or appropriate.

Library of Congress Cataloging-in-Publication Data

Names: Dreher, H. Michael, editor. | Glasgow, Mary Ellen Smith, editor. |
  Dahnke, Michael D., editor. | Cotter, Valerie T., editor.
Title: Dnp role development for doctoral advanced nursing practice /
  H. Michael Dreher, Mary Ellen Smith Glasgow, Michael D. Dahnke, Valerie
  T. Cotter.
Description: Third edition. | New York : Springer Publishing Company, 2024.
  | Includes bibliographical references and index.
Identifiers: LCCN 2023048551 (print) | LCCN 2023048552 (ebook) | ISBN
  9780826181367 (paperback) | ISBN 9780826181374 (ebook)
Classification: LCC RT75 (print) | LCC RT75 (ebook) | DDC
  610.73071/1--dc23/eng/20231215
LC record available at https://lccn.loc.gov/2023048551
LC ebook record available at https://lccn.loc.gov/2023048552

Contact sales@springerpub.com to receive discount rates on bulk purchases.

Publisher's Note: **New and used products purchased from third-party sellers are not guaranteed for quality, authenticity, or access to any included digital components.**

Printed in the United States of America.

Health care delivery systems are "held together,
glued together, enabled to function
... by the nurses."

—*Adapted from Lewis Thomas (Physician, Essayist, Researcher)*

To my lifetime companion of 25 years. Thank you for all
you do for me.
—*Heyward Michael Dreher*

This book is lovingly dedicated to my husband Tom.
Thank you for your love, support, and kindness. This book is also dedicated to
my dad, Frank Smith who passed away in 2021,
whose voice still guides me.
—*Mary Ellen Smith Glasgow*

To my loving husband who puts up with more than any husband should have to.
—*Michael Dahnke*

I dedicate this book to my three coeditors—Drs Dreher,
Smith-Glasgow, and Dahnke, who were inspirational and
supportive faculty in my doctoral program. I'm grateful for the
opportunity to work with each of you on this third edition.
—*Valerie T. Cotter*

Contents

Contributors xiii
Foreword xix
Preface xxi
Springer Publishing Resources xxv

SECTION I: HISTORICAL AND THEORETICAL FOUNDATIONS FOR ROLE DELINEATION AND PREPARATION IN DOCTORAL ADVANCED NURSING PRACTICE

1. **The Historical and Political Path of Doctoral Nursing Education to the Doctor of Nursing Practice Degree**   3
   H. Michael Dreher
   Reflective Response—Richard Cowling, III   **49**

2. **Professional and Doctor of Nursing Practice Roles in Nursing: A Theoretical and Historical Approach**   51
   H. Michael Dreher and Jeannine Uribe
   Reflective Response—Zane Wolf   **77**

3. **The Evolution of Advanced Practice Nursing Roles**   79
   Marcia R. Gardner, Bobbie Posmontier, Michael E. Conti, and Debra Hanna
   Reflective Response 1—Dana Pearlman   **109**
   Reflective Response 2—Michael Neft   **112**
   Reflective Response 3—Ksenia Zukowsky   **115**
   Reflective Response 4—Mary T. Bouchaud   **118**

4. **What Is Evidence?**   121
   Michael D. Dahnke
   Reflective Response—Graham J. McDougall, Jr.   **138**

5. **Engaging in Evidence-Based Practice to Maximize Healthcare Outcomes by the Advanced Practice Registered Nurse**   143
   Cindy Zellefrow and Bernadette Melnyk
   Reflective Response—Jennifer DeBerg   **165**

SECTION II: PRIMARY AND SECONDARY CONTEMPORARY ROLES FOR DOCTORAL ADVANCED NURSING PRACTICE

6. **The Role of the Practitioner**   169
   Diane C. Seibert
   Reflective Response—*Kymberlee Montgomery*   184

7. **The Role of the Clinical Executive**   187
   Barbara Wadsworth, Tukea L. Talbert, and Mary Ellen Smith Glasgow
   Reflective Response—*Diane S. Hupp and Mary Catherine Loughran*   209

8. **The Nurse Educator Role**   213
   Ruth A. Wittmann-Price and Dana Perlman
   Reflective Response 1—*Brittany Gaspar Nettles*   221
   Reflective Response 2—*Tiffany Pressley*   223
   Reflective Response 3—*Jennifer Lacy*   228

9. **The Clinical Scholar Role in Doctoral Advanced Nursing Practice**   229
   Brigit VanGraafeiland and Deborah Busch
   Reflective Response 1—*Brenda Douglass*   241
   Reflective Response 2—*Jessica L. Peck*   242
   Reflective Response 3—*Regena Spratling*   245

SECTION III: OPERATIONALIZING ROLE FUNCTIONS OF DOCTORAL ADVANCED NURSING PRACTICE

10. **Law and Ethics in Decision Making in the Doctoral Advanced Nursing Practice Role**   249
    Michael Dahnke
    Reflective Response—*Sharon Radzyminski*   260

11. **DNP as Applied Statistician**   263
    James Schreiber
    Reflective Response—*Maria Gilson deValpine and Matthew A. Jones*   282

12. **The Role of the DNP in Addressing Health Equity**   285
    Denise Lucas, Sr., Mary Meyers, and Janet Bischoff
    Reflective Response—*Roberta Waite and Deena A. Nardi*   304

13. **The DNP and Academic-Service Partnerships**   307
    Sandra Rader, Sandra Engberg, Shelley Watters, and Jacqueline Dunbar-Jacob
    Reflective Response—*Marie Ann Marino and Kate FitzPatrick*   317

14. **Coaching in the DNP Executive Role: Linking Personal Development and Performance Enhances Leadership Athleticism**   321
    Michael Smith and Rosalie Mainous
    Reflective Response—*Karen Kaufman and David Grad*   346

15. **Negotiation Skills in New Doctoral Advanced Nursing Practice Roles**   349
    H. Michael Dreher

    Reflective Response 1—*Tina Mertel*   365
    Reflective Response 2—*Catherine Paradiso*   367
    Reflective Response 3—*Rosemary Kunazcuk*   372
    Reflective Response 4—*Diane Maydick*   374
    Reflective Response 5—*Michael Conti*   378

16. **Three Real Career Role Trajectories From a Bedside Registered Nurse to a DNP-Prepared Family Nurse Practitioner**   379
    Veronica Quattrini, Courtney Hicks, Mary Grace Renfrow, Mary Marasa Radcliff, and Valerie T. Cotter

    Reflective Response—*Veronica Quattrini and Valerie T. Cotter*   387

17. **Interprofessional and Interdisciplinary Collaboration: Essential for the Doctoral Advanced Practice Nurse**   389
    Jihane Hajj, Kristen Nobles, and Mary Francis

    Reflective Response—*Bridgette Gourley*   399

18. **The DNP Graduate's Role in Health Policy and Advocacy**   401
    Sr. Rosemary Donley

    Reflective Response—*Deborah Dillon*   413

19. **The Role of the Doctoral-Prepared Nurse Leader During the COVID-19 Pandemic: Lessons Learned in Disruptive Times**   417
    Mary Beth Kingston and Claire Zangerle

    Reflective Response—*Cynthia Rost*   431

20. **Enhancing the Role of a Doctor of Nursing Practice Graduate: Two Models for Global Studies Experiences**   433
    Melanie T. Turk, H. Michael Dreher, Rick Zoucha, Manjulata Evatt, and Melissa A. Kalarchian

    Reflective Response—*Michele Bednarzyk*   459

21. **The Role of DNP-Prepared Nurses as Organizational and Clinical Preceptors**   461
    Yamini Teegala, Zyrene Marsh, Amanda Ambrosio, Laura O'Rourke, and Valerie T. Cotter

    Reflective Response 1—*Amanda Ambrosio*   466
    Reflective Response 2—*Laura O'Rourke*   467

22. **The Role of the DNP in Quality Improvement and Patient Safety Initiatives**   469
    Catherine Johnson and Eric Vogelstein

    Reflective Response—*Paula F. Coe*   497

23. **Stories of Successful Career Advancement Roles by DNP Graduates**   **499**
    Tammy Slater, Vanessa Battista, Jessica Peters, Laura O'Rourke, and Valerie T. Cotter
    Reflective Response—*Tammy Slater and Valerie T. Cotter*   **505**

24. **Analysis of the 2021 Essentials of Doctoral Education for Advanced Nursing Practice: Where Do We Go From Here?**   **509**
    Joan Rosen Bloch, Brenda Douglass, and Amanda Brock
    Reflective Response—*Mary F. Terhaar*   **542**

25. **Today, Tomorrow, and the Future: What Are the Critical Issues Facing Doctoral Advanced Practice Nursing?**   **545**
    Mary Ellen Smith Glasgow, David Campbell O'Dell, and H. Michael Dreher
    Reflective Response 1—*Janice M. Miller and Kathy Gray*   **559**
    Reflective Response 2—*Lorraine Frazier and Judy Honig*   **564**

Index   569

Contributors

Amanda Ambrosio, BS, CHW, Community Health and Social Impact Manager, Rocking Horse Communithy Health Center

Vanessa Battista, DNP, MBA, CPNP-PC, CHPPN, FPCN, FAAN, Senior Nursing Director, Palliative Care, Dana-Farber Cancer Institute

Michele Bednarzyk, DNP, FNP-BC, Associate Clinical Professor, University of North Florida

Janet Bischoff, PhD, RN, NE-Bc, CNE, Adjunct Faculty, Duquesne University

Joan Rosen Bloch, PhD, CRNP, FAAN, Emerita Faculty, Former Director of Global Health Initiatives, College of Nursing and Health Professions & School of Public Health, Drexel University

Mary T. Bouchaud, PhD, CNS, CCRN, Associate Professor, Thomas Jefferson University

Amanda Brock, MSN, MBE, RN, Associate Director of Clinical Research Nursing and Training, Perelman School of Medicine, University of Pennsylvania

Deborah Busch, DNP, CRNP, CPNP-BC, IBCLC, CNE, FAANP, FAAN, Director of the Pediatric Nurse Practitioner Tract, Associate Professor, School of Nursing, Johns Hopkins University

Paula F. Coe, DNP,MSN, RN, NEA-BC, FAONL, Vice President Nursing Education and Professional Practice, Allegheny Health Network

Michael E. Conti, PhD, CRNA, Staff Nurse Anesthesiologist, Dartmouth Hitchcock Medical Center Assistant; Clinical Professor, Geisel School of Medicine

Valerie T. Cotter, DrNP, AGPCNP-BC, FAANP, FAAN, Associate Professor, Johns Hopkins University

Richard Cowling III, RN, PhD, AHN-BC, SGAHN, ANEF, FAAN, Associate Professor, Department of Nursing Science, College of Nursing, East Carolina University

Michael D. Dahnke, PhD, Adjunct Assistant Professor at the College of Staten Island, City University of New York (CUNY) and teaches at Seton Hall University

Jennifer DeBerg, MLS, BS, OT, Clinical Education Librarian, University of Iowa Hardin Library

Maria Gilson deValpine, RN MSN PhD PMHNP-BC, James Madison University

Deborah Dillon, DNP, RN, CRNP, ACNP-BC, CCRN, CHFN, FAANP, FAAN, Clinical Associate Professor, AGACNP Program Director, Duquesne University

Sr. Rosemary Donley, PhD, APRM, BC, FAAN, Professor of Nursing and the Jacques Laval Chair for Justice for Vulnerable Populations, Duquesne University

H. Michael Dreher, PhD, RN, FAAN, ANEF, Professor of Nursing and Interim Dean of Health Sciences at the College of Staten Island, City University of New York (CUNY)

Brenda Douglass, DNP, APRN, FNP-C, CDCES, CTTS, Assistant Professor, Johns Hopkins University

Jacqueline Dunbar-Jacobs, PhD, RN, FAAN, Distinguished Service Professor and Dean Emerita, University of Pittsburgh

Sandra Engberg, PhD, RN, CRNP, FAAN, Professor Emeritus, School of Nursing, University of Pittsburgh

Manjulata Evatt, DNP, RN, CMSRN, Clinical Associate Professor, School of Nursing, Duquesne University

Kate FitzPatrick, DNP, RN, NEA-BC, FAAN, EVP/Connelly Foundation Chief Nurse Executive Officer; Professor and Associate Dean, Jefferson Health; Jefferson College of Nursing

Mary Francis, RN, PHD, ACNP-BC, Director of AGACNP Program; Associate Professor, Widener University

Lorraine Frazier, PhD, RN, FAHA, FAAN, Dean, School of Nursing, Columbia University

Marcia R. Gardner, PhD, RN, CPNP, CPN, ANEF, Dean, The Barbara H. Hagan School of Nursing and Health Sciences, Molloy University

Mary Ellen Smith Glasgow, PhD, RN, ACNS-BC, ANEF, FNAP, FAAN, Professor of Nursing and Interim Dean of Health Sciences at the College of Staten Island, City University of New York (CUNY)

Bridgette Gourley, DNP, CRNP, IBCLC, CNE, FAANP, FAAN, Assistant Professor, School of Nursing, Speciality Director FNP DNP, Department of Family and Community Health, University of Maryland

David Grad, MS, Executive Coach and Facilitator, The Kaufman Partnership

Kathy Gray, DNP, FNP-C, FAANP, Associate Professor, College of Nursing, Thomas Jefferson University

Jihane Hajj, DrNP, ACNP-BC, Associate Professor of Nursing, Widener University; Advanced Practice Provider - Neurosurgery and Neurocritical Care, Penn Presbyterian Medical Center

Debra Hanna, PhD, RN, ACNS-BC, Professor of Nursing, Coordinator of Clinical Nurse Specialist Program, The Barbara H. Hagan School of Nursing & Health Sciences, Molloy University

Courtney Hicks, DNP, FNP-C, CRNP, Nurse Practitioner, ENP/Plastic Surgery, Baltimore VA Medical Center

Judy Honig, EdD, DNP, CPNP, ANEF, FAAN, Dorothy M. Rogers Professor and Vice Dean, School of Nursing, Columbia University

Diane S. Hupp, DNP, RN, NEA-BC, FAAN, President, UPMC Children's Hospital of Pittsburgh

Catherine Johnson, PhD, CRNP, FNP-BC, FNP-BC, Clinical Associate Professor, Duquesne University

Matthew A. Jones, PhD, Principal Consultant, Northwest Emergent Solutions

Melissa A. Kalarchian, PhD, Professor & Associate Dean for Research, School of Nursing, Duquesne University

Karen Kaufman, MSOD, President, Co-Founding Partner, The Kaufman Partnership

Mary Beth Kingston, PhD, RN, FAAN, Executive Vice President, Chief Nursing Officer, Advocate Health

Rosemary Kunazcuk

Jennifer Lacy, DNP, APRN, GNP-BC, ANP-BC, Assistant Professor; CRNP, College of Nursing, Thomas Jefferson University

Mary Catherine Loughran, DNP, RN, MHA, Clinical Associate Professor, School of Nursing, Director, Doctor of Nursing Practice Program, Duquesne University

Denise Lucas, PhD, FNP-BC, FAANP, Chair, Advanced Practice Programs, Duquesne University

Rosalie Mainous, PhD, APRN, FNAP, FAANP, FAAN, Dean and Warwick Professor of Nursing, College of Nursing, University of Kentucky

Marie Ann Marino, EdD, RN, FAAN, Dean & Professor, Jefferson College of Nursing; Vice President for Academic Partnerships & Innovation, Jefferson Health, Thomas Jefferson University

Zyrene Marsh, DNP, APRN, FNP-C, Assistant Professor University of California Davis Betty Irene Moore School of Nursing

Diane Maydick, EdD, RN, ACNS-BC, CWOCN

Graham J. McDougall Jr, PhD, APRN, FAAM, FGSA, Affiliate Graduate Faculty, University of Alabama-Tuscaloosa

Bernadette Melnyk, PhD, APRN-CNP, FAANP, FNAP, FAAN, Vice President for Health Promotion, University Chief Wellness Officer, Dean and Helene Fuld Health Trust Professor of Evidence, The Ohio State University

Tina Mertel, MA, MCC, Executive and Leadership Coach, Meaningful Coaching

Sr. Mary Meyers, DNP, MSN, AGNP-C, BSN, RN, Director of Academic Support and NCLEX Success, Duquesne University

Janice M. Miller, DNP, CRNP, FAANP, Associate Professor and AACN Health Policy Fellow, Thomas Jefferson University

Kymberlee Montgomery, DNP, APRN, WHNP-BC, CNE, FAANP, FAAN, Vice Dean of Nursing & Student Affairs, Chief Academic Nursing Officer, College of Nursing & Health Professions, Drexel University

Deena A. Nardi, PhD, PMHCNS-BC, FAAN, Psychotherapist, Cathedral Counseling Center

Michael Neft, PhD, DNP, MHA, RN, CRNA, FNAP, FAANA, FAAN, Clinical Professor, Duquesne University

Brittany Gaspar Nettles, DNP, APRN, FNP-BC, Assistant Director, School of Nursing, Assistant Professor, University of North Florida

Kristen Nobles, DNP-EL, MSN, ACNP-BC, Lead Advanced Practice Provider, Department of Neurology, Hospital of the University of Pennsylvania

David Campbell O'Dell, DNP, APRN, FNP-BC, FAANP, President, Doctors of Nursing Practice, Inc.

Laura O'Rourke, DNP, APRN, ENP-C, FNP-C, CNE, Nurse Practitioner, Instructor of Emergency Medicine, and Assistant Program Director, NP/PA Emergency Medicine Fellowship, Mayo Clinic

Catherine Paradiso, DNP, ANP-BC, PMHNP-BC, Assistant Professor and Graduate Program Coordinator, The College of Staten Island, City University of New York

Jessica L. Peck, DNP, APRN, CPNP-PC, CNE, CNL, FAANP, FAAN, Clinical Professor, Louise Herrington School of Nursing, Baylor University

Dana Pearlman, DNP, CNM, FACNM, Doctoral Program Coordinator, Thomas Jefferson University

Jessica Peters, DNP, MSN, RN, ACNP-BC, Assistant Professor, Johns Hopkins School of Nursing

Bobbie Posmontier, PhD, CNM, PMHNP-BC, FAAN, Professor, Thomas Jefferson University

Tiffany Pressley, DNP, APRN, PMHNP-BC, CNE, CMSRN, Assistant Professor of Nursing, Psychiatric Mental Health Nurse Practitioner Program Coordinator, Francis Marion University

Veronica Quattrini, DNP, MS, FNP-BC, Senior Director, Doctor of Nursing Practice Program, Assistant Professor, University of Maryland School of Nursing, Baltimore

Mary Marasa Radcliff, DNP, FNP-BC, AOCNP, Nurse Practitioner, Johns Hopkins Hospital

Sandra Rader, DNP, MSA, RN, President, UPMC Presbyterian Shadyside

Sharon Radzyminski, PhD, JD, CNS, RN, Professor, University of Texas Rio Grande Valley

Mary Grace Renfrow, MS, DNP, FNP, Assistant Professor, School of Nursing, University of Maryland

Cynthia Rost, DNP, RN, CNE, HFQE, APNA Certified Suicide Prevention Nurse, Clinical Assistant Professor, School of Nursing, Duquesne University

James Schreiber, PhD, Professor, School of Nursing, Duquesne University, Editor-in-Chief, *Currents in Pharmacy Teaching and Learning*, Editor Emeritus, *The Journal of Educational Research*

Diane C. Seibert, PhD, WHNP-BC, FAANP, FAAN, Associate Dean for Academic Affairs, Uniformed Services University of the Health Sciences

Tammy Slater, DNP, MS, ACNP-BC, Assistant Professor, School of Nursing, Johns Hopkins University

Michael Smith, EdD, MBA, CEO & Founder, Huddle Advisory

Regena Spratling, PhD, RN, APRN, CPNP-PC, FAANP, FAAN, Professor, School of Nursing, Georgia State University

Tukea L. Talbert, DNP, RN, Chief Diversity Officer, University of Kentucky HealthCare

Yamini Teegala, MD, MPH, MBA, FAAFP, Chief Executive Officer, Rocking Horse Community Health Center

Mary F. Terhaar, PhD, RN, ANEF, FAAN, Associate Dean for the Graduate Program, M. Louise Fitzpatrick College of Nursing, Villanova University

Melanie T. Turk, PhD, RN, FTNSS, Associate Professor, School of Nursing, Duquesne University

Jeannine Uribe, PhD, RN, Associate Professor, School of Nursing and Health Sciences, La Salle University

Brigit VanGraafeiland, DNP, CPNP-PC, CNE, FAAN, FAANP, Associate Professor, Associate Director DNP, DNP/MBA, DNP/MPH, School of Nursing, Johns Hopkins University

Eric Vogelstein, PhD, Associate Professor and Director of Ethics, McAnulty College and Graduate School of Liberal Arts

Barbara Wadsworth, DNP, RN, MBA, NEA-BC, FAAN, FNAP, FACHE, Executive Vice President/Chief Operating Officer, Main Line Health

Roberta Waite, EdD, PMHCNS, ANEF, FAAN, Dean, Georgetown School of Nursing

Shelley Watters, DNP, RN, NE-BC, Senior Director Cultural Excellence, UPMC Presbyterian Shadyside

Ruth A. Wittmann-Price, PhD, RN, CNS, CNE, CNEcl, CHSE, ANEF, FAAN, Dean, W. Cary Edwards School of Nursing and Health Professions, Thomas Edison State University

Zane Wolf, PhD, RN, CNE, ANEF, FAAN, Dean Emerita, Professor, School of Nnursing and Health Sciences, La Salle University

Claire Zangerle, DNP, RN, MBA, NEA-BC, FAONL, FAAN, Chief Nurse Executive, Alleghany Health Network

Cindy Zellefrow, DNP, MSEd, RN, CSN, EBP-C, Assistant Clinical Professor, The Ohio State University College of Nursing Director, Academic Core; Helene Fuld Health Trust National Institute for Evidence Based Practice

Rick Zoucha, PhD, PMHCNS-BC, CTN-A, FTNSS, FAAN, Professor and Chair of Advanced Role and PhD Programs, School of Nursing, Duquesne University

Ksenia Zukowsky, PhD, CRNP, NNP-BC, Chair, Graduate Programs, Jefferson College of Nursing, Thomas Jefferson University

Foreword

This third edition of the classic text *DNP Role Development for Doctoral Advanced Practice* is a must read, both for students enrolled in the requisite coursework, and for faculty teaching the core courses to prepare nurse leaders with the professional doctorate. Dreher and colleagues have presented us with core knowledge across the spectrum of what is essential and requisite for the doctorally prepared advanced practice nurse. They share the historical perspective so important to the understanding of leaders within the discipline, they proceed to provide content that delves into both the foundation and the cutting edge issues for students embarking on doctor of nursing practice (DNP) education.

Particularly noteworthy is the attention to the various roles that can be assumed by the DNP graduate. The chapter authors provide in depth information, gleaned from years of experience in the identified roles. Attention is paid to the roles of practitioners, clinical executives, nurse educators, and clinical scholars, all prominent roles within nursing education and healthcare delivery. This attention to the specific roles is coupled with the comprehensive attention to the historical development of the advanced practice roles and the evolution of the DNP educational movement in the United States, and now globally.

Additionally, specific chapter content is included for development of the leadership skills of the students. These include negotiation skills, coaching, and interdisciplinary and interprofessional collaboration. The addition of a health policy and advocacy focus and negotiation skills are also extremely important as nurse leaders position themselves for key roles designing and implementing policy at local, national, and international levels. Also important is the attention to the role of DNP graduates in ethics and quality improvement and patient safety initiatives. While these components are most often considered within healthcare systems, it is important that the DNP graduates couple this understanding with a perspective of healthcare across the continuum of care, from community health to high-tech hospital settings.

One of the most important and comprehensive components of this book is the inclusion of stories from the field. These stories demonstrate for students the lessons learned not only from years of experience, but also from charting new initiatives and advancing the leadership roles of nurses. The stories shared by clinical nurses who transitioned to DNP-prepared advanced practice nurse will be of great insight to clinical nurses who are committed to the profession and wanting to assume a new role. We know that many clinical nurses are searching for opportunities to expand their knowledge and skills in healthcare, and the advanced practice role is particularly attractive. Career advancement opportunities are highlighted in several chapters, and present myriad experiences that will intrigue those committed to stretching beyond traditional boundaries. And, while we all hope that the recent pandemic experience is behind us, there are important lessons learned, and shared in a key chapter in this book, that can be instructive in future disruptive times.

One additional important hallmark of this book is its attention to the current and future challenges. The authors, Dreher, Glasgow, Dahnke, and Cotter, question our way forward in addressing the critical issues. They begin by debunking the statements made early in the launch of DNP programs and chart the course to today when DNP programs and enrollments far outpace other doctoral programs. In the past two decades we have witnessed monumental change in the landscape of graduate nursing education, and the subsequent changes in nursing professional practice and leadership. Key leadership positions within the profession are now held by those with DNP degrees, and preparation at this level has become the first choice for those advancing within clinical and leadership ranks. These chapter authors not only provide details about the essential elements of DNP curricula and the associated competencies but also challenge the current boundaries in thinking about the potential contributions of DNP graduates, for example, in translational research.

Too often nurse leaders in both professional practice and academia are bound by their understandings of beliefs and traditions of the past. This book and the authors of each of the chapters set a future course for the graduates of DNP programs, not only to think differently, but also to act differently. This book is refreshing in its future-oriented perspective, honoring the past while breaking down barriers of the present.

Joyce J. Fitzpatrick, PhD, MBA, RN, FAAN, FNAP, FAANP(H)

Preface

■ NAVIGATING AN UNCERTAIN DNP LANDSCAPE: WHERE IS THE EVIDENCE?

It has now been 20 years since the American Association of Colleges of Nursing (AACN) voted to require the doctor of nursing practice degree (DNP) as the highest level of preparation for clinical practice in 2004. In the press release, the AACN stated the vote was "to move the current level of preparation necessary for advanced nursing practice roles from the master's degree to the doctorate level by the year 2015" (p. 1). The referenced advanced practice nursing roles were nurse practitioners, clinical nurse specialists, nurse midwives, and nurse anesthetists. Chapter 1 discusses how the nurse executive role was later added as an advanced nursing practice role; however, the nursing educator role was not considered as advanced practice for reasons that are not fully understood and still debated by many. We are now some 20 years into a protracted nursing faculty shortage. Good nursing colleagues can disagree, but perhaps our colleagues should have shaped a DNP in nursing education as "nursing education practice" and comprehensively shaped and impacted all doctoral nursing education. It is widely documented that most DNPs go into academia for full-time faculty positions. Commonly, we see students get master's degrees as NPs and return for a DNP, and then enter academia, where we desperately need their expertise and credentials. In 2019, the AACN reported that in 2018, 60% of all DNP graduates went into full-time faculty positions, not clinical practice. This was not what was envisioned for the degree, but this data cannot be ignored.

As this book was going to press, the National Association of Clinical Nurse Specialists voted not to require the DNP for entry-level advanced practice by 2030 (2023). They did an extensive analysis of master's, DNP, and PhD CNS practice and found no measurable differences in patient or health outcomes. And while they endorse the DNP and support its refinement and progress, it is unlikely they will require it. The American College of Nurse-Midwives has held the same position statement since 2012: that the DNP is an option but that the master's degree will remain the entry-level degree for advanced midwifery practice (2019). Nurse anesthesia adopted a requirement for a doctorate for entry-level practice by 2025. They did not specify the degree, but it appears many programs have implemented the DNP and others the doctor of nurse anesthesia practice (DNAP).

The entry-level DNP for NPs is clearly the most likely advanced degree option to advance healthcare outcomes. They are the largest APRN specialty by far, with approximately 355,000 practitioners (American Association of Nurse Practitioners, 2022). But now DNP enrollment is flat for the first time, rising only 0.6% in 2021 to 2022 (AACN, 2023). DNP-prepared NPs cite a lack of salary increases, agency tuition reimbursement that supports master's study but not the doctorate, and limited or no scholarship time. DNP-NP graduates are educated to practice at the highest level, but often employers struggle with differentiating between master's-level versus doctoral advanced nursing practice. The DNP has been around for 20 years now, but the profession did not meet its ambitious goal to have all advanced practice nurses have an entry-level DNP degree by 2015. Nonetheless, the degree is now embedded in the profession. DNP programs and more graduates will continue. The challenges mentioned above will have to be resolved ultimately, but others will arise. Yes, the landscape for the DNP degree is uncertain, but it can be navigated. Graduates can and will have to make an impact on the health of the nation, however, for the DNP degree to thrive.

The next big question for nursing scholars, educators, and practitioners from all nursing specialties is: Where is the evidence that DNP-led practice improves health outcomes?

The DNP degree is recognized and accepted as one of two terminal doctoral degrees in the nursing discipline. Evidence is clear that many nurses seek the DNP degree as preparation for the highest level of nursing practice (AACN, 2020; Dreher & Glasgow, 2017). However, we have not seen ample evidence that patient outcomes have improved on a scale that corresponds with the increase in the number of doctoral-level-prepared nurses. The nursing discipline, practice setting, and higher education have failed to consistently demand academic rigor and the application of research to clinical practice in ways that improve patient care. The practice doctorate is sorely needed in the clinical environment, but advanced practice nurses have not been allocated the scholarly time and associated resources to address these concerning clinical problems, much less solve them and disseminate the findings.

What are the root causes of this disconnect? Nurse leaders have not invested in, advocated for, and/or insisted upon rigorous nursing research while simultaneously requiring nurses to implement evidence-based practice (EBP) standards into their daily practice as a national strategy. A strong investment in EBP will elevate nursing practice and demonstrate the impact of the DNP (Glasgow & Colbert, 2022). Presently, there is a lack of resources dedicated to EBP in the clinical setting.

The gap between academic nursing and clinical nursing practice needs to be closed. Academic-clinical service partnerships are critical to preparing a competent nursing workforce that meets society's needs. The concept of academic-clinical partnerships in nursing is not new; however, it has never been fully realized as a national strategy. While the evidence for partnerships is strong, the fact remains that there are many barriers to developing and sustaining them. A recent and more reoccurring barrier has emerged: the tidal wave of retirements of senior nurse leaders in both the academy and clinical sectors. Academic-clinical partnerships can play a fundamental role in building capacity for nursing schools via joint appointments while increasing the use of evidence-based practice and practice-based evidence in the clinical environment. A DNP program in both practice and academic settings is able to provide opportunities for collaboration that extend well beyond the traditional affiliation for clinical education. Academic-clinical partnerships provide an opportunity for a shared vision and resources, mutual problem-solving, and increased evidence for the profession. For many reasons (regulatory issues, faculty workload, ivory tower perceptions, fiscal resources, and decreased appreciation for intellectualism in nursing), nursing has not achieved this type of model (Glasgow & Colbert, 2022).

We would be remiss if we did not mention the uneven academic rigor, quality, and expectations of DNP curricula, which require equal attention from the nursing discipline. Also, positioning entry to advanced practice at the doctoral level will generally necessitate the revision of curricula for a younger student with less clinical practice and life experience. This new learner will require more faculty support and clinical mentoring and supervision, thus requiring more financial resources in a fiscally challenging time for institutions of higher education.

So where do we go from here? We need to fully embrace and implement academic-clinical practice service partnerships as a national strategy and advocate strongly for the requisite scholarly time and associated resources to support the DNP advanced practice nurse. Academic rigor needs to be at the forefront of the profession's minds. The national nursing shortage has resulted in uneven quality among many academic degree programs requiring intervention. We must review the evidence to determine if the new proposed curriculum changes are warranted and if they result in the desired effect.

We hope this book challenges your thinking but leaves you with optimism. It has a diverse spectrum of authors and unique Reflective Responses from practitioners, nurse executives, nurse educators, and experts from industry who respond to each chapter. There is probably no nursing book on the market that has so many DNPs in practice as authors.

It has only been 20 years since the DNP degree was founded. There is still a lot of work to do.

H. Michael Dreher
Mary Ellen Smith Glasgow

Note: As this book goes to press, the Commission on Collegiate Nursing Education (CCNE), the largest accreditation agency of baccalaureate or higher education degrees in nursing (PhD programs are not accredited), formed a Standards Committee and is proposing educator tracks in the DNP, among other changes. The deadline for public comment was November 16, 2023.

Our first thought is that maybe these are the first steps toward the recognition that over 20 years of strategies to increase PhD enrollments to solve the nursing faculty shortage have not worked. We look forward to seeing the outcome of this new dialogue (CCNE, 2023).

REFERENCES

American Association of Colleges of Nursing. (2004). *AACN adopts a new vision for the future of nursing education and practice: Position on the practice doctorate approved by AACN member schools.* https://www.aacnnursing.org/news-data/all-news/article/dnp-release

American Association of Colleges of Nursing. (2019). *Salaries of instructional and administrative nursing faculty in baccalaureate and graduate programs in nursing.* https://www.aacnnursing.org/Store/product-info/productcd/IDSR_19SALSINST

American Association of Colleges of Nursing. (2020). *DNP Fact Sheet.* https://www.aacnnursing.org/News-Information/Fact-Sheets/DNP-Fact-Sheet

American College of Nurse-Midwives. (2019). *Position statement: Midwifery education and the doctor of nursing practice.* https://www.midwife.org/acnm/files/acnmlibrarydata/uploadfilename/000000000079/PS%20Midwifery%20Education%20and%20Doctoral%20Preparation%20190927.pdf

American Association of Nurse Practitioners. (2022). *NP facts.* https://storage.aanp.org/www/documents/NPFacts__111022.pdf?_gl=1*rtq9dp*_gcl_au*NjQ1OTY2MzI1LjE2ODg0MTY2ODA

Commission on Collegiate Nursing Education. (2023, November 9). *Proposed CCNE standards for accreditation of baccalaureate and graduate nursing programs: A webinar for constituents.* https://www.aacnnursing.org/Portals/0/PDFs/CCNE/CCNE-Standards-Committee-Webinar-10-9-2023.pdf

Dreher, H. M., & Glasgow, M. E. S. (2017). *DNP Role Development for Doctoral Advanced Nursing Practice.* Springer Publishing.

National Association of Clinical Nurse Specialists. (2023). *Position Statement: Entry For CNS Practice,* Retrieved Entry-for-CNS-Practice-Position-Statement-FINAL.pdf (nacns.org)

Smith Glasgow, M. E., & Colbert, A. M. (2022). Nursing's Wicked Problems – A Path Forward through Transformative Academic Leadership and Collaboration. *Nursing Administration Quarterly, 46*(4), 275–282. https://doi.org/10.1097/naq.0000000000000545

Springer Publishing Resources

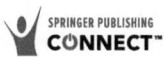 A robust set of instructor resources designed to supplement this text is located at http://connect.springerpub.com/content/book/978-0-8261-8137-4. Qualifying instructors may request access by emailing textbook@springerpub.com.

- **LMS Common Cartridge** With All Instructor Resources
- **Instructor PowerPoint Presentations**
- **AACN Essentials Mapping Grid**

SECTION ONE

Historical and Theoretical Foundations for Role Delineation and Preparation in Doctoral Advanced Nursing Practice

CHAPTER ONE

The Historical and Political Path of Doctoral Nursing Education to the Doctor of Nursing Practice Degree

H. MICHAEL DREHER

■ INTRODUCTION

This opening chapter examines the history of the Doctor of Nursing Practice (DNP) degree in the United States. It is the historical and sociological efolution of the degree and its reception in our health system labor market that will ultimately shape the role of this still evolving doctoral advanced practice nurse, or the nurse who engages in doctoral advanced nursing practice (Dreher & Montgomery, 2009). The chapter draws on contexts, both historical and political, that illustrate the progress of the degree, from the earliest attempts, including the failures and successes in our discipline to the first doctorate to prepare nursing faculty, an EdD in Education from Teacher's College of Columbia University, which offered little, if any, coursework in nursing (Carter, 2013); a research doctorate (PhD); a DNSc—an impactful research doctorate sometimes founded where some institutional academic forces prohibited the constitution of a PhD in nursing. Other iterations of the DNSc were constructed along the way: a doctor of science in nursing (DSN); doctor of nursing science (DNS); the first professional doctorate, a doctor of nursing (ND), started at only four institutions and closed; and two early doctor of nursing practice models (DrNP) at Columbia University School of Nursing and Drexel University, which did not survive. The DNP became the chosen professional doctorate degree model for the profession and transformed advanced practice nursing and graduate education. Some of the positive outcomes and still-not-fully-resolved issues with the DNP degree are also summarized. The 2021 American Association of Colleges of Nursing's (AACN's) *The Essentials: Core Competencies of Professional Nursing Education* is not discussed since doctoral advanced practice nurse education does not have a singular emphasis but is considered advanced-level nursing education. In Chapter 24, Bloch, Douglass, and Brock attempt this. This chapter concludes with points on how the American iteration of the DNP degree interfaces with the prevalent international professional doctorate degree model. With the publication of this book, the UK Council for Graduate Education will have convened in March 2023 its *8th International Conference on Professional and Practice Based Doctorates*, where the degree model for doctoral practice in nursing education is very different. The internationalization of practice doctorates in any health-related field highlights how today's global health issues can impact anyone anywhere and the need for highly advanced health professions' education that advances health for all.[1]

BACKGROUND

A new doctorate in any discipline is rarely created without some controversy. The origins of the pharmacy doctorate (PharmD) began in 1992 and the degree was not required by the American Association of Colleges of Pharmacy until 2000 to replace the BSc degree (Evans, 2019; McLeod, 1992). More recently, physical therapy moved from the requirement of a master's in physical therapy to a doctorate of physical therapy (DPT) in 2016. As Creighton University created the first DPT program in 1993, this transition took 23 years (Plack & Wong, 2002). The Council of Social Work Education still considers the master's of social work (MSW) as the terminal degree. There has been some discussion of the doctor of social work (DSW) as the requirement for entry-level practice, but although the value of the degree to the profession is acknowledged, the chances of this happening seem bleak (Coyle, 2019). Additionally, the DSW is not an entry-level practice degree option, and all DSW programs require some previous MSW social work practice for admission. In our profession, the American College of Nurse-Midwives (ACNM) has also resisted doctoral-level entry practice. While the Accreditation Commission of Midwifery Education (ACME) accredits master's, DNP, and doctor of midwifery (DM) degrees, a doctorate is not required.

The DNP degree, at its founding in 2001 at the University of Kentucky College of Nursing and endorsement as the entry-level degree for advanced nursing practice (ANP) by the AACN in 2004, was not immune to impending controversy (Dreher et al., 2005). There grew significant and sometimes impassioned divisions both as the entrylevel to advanced nursing practice degree (master's versus DNP) and as the terminal doctorate for the profession (the DNP versus the PhD). However, the controversies have largely subsided, and the central questions now are more about a thorough assessment of where we are now and about "where do we go from here?" Some speculation and recommendations are exceptionally well written by McCauley and colleagues in their 2020 article, *"Doctor of Nursing Practice (DNP) Degree in the United States: Reflecting, Readjusting, and Getting Back on Track."* Some of the earliest programs are now about 20 years old, and much curriculum evaluation and revision have been completed since the publication of the AACN's 2006 *The Essentials of Doctoral Education for Advanced Nursing Practice*. Under the influence of the AACN, the new *Essentials: Core Competencies for Professional Nursing Education* (2021a) and other specialty advanced practice documents will now shape the next evolution of this degree.

Different from most historical analyses in nursing education, this chapter attempts to provide an honest and objective (as much as possible) narrative critique of both the problems and progress of the DNP degree as it emerged and has evolved over two decades. This author was not at the table of the AACN when members (restricted to colleges, schools of nursing deans, and/or the chief nursing administrator in any given AACN-affiliated program) cast a very narrow vote in 2004 to require the DNP degree instead of the MSN degree for advanced practice nurses (APNs) by 2015. Ultimately, it did not happen. Nor will it happen in 2025, which is the goal for entry-level nurse practitioners set by the National Organization of Nurse Practitioner Faculty (NONPF, 2021). However, I have been a keen observer of the practice doctorate movement from the beginning and was the only non-UK citizen on the 2011 UK *Second Commissioned Report on the Professional Doctorate* (Armsby & Dreher, 2011).

In a previous academic appointment, my own university sponsored what was the very first national conference on the practice nursing doctorate in Annapolis, Maryland, in 2007 titled *Practice Doctorate: Where Is It Headed? The First National Conference on the Doctor of Nursing Practice: Meanings and Models* and the second held in Hilton Head Island, South Carolina, in 2009, titled *Doctor of Nursing Practice: The Dialogue Continues ...*" At each of these venues, many of the contemporary discussion points were highly visible in the podium papers, poster sessions, and conversations and networking that took place among faculty, some of the first graduates with the degree in the country, current students, and various stakeholders, including the AACN at the first conference. Actually, as the chair for each of those conferences, one of the primary objectives of the organizing committee was to attempt to provide a safe platform for nursing scholars with diverse points of view. We thought the profession needed more critical discourse about the DNP degree, especially from a broader subset of doctoral nursing faculty who were not necessarily academic administrators or tied more publicly to the mission or position statements of various nursing organizations. We even invited a very prominent anesthesiologist (herself a former certified registered nurse anesthesiologist) who had been publicly criticizing the certified registered nurse anesthetist (CRNA)-to-doctorate movement to share her professional perspective.

Internal debate and idealism have always been part of the history of our profession. We only have to look at our profession's failure, now 40 years old and counting, to require the bachelor of science in nursing degree for entry into professional nursing, for example (Donley & Flaherty, 2008). Only New York State requires a BS degree in nursing. The "BSN in 10" law mandates each associate degree–prepared RN to obtain the BS degree in nursing within 10 years from initial licensure (New York State Senate, S2145, 2015–2016). Labor historian Barbara Melosh (1982), in her sociological analysis of nursing in *The Physician's Hand: Work, Culture, and Conflict in American Nursing*, calls the history of nursing a battle between the "professionalizers" and the "traditionalists." The battle lines again appear to be drawn (perhaps less visibly these days) between those perceived to be the most in favor of replacing the master's degree with the practice doctorate for entry-level practice (BSN to DNP)—the professionalizers (nursing academics)—and those who prefer the post-master's DNP (against phasing out the master's)—the traditionalists (and the masses of advanced practice registered nurses [APRNs] with a master's degree who do not want a DNP, as well as many nursing academics). This divide exists because APRNs, despite being only master's prepared, are confident in their knowledge, skills, and expertise to practice at a high level. They may not know that the literature touts their outstanding primary healthcare delivery outcomes (American College of Nurse-Midwives [ACNM], 2012; Horrocks et al., 2002; Malina & Izlar, 2014; Mundinger et al., 2000).

Now, we have the American Medical Association (AMA) back in full throttle to interfere and limit the autonomy of APRN practice. At their meeting on June 14–19, 2023, their House of Delegates voted for a policy amendment to require that the licensing and regulation of APRNs be jointly regulated by state nursing and medical boards.[3] The NCSBN (2023) and American Nurses Association (June 17, 2023) immediately put out press releases to voice their opposition. This is another example of the historical founding of physician dominance in nursing in the United States, from the 1910 Flexner Report to the physician-anesthesiologist opposition to the scope of the CRNA (Vitale, 2021) and nurse practitioner (AMA, 2018). Of course, this description is partly an oversimplification, as these lines are not so black and white. There are still nursing faculty who oppose the DNP degree (increasingly fewer, it seems) and APRNs who support it (increasingly more, it seems). And of course, if you are a DNP student reading this book, you are likely matriculating in a DNP program of your own volition and are therefore likely not a traditionalist.

Nonetheless, discourse, debate, and critique are very healthy for our discipline. Absolute division is not. But maybe with the surge of the DNP degree (and make no mistake, nursing education has never seen a degree captivating the profession so quickly), professionalizers and traditionalists can learn from each other. It would be helpful in the spirit of egalitarianism (not elitism) and continuous improvement, however, if the nursing profession's members could work more cohesively toward the broader benefit of increased access to health services and ultimately to the improvement of health in our nation and globally. As we reflect on where we have come, we can emphasize graduate nursing education policy that is both evidence-based and does not do what Melosh says happened in our earlier history when "Nurses on the job were sometimes threatened by the strategies leaders adopted, for the rising standards of professionalization often meant downgrading or even eliminating current practitioners" (1982, p. 5). Dracup and Bryan-Brown (2005) also expressed these concerns, stating, "We also worry that the current advanced practice nurses who hold MS degrees will feel disenfranchised" (p. 280). And in very frank language, they also echoed much of Melosh's early analysis:

> When nursing education moved from the hospital to the university or college setting, diploma nurses found themselves with an education that provided little or no college credit. We had an entire generation of embittered nurses who saw nursing academics as out of touch with clinical practice. (p. 280)

We implore the nursing profession not to forget its history and, this time, to learn from some of these very painful growing pains in our discipline, and respond differently in the future. As Dracup and Bryan-Brown beseech, we must avoid disenfranchising a large number of nurse practitioners, nurse-midwives, nurse anesthetists, and clinical nurse specialists who believed they were properly prepared for their roles when they entered advanced practice with a master's degree. However, even though they must acknowledge the landscape for advanced practice nursing is changing, the increasing complexity of their own work environment must be obvious, and so the rise of the DNP must be structured so they see value in returning to obtain this degree.

■ THE EARLY BEGINNING OF DNP DEGREE DIFFERENTIATION

How might we today classify or categorize the first doctoral degree in nursing, an EdD in nursing education, founded at Teachers College, Columbia University, in 1933? Might it have been the "seeds" of a PhD nursing research-based inquiry? After all, New York University founded the first PhD program in nursing the following year. Perhaps it was more of a professional (or practice) doctorate, but those terms didn't exist. My guess is that it was partly both. Globally, the EdD degree is viewed as the professional doctorate in education, but herein lies the problem. Research is part of every professional doctorate degree; it is less theoretical, however. Hawkes and Taylor identify that a thesis is completed in the UK for the EdD (2016). But herein lies one of the issues that still plagues the nursing academy with the DNP degree. In the United States, the EdD graduate also completes a dissertation (like the PhD graduate), but the EdD dissertation is more practice-oriented and work-based. Some even view the EdD as a research degree analogous to the PhD. The first EdD degree in the United States was offered by the School of Education at Harvard in 1921, and it did not convert to a PhD until 2012 (*Inside Higher Education*, 2012; Kaustuv, 2012). Harvard also created the first doctor of business administration (DBA) in 1953 and transitioned to a PhD in 2018–2019. Both were viewed as professional doctorates but included practice-oriented, rigorous research in a dissertation project or the equivalent. However, the EdD succumbed to the pressures of the more prestigiously recognized PhD and the DBA to the pressures of identity. What is a "DBA?" Even a Harvard pedigree could not save them. Will the DNP suffer the same fate (very unlikely)? However, the length of time before it has its own "degree identity" may be long.

The DNP degree, however, is very similar to other professional doctorates that do not normally include an original research project—the doctor of medicine (MD), the doctor of pharmacy (PharmD), and the doctor of physical therapy (DPT), for example. Nonetheless, even now, in 2023, this question remains a point of contentious discussion among doctoral nursing educators (both DNP and PhD): What is the role of research in the DNP degree, and should DNP students and graduates generate new nursing knowledge or be restricted to expertly translating and disseminating what is currently known? Why is there a line of demarcation for clinical scientific knowledge generation? It seems inegalitarian. One "generates." Another "translates." But they both disseminate. In 2015, the AACN published a white paper that clarifies some of this knowledge production role (AACN, 2015a). This clarification will be revisited in this chapter, as the term "research" became a serious discussion issue at the founding of the degree and still is.

Nevertheless, maybe what we are pursuing now with the DNP degree is simply a return to nursing's orientation as a practice discipline in the same way the EdD was first created to advance nursing education practice. Some would applaud this return to our disciplinary roots, whereas others would see this as a diversion.

■ DOCTORAL NURSING EDUCATION STARTS A 100-YEAR JOURNEY

As there was a very sluggish growth of doctoral programs in nursing after the Teachers College experiment in 1933, it is noteworthy that three of the next four doctoral nursing programs were aimed at clinical specialization in the discipline rather than a doctorate awarded in the general discipline of nursing itself. The first doctor of philosophy (PhD) program in nursing was started at New York University in 1934. There is not a lot written about this very early PhD, and I have wondered, "Who taught in this program?" Furthermore, because nursing was often not allowed to offer a PhD degree by many university faculties beginning in the 1960s and into the 21st century, with other disciplines arguing, "Is nursing a real science?" it is remarkable that the New York University faculty was progressive enough to position itself at the literal forefront of nursing as a recognized academic discipline (Meleis & Dracup, 2005). However, it would take until the mid-1980s, at least 50 years after NYU, before nursing science would clearly evolve into a scientific discipline.

In late 1985, in nursing schools where faculty were active in moving the profession forward, research was now becoming a significant part of the academic role, while at the same time faculty clinical practice was falling out of favor. The third and fourth doctorates in nursing were developed with a clinical focus. The PhD in nursing at the University of Pittsburgh was started in 1954 with a clinical nursing and clinical research emphasis, and the DNSc at Boston University was started in 1960 with a psychiatric-mental health focus (Grace, 1989; Nichols & Chitty, 2005). Two important distinctions should be made about these two programs, as they both (PhD and DNSc) created two distinctive pathways to nursing science knowledge development and shaped doctoral nursing education differently.

First, perhaps it is the historic inability to develop a widely viewed "clinical doctorate" for the profession as an alternative to the research-intensive PhD that has led

TABLE 1.1 The First Quests for an Alternative Nursing Doctorate to the PhD

Iteration #1: The "Doctor of Nursing Science" degree: DNSc	First at Boston University in 1960, later at the University of California, San Francisco (UCSF), Columbia, Yale, Catholic, Rush, Widener, etc., all converted to the PhD.
Iteration #2: The "Doctor of Science in Nursing" degree: DSN	First at the University of Alabama-Birmingham in 1975, later at East Tennessee State, U. Texas Health Sciences-Houston, West Virginia, etc., all converted to the PhD.
Iteration #3: The "Doctor of Nursing Science" degree: DNS	First at Indiana University in 1976, later at the University of Pennsylvania, Arizona State, Louisiana State University Health Sciences Center (LSUHSC), University of Buffalo, etc., all converted to the PhD except the Sage Colleges (DNS in Nursing Education & Leadership) and Kennesaw State University, which closed the DNS and no longer offers a doctoral program.

to the opening for the DNP degree. Fitzpatrick (2003) made a very strong case for the clinical doctorate in nursing in 2003 (prior to the 2004 AACN vote), even advocating a clinical doctorate for teachers of nursing. Over the years, much has been written about the DNSc, DSN, and DNS degrees. Although the last two were initially designed to be clinical research-oriented doctorates, the profession ultimately came to view them all as de facto PhD degrees (AACN, 2006; Carlson, 2003). To that measure, by 2016, almost all of them had been converted to a PhD (except for one DNSc degree at the University of Tennessee Health Sciences Center, which oddly converted to a DNP program perhaps because they already had a PhD degree). Table 1.1 lists most of the schools that attempted the clinical doctorate and also traces one school's history from its earliest nursing education to the conversion of its clinical doctorate (DNS) to a PhD, and finally to the approval of the DNP degree (Exhibit 1.1).

The unanswered question is: Why did the profession ultimately abandon the idea of a clinical doctorate? The discipline of psychology faced this very issue in the 1960s, when many felt the PhD in psychology had become too research oriented, too experimental, and not client-focused. As a result, the doctor of psychology degree (PsyD) was first started in 1968 as a clinical doctorate (Murray, 2000). The PsyD degree, however, did not eliminate the research enterprise in the new degree; it only deemphasized it, and its founders developed a clinical dissertation model in lieu of the traditional PhD dissertation, which is still integral to the degree (Sayette et al., 2010). Peterson (1997),

EXHIBIT 1.1 The Indiana University Nursing History

University-based nursing education began in 1914.
Sigma Theta Tau was founded in 1922 by six educators from the Indiana University Training School for Nurses.
BSN curricula was first established in 1932.
MS was first offered in 1945.
MSN was first offered in 1966.
DNS approved in 1976.
The first DNS degree was awarded in 1981.
Planning for a PhD began in 1990.
DNS converts to PhD in 1996.
DNP degree approved in 2009.

BSN, bachelor of science in nursing; DNP, doctor of nursing practice; DNS, doctor of nursing science; MS, master of science; MSN, master of science in nursing; PhD, doctor of philosophy.

in referring to the PsyD degree versus the PhD, succinctly said that it is not that science and practice do not belong in the same program, but that it is a matter of emphasis. The AACN, however, was quite precise in stating that the DNP degree should not be described as a clinical doctorate but a "practice doctorate," stating: "The Task Force recommended that the terminology, practice doctorate be used instead of clinical doctorate" (2004a, p. 4). Is the reason for this distinction (i.e., calling the DNP a "practice" doctorate and not a "clinical" doctorate) the realization that our earlier clinical doctorate nursing models did include both a clinical and research emphasis (and the desire, at least by the AACN leadership at the time, was to move away from this type of degree model)? We will later revisit two universities that tried to offer different models of the "doctor of nursing practice" in 2005, but their curricular innovations were not adopted by others and ultimately not endorsed by the AACN (Dreher et al., 2005; Mundinger, 2009).

Second, the arrival of the PhD at the University of Pittsburgh in 1954 was perhaps better timed than the PhD at New York University in 1934 due to the slow maturation of the field of nursing as a discipline. The profession's first research journal, *Nursing Research*, was founded in 1952, and elsewhere I discuss at length the early struggles of the journal to attract enough high-level, true research-oriented submissions (Dreher, 2011, 2016a). The profession also benefited, especially the specialty of psychiatric-mental health nursing, with the publication and work of Dr. Hildegard Peplau's *Interpersonal Relations in Nursing* in 1952. Her work spurred interest in this specialty, and the editor of *Nursing Research* at one point emphasized (or complained about?) the overrepresentation of articles specific to psychiatric-mental health nursing (Bunge, 1962). Nevertheless, momentum was slowly growing toward nursing as a scientific discipline.

The first federal research grants in nursing were established in 1955 through a new research and fellowship branch within the federal Division of Nursing Resources (founded in 1948). In 1961, with the implementation of the Nurse-Scientist Graduate Training Grants Program, the growing need for nurses with a doctorate emerged (Gortner, 1986, 2000). With so few doctoral programs in nursing in 1961 (there were only three), this innovative research training program prepared nurses for PhDs in other fields besides nursing. The idea was that hopefully these early nurse scientists from the fields of sociology, anthropology, and psychology, for example, would graduate and then pursue nursing scientific inquiry and establish new doctoral programs in nursing. The universities that received these first training grants were:

Boston University School of Nursing

UCSF California School of Nursing

UCLA School of Nursing

University of Washington School of Nursing

Western Reserve University School of Nursing

University of Kansas

Teacher's College, Columbia University

University of Pittsburgh

University of Arizona

University of Colorado

University of Illinois

New York University (briefly)

TABLE 1.2 The First Doctoral Nursing Programs in the United States

Rank	Institution	Degree	Year
1	Teachers College, Columbia University	EdD	1933
2	New York University	PhD	1934
3	University of Pittsburgh	PhD	1954
4	Boston University	DNSc	1960
5	University of California, San Francisco	DNSc	1964
6	Catholic University	DNSc	1967
7	Texas Woman's University	PhD	1971
8	Case Western Reserve University	PhD	1972
9	University of Pennsylvania	DNS	1978
	University of Texas at Austin	PhD	1974
10	University of Alabama-Birmingham	DSN	1975
	University of Illinois—Chicago	PhD	1975
	University of Michigan	PhD	1975
	Wayne State University	PhD	1975
	University of Arizona	PhD	1975

From this list, many of the first PhD programs in nursing began. Table 1.2 lists the next doctoral programs in nursing founded mostly after the Nurse-Scientist Graduate Training Grant era. The prevalence of the DNSc and the absence of another EdD degree should be noted.

Vreeland believed that nursing was aiming toward a scientific orientation (1964). Whether that would evolve at the expense of the discipline's original practice orientation is another question. I would add that it is the failure of the discipline to bridge its two disciplinary orientations, what Peplau aptly called the "art and science [or art versus science] of nursing" (1988, p. 8), that has led many practicing nurses (both professional and advanced) to view the "nursing ivory tower" as too removed from practice (and its realities) and, in some eyes, even irrelevant.

One final point on the EdD: Why was the Teachers College degree model of an EdD in nursing education never replicated over many decades? An extensive review of the web identified only two: 1) joint Western Connecticut State University and Southern Connecticut State University EdD in Nursing Education program founded in 2012 and enrolling its seventh cohort in 2023; and 2) University of West Georgia founded in 2012, both cohort models. Programs that were not specifically stated to be an EdD in nursing education, such as an EdD with a specialization in nursing education, were excluded. At institutions where there is already a school of education or an EdD, it may be unlikely that a free-standing EdD in nursing education could be established. That would likely be the case for my college.

THE EVOLUTION OF THE NEED FOR THE NURSE WITH A DOCTORATE

With the first step in the movement of nursing into the university setting—which included various landmark events such as (a) the first constituted nursing school in a university (albeit under medicine) at the University of Minnesota in 1909; (b) the first individual (Professor Adelaide Nutting) appointed as a nursing professor at Teachers College in 1910; and (c) the first independent nursing school at Yale University in 1924—nursing began its slow path to perceiving the need for the profession to produce nurses with doctorates (Donohue, 1996). If nurses were indeed going to be full members of the academy (a rather oblique term that includes members of the formal academic community) with other disciplines, this would be essential. The Flexner Report on the state of medical education in 1910 also had implications for nursing education. Although this report was in many ways very critical of institutionalized medicine, medicine's dominance over nursing was under way (Hiatt, 1999). Further, and perhaps most importantly, the derision of medicine did not elevate nursing or the status of nurses. Examples of his critique of institutionalized medicine among the 155 graduate and 12 postgraduate medical schools in the United States and Canada that he claimed to have visited included findings of equipment at one school "dirty and disorderly beyond description" (Flexner, 1910, p. 190), and another institution had "in place of laboratories, laboratory signs" (p. 165). Additionally, Flexner was actually criticized for being too critical, and his methods of data collection came under heavy fire (Hiatt, 1999).

This widely publicized report on medicine also made it obvious to nursing leaders that they would likewise need to evaluate the state of nursing education even as the profession was in its early formative years. A subsequent 1912 report titled *The Educational Status of Nursing* (Nutting, 1912), which became the first comprehensive survey of schools of nursing, was likewise critical of the about 1,100 schools of nursing that responded. In this report, Melosh (1982) writes, "315 schools, or nearly 45%, reported that they did not have a single paid instructor, and 299 did not maintain a library. Instead, the nursing 'curriculum' in many hospitals consisted of two or three years of ward work" (p. 41).

THEN: THE DOCTORAL-PREPARED NURSE EMERGES FROM A FRAGILE POOL, DIVERGING FACTORS

The ultimate movement of nursing into college and university settings from hospital-based diploma settings has taken place ever so slowly in the past 100 years or so. There are even 28 RN Diploma programs currently accredited by the Accreditation Commission for Educators in Nursing (2023) across nine states, with three states having more than one (Pennsylvania 15, New Jersey 5, and Ohio 2). To indicate the progression of nurses with the BSN, among the 1.4 million nurses who entered the profession between 1970 and 1994 with either an associate degree (AD) or BSN, 59% entered with an AD and 41% with a BSN (Aiken et al., 2009). There has been a steady indication of the progression of RNs with the BSN degree. It is certain that the many early nursing leaders who sought the increasing professionalism of nursing at the baccalaureate level in the 1960s and beyond did not intend that associate degree technical nursing education from a community college rather than from a university or other 4-year degree granting institution would predominate (Haase, 1990; Mahaffey, 2002).

Only in 2011 did BSN-prepared nurses become predominant over associate degree-prepared nurses (ADN/diploma-prepared nurses), and data from 2013 indicated that the BSN degree was proliferating, with between 55% and 61% of nurses now having a BSN degree or higher (Budden et al., 2013; Health Resources & Services Association [HRSA], 2013; Robert Wood Johnson Foundation, 2015). Now, national data from the Center to Champion Nursing in America and the Future of Nursing: Campaign for Action and data between 2010 and 2018 indicate the percentage of nurses who hold a bachelor of science degree or higher is 56%, up from 49% in 2010 (Campaign for Action, 2021). The most recent 2020 National Council of State Boards of Nursing (NCSBN) report states that over 70% of RNs have a BSN degree. Because data from Aiken, Cheung, and Olds in 2009 indicated that only 6% of nurses who first get an ADN go on to advanced practice (the master's degree or higher), this trend away from an initial community college nursing education may have an important impact on the profession toward more nurses pursuing a graduate degree.

The rise in the number of new DNP programs aligned closely with the Great Recession of 2007–2009 (Krugman, 2009). With the retirement of many older nurses, a continuing shortage of nursing faculty (with doctorates), and a shortage of nurse scientists (with the projected retirements of so many senior faculty), the prospects for an adequate supply of nurses in different sectors remained predictably uneven. Furthermore, the movement to end advanced practice at the master's degree, or at least the transition away from the master's to the DNP, caused some to warn that this move would cause a drop in the number of new NPs each year out of fear their degree would be devalued and harm their job prospects (Bloch, 2007; Dreher & Gardner, 2009; Ford, 2008). There is no evidence of this, as the AACN reported that the number of APRN students (likely the largest APRN specialty, nurse practitioners) opting for master's-level practice entry continued to rise from 10,737 in 2004 to 46,622 in 2018 (2019).

Aligned with the prediction that master's-level NP enrollments may decline, according to the Society for Human Resource Management (2013), some 61% of employers offered undergraduate tuition assistance in greatly varying amounts. But while graduate tuition assistance was slightly less prevalent (59%), I have had doctoral students whose employers specifically did not support doctoral tuition reimbursement. However, economic conditions both external and internal to the lives of nurses at this particular time must be placed in this context. Would the 2004 AACN vote have occurred during this substantial economic downturn of the Great Recession, and would it still pass today? Similarly, and why a critique of the new AACN's *The Essentials: Core Competencies for Professional Nursing Education* (2021) is not the focus of this chapter, it cannot be overemphasized that this document, which may ultimately be transformative to nursing education (in DNP education too), was released in April 2021, during a pandemic and a "persistent" (AACN, 2021b, p. 1), "worsening" (Freund, 2021, p. 1) nursing faculty shortage. Grainger (2022) has written, "The issue of nursing faculty shortages predates the COVID-19 pandemic, but the pandemic has added new weight to this reality" (p. 1). It is too soon to assess the impact of the timing of this change by the largest organizing (and most influential) body of nursing education, but I have already had a colleague say, "Why now? Our nursing faculty are exhausted." The *Essentials* and competency-based nursing education are indeed paradigm shifts in nursing education, and a three-year or longer transition period is expected (2021).

The number of DNP programs grew from approximately 50 in 2007 to 424 in 2021, and the number of enrolled DNP students increased from 6,599 to 40,384 (AACN, 2022b). Still, 90% of NPs graduated from master's-level programs between 2019 and 2020 (AACN, 2021b). Nevertheless, while more schools are offering the post-master's DNP degree, the AACN reports the BSN to DNP has had larger enrollments than the post-master's DNP since 2010 (AACN, 2022). This perspective is not fully supported by Auerbach and colleagues (2015), who document problems with BSN-to-DNP education in the RAND Report sponsored by the AACN. McCauley et al. (2020) report that the overwhelming majority of institutions are still reticent about closing their master's-level advanced practice tracks out of fear of potential declining enrollments and loss of tuition revenue. Data reported by the AACN in 2019 demonstrated the continued popularity of students pursuing APRN entry-level master's programs, from 10,737 enrolled in 2004 to 46,622 in 2018 (AACN, 2019a), and only 152 master's programs closed between 2008 and 2018. I was a consultant to two state nursing boards of education at the beginning of the DNP movement, and expressed skepticism that the DNP would replace the master's degree as the required entry-level to advanced nursing degree. The author also counseled provosts and nursing deans to start BSN-to-DNP degrees but not eliminate the MS-entry degree unless their enrollment models supported such a transition. Colleges or schools of nursing with large resources and student enrollment can drop their MS-entry-level degree for the BSN-to-DNP with little financial risk. But the majority of small to medium-sized nursing programs across the country cannot. It is well established that many colleges and schools will offer both options (MS-entry and a post-master's DNP) permanently. The slow rate of actual conversions of master's-level advanced practice programs to the DNP was actually another reason the AACN commissioned the RAND Corporation to study this problem (Auerbach et al., 2015). The four most important conclusions from their report are:

- The DNP continues to expand steadily.
- The MSN remains the dominant pathway for APRN entry-into-practice education, though there is some limited movement toward replacement with the BSN-to-DNP.
- There will likely be two tracks toward the DNP in the near future (defined by schools' planning horizons): a single-step process (BSN-to-DNP) and a two-step process (BSN to MSN followed by an MSN-to-DNP at a later date).
- The value of the added content of DNP education is almost universally agreed upon.

In reflecting back, at the 2010 National Organization of Nurse Practitioner Faculties (NONPF) meeting, the sense was that both degrees would continue and be supported at least for the time being (Academic Nurse, 2010). That characterization was prescient, as the NONPF still supports master's-level practice, but they have now set a *commitment* to move all entry-level nurse practitioner education to the DNP degree by 2025 (Idzik et al., 2021), a goal that will not be met. Several years after the AACN's endorsement of the DNP for entry-level advanced-level practice, discussions of APRN master's level practically disappeared at that annual AACN Masters Education Conference (the entry-level NP (in particular). It was if they accepted it, but did not want to promote it at the expense of the growing DNP degree. The release of the 2021 *Essentials* document (AACN) likely spurred these concerns (probably from nursing programs that only had master's degrees and maybe could not afford to start baccalaureate entry-level APRN practice programs) for them to publish a later document *"AACN Statement Supporting the Masters Degree in Nursing"* (2022) supporting the master's degree for advanced level nursing education for master's-level APRN practice. As previously noted, this disconnect was recognized by the RAND Corporation, but attention to quality master's-level advanced practice nursing programs needs to continue with a higher level of visibility and support, despite the politics of the profession. In this way, the *Essentials* does this.

One of my previous employers still has robust enrollments in all its online master's NP programs, has had a doctor of nursing practice degree for over a decade, but still has no BSN-to-DNP program offered. At another previous institution, the enrollment as late as 2019 in the Master's Family Nurse Practitioner (FNP) program was at capacity and challenged like many institutions to secure a steady supply of master's-prepared FNP preceptors. This is one barrier to all types of DNP education that has not been given enough attention, particularly to APRN practice across all specialties (NP, CNS, CNM, and CRNA). A federal, comprehensive 17th Report to the Secretary of Health and Human Services and the U.S. Congress written by the National Advisory Council on Nurse Education and Practice (NACNEP) titled "Preparing Nurse Faculty, and Addressing the Shortage of Nurse Faculty and Clinical Preceptors" (2021) did not mention any new preceptor challenges by the introduction of DNP entry-level degree students. However, there are substantial barriers for NP students to obtain qualified preceptors today that are beyond the scope of this chapter. McIness and colleagues

(2021) cite the COVID-19 pandemic and opposition to practice autonomy as barriers to access for NP preceptors, not the DNP. Finally, what happens when the DNP NP student cannot secure a "qualified" preceptor when they have to pay for it, now an increasingly common practice that has been long practiced by physician assistant and CRNA students. This is now an extra financial burden McCauley and colleagues (2020) assign to the cost of the BSN-to-DNP student education that slows its expansion.

The question remains: Does the profession really need nurses with doctorates? What would the associate degree nursing student say? The answer is unequivocally "yes." In our history, the burden of a burgeoning discipline has always necessitated that nurses possess doctorates to achieve parity with other faculty in other disciplines in colleges and universities (the academy). Superimposed on this need for nurses with doctorates with research skills was the realization that if the scientific basis of nursing was going to grow, the profession would need such nurses in larger numbers, and thus we saw mostly new PhD and DNSc programs opening in the 1970s. Certainly, this supply would have to grow for more rigorous nursing science to be conducted and for our science to be perceived more as a "real science" by others. We should mention that as the science of nursing slowly evolved, there was initially a focus on nursing administration and nursing education research and an absence of focus on clinical research. Indeed, with the founding of the Association of Collegiate Schools of Nursing in 1935, with its mission to promote nursing education in the collegiate/university environment and away from the hospital-based programs, one of the aims of the new organization was "to promote study and experimentation in nursing service and nursing education" (Goodrich, 1936, p. 767). This may very well have been one of the earliest visible policy statements to encourage nursing research. Yet, over time, although nursing administration research has been aligned with health services research, the predominance of clinical research over all other types (with the devaluation of nursing education research), has happened. Clinical research, favoring quantitative methods (and some occasional mixed methods), is now the expected format, as it has more and more extensive funding sources (Guetterman et al., 2019; Hutchinson, 2001; Werley & Westlake, 1985). A very informal review of Google Scholar of qualitative methodology grants awarded by the National Institute of Nursing Research (NINR) that had a peer-reviewed publication since 2020 showed three total. Likely there are more.

Despite significant advances in nursing education, however, education-focused research in the discipline has unfortunately suffered, and I believe that this did not need to happen. For example, nursing health systems research (oriented toward the administrative indirect care role in nursing) has grown in sophistication over the decades. One only has to look at the extensive work of Dr. Linda Aiken, professor in nursing, professor of sociology, and founding director of the Center for Health Outcomes and Policy Research at the University of Pennsylvania School of Nursing, to see the kind of high impact that nursing health system research can make. Nursing education research, however, has suffered from a lack of innovation and too many education-oriented dissertations that have focused on minor issues of importance inside and outside the profession. Maybe this will change as the National League for Nursing (NLN) continues to support nursing research and education funding, and if DNP faculty scholars and graduates conduct and publish high-impact outcome data. The AACN reported that in 2018 60% of DNP graduates went into full-time faculty roles and the AACN made a clear position statement that the educator role was not advanced nursing practice. That meant that only 40% of DNP graduates were employed in roles the DNP designed the degree for. This is probably the most unforeseen miscalculation by nursing leadership since the 1965 ANA proclamation to call for the BSN degree for entry level into the profession.

Severely complicating this early drive to the doctorate were data in 1965 indicating that only approximately 22% of all nurses had been prepared in academic programs (this included associate degree graduates; Nelson, 2002). As mentioned earlier, the ANA in 1965 first tried to change this percentage by mandating that nursing education should take place in a college or university setting, and that the BSN be required for entry into professional nursing (Donley & Flaherty, 2008). Today, this percentage exceeds 50%; hence, although the mandate was never realized, perhaps we can recognize there has been success at upgrading the overall preparation of RNs. Next, the emergence of the NP role at the University of Colorado, Denver, in 1965 and the rise of NP programs offering MSN degrees in the 1970s increased the need for the doctoral credential for faculty NPs, as nurses without common university credentials (typically the PhD) were marginalized in academia (Dunphy et al., 2009; Silver et al., 1968). What is not known, however, is how broadly current NP faculty (or other APN faculty) are prepared at the doctoral level. A cursory review of many nursing school websites across the country indicates that there is still a plethora of NP track coordinators, who do not possess the doctorate. Perhaps the DNP degree will help alleviate this. In the summary of this chapter we now see more than 80,500 new nurses with the doctorate in the 17 years since the AACN's 2004 position to require the doctor of nursing degree for entry-level practice.

■ NOW: THE DWINDLING SUPPLY OF NURSING FACULTY WITH THE PHD

In 2008, the AACN published a white paper *The Preferred Vision of the Professoriate in Baccalaureate and Graduate Nursing Programs* indicating that nurses who teach in university settings (not the community college) should have a doctorate degree at minimum (AACN, 2008). Unfortunately, in challenging economic times, the profession faced two issues on this front to accomplish this: (a) how to attract more nurses to doctoral study and to the educator role and (b) how can we help the masses of MSN-prepared faculty across the country complete a doctorate? These two issues were critically important because it is the nursing faculty role that most drives the need for nurses with doctorates. For instance, DNP programs would not be offered, nor would you be sitting in your classroom (or behind your computer), if there were not a faculty member in front of you or online with a doctorate. Similarly, it will likely take considerable time (honestly if ever) for the consumer healthcare market to expect the nurse clinician (NP, CRNA, CNM, CNS) to have a doctorate in the same way that it is expected in academia. What is essential, however, is that an increasing number of DNP graduates will have a growing impact. That could accelerate change.

The complete answer to the first question previously mentioned—how to attract more nurses to doctoral study and to the educator role—is beyond the scope of this chapter. There is, however, a protracted nursing faculty shortage that has now existed for more than a decade and is predicted to persist (AACN, 1999, 2005a, 2015a; Aiken et al., 2009). The reasons why the shortage is likely to continue include the following factors that were prevalent in 2017 when the second edition of this text was published and now in 2024 as this third edition goes to press:

1. *2017*: A predicted surge in faculty retirements that will exceed predicted replacements (AACN, 2021b; Fang & Kesten, 2017; Smith Glasgow & Dreher, 2010); Fang and Lang summarized the following:

   The percentage of full-time nursing faculty aged 60 and older increased from 17.9% in 2006 to 30.7% in 2015.

   The mean age at retirement increased from 62.2 to 65.1 years

The projected faculty retirements for the next 10 years equal roughly one-third of the total faculty in 2015.

The retiring faculty are likely to come from faculty aged 60 or older in 2015, and faculty aged 50–59 in the same year are likely to be the replacements for the retiring faculty.

The impact of the retiring faculty on the faculty workforce will be huge given their overrepresentation in doctoral attainment, senior rank, and ability to teach at the graduate level.

Younger faculty who are likely to replace the retiring faculty possess fewer doctoral degrees, lower senior faculty ranks, and are more limited in their ability to teach at the graduate level.

2022/2023 According to an AACN 2022 *Special Survey on Vacant Faculty Positions* of 909 nursing schools (84.4% response rate), there were 2,166 full-time faculty vacancies where a candidate with a doctoral degree was preferred. Part of this shortage can also be attributed to there not being enough faculty to meet student demand, all due to and exacerbated by faculty retirements and especially at the senior ranks (Fang & Kesten).

2. *2017*: Lack of competitive salaries for nursing professors versus what they can earn in industry (Bakwell-Sachs et al., 2022; Ingeno, 2013; Smith & Dreher, 2003;

    2022: While it is widely known that nursing faculty are paid significantly less than nurses who work in hospitals (or related healthcare agencies), there is also wide variability in salaries based on region of the country, urban versus rural, and with a master's or doctorate. In 2002 the AACN reported a national mean salary of $87,523 with a master's degree, but the mean salary reported by the National Advisory Council on Nurse Education and Practice (2021) was $57,454.

3. *2017*: Lack of adequate role modeling in undergraduate nursing education to foster pursuing the doctorate and a teaching career (Potempa et al., 2008).

    2023: Although there has been no further peer-reviewed research in this area, it is strategic to invite students to consider higher education and encourage them at some point to become a nursing professor. But at this time, they are almost only wanting to focus on graduating and practicing as a registered nurse. However, planting the seeds and good role modeling is a better strategy than none all.

One example of the previously mentioned gender bias is the low comparative research start-up packages reported for tenure-track nursing faculty versus start-up packages for business, law, medicine, and engineering faculty (Valian, 2005). Although Rudy and Grady (2005) reported that among 31 biological nurse scientists engaged mostly in animal-model research (48% had formal postdoctoral training and all had received previous National Institute of Nursing Research funding), their mean research start-up package was for $50,000 (in the range from $2,000 to $105,000); I heard from several doctoral faculty at one annual AACN Doctoral Nursing Education meeting complain about their comparative research start-up packages in their own universities. Furthermore, administrative stipends for nursing administrators pale in comparison to stipends for faculty administrators from the disciplines mentioned previously and perhaps others (Kirkpatrick, 1994). Although Kirkpatrick reported stipends as low as $1,000 for the nursing department chair, this type of data admittedly is hard to substantiate, because the university power structure that favors one discipline (for whatever reason) over another has reason to keep these data hidden. Nevertheless, I (and others) have had multiple confirmations of this practice, and there is no reason to believe that this inequity has been rectified in the past 20 years. It is also not unusual for colleges or universities to internally cap permanent administrative promotions to 10% of the base salary, thus exposing an internally imposed salary compression that can generally be circumvented by an external candidate who may have more salary negotiation opportunities on the front end of the hire (University of South Florida, 2015). One major salary equity document that the AACN provides is the publication of annual salary ranges that can be used to guide faculty and administrator salary offers. This critique of the "status of the nurse in the academy" is not meant to discourage readers from the professoriate or from taking academic nursing administrator positions, but to identify some of the challenges that the current and next generation of nursing professors will face. A critical mass of DNP, largely nontenure-track faculty educators in particular, whose own entrance into the academy is going to spark a multitude of additional issues, may be particularly vulnerable. It may also be encouraging that if 60% of DNP graduates are entering full-time faculty positions, tenure-track options may become prevalent, especially at small colleges. Finally, the Medscape 2020 APRN Compensation Report stated that male CRNAs made an annual salary of $217,000 and female CRNAs made $189,000.

Encouraging MSN-prepared faculty to pursue the doctorate is equally problematic. This is a reminder of Melosh's (1982) and Dracup and Bryan-Brown's (2005) critiques of the disenfranchisement of nurses in an earlier generation (and the risk to current MSN-prepared APRNs), and of the current lack of flexible transitioning to the next degree as the profession suddenly mandates a doctorate for all university nursing professors (AACN, 2008). On the surface, is this not an expectation if you are teaching at minimum in a BSN program? Shouldn't nurses who teach in a university setting possess a doctorate, as other colleges and universities do? But again, as a practice profession, is this realistic? Foremost, what is needed most in undergraduate and APN education is to have faculty who are current and competent in the nursing practice they are teaching. I recall very vividly while in a master's of nursing graduate course in the late 1980s how a very talented pathophysiology instructor (with an MSN) was removed from the teaching roster in favor of a faculty member with a doctorate who had very little background or currency in the topic. This class was literally taught by the students themselves each week with class presentations. Most current MSN-prepared nursing faculty have no aim to be nurse scientists, and thus the PhD option (which takes an average of 8.3 years to complete after obtaining a master's degree) for many reasons is not attractive (Valiga, 2004). An AACN study of 5,391 nursing PhD students from 2001 to 2010 matriculating cohorts reported reported the average time to degree completion was 5.7 years. Students who were part-time or full-time faculty had higher attrition rates (Fang & Zhan, 2021). Many nursing schools prohibit their own master's-prepared faculty from matriculating internally in their own doctoral nursing programs due to potential conflicts of interest (Anselmi et al., 2010). Instead, they must go to another university for the nursing doctorate or attend a non-nursing, internally offered doctorate where they might get tuition support as an employee benefit. And even in those universities that do permit internal matriculation, "faculty-as-students" face conflicts of interest when nursing faculty attend classes taught (and graded) by their peers and colleagues. If the PhD is not an option, then what other nursing degree program can faculty attend? One option is an online DNP or PhD faculty exchange where one nursing program allows DNP/PhD matriculation from one institution to attend the other for essentially "free," and increase the number of each faculty at each institution with the doctorate. Duquesne University has used this strategy successfully with Saint Louis University and Catholic University.

The DNP degree is being increasingly suggested as a de facto solution to the nursing faculty shortage. But despite internal disagreements within the profession on this issue, the nursing educator role was not a role supported by the AACN within the confines of the normal DNP curriculum (AACN, 2006; Fitzpatrick, 2008). The fear was that these graduates would be unprepared for the faculty role and would experience even more inequities in the academy (AACN, 2005a,b). But the logic then and now remains that it is the DNP FNP in the faculty role, for example, who we need to teach the next generation of NPs. It is essential that they have nursing educator skills, too. The AACN (2006) suggested that DNP graduates may take extra courses to add the educator role to the DNP degree. Again, this seems reminiscent of Melosh's (1982) earlier critique of nursing leadership's professionalizers. In 2010 the National League for Nursing held a stakeholder Forum on the Master's in Nursing Education. It appears to be the first time they indirectly weighed in on the new AACN's 2004 call for the entry-level DNP for APNs, although the AACN chose not to recognize nursing education as an advanced practice specialty. The National League for Nursing chose to respond (at their own time period) with the following summary:

1. Every program does *not* have to be the same.
2. Now is *not* the time to exercise a restrictive control of education development.
3. Now is *not* the time to rapidly lengthen the only route to advanced practice nursing education which may not be in the best interest of our patients.
4. Data are needed to make evidence-based decisions about workforce projections to meet future practice imperatives.
5. An appreciation of the discipline of nursing is imperative as new specialized roles for advanced practice nursing emerge.

They pronounced that "Advanced practice nurses must have in-depth clinical knowledge of nursing practice; similarly, both part- and full-time faculty must have an in-depth knowledge of nursing education and nursing practice" (p. 1). They indicated that the proper preparation for the nursing faculty role is to have coursework and practica in the teaching role to ensure the effectiveness of the graduate. This still remains their concern, but while not endorsing a particular degree, continued concern is whether the move to properly and expertly prepare the DNP graduate for the academic role will nonetheless result in the burden of extra coursework at an additional cost. Instead, in preparation for the nurse educator (whether with a DNP degree or not), eight competencies must be attained (Keating et al., 2021).

1. Facilitate Learning
2. *Facilitate Learner Development and Socialization*
3. *Use Assessment and Evaluation Strategies*
4. *Participate in Curriculum Design and Evaluation of Program Outcomes.*
5. *Function as a Change Agent and Leader*
6. *Pursue Continued Quality Improvement in the Nurse Educator Role*
7. Engage in Scholarship
8. Function Within the Educational Environment

What, then, is the solution? Certainly, the answer is not to create easy or quick doctorates that MSN-prepared nurse educators can complete. In 2014, I conducted a survey for external feedback on the development of the DNP, and one respondent wrote that the best program would take less than a year to complete and be totally online and that work experience should be credited to the awarding of the doctorate. In 2015 AACN (2015a) a white paper on the DNP suggested that DNP students who are nationally certified should be considered for automatic credit toward their 1,000 total practice hours post the awarding of the BSN:

One commonly used process adopted by programs is to award credit to students who hold national certification in an area of advanced nursing practice, most commonly for national certification in one of the four APRN roles. Some programs also currently waive practice hours for other national advanced nursing practice certifications e.g. ANCC's [American Nurses Credentialing Center] Advanced Public Health Nursing certification and ANCC's Advanced Nurse Executive certification. (pp. 8–9)

That strategy was quickly abandoned to avoid opening Pandora's box for DNP programs in which one program would waive a certain percentage of practice hours and the next program might attempt to attract more students by waiving even more practice hours. This was a new early element of the DNP that had the potential to be detrimental to the rigor of the DNP degree to many stakeholders.

Large numbers of the current nursing professoriate are pursuing the DNP and many schools of nursing have more applicants for vacant teaching positions with the DNP instead of the PhD or EdD. What is one to do? This is where nursing innovation is needed and where accreditors too often become the barriers to innovation (Dreher, 2008a; Melnyk & Davidson, 2009; Neal, 2008; Stewart, 2009). It is beyond the full scope of this chapter to emphasize AACN's consequential miscalculation and not foresee the impending nursing faculty shortage. There was no data that rising numbers of PhD nursing students might be a purposeful strategy or solution. Further compounded by this was a secondary distraction to the nursing faculty with the launching of the clinical nurse leader (CNL) role and degree in 2007.

Finally, large numbers of MSN faculty are not going to return for the doctorate with the likelihood of only marginal increases in compensation. It is disturbing that in a report from the Texas Higher Education Coordinating Board (2013) there was limited upward mobility of graduates, with only 37% achieving higher levels of compensation after the DNP. Certainly, Texas is just one market and every individual DNP graduate has the ability to negotiate new employment terms, including compensation. I have seen significant upward career mobility with DrNP graduates and in other DNP graduates as well. But all three nursing accreditor agencies, the Commission on Collegiate Nursing Education (CCNE), Accrediting Commission for Education in Nursing (ACEN), and the NLN Commission for Nursing Education need to be more proactive in adding nursing faculty salary review in their accreditation criteria but they have not done so. Many believe it is because it is because nursing is a female-dominated profession. The Association to Advance Collegiate Schools of Business includes adequate faculty compensation in their accreditation review criteria. A 2010 report found that female law partners at elite law firms made on average $66,000 less than their male counterparts, and this disparity was largely attributed to stereotyping, gender bias, and even bullying and intimidation (Williams & Richardson, 2010). Seven years ago, *The Guardian* reported that global economic disparity between men and women is rising, with levels now similar to those during the 2008 financial crisis. At this pace of sustained gender pay inequity, it will take 170 years to achieve pay equity, according to data from the World Economic Forum (Treanor, 2016). The AACN does publish extensive salary data each year and it is an excellent resource when academic nursing administrators need to negotiate internal salary adjustments and external competitive offers to new faculty.

■ BEFORE THE DNP: THE FIRST PROFESSIONAL NURSING DOCTORATE: THE ND, SHORT-LIVED, AND TOO INNOVATIVE?

To be completely true to history, Case Western Reserve University's (CWRU's) initiation of the extraordinarily innovative ND degree in 1979 was never called nor classified as a "practice" doctorate. Indeed, it was called a "professional doctorate" (p. 308) by its founder Dean Rozella Schlotfeldt (1978) of the Frances Payne Bolton School of Nursing at CWRU. Only now do revisionists call it the "first practice doctorate" (AACN, 2006; Case Western Reserve University, 2016; Hathaway et al., 2006; Lenz, 2005). Again, the 1970s was a time of rapid growth in nursing education. The DSN and DNS clinical doctorates were initiated, more PhD and DNSc programs were founded, MSN NP programs began to flourish, and the ANA was still battling to require the BSN for professional nursing (Nelson, 2002). Then Schlotfeldt (1978), followed by Dean Luther Christman (1980) of the Rush University School of Nursing in Chicago, affirmed this vision that the doctorate should be the entry-level degree for nursing (Nelson, 2002). If there was ever a larger gap in the nursing profession between the professionalizers and the masses of practitioners or traditionalists, it was at this time. The ND degree at CWRU was designed after the MD degree. Students entered the doctoral nursing program with any basic college degree (just like medicine) and then completed a 3-year full-time curriculum including the completion of an ND thesis (somewhat differentiated from the university's PhD dissertation). Without a doubt, this was a professional doctorate model, and graduates initially were not prepared for advanced practice roles. This changed in 1990 when alternate pathways to the ND were created, including a post-master's option for nurses with an MSN, and indeed graduates at this time were prepared for advanced practice roles (Dr. Joyce Fitzpatrick, personal communication, April 13, 2010). Technically, this degree modification could be termed "a practice doctorate" (entry level vs. advanced practice), but again the term practice doctorate was not yet part of the nursing vernacular.

In the end, the ND degree failed and only three other schools ever adopted the degree model (Rush University in 1987, the University of Colorado in 1990, and the University of South Carolina in 1999). All four of these programs subsequently closed and transitioned to DNP programs in 2004 and 2005. One day someone will write the history of the ND degree and why it failed. Was it the unrealistic initial concept that any nurse needed a doctorate for entry into practice? In hindsight, and with apologies to Christman, a true pioneer in nursing, retrospectively this idea seemed extremely idealistic. For whatever reason, the first working group on the clinical doctorate established by the AACN in 2002 did not see much of a future for the degree. Were the initials "ND" perhaps too foreign? Was the degree confusing to some outside the discipline who thought it was a doctor of naturopathy—also an ND degree as the AACN has noted (AACN, 2004a)? Certainly, the post-master's ND model was an alternative doctorate model to the PhD. But I think it was more properly a "second generation clinical doctorate" (the DSN, and DNS degrees were the first generation), in that its graduates did complete an ND thesis and were generating evidence for the discipline. In other words, this post-master's model emphasized practice and practice-based research. And in the transition from the ND to the DNP, it is perplexing why the practice mission of the degree was retained but the practice–evidence-generating mission eliminated (at least until the current DNP white paper; AACN, 2015).

SETTING THE STAGE FOR THE DNP MODEL

The contemporary practice doctorate movement can be largely attributed to the innovators at Columbia University School of Nursing and its dean, Mary Mundinger (who retired in 2010). In the late 1990s, a team of investigators conducted a randomized clinical trial to determine whether, under comparable primary care protocols, MSN-prepared NPs and doctorally prepared physicians would have similar or different patient outcomes? In 2000, Mundinger et al. published their findings in the prestigious *Journal of the American Medical Association* (JAMA) and indeed reported that the outcomes were equivalent. This was certainly a landmark study for the nursing profession and caused quite a controversy in medicine. If possible, I would give a special courage award to the physician investigators and participants who even agreed to participate in the study (at seemingly some risk to the prestige of their discipline and the superiority of physician practice). The first outcome of this study set the stage for an innovative comprehensive care practice by Columbia University faculty NPs (Rubenstein, 2009). With this evidence, they gained admitting privileges (albeit with great passionate, political maneuvering by Dean Mundinger) to hospitals, and participated in the first model of comprehensive care where the NP sees and follows patients throughout their hospital stays, and not just seen by the APRN in the confines of a primary care clinic (Mundinger, 2005).

The second outcome of this study was the initiation of the doctor of nursing practice (DrNP) degree model. Although the inventors first described this as a "clinical doctorate" and a "Doctor of Nursing Practice in Primary Care," they later dropped the primary care emphasis, largely out of the realization that many of their APRNs were not practicing only primary care and they embraced their comprehensive care model more explicitly (Dreher et al., 2005; Mundinger, 2005). They later retained the idea that their degree was a clinical doctorate, as the overwhelming emphasis in their curriculum was on direct clinical practice and focused on Essential VII: Advanced Practice from the AACN's Essentials of Doctoral Education for Advanced Nursing Practice (2006; Dr. Janice Smolowitz, personal communication, June 25, 2010). At the time I was in a quandary about whether this iteration was really a clinical doctorate It did not have the thesis or dissertation knowledge generation model that the earlier clinical doctorates all had. Instead, they implemented a DNP portfolio that was innovative, but did not have an emphasis on generating new practice knowledge; rather, it emphasized translation of evidence to practice (which was technically more in line with the AACN conception of the DNP degree as a nonresearch degree [Honig & Smolowitz, 2009]). Nonetheless, there was no DrNP/DNP program in the United States that had more emphasis on clinical practice, and it even included a 1-year full-time practicum in the second year of study. The Columbia DrNP degree model was never replicated. Its initials were changed to "DNP" in 2009, probably in order to be accredited by the CCNE, which elected to only accredit DNP programs that subscribe to the "DNP" initials (AACN, 2005b). Consequently, is this degree model a clinical doctorate as the profession has traditionally defined this term? As I am aware that some Columbia graduates actually assumed primary investigator roles and the degree model students and graduates to generate new evidence for the profession, the conclusion is yes. The Columbia DNP model with its intensive emphasis on clinical practice was (albeit very briefly), a new type of third-generation clinical doctorate (despite the use of the DNP degree initials). This was further confirmed by the New York Department of State Office of the Professions, which has only recognized the DNP as a Clinical Doctorate and has never approved a DNP in Leadership, Education or Informatics, etc.

Historically, credit for the first DNP degree in 2001 belongs to the faculty of the University of Kentucky. However, this DNP focused on the clinical/executive management role and not advanced practice. It is perplexing why the AACN membership chose to endorse the Kentucky DNP model that did not emphasize advanced clinical practice, instead of the Columbia DrNP degree model that did. It is also unfortunate that the inventors of the Kentucky DNP model did not publish the reasoning behind their new degree in the peer-reviewed literature. Thus, we were left only with the dean's deliberations at the AACN membership to ascertain why the DNP degree model was preferred and why it was altered (from the Kentucky degree model) to include the traditional advanced practice role in the organization's first endorsement of the degree (AACN, 2004a). Interestingly, the addition of the clinical executive role (termed aggregate/systems/organizational focus) was only done after minor language in the AACN draft document was changed from the January 2004 AACN Draft Position Statement on the Practice Doctorate in Nursing (AACN, 2004b). From the January 2004 draft, it is stated in Recommendation 8 that:

> The practice doctorate should eventually be identified as the preferred graduate degree for APN preparation in the four current roles: clinical nurse specialist, nurse anesthetist, nurse midwife, and nurse practitioner. (2004b, p. 10)

Two months later, in March 2004, in the AACN Draft Position Statement on the Practice Doctorate in Nursing, in Recommendation 10 (originally Recommendation 8), the language changed to:

> The practice doctorate should eventually be identified as the preferred graduate degree for advanced nursing practice preparation, *but not limited to* [*italicized for emphasis*] the four current roles: clinical nurse specialist, nurse anesthetist, nurse midwife, and nurse practitioner. (AACN, 2004c, p. 12)

The change in language from APN to ANP is important, because the administrative role could never technically be equated with the advanced practice roles of the four traditional APRN roles. But if it were under the umbrella of ANP, it could. This inclusion of the clinical executive role, however, was not widely realized or perhaps promoted (again we reaffirm the clinical executive has been granted an advanced role by this definition, but not the advanced role of the educator). Even in the October 27, 2004, press release by the AACN titled "AACN Adopts a New Vision for the Future of Nursing Education and Practice", the AACN stated:

> In a historic move to help shape the future of nursing education and practice, the American Association of Colleges of Nursing (AACN) has adopted a new position which recognizes the Doctor of Nursing Practice degree as the highest level of preparation for clinical practice" [italics my emphasis]. (AACN, 2004d, p. 1)

Further in the press release, the AACN stated:

> Currently, advanced practice nurses (APNs), including Nurse Practitioners, Clinical Nurse Specialists, Nurse Mid-wives, and Nurse Anesthetists, are prepared in master's degree programs that often carry a credit load equivalent to doctoral degrees in the other health professions. AACNs newly adopted Position Statement on the Practice Doctorate in Nursing calls for educating APNs and *other nurses seeking top clinical roles* [*italics for emphasis*] in Doctor of Nursing Practice (DNP programs). (AACN, 2004d, p. 1)

Certainly, this is was just a press release and not the official policy of the AACN, but the reader is left to believe that APRNs are the target and who are the "other nurses seeking top clinical roles?" That is indeed a very odd way to describe the job of a chief nursing officer or vice president for nursing. These are not clinical roles. All the indirect functions in nursing (e.g., administration, teaching, clinical trials management) are classified differently from direct care roles, and the point made here is that the nursing professor who oversees students in the clinical area is as close to clinical as the administrator in charge of clinical services. Ultimately, the clinical executive role was made explicit in the AACN's (2006) Essentials of Doctoral Education for Advanced Nursing Practice and became an official ANP specialty.

A further examination of the final 2004 AACN position statement document does indicate that there was no consensus over endorsing only the DNP degree initials, but the argument that multiple degree initials would create confusion and perhaps lead to the DNSc, DNS, and DSN conundrum again apparently won (AACN, 2004a). It is largely unknown, however, how the practice of the nurse executive was deemed "advanced practice" by the AACN in 2006, but the practice of the nurse educator was excluded. I have covered this unfolding history in detail, mostly because it was unrealistic to assume that PhD enrollment was positioned to alleviate the nursing faculty shortage. It was later exacerbated with a 3.1% decline in PhD enrollment (and a 19.1% increase in DNP enrollments) in 2015 to 2016 (Fang et al., 2016). Since 2004 enrollments have been very erratic and graduations from PhD programs did not look promising. For instance, in 2008, there were only three net new PhD graduates in the United States, with an overall increase of 0.1%, while there was an increase of 5.1% in 2009, with 201 net new graduates (AACN, 2009a; Fang, Tracy, & Bednash, 2010). Eight years later in 2016, enrollment in doctoral, research-focused programs decreased by 3.2% (minus 168 students) and graduations decreased by 3.5% (net loss of 26 graduates; Fang, Li, Stauffer, & Trautman, 2016). Nevertheless, what was worrisome then was that these stagnant enrollments and the decline in graduation from PhD programs represented a very obvious trend that would adequately resupply the number of PhD-prepared, senior faculty teaching in the academy. The AACN now confirms this in their 2022 Data Report, with PhD enrollment down 4.14%. Over two decades, the problem looks worse.

The U.S. Bureau of Labor Statistics (BLS) expects that by the year 2022, the number of practicing RNs will grow by 19% and that employment of NPs, CRNAs, and CNMs will grow by 31%. Moreover, a 2013 HRSA report anticipates that waves of retirements in the nursing workforce will leave a significant burden on the pipeline. Over the next 10 to 15 years, the nearly one million RNs over age 50 (comprising approximately one-third of the current workforce), will reach retirement age (p. 1).

The current BLS projection of increase in the number of RNs needed between 2021 and 2031 is 6%. BLS statistics are known to be underestimated or overestimated. Even the BLS 10-year growth rate for CRNAs is 40% while a more reliable source reports 13.6% over 10 years. The following APRN job data is listed below chiefly because graduates from these programs who obtain the DNP or other doctorate are the pool of our next generation of DNP faculty (mostly). However, current AACN data released May 2, 2023, raises concerns about the entire U.S. nursing workforce from undergraduate (BS) to graduate (MS, PhD and even DNP) enrollment.

NPs Increase by 52% 2020–2030; current 2022 workforce is 2020, need 336,200 by 2030.
BLS https://www.nursingprocess.org/nurse-practitioner-job-outlook.html#:~:text=Over%20the%20next%20decade%2C%20there,acuity%20you%20choose%20to%20pursue.

CRNAs Projection 2020–2030 growth projection 13.6: average male CRNA salary $202,779; female CRNA $153,500. https://datausa.io/profile/soc/nurse-anesthetists

CNMs American College of Nurse Midwives (2023) website:

> Currently, the United States has approximately 4 midwives employed per 1,000 live births. With over 3.7 million live births a year, at least 22,000 midwives are needed in the midwifery workforce to meet the World Health Organization goal of at minimum 6 midwives per 1,000 live births. Currently, there are about 14,000 midwives in the United States including those not in clinical practice, resulting in a gap of at least 8,200 midwives.

In early 2023 the AACN released the following 2022 program enrollment data:

> In 2022, for the first time since 2000, enrollment in generic baccalaureate programs declined slightly compared to the previous year. When comparing the schools that reported in both 2021 and 2022, enrollments decreased by 3,518 students (1.4%), contrasting with the 2.8% increase between 2020 and 2021.

But this book and chapter are about the DNP degree. What has slowly begun to happen with the significant progress of the DNP? Will the sudden retraction in enrollments persist or is it time to ponder new strategies to strengthen it? I adopt an "all hands-on board" strategy to review what is working, what is not, and think strategically and even innovatively as we create a new path/vision for the DNP for the next 5 years or its third decade.

THE AACN ORGANIZES FOR THE DNP DEGREE

While Columbia started down one track toward what it called a new clinical doctorate (DrNP), which would ultimately become a practice doctorate, and with Kentucky earlier and boldly introducing a practice doctorate (DNP) that did not actually emphasize clinical practice, we should trace the third track by the AACN that in the end had the most influence. In March 2002, the AACN Board of Directors charged a task force to examine the current status of clinical or practice doctoral programs and other related charges (AACN, 2004b). What is interesting about this 2004 document is that the task force reported that it had established a collaborative relationship with NONPF, and therefore there was a strong faculty–NP connection in these early deliberations. Yet, there was also no liaison with the major practicing APRN organizations, including the ACNM, the American Association of Nurse Anesthetists (AANA), the National Association of Clinical Nurse Specialists (NACNS), the American Academy of Nurse Practitioners (AANP), or the American College of Nurse Practitioners (ACNP). Further, none of the 10 external reaction panel members invited by the AACN to comment on deliberations represented these organizations, and the formal exclusion of the ANA is noteworthy (AACN, 2004c). This lack of diversity of decision makers and formal consultants to the exclusion of organizations representing members (and future members) who would be the most impacted by any proposed change in educational requirements led to early criticism of the AACN for not fully vetting its proposal with audiences not inclined to agree with them. As Fulton and Lyon wrote back in 2005, "In proposing the practice doctorate AACN has engaged only a limited number of stakeholders in meaningful dialogue" (Fulton & Lyon, 2005, p. 3).

At the writing of the chapter in 2017, the only national groups representing Nurse Anesthesia and CNSs (two of the four traditional APRN specialties) had endorsed mandatory doctoral entry. The Council on Accreditation (COA), which accredits nurse anesthesia programs), announced in 2017 the requirement that doctoral entry be required by 2025 and they are on track to accomplish this. However, the DNP degree is not a requirement. Some pursue the doctor of nurse anesthesia practice (DNAP). There are two CRNA contributors to this book. One has a PhD and the other has a DNP and a PhD. In 2015, the NACNS called for the DNP requirement for entry-level practice by 2030. The NACNS had remained neutral on the DNP degree, neither endorsing it nor discouraging it for future CNSs (NACNS, 2015). Part of the NACN's argument was a study presented at the 2007 DNP Conference in Annapolis, Maryland, indicating significant duplication of curriculum outcomes between MSN and DNP degrees, and thus the need for another degree was questioned (Jacobson et al., 2007). Furthermore, because many CNS positions had a strong research role component (and many had a PhD), a degree that deemphasized the conduct of research was seen as problematic (Fulton, 2010; McNett, 2006). Just this past March 2023, the NACNS revised its entry level to practice as follows:

> NACNS's Revised Position: Entry for CNS Practice: The NACNS endorses three academic degree options as minimum entry to CNS practice: a master's degree, post-graduate certificate, or DNP degree from an accredited academic program that prepares graduates as a CNS.

Part of this decision-making was (a) a thorough cross-walk with the *Essentials* and the determination that graduate level 2 competencies and subcompetencies aligned with the NACNS core practice competencies, and were being achieved through MSN, DNP, and postgraduate certificate levels of CNS education; (b) NACNS embraces educational options for CNSs and all APRNs seeking academic preparation beyond the master's degree and views both the DNP and PhD as terminal nursing degrees; (c) the additional costs and time associated with obtaining a DNP degree over a master's degree, and the barrier (larger or small) to leave the CNS workforce resulting in fewer CNSs supporting quality and safety at a time of post-pandemic rebuilding the presence of the CNS role. The NACNS did state that it fully embraces the 2022 recommendation put forth by the AACN that academic and practice leaders clarify the purpose and goals of the DNP degree, identify hallmarks of high-quality DNP programs, educate employers about the unique competencies of DNP graduates, collect systems-level data on DNP CNS role; and finally, (d) using all the best evidence possible, they found no demonstrable difference in outcomes between master's and DNP practice. Their Position Statement did conclude with the following:

> NACNS fully embraces the 2022 recommendation put forth by AACN that academic and practice leaders clarify the purpose and goals of the DNP degree, identify hallmarks of high-quality DNP programs, educate employers about the unique competencies of DNP graduates, collect systems-level data on DNP effectiveness, and conduct research on the impact of DNP-prepared nurses on patient outcome. (pp. 1–2)

A TWO-DECADE-LONG, STILL UNRESOLVED ISSUE OF THE DOMAIN OF "RESEARCH" IN THE DNP DEGREE

As we reflect on the history that both Columbia University and the University of Kentucky have provided for the contemporary practice doctorate, it is also important to examine the first critical mass of schools that began DNP programs in 2005. At the time, despite the October 25, 2004, vote by the AACN to require the DNP degree for all advanced practice nurses—NPs, CRNAs, CNMs, and CNSs—by 2015, the landscape and the curricula of the DNP degree had not yet evolved. Table 1.3 lists the DNP programs (both DNP and DrNP) that existed on August 1, 2005, the first critical mass of DNP programs.

Right after Columbia University introduced its DrNP mode in early 2005, Drexel University in Philadelphia launched its own doctor of nursing practice degree model in March 2005, labeling it also with the DrNP. It was labeled as a "clinical research doctor of nursing practice degree." It combined both advanced practice and the conduct of practical clinical research, concluding with a clinical dissertation. The degree was modeled after the PsyD and DrPH degrees (both professional doctorates that include

TABLE 1.3 Inaugural Doctor of Nursing Practice Programs in the United States (as of August 1, 2005)

University	Year Founded	Type of Program	Notes
Case Western Reserve University	2005	DNP	Founded as ND and converted to DNP.
Columbia University	2005	DrNP	Founded as DrNP and converted to DNP in 2008. Founders still refer to the degree as a "clinical doctorate."
Drexel University	2005	DrNP	A hybrid professional doctorate combining the practice doctorate and the academic research doctorate. Founders refer to the degree as a "clinical research Doctor of Nursing Practice degree"; it converted to a DNP in 2014.
Rush University	2005	DNP	Founded as an ND and converted to a DNP in Leadership and the Business of Health Care (only).
Tri-College University Nursing Consortium	2005	DNP	NDSU left the consortium in 2007; the consortium disbanded in 2008.
University of Colorado, Denver	2005	DNP	Founded as ND and converted to DNP.
University of Kentucky	2001	DNP	First DNP—Clinical Leadership (only).
University of South Carolina	2005	DNP	Founded as ND and converted to DNP. First school to offer the BSN-to-DNP option to prepare entry-level NPs.
University of Tennessee, Memphis	2005	DNP	Founded as DNSc and converted to DNP.

Concordia College; Minnesota State University, Moorhead; and North Dakota State University.

BSN, bachelor of science in nursing; DNP, doctor of nursing practice; DrNP, doctor of nursing practice; DNSc, doctor of nursing science; ND, doctor of nursing; NDSU, North Dakota State University; NPs, nurse practitioners.

a research emphasis), and the authors detailed their new degree model in the *Journal of Online Issues in Nursing* in 2005 (Dreher et al., 2005). As the founding chair of the Doctoral Nursing Department, I and a talented group of faculty (some of them NPs and one nurse midwife) started a doctoral nursing program development committee. Before this committee was formed, there had already been a faculty working group contemplating a degree model in 2000 in a quest to find a practice-oriented degree as an alternative to the PhD. However, the Drexel nursing faculty felt very strongly that the research mission of the degree should only deemphasize the PhD degree's focus on conducting research and creating new knowledge, not eliminate it. The College of Nursing and Health Professions also had a Department of Public Health, which offered the PhD and DrPH. A clearer understanding of those two degrees' differences certainly impacted our thinking. Certainly, since the Drexel program was an obvious outlier, other programs using the DNP initials quietly let their students engage in clinical research, as this was probably what the faculty felt more comfortable mentoring their students to perform.

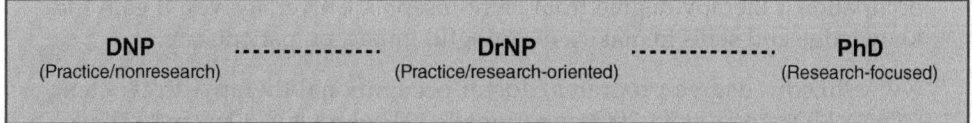

FIGURE 1.1 Practice/nonresearch, practice/research-oriented, and research-focused nursing doctorates.

DNP, doctor of nursing practice; DrNP, doctor of nursing practice.

The DrNP actually modeled its clinical research dissertation on the PsyD clinical dissertation. The department invited the chair of a local PsyD program. They chose not to start a PhD but instead a professional doctorate emphasizing the clinical practice of psychology and some different pathways of scholarship for the student (Murray, 2000). A few students still wanted to conduct experimental research. The professional psychology doctorate is a "hybrid doctorate."

Some thought that the AACN in 2004 had not seriously considered hybrid doctorates like the PsyD. All hybrid doctorates in the health professions require completion of a research project, usually in the form of a dissertation (in the UK, the words "thesis" and "dissertation" are used interchangeably and mean the same thing; Dreher et al., 2008; Hawkins & Nezat, 2009; Smith-Glasgow & Dreher, 2010). Figure 1.1 indicates that the DrNP degree was theoretically designed to fall in between the PhD and the DNP degrees, and Figure 1.2 indicates how this is approached similarly (from a practice doctorate with the smallest emphasis on research to the most, the PhD) in occupational therapy. Finally, as the DrNP degree model at the time included four roles (practitioner, clinical executive, educator, and clinical scientist), it is noted that 50% of the first 16 current graduates who entered the doctoral program in a role other than that of an educator (most were full-time practicing certified NPs) went into academia postgraduation, and 56% of these graduates were in full-time academic appointments. We suggested that at that time this degree model had a high rate of producing new full-time nursing faculty (three of whom have even procured tenure-track positions), and the average time from matriculation to graduation was approximately 3.29 years.

DOT, doctor of occupational therapy; DrOT, doctor of occupational therapy; OTD, occupational therapy doctorate: Some current active DrOT programs are at Nova Southeastern University in Florida, St. Joseph's University in Philadelphia, Valparaiso University in Indiana, and Grand Valley State University in Michigan. Most (but not all) are postprofessional programs for licensed occupational therapists who already have a master's degree.

St. Joseph University's DrOT has program for entry-level occupational therapists:

> The Doctor of Occupational Therapy (DrOT) is a doctorate degree that prepares you to become a successful OT practitioner, researcher, or leader in a variety of medical and community settings. It's the highest level of formal education available to entry-level occupational therapists. By earning your

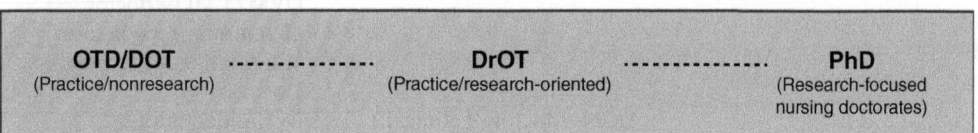

FIGURE 1.2 Practice/nonresearch, practice/research-oriented, and research-focused occupational therapy doctorates.

occupational therapy degree from Saint Joseph's University, you'll gain the knowledge and skills to make a meaningful impact on patient care.

www.sju.edu/degree-programs/doctor-occupational-therapy-drot#:~:text
=The%20Doctor%20of%20Occupational%20Therapy,to%20entry%2Dlevel
%20occupational%20therapists.

The hybrid degree is particularly facile in academia because all students complete some research training, culminating in a variety of research formats, and therefore have some common research skills with the PhD. In my discussion of the DrPH and PhD degrees, the DrPH faculty made it clear that there was no difference in research skill preparation. It was the focus of their research. One PhD example may be a career trajectory emphasizing longitudinal epidemiology on some subject or, for a DrPH, the study of the efficacy of a field intervention for a public health problem. Other health professions have also dealt with the realities of professional doctorates (only nursing uses the term "practice doctorate") and the difficult transition of their graduates into academic roles, particularly when the degree emphasis was on practice, not scholarly productivity. Table 1.4 identifies other health professions that have hybrid doctorates and indicates the differences among the research, hybrid professional, and professional doctorates.

Previously, the National Institutes of Health (NIH) opened up research funding (at least in the Parent K23 mechanism) to both graduates of "doctoral nursing research and nursing practice" programs (NIH, 2009a, section 1.B), It seems unegalitarian to say that one doctoral nursing graduate will create the evidence and the other will then translate and disseminate it. Good science, especially science grounded in practice, is not really conducted that way. That is part of the critique that Florczak (2010) made, querying "just how and where one could arbitrarily uncouple the practice of nursing from nursing

TABLE 1.4 Types of Doctorates for Health Professions Disciplines in the United States

Academic Research Doctorates (Research-Intensive Emphasis)	Hybrid Professional Doctorates (Practice/Research-Oriented Emphasis)	Professional Doctorates (Practice/Nonresearch Emphasis)
PhD—doctor of philosophy	DrPH—doctor of public health	MD/DO—doctor of medicine, doctor of osteopathy
ScD—doctor of science	DSc—doctor of science	DPT—doctor of physical therapy
	PsyD—doctor of psychology	PharmD—doctor of pharmacy
	DSW—doctor of social work	DNP—doctor of nursing practice
	DScPT—doctor of science in physical therapy	DDS/DMD—doctor of dental surgery, Dentariae Medicinae Doctoris
		DVM/VMD—doctor of veterinary medicine, Veterinariae Medicinae Doctoris
	DCN—doctor of clinical nutrition	DOT—doctor of occupational therapy AuD – doctor of audiology

research" (p. 16). The "DNP Project" title was not so easily embraced. The University of Washington School of Nursing faculty initially promoted the concept of "practice inquiry" (which some schools adopted; Magyary et al., 2006). Although this scholarly approach did not prohibit the conduct of nursing research, it was designed to frame their DNP scholarly end product with a practice orientation and called it a clinical investigative project. The call to revisit the particular "scholarly/research mission" of the DNP was heard over the last decade (Radzyminski, 2023; Root et al., 2018; Terry, 2014; Vincent et al., 2014) and again with the white paper on the DNP (AACN, 2015). What lies ahead is hopefully a maturing of scholarship from DNP graduates and more precise mentoring and supervision from their DNP faculty. I have studied DNP curricula intensely for years. Having chaired two national conferences on the practice doctorate and presented at several International Conferences on Professional Doctorates in the UK, Scotland, and Italy, and in dialogue with largely European and Australian colleagues, I have come to hypothesize that the DNP graduate may be best positioned to create "Practice Knowledge" for the profession (Dreher, 2010b, 2016). It is in the focus on creating practice-based evidence that DNP graduates may excel, even beyond the PhD graduate.

In the mid-1900s, a group of scholars wanted to find a new theoretical way to distinguish among different kinds of technological and scientific knowledge that could be aligned with knowledge produced in the social and behavioral sciences in the same way (Gibbons et al., 1994; Nowotny et al., 2001). They categorized all forms of knowledge into two different modes. Mode 1 knowledge is mostly traditional, empirical, theoretical, and disseminated very typically according to academy norms (not the focus of this book). Mode 2 knowledge, which is work-based and practice-oriented, is derived and disseminated differently than mode 1 knowledge. I view mode 2 knowledge as *DNP-generated knowledge* and analogous to practice evidence.

In my own proposed model of scientific inquiry in nursing, shown in Figure 1.3, it is suggested that it is practice knowledge, or mode 2 knowledge (represented by the right circle of the Venn diagram), that the DNP graduate is most prepared to conduct (Dreher, 2010b, 2016). This knowledge is created through practice-based research and inquiry that leads to practice-based evidence (Barkham & Mellor-Clark, 2003; Hellerstein, 2008; San Francisco AIDS Foundation, 2008). The left circle represents theoretical knowledge, or mode 1 knowledge, and it is here that the PhD student is more prepared to conduct theoretical knowledge and generate evidence-based practice knowledge generally using larger data sets. The mode 2 knowledge emanating from DNP programs, however, would be more practice-oriented and closely connected to the work or clinical environment. It could be conducted in real time or even through the measurement of observations. Then, after rigorous and efficient analysis, the findings could be refined and translated into practice on a smaller scale (e.g., a feasibility study first, followed by a pilot test). It is likely some degree of practice-based evidence has been generated. Next, there must be decisions about the cost/impact determination of a more standardized research process on a larger scale toward possibly generating evidence-based practice knowledge. However, this drive for practice-based evidence should not be construed as a lesser research function. Some new or novel phenomena are just not ready for multisite, double-blind, clinical trial investigation. Most nursing-sensitive healthcare problems will never be funded at that level. The practitioner or clinical executive scholar closest to practice is in the best position to identify new or intransigent clinical problems that need investigation. The intersection of the two circles in the Venn diagram represents research that is highly contextualized in both practice-based evidence and evidence-based practice domains. Here, the final research project

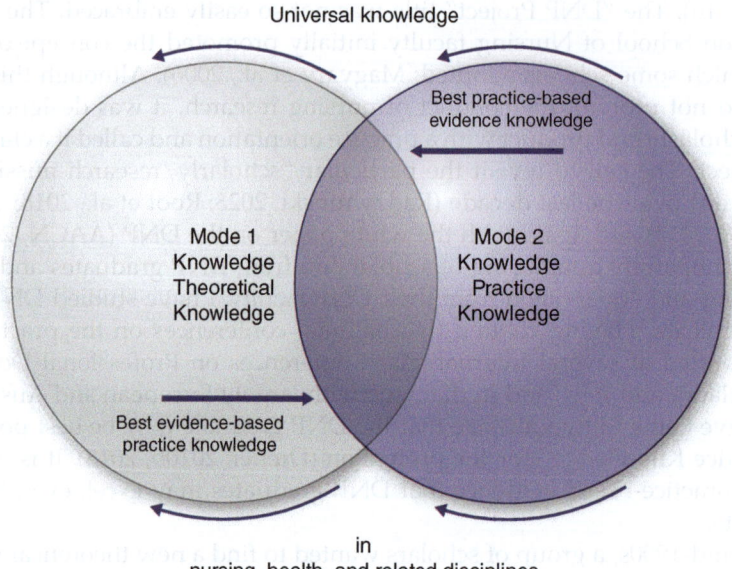

FIGURE 1.3 A model of scientific inquiry in nursing.

Sources: Dreher, H. M. (2011b). The path to nursing science today, 1910–2010. In M. D. Dahnke & H. M. Dreher (Eds.), *Philosophy of science for nursing practice: Concepts and applications* (pp. 269–300). Springer Publishing; Dreher, H. M. (2016b). Next steps toward practice knowledge development. In M. D. Dahnke & H. M. Dreher (Eds.), *Philosophy of science for nursing practice: Concepts and applications* (2nd ed., pp. 353–391). Springer Publishing.

(whatever it is called), whether PhD or DNP, is simply indistinguishable. Herein lies the rigor of the best DNP and PhD programs, where clinical practice problem solving is the overwhelming emphasis. I conclude that this is where knowledge development is most highly developed and relevant to the discipline. I further believe this conceptualization of the intersection of the Venn diagram and its integrated model of mode 1 and mode 2 nursing knowledge is unique. In 2016, Greenhalgh, Jackson, Shaw, and Janamian clearly rejected the idea that a separation of mode 1 and mode 2 knowledge has a beneficial research impact:

> Context: Co-creation—collaborative knowledge generation by academics working alongside other stakeholders—reflects a "Mode 2" relationship (knowledge production rather than knowledge translation) between universities and society. Co-creation is widely believed to increase research impact. (p. 1)

I would make a legitimate analogy that mode 1 nursing scholarship (PhD student knowledge production/generating) and mode 2 nursing scholarship (DNP knowledge translation) are harmful to a profession with limited resources to advance clinical care. Aside from there being no equality, the PhD student's "I generate" and the DNP's "then I translate and disseminate" are just not the way science is produced.

These indistinguishable particular studies represented at the intersection of both circles, whether DNP or PhD student-led studies, include both large and small data sets. There is no logic why the DNP Project cannot have a larger sample size than PhD Study X. Some DNP projects/clinical dissertations/DNP theses (you name it!) are naturally more focused on practice-based evidence (problems that need more initial inquiry), and

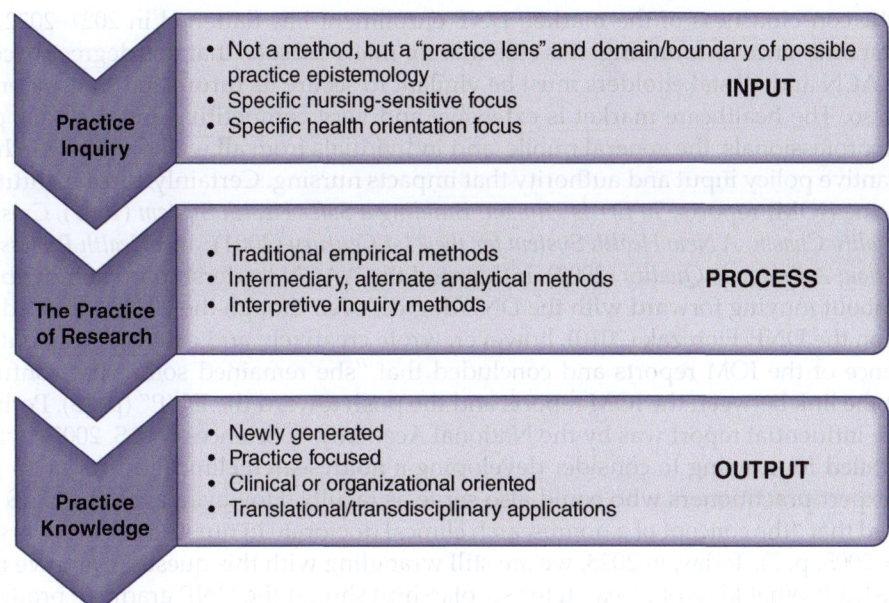

FIGURE 1.4 Path of practice knowledge generation in an emerging nursing epistemology.
Sources: H. Michael Dreher (2011, 2017)

large data sets usually have already documented studies with useful outcome data. The PhD student interested in building a research focus within their academic role will seek research mentors to collaborate with. It is critical for them to have at least one non-nurse on the research team to indicate they are collaborating interprofessionally. It should be no different for DNP students, who need mentors too. It is likely that most DNP programs are located in colleges or universities with other clinical disciplines that have hybrid doctoral programs and faculty there who would be honored (even flattered) that you sought them out with the potential to collaborate with and be mentored by them. One exciting collaborative dyad would be between an experienced post-master's NP (who could benefit from more research skills exposure) and the other student benefiting from the NP's clinical knowledge. A more complete description of this model (Figure 1.3) can be found in Chapter 16, "Next Steps Toward Practice Knowledge Development: An Emerging Epistemology in Nursing," in Dahnke and Dreher's (2016) second edition of *Philosophy of Science for Nursing Practice: Concepts and Applications*.

Mode 2 knowledge generation is where the professional/practice doctorate graduate should excel. Figure 1.4 is a diagram identifying the different paths/choices the DNP student can take to generate practice knowledge.

■ POSITIVE OUTCOMES AND UNRESOLVED ISSUES: THEN AND NOW STILL MEANS PROGRESS

This section of this chapter provides a short overview of some of the positive outcomes and central challenges or unresolved issues that the DNP degree faced in 2017 (just after a decade of the launch of the DNP) and now in 2023, 20 years after its implementation. Resolving these is essential as this still relatively new doctoral degree (we can revisit the DPT and PharmD histories) tries to gain a foothold in academic nursing circles and into the consciousness of the market. DNP enrollment has flattened in 2021–2022, for the first time since its founding. It is essential for many reasons that this degree succeed. The AACN and all stakeholders must be vigilant to secure its future and transparent in doing so. The healthcare market is extensive and very competitive and includes peer health professionals, the general public, and individuals from all walks of life who have substantive policy input and authority that impacts nursing. Certainly, three Institute of Medicine (IOM) reports, *To Err Is Human: Building a Safer Health System* (1999), *Crossing the Quality Chasm, A New Health System for the 21st Century* (2001), and *Health Professions Education: A Bridge to Quality* (2003), influenced the AACN leadership in their deliberations about moving forward with the DNP degree, even though the 2003 report did not mention the DNP. Florczak (2010), however, wrote creatively and extensively about the influence of the IOM reports and concluded that "she remained somewhat confused about the link between the IOM reports and the push toward the DNP" (p. 15). Perhaps a more influential report was by the National Academy of Sciences (NAS, 2005), which then called for nursing to consider developing a nonresearch clinical doctorate to prepare expert practitioners who could also serve as faculty. However, even the NAS recognized that "the concept of a nonresearch clinical doctorate in nursing is controversial" (NAS, 2005, p. 7). Today, in 2023, we are still wrangling with this question, and we now ask instead: What kind of research (or scholarship) should the DNP graduate produce?

The first of the chief positive outcomes of the DNP degree is the realization that, with the complexity of healthcare today, there is indeed curricular content and specialized knowledge beyond the MSN to give DNP graduates additional, enhanced skills. This has been detailed earlier, by both the AACN (2004a) and the National Panel for Nurse Practitioner Practice Doctorate Competencies (2006). In 20212, the NONPF (2012) abandoned specific DNP-only competencies, in the realization that the competencies for nurse practitioner practice for initial licensure for the NP at the master's level could not be different from the DNP. In 2022, the National Task Force (NTF) on Quality Nurse Practitioner Education called for the current minimum clinical hours for NP education to be raised from 500 to 1000 hours. However, that was rejected in favor of 750 hours with a 2-year transition period. In 2020, the *Essentials* made the same calculation. You cannot disenfranchise the overwhelming numbers of APRNs who have master's degrees without outcome data on a clear differentiation of role and practice and without regulatory changes at the state level (McCauley et al., 2022). But the AACN has made the correct move to require the same competencies in the domains for advanced-level practice (MS and DNP), but add some subdomains for the DNP. It is unclear whether they will be required during their three-year transition to the *Essentials* curriculum. There is likely to be continued resistance at the academic and state regulatory levels even if one fully supports doctoral-level advanced practice, as I, like many others, do. The literature needs lots more evidence. Whether the DNP degree ultimately changes the scope and practice of the advanced practice nurse is another question. Although the AACN (2009b) says, "No, transitioning to the DNP will not alter the current scope of practice for APRNs" (p. 1), it is somewhat illogical to require additional skills and competencies for more ANPs and then assume that the scope of practice will not change. Maybe that is actually what the American Medical Association (AMA) fears the most: not nurses using the title "Dr." but real fears about the possibility that the scope and boundaries of their practice will expand (AMA, 2009, 2023). Nevertheless, if there was ever an argument against the DNP, it would be a situation in which MSN programs simply added a few credits and called the degree a "doctorate" without any forthright attention to educating a more highly prepared practitioner.

A second positive outcome is that there is now a widely established nursing doctorate that gives nurses an alternative to the PhD (Buchholz et al., 2015; Sperhac &

Clinton, 2008). For decades, nurses only had a research-intensive degree, clinical doctorates that were de facto research-intensive degrees, four NDs, and one lone EdD—degree models that never gained a foothold within the profession. Whether it really is in the interest of nursing for there to be only one alternative to the PhD, the DNP, with the CCNE's refusal to recognize any form of the practice doctorate except the initials "DNP," is still debatable (AACN, 2005b). However, because of the power and influence of the AACN and CCNE, they are not likely to endorse a third doctorate. But the CRNAs did with their doctor of nurse anesthesia practice (DNAP) degree. And perhaps CNMs are on their way too, with Jefferson University's new doctor of nurse midwifery (DM) degree. From Dana B. Perlman, DNP, CNM, FACNM, Program Coordinator, Doctorate in Midwifery:

> The Doctorate of Midwifery (DM) degree is the first doctoral degree in the US specifically in the discipline of midwifery. It is post-professional in line with the articulated ACNM position statement that a graduate degree, not a doctorate, is the minimum degree for midwifery practice by CNMs and CMs. We do have a dual MS+DM program where entry-to-practice students are able to "front-load" selected DM courses while they complete their graduate education in midwifery. They must pass the comprehensive exam for the midwifery education program and their national board certification prior to matriculation into the doctoral phase and are awarded an MS degree. Just as MDs and MPH students do not limit their research to QI, we do not either. We do envision the DM as an implementation, translational, or action research degree rather than a knowledge development degree. The DM does not confer a scope of practice. Qualified midwives who have earned a graduate degree in midwifery, nursing, public health, or another relevant degree, are eligible to apply.

This comprehensive degree describes itself as a "professional" doctorate. But is it scalable to the largest APRN group by far, nurse practitioners? The answer is no. So, herein lies the problem. From the PsyD, PharmD, DNP, DOT/OTD, MD, DPT, etc., all the programs require some form of research, even original research. There are simply too many articles in the literature to cite on problems with the DNP Project. It began with the AACN saying the DNP should not include original research, and there was no compromise.

I suggest the following (why not?):

> The AACN, which represents all collegiate faculty, convenes a forum from all APRN specialty groups, including nursing executive leadership (now AONL) as an endorsed DNP degree advanced practice role *and* from nursing education. The AACN does not recognize nursing education as an advanced practice role, and they still don't have to. But they do award the DNP degree. We know from their early deliberations that they considered it. If the nurse educator leadership were not invited, immense harm to the profession could be done. The group should not just be elite leaders in the profession but also comprise a diverse group of academic stakeholders. Diversity, inclusivity, and equity should be core principles of the selection of stakeholders at the forum. It could be called "A National Forum on DNP Student Scholarship Needed in the Nursing Profession." The objective should be to have discussions around core principles of scholarship that can cross our APRN, nurse executive, and educator specialties. I mentioned this earlier in this chapter: Nursing education scholarship at the undergraduate and graduate levels

should be team-based as the lone investigator model in science is practically nonexistent. Another core principle for DNP students (and our course faculty), could be that interdisciplinary and interprofessional scholarship begin early, particularly for DNP Projects and research studies. At my college, research funding will not be awarded unless there is one faculty member from another department. The core principles would be turned over to the nursing APRN organizations, including specialty organizations such as the AONL and NLN. They would then be asked to devise five forms of scholarship acceptable for DNP students and the standards they must meet for each one of them, from the highest (exceptional, knowledge-generating) to the lowest (but still acceptable). Refer to Figure 1.3: A Model of Scientific Inquiry in Nursing.

A third positive outcome of this doctoral option gives doctoral advanced practice nurses more parity with other health professionals (Flanagan et al., 2021; O'Sullivan, 2005). Although this was one of the goals for the creation of this degree, it really should not be the leading reason for individuals to seek it. The incentive to be called "Dr." ought to be driven more by what the doctorate adds to the master's-prepared practitioner to warrant the higher degree. Furthermore, the doctorate ought to be credible, have rigor, and be seen by others as legitimate. This happens with every new doctorate: Public critical analyses by degree supporters, detractors, and skeptics, and not just toward the DNP. Furthermore, with a new degree, some DAPRNs are going to experience some difficulty in the workplace while working alongside master's-prepared APRNs who may feel resentment or deny that there is any difference in practice. Doctoral-prepared physical therapists, working alongside masters-prepared physical therapists, have already experienced this, and it is likely to happen in nursing, too (Salzman, 2010). But parity is important. It allows us to sit at the table as equal contributors. Noted healthcare and nursing journalist Suzanne Gordon (2006) has written about the "invisibility of nursing" (p. 184). Maybe the DNP degree can help increase our visibility and permit our practitioners and clinicians (and others) to be seen as full partners in both practice and policy.

A fourth positive outcome is that this degree was designed to emphasize the translation and dissemination of research findings (AACN, 2006). To others, this may be an unresolved issue or one that is slowly evolving. It is evolving, as the AACN published on it in 2015 and again in 2018. Although I and others believe that generating practice knowledge through practice inquiry (Flanagan et al., 2021; Dreher, 2010b; Magyary et al., 2006) should be incorporated into the degree, the opportunity this degree presented the profession was nonetheless unique for DNP to generate knowledge for our discipline. Magyary et al. (2006) write of the DNP student's role in practice inquiry:

> How to frame researchable questions generated from clinical observations and discourse is an essential practice inquiry competency. Clinical observations discrepant with habitual ways of knowing and doing may reveal new insights into clinical phenomena that have received limited or no empirical inquiry. These types of revelations may generate questions that beg to be answered through rigorous scientific investigation. DNP graduates should also help broaden the definition of evidence through their work-based problems. (p. 144)

One problem with evidence-based practice is that the concept of what is "evidence" must be understood first before discussions of what is evidence-based practice or practice-based evidence can take place and be understood. Dahnke does this in Chapter 4, "What Is Evidence?" A very traditional definition of "what is evidence in the health professions" was challenged by Pearson et al. (2007) at the Joanna Briggs Institute at the University of Adelaide in Adelaide, Australia, and American DNP (and PhD) nursing faculty would benefit from exploring this literature. Initially, Pearson and colleagues describe four different types of clinical evidence that are posited based on a clinical question: (a) evidence of feasibility, (b) evidence of appropriateness, (c) evidence of meaningfulness, and (d) evidence of effectiveness. Later, the Joanne Briggs Institute expanded its taxonomy of evidence and offered a more detailed, descriptive reorganization of levels of evidence based on: (a) levels of evidence for effectiveness, (b) levels of evidence for diagnosis, (c) levels of evidence for prognosis, (d) levels of evidence for economic evaluations, and (e) levels of evidence for meaningfulness (Joanna Briggs Institute Levels of Evidence and Grades of Recommendation Working Party, 2013). It is highly recommended that both DNP faculty and students review this document in which the clinical problem is identified and the methodology is developed.

The first three chief unresolved issues surrounding the DNP degree from its inception remain to this day to a greater or lesser extent and are summarized as follows:

- Continuing controversy over the domain of knowledge development within the DNP degree and whether empirical research should be generally acceptable or not.
- Early debate on the required minimum clinical hours for the degree (NP) has now mostly subsided with the 2022 NTF Standards, but there are still those who want 1,000 hours (not the current compromise of 750). Initially, most programs interpreted the statement from the AACN's Essentials of Doctoral Education for Advanced Nursing Practice (2006), "In order to achieve the DNP competencies, programs should provide a minimum of 1,000 hours of practice post-baccalaureate as part of a supervised academic program" (p. 19) very, very liberally. Even the usually supportive NONPF never fully endorsed the mandate that every post-master's clinical DNP student needs 400 more hours of actual practice (if the original MSN degree in pediatrics, e.g., had 600 hours). According to the NONPF (2006), "The evidence for the AACN recommendation for 1,000 clinical hours for all practice doctorate students has not been presented" (p. 1). Additionally, for the Nurse Executive Track, it was the "wild, wild West!" These students did not complete hundreds of hours of precepted time during their MSN degrees in nursing administration, and therefore it seemed exorbitant to require them to complete 1,000 total hours for the degree. This was not logical. All DNP tracks required 1,000 hours, and even if the requirement was there, it may not have been tacitly enforced. There was inequity there.

This last issue was debated at length at the 2007 DNP Conference in Annapolis, Maryland. For some, it seemed unrealistic that part-time students (who work full-time) would need a total of 1,000 clinical hours (including whatever was earned for the master's degree), plus coursework (and still remain fully employed, particularly if they were receiving employer-based tuition benefits), to complete the degree. At Drexel, almost all of the students worked full time and attended doctoral study as part-time students, and they barely seemed able to complete the rigorous, intense curriculum that was structured year-round (four quarters) over 3 years (the third year was devoted exclusively to the completion of the clinical dissertation). The Drexel program did not require 1,000 hours, but it focused more on the quality of the two required doctoral practice practica and not the quantity of hours.

- Controversy by the CCNE that an "accredited" DNP degree may not formally prepare nurse educators. This was a serious, consequential decision. Most nursing faculty in my experience want to teach nursing. Many want to participate in pursuing scholarship too. However, there are many factors, including cost, raising families, and the immense labor-intensive workload of teaching nursing (not history or psychology), that prevent them from pursuing a PhD in nursing. With the narrow vote, it was clear it was a divisive issue. Leadership should have found a way to reach more consensus. For some, it seemed too tactical.
- An ongoing discussion over whether PhD and DNP students should share any common coursework. Early on, this was a very divisive issue. "DNP students should not be in PhD courses!" I would hear this at AACN Doctoral Conferences. Now the tone is more about collaboration between the two. But most articles are about "how they can/should" collaborate with no real-world examples. And moreover, I wonder, how often who is leading who?

The issue over the role of research in the DNP degree may never end. The NACNS has just taken a different stance because, in their pre-DNP world, many of them were already operating in the world of empirical research. Our inclination is to predict that ultimately the DNP degree may look different at research-intensive and research-extensive universities where knowledge generation and scholarship are central to the mission. DNP programs that reside in colleges where the teaching mission and scholarship are emphasized, however, may be less inclined to design curricula that generate practice knowledge. However, these generalizations need not be used indiscriminately to prevent practice inquiry or even formal empirical inquiry by any DNP student anywhere. If we are honest, the same reality is present in PhD nursing/nursing science programs all across the country. Although some PhD programs emphasize the nurse scientist model (with a focus on generating nursing science), other PhD programs emphasize teaching and education research and are less focused on producing graduates for research careers. The DNP degree should be no different. It will continue to evolve, and it will evolve best when both doctoral advanced nursing practitioners who simply want to practice and those who want to practice and generate practice knowledge (e.g., generate primary care, clinical, or organizational nursing knowledge) are both seated at the table and can respect the role each wants to play as stewards of the discipline. Medicine is actually no different, as many practicing physicians are not involved in research or have no interest in it. They simply want to practice the art of medicine. Other physicians, however, see problems in their practice and are interested in initiating or participating in research related to these problems.

The other previously discussed issue—the role of the DNP degree in the preparation of nurse educators—is now led by the National League for Nursing, and all three other nursing accreditors accredit DNP programs. In the 2017 edition of this book, I wrote the following, which is worth replicating:

> ...there are unfortunately no aggressive strategic plans by nursing's current leadership to adequately replenish the supply of retiring nursing professors and nurse scientists. This is most unfortunate, because, without nursing faculty, we cannot admit more nursing students and help alleviate the long-term nursing shortage. It seems highly unlikely, however, that we can increase the number of PhD students and graduates in the critical mass that is needed. The only solution that seems plausible is to reengineer the DNP graduate, especially those interested in teaching in MSN and DNP programs, for pathways that include a specific curriculum focus on teaching doctoral advanced practice. (p. 37)

How much has changed and worsened with the pre-and post-COVID-19 pandemic? Very little.

- At the January 2009 AACN Doctoral Nursing Education Conference in Coronado Island, California, attendees engaged in a lengthy discussion about the final issue—shared coursework between the two degree programs. From my point of view, there seemed to be two camps of nursing faculty perspectives. One camp firmly believed that students from both degrees could learn from each other and therefore supported some joint coursework between the two programs. The other camp was firmly against crossover between the two curricula, fearing dilution of the PhD degree and the slow trajectory to one day "the DNP becoming the same as the PhD." Interestingly, I had not heard DNP faculty similarly state they did not want their DNP students taking courses with PhD students. It appears, however, that across the country, there is already some minimal coursework that students in the two degrees share. For faculty administrators, it also seemed more cost-effective to offer some courses to both groups, especially if the class size (usually the PhD classes) was small. Sometimes this is still heard from RNs who share coursework with generic BSN students. It was good to see in the white paper (AACN2, 2015) that more collaboration between DNP and PhD students is encouraged. The comments I heard, however, came from post-master's DNP graduates who took some common coursework with BSN-to-DNP students and who complained of the level of the content and its appropriateness for experienced master's-prepared APRNs. "DNP and PhD graduates will [should] have the opportunity to collaborate and work synergistically to improve health outcomes" (p. 3). Absolute separatism, which I am aware exists in some schools where there is a PhD and a DNP program might foster elitism in PhD students and in PhD programs (or even among faculty), deans and chairs need to actively promote collegiality among students (and faculty) in both cohorts, and if these students are going to be involved in PhD/DNP translational research teams, as some are now suggesting, then what better time to begin to work together than during doctoral study (Cacchione, 2007; Hastings et al., 2010)?

One important point, however, needs to be emphasized. "Translation of research" and "translational research" are not the same thing. The NIH (2009b) has very clear definitions of what constitutes translational research, indicating:

> Translational research includes two areas of translation. One is the process of applying discoveries generated during research in the laboratory, and in preclinical studies, to the development of trials and studies in humans. The second area of translation *concerns research* [italics mine] aimed at enhancing the adoption of best practices in the community. The cost-effectiveness of prevention and treatment strategies is also an important part of translational science. (Section 1.1)

The AACN *Essentials of Doctoral Education for Advanced Nursing Practice* (2006) document makes it clear that "translational research" is not what it is referring to when it states:

> The scholar applies knowledge to solve a problem via the scholarship of application (referred to as the scholarship of practice in nursing). This application involves the *translation of research* [italics mine] into practice and the dissemination and integration of new knowledge, which are key activities of DNP graduates. (p. 11)

The nuance is nevertheless very clear. Translational research involves very formal, traditional methods of scientific inquiry (Rubio et al., 2010). Supporting this in their description of practice inquiry, Magyary and colleagues (2006) indicate, "Practice inquiry entails a wide spectrum of designs, methods, and statistical approaches. Emerging conceptual and technological advances in clinical epidemiology and informatics provide APNs with the instruments to identify and monitor clinical patterns over time" (p. 145). In my view, the skill set of the DNP graduate described here is different from the more narrow focus of the scholarship of application. Therefore, until there is more clarity about the direction of the scholarship focus of the DNP degree, we are likely to see individual DNP programs undertaking very different forms of scientific and practice inquiry.

INTERNATIONAL IMPLICATIONS FOR THE DNP DEGREE

Finally, this chapter concludes with some thoughts about the DNP degree in the larger professional doctorate and universal doctoral nursing communities. With the exception of medicine, dentistry, and veterinary medicine, there are no doctoral programs outside of the United States that do not include the conduct of research. Indeed, the European Union (EU) in their Bologna Third Doctoral Cycle deliberations is trying to establish some uniformity among EU nations to better standardize both the PhD and the professional doctorate so that the transferability of scholars' credentials across borders is not an issue (Bologna Process, 2010; Davies, 2008). First, it may not be common knowledge, but professional nursing doctorates have existed globally, particularly in Australia, Northern Ireland, and Great Britain, since the 1990s (Ellis & Lee, 2005; McKenna & Cutcliffe, 2001). What is common among them (and professional doctorates in all other disciplines aside from those disciplines identified previously) is that the conduct of research is an integral part of their core competencies. Stew (2009) and his colleagues from the University of Brighton indicate that the difference between the PhD and the professional doctorate is that the PhD prepares the "professional researcher" and the professional doctorate prepares the "researching professional." But does the DNP degree fit into this international professional nursing doctorate degree model? The answer is that some do, but most do not. However, what the DNP and other U.S.-based professional doctorates do that the international professional doctorates largely do not is emphasize and actually require additional practice hours beyond the MSN or other health professions master's degree.

Even as I attended the first Professional and Practice-Focused Doctoral Research Special Interest Group meeting in London in July 2010 as the only U.S. attendee, I queried a fellow colleague who indicated that their professional doctorate graduates do gain advanced practice hours at their work site, although absolute hours are not required. I argued that it would be controversial (even open the university to liability, which I understand is less prevalent in the British legal system) to award credit in the United States for actual work the student completed as the agent of the employer (hospital) and not primarily as the agent of the university. Further, I am skeptical that one can prepare a more advanced practitioner just by gaining more clinical research skills that can be applied in the practice environment.

Nevertheless, especially with the emerging codified language from the Bologna Third Cycle, it is very unlikely that a nursing doctorate without a research project would be accepted outside the United States. The Bologna Process is designed to develop common, transferable higher education standards across the European Union and a few other affiliated countries (2024). Therefore, any American DNP nurse who might seek a teaching position outside the United States should be aware of this expectation. On the other hand, the proximity of Canada to the United States has already got Canadian nursing scholars wondering how the DNP might impact the Canadian nursing educational system (Brar et al., 2010; Joachim, 2008), but the DNP degree is still absent outside the United States. I conclude by writing humorously that I did warn my mostly British colleagues in London once that they should not ignore what is happening "across the pond" in the United States with the professional doctorate or with the DNP degree. Our ideas, both good and bad, can easily make a transatlantic voyage or flight.

SUMMARY

As the DNP degree continues to evolve, some 20 years after the first DNP degree was developed in 2004 and many launched in 2005, it is now time to take a deep breath and evaluate how far we have come and what direction this degree should now take. The idea that all advanced practice registered nurses will one day have an entry-level DNP now seems unrealistic. The CNSs and CNMs, while supporting the degree, are not going to fully embrace it. The CRNAs have been more supportive, and they still have options with the DNAP (or another doctorate). DNP-educated nurse practitioners seem best positioned to make an impact with a DNP degree as the largest APRN specialty. Good people can disagree, but I believe the AACN made a miscalculation and a mistake by not allowing nursing faculty to become APNs but allowing the nurse executive APN role. The CCNE could have been very innovative and reinvented the nursing faculty role. Maybe they could have found a solution to this intransigent nurse faculty shortage. I am not a pessimist by nature, but I believe this was a lost opportunity with serious consequences.

However, the DNP degree first arrived, then survived, and has thrived for almost 20 years. Graduates are going out into the professional workforce and making a mark. New DNPs are working in roles that the healthcare system has never seen before. Some PhD nursing graduates have unfairly, but sometimes fairly, had their relevance to the clinical practice environment questioned (Wilkes & Mohan, 2008). The clinical practice environment, however, is fertile ground for the DNP graduate, and it is here that you are educated to excel.

I have tried to provide a descriptive analysis and commentary on the trajectory of this degree, particularly in the context of doctoral nursing education. Sometimes history and one's analysis and commentary are not pretty, especially as an author may suggest or affirm views a reader may disagree with. But mostly, history and its politics, seen through a human lens, are complex. In the end, the history of the DNP degree can be summarized as follows: Initially, there was great opposition to the DNP degree, but the opposition was largely quelled quickly. Now what we have left is the fine-tuning of the degree and a need to generate outcome data that will help enable our graduates to better define and "live" this new role so that nursing's mission to improve health and alleviate suffering can advance.

CRITICAL THINKING QUESTIONS

1. How do you view the state of critical discourse in nursing? Do we debate enough? Do we need more agreement and more consensus? Or should we embrace difference more and be less concerned with conformity?
2. The nursing profession appears to have abandoned the idea of a clinical doctorate as an alternative to the PhD and has embraced the title "practice doctorate" to describe the DNP. Discuss whether you think the profession needs a research doctorate (PhD), a practice doctorate (DNP), and a clinical doctorate.

3. Why do you think the EdD in nursing education degree model at Teachers College is suddenly being replicated after decades (since its founding) passed by in which it was never replicated?
4. What can be done to combat the aging nursing workforce, which faces imminent retirements that will not be replaced by the current pool of those entering the profession at all levels?
5. Debate the following: "Resolved, nursing is a profession."
6. The ND degree and now the DNP were partly modeled after the MD degree. What are your thoughts about this?
7. Discuss whether you think 1,000 total clinical hours should be required for the DNP degree, including practice and clinical executive tracks.
8. Discuss whether original research ought to be part of the formal DNP curriculum.
9. Do you agree that the DNP degree might offer something the PhD degree cannot? Provide your rationale.
10. Discuss why you have chosen the particular DNP program you are currently matriculating in.

NOTES

1. In a historical-oriented chapter, through an interpretive lens, some important points must be made. In the first edition of this book in 2011, the history of the doctor of nursing practice degree was fresh, and there was a lot of debate about a number of issues. All links were previously verified by me and the editors. Over the past 20 years, some access to these documents has not been possible. Some organizations have limited access to only those with membership, and it is likely some are deeply buried in archives. The digital archivists probably believe no one is any longer interested in a position statement their organization published 15 to 20 years ago. But I am. Every American Association of Colleges of Nursing and National Organization of Nurse Practitioner Faculty citation (and some new ones) from the first and second editions return. These two organizations' influence and leadership were central to the development of the degree. The DNP has transformed our profession. Let's talk about it.
2. The actual vote was 162 yes, 101 no, 13 abstentions, and no proxy or in absentia votes were permitted. Indeed, the power and influence of 162 individuals was substantial (Dreher et al., 2005).
3. These actions by the AMA occurred as recently as June 2023. But there is one lesson for APRNs: Keep your eye on your long-fought battles to advance your scope of practice. NCSBN: https://www.ncsbn.org/news/ncsbn-opposes-ama-amendment-on-aprns, American Nurses Association (ANA) (2023, June 17) ANA Refutes Recommendations that APRN Roles Should Be Licensed and Regulated by State Medical Boards (nursingworld.org).

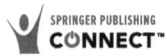

A robust set of instructor resources designed to supplement this text is located at http://connect.springerpub.com/content/book/978-0-8261-8137-4. Qualifying instructors may request access by emailing textbook@springerpub.com.

REFERENCES

Academic Nurse. (2010). Ten years of progress: The council for the advancement of care: The academic nurse. *The Journal of Columbia University School of Nursing and its Alumni, Spring,* 21–27. https://doi.org/10.1891/1939-2095.3.2.80

Accreditation Commission for Education in Nursing (2023). *Diploma nursing programs.* https://www.acenursing.org/search-programs/

Aiken, L. H., Cheung, R. B., & Olds, D. M. (2009). Education policy initiatives to address the nurse shortage in the United States. *Health Affairs, 28*(4), 646–656. https://doi.org/10.1377/hlthaff.28.4.w646

American Association of Colleges of Nursing. (1999). *Faculty shortages intensify nation's nursing deficit.* http://www.aacn.nche.edu/publications/issues/IB499WB.htm

American Association of Colleges of Nursing. (2004a). *AACN position statement on the practice doctorate in nursing October 2004.* http://www.aacn.nche.edu/DNP/pdf/DNP.pdf

American Association of Colleges of Nursing. (2004b). *AACN draft position statement on the practice doctorate in nursing January 2004.* Author.

American Association of Colleges of Nursing. (2004c). *AACN position statement on the practice doctorate in nursing March 2004.* Author.

American Association of Colleges of Nursing. (2004d). *AACN adopts a new vision for the future of nursing education and practice.* http://www.aacn.nche.edu/Media/NewsReleases/DNPRelease.htm

American Association of Colleges of Nursing. (2005a). *Faculty shortages in baccalaureate and graduate nursing programs: Scope of the problem and strategies for expanding the supply.* http://www.aacn.nche.edu/publications/pdf/05FacShortage.pdf

American Association of Colleges of Nursing. (2005b). *Commission on collegiate nursing education moves to consider for accreditation only practice doctorates with the DNP degree title.* http://www.aacn.nche.edu/Media/NewsReleases/Archives/2005/CCNEDNP.htm

American Association of Colleges of Nursing. (2006). *The essentials of doctoral education for advanced nursing practice.* http://www.aacn.nche.edu/DNP/pdf/Essentials.pdf

American Association of Colleges of Nursing. (2008). *The preferred vision of the professoriate in baccalaureate and graduate nursing programs.* http://www.aacn.nche.edu/Publications/pdf/PreferredVision.pdf

American Association of Colleges of Nursing. (2009a). *2008–2009 Enrollment and graduations in baccalaureate and graduate programs in nursing.* Author.

American Association of Colleges of Nursing. (2009b). *Frequently asked questions, position statement on the practice doctorate in nursing.* http://www.aacn.nche.edu/DNP/dnpfaq.htm

American Association of Colleges of Nursing. (2015). *The doctor of nursing practice: Current issues and clarifying recommendations, report from the task force on the implementation of the DNP.* http://www.aacn.nche.edu/aacn-publications/white-papers/DNP-Implementation-TF-Report-8-15.pdf

American Association of Colleges of Nursing. (2019). *2018–2019 Enrollment and graduations in baccalaureate and graduate programs.* Author. https://www.aacnnursing.org/News-Information/Research-Data-Center/Standard-Data-Reports

American Association of Colleges of Nursing. (2020). *Data spotlight: Trends in graduate nursing program areas of study, data spotlight: Trends in graduate nursing program areas of study* (aacnnursing.org)

American Association of Colleges of Nursing. (2021a). *The essentials: Core competencies for professional nursing education.* The Essentials: Competencies for Professional Nursing Education (aacnnursing.org)

American Association of Colleges of Nursing. (2021b). *Data spotlight: Insights on the nursing faculty shortage.* Retrieved August 2021, from Data Spotlight: Insights on the Nursing Faculty Shortage (aacnnursing.org)

American Association of Colleges of Nursing. (2021c). *Understanding the re-envisioned essentials: A roadmap for the transformation of nursing education.* https://www.aacnnursing.org/Portals/42/AcademicNursing/pdf/Roadmap-to-New-Essentials.pdf

American Association of Colleges of Nursing. (2022a). *AACN Statement supporting the masters degree in nursing, retrieved from* AACN Statement Supporting the Masters Degree in Nursing (aacnnursing.org). The State of Doctor of Nursing Practice Education in 2022. State-of-the-DNP-Summary-Report-June-2022.pdf (aacnnursing.org)

American Association of Colleges of Nursing. (2023, May 2). *New data show enrollment declines in schools of nursing, raising concerns about the nation's nursing workforce.* https://www.aacnnursing.org/news-data/all-news/new-data-show-enrollment-declines-in-schools-of-nursing-raising-concerns-about-the-nations-nursing-workforce

American College of Nurse-Midwives. (2012). *Midwifery: Evidence-based practice: A summary of research on midwifery practice in the United States.* http://www.midwife.org/acnm/files/cclibraryfiles/filename/000000002128/midwifery%20evidence-based%20practice%20issue%20brief%20finalmay%202012.pdf

American Medical Association. (2009). *AMA scope of practice data sets: Nurse practitioners*. Author.
American Medical Association. (2018). Physician-led health care teams, 1–31. https://www.ama-assn.org/system/files/2018-09/physician-led-teams-campaign-booklet.pdf
American Nurses Association. (2023, June 17). *ANA Refutes recommendations that APRN roles should be licensed and regulated by state medical boards*. https://www.nursingworld.org/news/news-releases/2023/ana-refutes-med-board-aprn-oversight
Anselmi, K. K., Dreher, H. M., Smith Glasgow, M. E., & Donnelly, G. F. (2010). Faculty colleagues in your classroom as doctoral students: Does a conflict of interest exist? *Nurse Educator, 35*(5), 213–219. https://doi.org.10.1097/NNE.0b013e3181ed83c7
Armsby, P., & Dreher, H. M. (2011). Towards a metric for measuring the value of professional doctorates. In T. Fell, K. Flint, & I. Haines (Eds.), *Professional doctorates in the UK 2011* (pp. 71–78). UK Council for Graduate Education, April 2011, (second *commissioned report on Professional Doctorate in UK, first in 2002*).
Auerbach, D. I., Martsolf, G. R., Pearson, M. L., Taylor, E. A., Zaydman, M., Muchow, A. N., Spetz, J., & Lee, Y. (2015). *The DNP by 2015: A study of the institutional, political, and professional issues that facilitate or impede establishing a post-baccalaureate doctor of nursing practice program*. RAND. http://www.rand.org/pubs/research_reports/RR730.html
Barkham, M., & Mellor-Clark, J. (2003). Bridging evidence-based practice and practice-based evidence: Developing a rigorous and relevant knowledge for the psychological therapies. *Clinical Psychology and Psychotherapy, 10*(6), 319–327. https://doi.org/10.1002/cpp.379
Bloch, J. R. (2007, March 28–30). *The DNP/DrNP degree as entry into NP practice: Is this nursing's answer to eliminate disparities in health care access for vulnerable populations?* Paper presented at the First National Conference on The Doctor of Nursing Practice: Meanings and Models, Annapolis, MD.
Bologna Process. (2010). *Third cycle: Doctoral education*. http://www.ond.vlaanderen.be/hogeronderwijs/bologna/actionlines/third_cycle.htm
Brar, K., Boschma, G., & McCuaig, F. (2010). The development of nurse practitioner preparation beyond the Masters level: What is the debate about? *International Journal of Nursing Education Scholarship, 7*(1), Article 9, 1–15. https://doi.org/10.2202/1548-923X.1928
Buchholz, S. W., Yingling, C., Jones, K., & Tenfelde, S. (2015). DNP and PhD collaboration: Bringing together practice and research expertise as predegree and postdegree scholars. *Nursing Educator, 40*(4), 203–206. https://doi.org/10.1097/NNE.0000000000000141
Budden, J. S., Zhong, E. H., Moulton, P., & Cimiotti. J. P. (2013). The national council of state boards of nursing and the forum of state nursing workforce centers 2013 National workforce survey of registered nurses. *Journal of Nursing Regulation, 4*(2), S1–S72. https://doi.org/10.1016/S2155-8256(15)30151-4
Bunge, H. (1962). The first decade of "nursing research." *Nursing Research, 11*(3), 132–138.
Cacchione, P. Z. (2007). What is clinical nursing research? *Clinical Nursing Research, 16*(3), 167–169. https://doi.org/10.1177/1054773807305870
Campaign for Action. (2021, May 6). *6 May 2021: Change in percent of registered nurses with a bachelor's in nursing or higher, 2010–2018*. https://publichealthmaps.org/motw-2021/2021/5/6/6-may-2021-change-in-percent-of-registered-nurses-with-a-bachelors-in-nursing-or-higher-2010-2018#:~:text=The%20percentage%20of%20registered%20nurses%20who%20hold%20a,percent%2C%20up%20from%20about%2049%20percent%20in%202010
Carlson, L. H. (2003). The clinical doctorate—asset or albatross? *Journal of Pediatric Health Care, 17*(4), 216–218. https://doi.org/10.1067/mph.2003.61
Carter, M. (2013). The Evolution of Doctoral Education in Nursing. In S. DeNisco & A. M. Barker (Eds.), *Advanced practice nursing: Evolving roles for the transformation of the profession* (2nd ed., pp. 28–35). Jones & Bartlett.
Case Western Reserve University. (2016). *The next level in nursing*. https://nursing.case.edu/dnp
Christman, L. (1980). Leadership in practice: Image. *Journal of Nursing Scholarship, 12*, 31–33.
Coyle, S. (2019). Evolving education: Defining the terminal degree. *Social Work Today, 19*(2), 10.
Dahnke, M. D., & Dreher, H. M. (2016). *Philosophy of science for nursing practice: Concepts and applications* (2nd ed.). Springer Publishing Company.
Davies, R. (2008). The Bologna process: The quiet revolution in nursing higher education. *Nurse Education Today, 28*, 935–942. https://doi.org/10.1016/j.nedt.2008.05.008
Donley, R., & Flaherty, M. J. (2008). Revisiting the American Nurses Association's first position on education for nurses: A comparative analysis of the first and second position statements on the education of nurses. *The Online Journal of Issues in Nursing, 13*(2). http://www.nursingworld.org/MainMenuCategories/ANAMarketplace/ANAPeriodicals/OJIN/TableofContents/vol132008/No2May08/ArticlePreviousTopic/EntryIntoPracticeUpdate.aspx

Donohue, P. (1996). *Nursing the finest art: An illustrated history* (2nd ed.). Mosby.

Dracup, K., & Bryan-Brown, C. (2005). Doctor of nursing practice—MRI or total body scan? *American Journal of Critical Care*, 14(4), 278–281. https://doi.org/10.4037/ajcc2005.14.4.278

Dreher, H. M. (2005). The doctor of nursing practice: Has this train left the station? If so, just where is it going? *The Pennsylvania Nurse*, 60, 17–19. https://doi.org/10.1155/2016/1846178

Dreher, H. M. (2008a). Innovation in nursing education: Preparing for the future of nursing practice. *Holistic Nursing Practice*, 22(2), 77–80. https://doi.org/10.1097/01.HNP.0000312655.68147.a4

Dreher, H. M. (2008b). A dearth of geriatric specialists: Will invention and gerotechnology save us? *Holistic Nursing Practice*, 22(5), 255–260. https://doi.org/10.1097/01.HNP.0000334918.39057.5d

Dreher, H. M. (2009). How do RNs today best stay informed? Do we need "knowledge management?" *Holistic Nursing Practice*, 23(5), 263–266. https://doi.org/10.1097/HNP.0b013e3181b66c68

Dreher, H. M. (2011). The path to nursing science today, 1910–2010. In M. D. Dahnke & H. M. Dreher (Eds.), *Philosophy of science for nursing practice: Concepts and applications* (pp. 269–300). Springer Publishing Company.

Dreher, H. M. (2013). Differentiating "clinical evidence" and "clinical knowledge." *Clinical Scholars Review: The Journal of Doctoral Nursing Practice*, 6(1), 9–12.

Dreher H. M. (2014). Unpublished Manuscript.

Dreher, H. M. (2016). Next steps toward practice knowledge development. In M. D. Dahnke & H. M. Dreher (Eds.), *Philosophy of science for nursing practice: Concepts and applications* (2nd ed., pp. 353–391). Springer Publishing Company.

Dreher, H. M., & Gardner, M. (2009, March 24–27). *With the rise of the DNP, who will conduct primary care research?* Paper presented at the Second National Conference on the Doctor of Nursing Practice: The Dialogue Continues, Hilton Head Island, SC.

Dreher, H. M., & Montgomery, K. E. (2009). Let's call it "doctoral" advanced practice nursing. *The Journal of Continuing Nursing Education*, 40(12), 530–531.

Dreher, H. M., & Smith Glasgow, M. E. (2011). Global perspectives on the professional doctorate. *International Journal of Nursing Studies*, 48, 403–408.

Dreher, H. M., Donnelly, G., & Naremore, R. (2005). Reflections on the DNP and an alternate practice doctorate model: The Drexel DrNP. *The Online Journal of Issues in Nursing*, 11(1). www.nursingworld.org/ojin/topic28/tpc28_7.htm

Dreher, H. M., Fasolka, B., & Clark, M. (2008). Navigating the decision to pursue an advanced degree. *Journal of Men in Nursing*, 3(1), 51–55.

Dunphy, L. M., Smith, N. K., & Youngkin, E. Q. (2009). Advanced practice nursing: Doing what has to be done—Radicals, renegades, and rebels. In L. Joel (Ed.), *Advanced practice nursing: Essentials for role development* (2nd ed., pp. 2–22). F. A. Davis.

Ellis, L. B., & Lee, N. (2005). The changing landscape of doctoral education: Introducing the professional doctorate for nurses. *Nurse Education Today*, 25(3), 222–229.

Evans, A. (2019). PharmD or RPh: Does it matter? *Pharmacy Times*, PharmD or RPh: Does It Matter?

Fang, D., & Kesten, K. (2017). Retirements and succession of nursing faculty in 2016 to 2025. *Nursing Outlook*, 65, 633–642.

Fang, D., & Zhan, L. (2021). Completion and attrition of nursing PhD students of the 2001 to 2010 matriculating cohorts. *Nursing Outlook*, 69(3), 340–349.

Fang, D., Li, Y., Stauffer, D. C., & Trautman, D. E. (2016). *2015–2016 Enrollment and graduations in baccalaureate and graduate programs in nursing*. American Association of Colleges of Nursing.

Fang, D., Tracy, C., & Bednash, G. D. (2010). *2009–2010 enrollment in baccalaureate and graduate programs in nursing*. American Association of Colleges of Nursing.

Fitzpatrick, J. (2003). The case for the clinical doctorate in nursing. *Reflections on Nursing Leadership, First Quarter*, 8–9, 37, 52.

Fitzpatrick, J. (2008). Doctor of nursing practice programs: History and current status. In J. Fitzpatrick & M. Wallace (Eds.), *The doctor of nursing practice and clinical nurse leader: Essentials of program development and implementation for clinical practice* (pp. 13–30). Springer Publishing Company.

Flanagan, J., Turkel, M. C., Roussel, L., & Smith, M. (2021). Nursing knowledge in the doctor of nursing practice curriculum. *Nursing Science Quarterly*, 34(3), 268–274. https://doi.org/10.1177/08943184211010458

Flexner, A. (1910). *Medical education in the United States and Canada: A report to the Carnegie foundation for the advancement of teaching. Bulletin No. 4.* Carnegie Foundation for the Advancement of Teaching.

Florczak, K. L. (2010). Research and the doctor of nursing practice: A cause for consternation. *Nursing Science Quarterly*, 23(1), 13–17.

Ford, J. (2008). *Editorial: DNP a bad idea*. http://community.advanceweb.com/blogs/np_1/archive/2008/07/23/editorial-on-dnp.aspx

Freund, C. (2021, February 4). "I took a paycut": Nursing faculty shortage worsening, low pay a major factor. WHQR Public Media.

Fulton, J. S. (2010). Evolution of clinical nurse specialist role and practice in the United States. In J. S. Fulton, B. L. Lyon, & K. A. Goudreau (Eds.), *Foundations of clinical nurse specialist practice* (pp. 3–14). Springer Publishing Company.

Fulton, J., & Lyon, B. (2005). The need for some sense making: Doctor of nursing practice. *The Online Journal of Issues in Nursing, 10*(3), Manuscript 3. www.nursingworld.org/MainMenuCategories/ANAMarketplace/ANAPeriodicals/OJIN/TableofContents/Volume102005/No3Sept05/tpc28_316027.aspx

Gibbons, M., Lomoges, C., Nowotny, H., Schwartzman, S., Scott, P., & Trow, M. (1994). *The new production of knowledge*. Sage.

Goodrich, A. A. (1936). Modern trends in nursing education. *American Journal of Public Health, 26*, 764–770.

Gordon, S. (2006). *Nursing against the odds: How health care cost cutting, media stereotypes, and medical hubris undermine nurses and patient care*. Cornell University Press.

Gortner, S. R. (1986). Impact of the division of nursing on nursing research development in the U.S.A. In S. M. Stinson & J. Kerr (Eds.), *International issues in nursing research* (pp. 113–130). Charles Press.

Gortner, S. R. (2000). Knowledge development in nursing: Our historical roots and future opportunities. *Nursing Outlook, 48*(2), 60–67.

Grace, H. (1989). Issues in doctoral education in nursing. *Journal of Professional Nursing, 5*(5), 266–270.

Grainger, L. (2022). Nursing faculty shortage in the U.S.: Has a pandemic compounded an existing problem? *wolterskluwer.com*, Retrieved from Nursing faculty shortage in the U.S.: Has a pandemic compounded an existing problem? | Wolters Kluwer.

Greenhalgh, T., Jackson, C., Shaw, S., & Janamian, Y. (2016). Achieving research impact through co-creation in community-based health services: Literature review and case study. *The Milbank Quarterly, 94*, 392–429. https://doi.org/10.1111/1468-0009.12197

Guetterman, T. C., Sakakibara, R. V., Plano Clark, V. L., Luborsky, M., Murray, S. M., Castro, F. G., Creswell, J. W., Deutsch, C., & Gallo, J. J. (2019) Mixed methods grant applications in the health sciences: An analysis of reviewer comments. *PLoS ONE 14*(11), e0225308. https://doi.org/10.1371/journal.pone.0225308

Haase, P. T. (1990). *The origins and rise of associate degree nursing*. Duke University Press.

Hastings, C. E., Mitchell, S. A., & Loud, J. T. (2010, April 5–7). *Advancing nursing roles in clinical and translational science*. Paper presented at the 2010 Clinical and Translational Research and Education Meeting, ACRT/SCTS Joint Annual Meeting, Washington, DC.

Hathaway, D., Jacob, S., Stegbauer, C., Thompson, C., & Graff, C. (2006). The practice doctorate: Perspectives of early adopters. *Journal of Nursing Education, 45*(12), 487–496.

Hawkes, D., & Taylor, S. (2016). Redesigning the EdD at UCL Institute of Education: Thoughts of the Incoming EdD program leaders. In V. A. Storey, (Ed.), *International perspectives on designing professional practice doctorates* (pp. 115–125). Palgrave Macmillan. https://doi.org/10.1057/9781137527066_7

Hawkins, R., & Nezat, G. (2009). Doctoral education: Which degree to pursue? *American Association of Nurse Anesthetists Journal, 77*(2), 92–96.

Hellerstein, D. (2008). Practice-based evidence rather than evidence-based practice in psychiatry. *Medscape Journal of Medicine, 10*(6), 141.

Hiatt, M. D. (1999). Around the continent in 180 days: The controversial journey of Abraham Flexner. *The Pharos, 62*(1), 18–24.

Honig, J., & Smolowitz, J. (2009). Clinical doctorate at Columbia University School of Nursing: Lessons learned. *Clinical Scholars Review, 2*(2), 51–59.

Horrocks, S., Anderson, E., & Salisbury, C. (2002). Systematic review of whether nurse practitioners working in primary care can provide equivalent care to doctors. *British Medical Journal, 324*, 819–823.

Hutchinson, S. A. (2001). The development of qualitative health research: Taking stock. *Qualitative Health Research, 11*, 505–521.

Idzik, S., Buchholz, S. W., Kelly-Weeder, S., Finnegan, L., & Bigley, M. B. (2021). Strategies to move entry level nurse practitioner education to the doctor of nursing practice degree by 2025. *Nurse Educator, 46*(6), 336–341.

Ingeno, L. (2013). *Who will teach nursing?* https://www.insidehighered.com/news/2013/07/22/nursing-schools-face-faculty-shortages

Inside Higher Education. (2012, April 12). *Ending the first Ed.D. program.* Insidehighered.com. https://www.insidehighered.com/news/2012/03/29/country%E2%80%99s-oldest-edd-program-will-close-down

Institute of Medicine. (1999). *To err is human: Building a safer health system.* National Academies Press.

Jacobson, A., Stern, C., Gaspar, P., Spross, J., Heye, M., France, N., ... Sedhorn, L. (2007, March 28–30). *Comparison of national association of clinical nurse specialist statement competencies with DNP Essentials: What is the fit?* Paper presented at the First National Conference on The Doctor of Nursing Practice: Meanings and Models, Annapolis, MD.

Joachim, G. (2008). The practice doctorate: Where do Canadian nursing leaders stand? *Nursing Leadership, 21*(4), 42–51.

Joanna Briggs Institute Levels of Evidence and Grades of Recommendation Working Party. (2013). *New JBI levels of evidence.* http://joannabriggs.org/assets/docs/approach/JBI-Levels-of-evidence_2014.pdf

Kaustuv, B. (2012, March 29). *Ending the first Ed.D. degree. Inside Higher Education. The country's oldest Ed.D. program will close down.* (insidehighered.com)

Keating, S. A., Berland, A., Capone, K., & Chickering, M. J. (2021). Global nursing education: International resources meet the NLN Core competencies for nurse educators. *Online Journal of Issues in Nursing, 26.* (nursingworld.org)

Kirkpatrick, M. (1994). The department chair position in academic nursing. *Journal of Professional Nursing, 10*(2), 77–83.

Krugman, P. (2009). The Great Recession versus the Great Depression. *New York Times.* http://krugman.blogs.nytimes.com/2009/03/20/the-great-recession-versus-the-great-depression

Lenz, E. R. (2005). The practice doctorate in nursing: An idea whose time has come. *The Online Journal of Issues in Nursing, 10*(3), Manuscript 1. www.nursingworld.org/MainMenuCategories/ANAMarketplace/ANAPeriodicals/OJIN/TableofContents/Volume102005/No3sept05/tpc28_116025.aspx

Magyary, D., Whitney, J. D., & Brown, M. A. (2006). Advancing practice inquiry: Research foundations of the practice doctorate in nursing. *Nursing Outlook, 54*(3), 139–151.

Mahaffey, E. H. (2002). The relevance of Associate Degree nursing education: Past, present, future, *Online Journal of Issues in Nursing, 7*(2). (nursingworld.org)

Malina, D. P., & Izlar, J. J. (2014). Education and practice barriers for CRNAs. *The Online Journal of Issues in Nursing, 19*(2), Manuscript 3. http://www.nursingworld.org/MainMenuCategories/ANAMarketplace/ANAPeriodicals/OJIN/TableofContents/Vol-19-2014/No2-May-2014/Barriers-for-Certified-Registered-Nurse-Anesthetists.html

McCauley, L. A., Broome, M. E., Frazier, L., Hayes, R., Kurth, A., Musil, C. M., Norman, L. D., Rideout, K. H., & Villarruel, A. M. (2020). Doctor of nursing practice (DNP) degree in the United States: Reflecting, readjusting, and getting back on track. *Nursing Outlook, 68,* 494–503.

McKenna, H., & Cutcliffe, J. (2001). Nursing doctoral education in the United Kingdom and Ireland. *The Online Journal of Issues in Nursing, 6*(2). www.nursingworld.org/MainMenuCategories/ANAMarketplace/ANAPeriodicals/OJIN/TableofContents/Volume62001/No2May01/ArticlePreviousTopic/UKandIrelandDoctoralEducation.aspx

McLeod, D. C. (1992). All-Pharm.D. degree will not significantly alter the pharmacy profession. *The Annals of Pharmacotherapy, 22,* 998–1000.

McNett, M. (2006). The PhD-prepared nurse in the clinical setting. *Clinical Nurse Specialist, 20*(3), 134–138.

Medscape.com. (2020). *Medscape APRN Compensation Report 2020.*

Meleis, A., & Dracup, K. (2005). The case against the DNP: History, timing, substance, and marginalization. *The Online Journal of Issues in Nursing, 10*(3), Manuscript 2. www.nursingworld.org/MainMenuCategories/ANAMarketplace/ANAPeriodicals/OJIN/TableofContents/Volume102005/No3Sept05/tpc28_216026.aspx

Melnyk, B., & Davidson, S. (2009). Creating a culture of innovation in nursing education through shared vision, leadership, interdisciplinary partnerships, and positive deviance. *Nursing Administration Quarterly, 33*(4), 288–295.

Melosh, B. (1982). *The physician's hand: Work culture and conflict in American nursing.* Temple University Press.

Mundinger, M. O. (2005). Who's who in nursing: Bringing clarity to the doctor of nursing practice. *Nursing Outlook, 53,* 173–176.

Mundinger, M. O. (2009). The clinical doctorate 15 years hence. *Clinical Scholars Review, 2*(2), 35–36.

Mundinger, M. O., Kane, R. L., Lenz, E. R., Totten, A. M., Tsai, W. Y., Cleary, P. D., Friedewald, W. T., Siu, A. L., & Shelanski, M. L. (2000). Primary care outcomes in patients treated by nurse practitioners or physicians: A randomized trial. *Journal of the American Medical Association, 283*, 59–68.

Murray, B. (2000). The degree that almost wasn't: The PsyD comes of age. *The Monitor, 31*(1), 52.

National Academy of Sciences. (2005). *Advancing the nation's health needs: Committee for monitoring the nation's changing needs for biomedical, behavioral, and clinical personnel.* National Academies Press.

National Advisory Council on Nurse Education and Practice (NACNEP). (2021). Preparing nurse faculty, and addressing the shortage of nurse faculty and clinical preceptors, *17th Report to the Secretary of Health and Human Services and the U.S. Congress.* Author. (hrsa.gov)

National Association of Clinical Nurse Specialists. (2009). *Statement on the nursing practice doctorate.* https://nacns.org/docs/PositionOnNursingPracticeDoctorate.pdf

National Association of Clinical Nurse Specialists. (2015). *NACNS position statement on the doctor of nursing practice.* http://www.nacns.org/docs/DNP-Statement1507.pdf

National Association of Clinical Nurse Specialists. (2023). *Position Statement: Entry For CNS Practice.* https://nacns.org/wp-content/uploads/2023/05/Entry-for-CNS-Practice-Position-Statement-FINAL.pdf

National Council of State Boards of Nursing. (2012). *Model rules.* https://www.ncsbn.org/17_Model_Rules_0917.pdf

National Council of State Boards of Nursing. (2020). The 2022 National Nursing Workforce Survey. Table of Contents page: *Journal of Nursing Regulation.*

National Council of State Boards of Nursing. (2023, June 6). NCSBN opposes American Medical Association amendment on APRNs I NCSBN.

National Institutes of Health. (2009a). *Mentored patient-oriented research career development award (Parent K23), program announcement (PA) Number: PA-10-060.* http://grants2.nih.gov/grants/guide/pa-files/PA-10-060.html

National Institutes of Health. (2009b). Part II full text of announcement. Section I. Funding opportunity description. 1. Research objectives. In: Institutional Clinical and Translational Science Award (U54), RFA-RM-07-007. http://grants.nih.gov.ezproxy2.library.drexel.edu/grants/guide/rfa-files/RFA-RM-07-007.html

National League for Nursing. (2010). Masters education in nursing June 2010. Reflection & Dialogue #6 - Master's Education in Nursing, June 2010 (nln.org)

National Organization of Nurse Practitioner Faculty. (2006). *Doctor of Nursing Practice (DNP) Related Statements: Response to recommendations on clinical hours & degree title.* http://www.nonpf.com/displaycommon.cfm?an=1&subarticlenbr=16 [Historical document, verified 11/29/2016, under Protected View

National Organization of Nurse Practitioner Faculty. (2012). *Nurse practitioner core competencies, amended 2012.* http://c.ymcdn.com/sites/www.nonpf.org/resource/resmgr/competencies/npcorecompetenciesfinal2012.pdf

National Organization of Nurse Practitioner Faculty. (2021). *NONPF Statement–Reaffirming DNP: Entry to nurse practitioner practice by 2025.* https://www.nonpf.org/news/638126/NONPF-Statement---Reaffirming-DNP-Entry-to-Nurse-Practitioner-Practice-by-2025-.htm

National Organization of Nurse Practitioner Faculty. (2023). *Reaffirming the Doctor of Nursing Practice Degree: Entry to Nurse Practitioner Practice by 2025.* https://www.nonpf.org/news/638126/NONPF-Statement%EF%BF%BD-Reaffirming-DNP-Entry-to-Nurse-Practitioner-Practice-by-2025-.htm

National Panel for Nurse Practitioner Practice Doctorate Competencies. (2006). *Practice doctorate nurse practitioner entry-level competencies.* http://c.ymcdn.com/sites/www.nonpf.org/resource/resmgr/competencies/dnp%20np%20competenciesapril 2006.pdf

National Task Force Standards (NTF). (2022). *Standards for quality nurse practitioner education, 6th Edition.* https://cdn.ymaws.com/www.nonpf.org/resource/resmgr/ntfstandards/ntfs_final.pdf

Neal, A. (2008). Seeking higher-ed accountability: Ending federal accreditation. *Change: The Magazine of Higher Education Regulation*, 25–29.

Nelson, M. (2002). Education for professional nursing practice: Looking backward into the future. *The Online Journal of Issues in Nursing, 7*(3), Manuscript 3. www.nursingworld.org/MainMenuCategories/ANAMarketplace/ANAPeriodicals/OJIN/TableofContents/Volume72002/No2May2002/EducationforProfessionalNursingPractice.aspx

New York State Senate. (2015–2016). S2145. Retrieved from NY State Senate Bill S2145 (nysenate.gov)

Nichols, E. F., & Chitty, K. K. (2005). Educational patterns in nursing. In K. K. Chitty & B. P. Black (Eds.), *Professional nursing: Concepts and challenges* (3rd ed., pp. 31–62). Saunders.

Nowotny, H., Scott, P., & Gibbons, M. (2001). *Re-thinking science: Knowledge and the public in an age of uncertainty.* Polity Press.

Nutting, M. A. (1912). *The educational status of nursing: U.S. Bureau of Education Bulletin. No. 7.* U.S. Government: Printing Office.

O'Sullivan, A. L. (2005). The practice doctorate in nursing. *The Mentor: The NONPF Newsletter, 16*(1), 1–2, 12.

Pearson, A., Wiechula, R., Court, A., & Lockwood, C. (2007). A re-consideration of what constitutes "evidence" in the healthcare professions. *Nursing Science Quarterly, 20*(1), 85–88.

Peplau, H. E. (1988). The art and science of nursing: Similarities, differences, and relations. *Nursing Science Quarterly, 1*(1), 8–15.

Peterson, D. R. (1997). *Educating professional psychologists: History and guiding conception.* American Psychological Association.

Plack, M. M., & Wong, C. K. (2002). The evolution of the doctorate of physical therapy: Moving beyond the controversy. *Journal of Physical Therapy Education, 16*(1), 48–59.

Potempa, K. M., Redman, R. W., & Anderson, C. A. (2008). Capacity for the advancement for nursing science: Issues and challenges. *Journal of Professional Nursing, 24,* 329–336.

Radzyminski, S. (2023). DNP: Research or not – that is the question. *Journal of Professional Nursing, 44,* 33–37.

Robert Wood Johnson Foundation. (2015). *In historic shift, more nurses graduate with bachelor's degrees.* http://www.rwjf.org/en/library/articles-and-news/2015/09/more-nurses-with-bachelors-degrees.html

Root, D. E., Diane E., Nuñez, D. V., Malloch, K., & Timothy Porter-O'Grady, T. (2018). Advancing the rigor of DNP projects for practice excellence, *Nurse Leader, 16*(4), 261–265

Roper, R. (2020). U.S. midwife workforce far behind globally. *statistica.com.* https://www.statista.com/chart/23559/midwives-per-capita

Rubenstein, D. (2009). The nurse-crusader goes to Washington. *New York Observe.* http://www.observer.com/2009/nurse-crusader-goes-washington

Rubio, D. M., Schoenbaum, E. E., Lee, L. S., Schteingart, D. E., Marantz, P. R., Anderson, K. E., & Platt, L. D. (2010). Defining translational research: Implications for training. *Academic Medicine, 85*(3), 470–475.

Rudy, E., & Grady, P. (2005). Biological researchers: Building nursing science. *Nursing Outlook, 53,* 88–94.

Salzman, A. (2010). The DPT degree: Our destiny or a cosmetic change? *Advance for Physical Therapy & PT Assistants, 14*(4), 55.

San Francisco AIDS Foundation. (2008). Confronting the "evidence" in evidence-based HIV prevention: Summary report. *HIV Evidence-Based Prevention,* 1–5.

Sayette, M. A., Mayne, T. J., & Norcross, J. C. (2010). *Insider's guide to graduate programs in clinical and counseling psychology.* Guilford.

Schlotfeldt, R. M. (1978). The professional doctorate: Rationale and characteristics. *Nursing Outlook, 26,* 302–311.

Silver, H. K., Ford, L. R., & Day, L. R. (1968). The pediatric nurse–practitioner program: Expanding the role of the nurse to provide increased health care for children. *Journal of the American Medical Association, 204*(4), 298–302.

Smith, M. E., & Dreher, H. M. (2003). Wanted, nursing faculty! If you think the nursing shortage is bad, the nursing faculty shortage is worse. *Advance for Nursing, 5,* 31–32.

Smith-Glasgow, M. E., & Dreher, H. M. (2010). The future of oncology nursing science: Who will generate the knowledge? *Oncology Nursing Forum, 37*(4), 393–396.

Society for Human Resource Management. (2013). *2013 Employee benefits: An overview of employee benefits offerings in the U.S.* https://www.shrm.org/research/surveyfindings/articles/documents/13-0245%202013_empbenefits_fnl.pdf

Sperhac, A. M., & Clinton, P. (2008). Doctorate of nursing practice: Blueprint for excellence. *Journal of Pediatric Health Care, 22*(3), 146–151.

Stew, G. (2009, March 24–27). *The professional/practice nursing doctorate in the United Kingdom.* Paper presented at the Second National Conference on the Doctor of Nursing Practice: The Dialogue Continues, Hilton Head Island, SC.

Stewart, D. (2009, November 5–6). *Challenges and opportunities for the professional doctorate: A North American perspective.* Paper presented at the European Conference on the Professional Doctorate, London, England.

Terry, A. J. (2014). *Clinical research for the doctor of nursing practice degree* (2nd ed.). Jones & Bartlett.

Texas Higher Education Coordinating Board. (2013). *White paper: The doctor of nursing practice degree.* http://www.thecb.state.tx.us/reports/PDF/2963.PDF?CFID=41003217&CFTOKEN=99921138

Treanor, J. (2016, October 25). *Gender pay gap could take 170 years to close, says World Economic Forum.* The Guardian. https://www.theguardian.com/business/2016/oct/25/gender-pay-gap-170-years-to-close-world-economic-forum-equality

University of South Florida. (2015). *Faculty salary adjustment.* http://health.usf.edu/facultyaffairs/facultysalary

Valian, V. (2005). Beyond gender schemas: Improving the advancement of women in academia. *Hypatia, 20*(3), 198–213.

Valiga, T. (2004). *The nursing faculty shortage: A national perspective.* Congressional briefing presented by the A. N. S. R. Alliance, Hart Senate Office Building.

Vincent, D., Johnson, C., Velasquez, D., & Rigney, T. (2014). DNP-prepared nurses as practitioner-researchers: Closing the gap between research and practice. *Web NP Online.* http://www.doctorsofnursingpractice.org/wp-content/uploads/2014/08/Vincet_et_al.pdf

Vitale, C. M. (2021). The state of nurse anesthetist practice and policy: An integrative review. *AANA Journal, 89*(5), 403–412.

Vreeland, E. M. (1964). Nursing research programs of the public health service: Highlights and trends. *Nursing Research, 13*(2), 148–158.

Werley, H. H., & Westlake, S. K. (1985). Impact of nursing research on public policy: An examination of ANA research priority statements. *Journal of Professional Nursing, 1*(3), 148–151, 154–156.

Wilkes, L. M., & Mohan, S. (2008). Nurses in the clinical area: Relevance of a PhD. *Collegian, 15,* 135–141.

Williams, J. C., & Richardson, V. T. (2010). New millennium, same glass ceiling? The impact on law firm compensation systems on women. A joint report of the Project for Attorney Retention, Minority Corporate Counsel Association. http://www.pardc.org/Publications/SameGlassCeiling.pdf

CHAPTER ONE   Reflective Response

RICHARD COWLING, III

Dr. Dreher has made significant contributions to the evolution of the doctor of nursing practice degree throughout his career, as reflected in his chapter. His voice has been vital to the disciplinary discourse regarding the meaning, purpose, and value of the degree. His career contributions as a major thought leader in the DNP movement include convening the first two national conferences on the doctor of nursing practice degree; launching one of the first doctor of nursing practice degrees in the United States in 2005 at Drexel University modeled after the Columbia University School of Nursing Doctor of Nursing Practice Degree; served as the only non-United Kingdom citizen as a contributing author to the 2011 United Kingdom Council for Graduate Education's *Second Commissioned Report on the Professional Doctorate in the UK*; and, with colleagues, published *Role Development for Doctoral Advanced Nursing Practice*, which in 2011 won first place in the *American Journal of Nursing* Book-of-the-Year awards. These contributions position the author to provide a major historical and political commentary on the DNP degree as it fits into the broader evolution of doctoral nursing education represented in this chapter.

The launch of the doctor of nursing practice was bold and innovative, following the original conception of a professional doctoral education envisioned by Rozella Schlotfeldt. That doctorate was conceived as a way of advancing the discipline of nursing through awarding a doctor of nursing (ND), a postbaccalaureate professional doctorate, as preparation for entry into nursing practice, referred to by Dreher in this chapter. I had the joy of working with students in that program between the years of 1983 and 1986 at Case Western Reserve University's Frances Payne Bolton School of Nursing. Dreher quite accurately portrays that degree as a professional doctorate rather than a practice doctorate, which is a significant distinction. I was impressed with the curriculum and courses that helped new entrants to the profession understand the scope and value of nursing knowledge as a foundation for professional practice. In the light of the predominance of BSN education, unfortunately it never gained the traction to become viable beyond a few schools.

As pointed out in this chapter, one of the most compelling issues that has lingered throughout the evolution of the DNP is what kind of knowledge should comprise the base of curricula in the degree preparation. There is widespread variation across programs, in spite of efforts to clearly distinguish the DNP from the PhD by professional education organizations. Perhaps it is time to contextualize this debate in an entirely new way, dropping the discourse around the differences between these two degrees. For instance, might we ask, what is the knowledge base required of a nurse practicing at the doctoral level that would most effectively serve the betterment of people? While this seems too broadly conceived, for me it is at the heart of what nursing is about. We might find overlays between research and practice that should not be avoided but embraced in moving the discipline forward. I would argue that nursing care is fundamentally fragmented and over-medicalized to the disadvantage of the well-being of humans in general. The development and use of nursing knowledge based on the wholeness of human beings needs attention. This kind of knowledge discovery and generation requires an active, meaningful, and appreciative stance among nurses in research and practice, but more importantly, with the participation of people, families, groups, and communities. Who will attend to these broader areas of disciplinary knowledge development? As Dreher accurately points out, the issue of what kind of knowledge belongs in the curricula of DNP programs is likely to remain unresolved and may never garner consensus. I suggest that the question of what nurses need to know and what people deserve from us that distinguishes us as a discipline, worthy of doctoral degree attainment, merits our attention regardless of the challenges it presents.

This chapter provides a broad, sweeping overview of the evolution of the DNP, described along with the discourses on knowledge development, identification, and inclusion in education programs, that have surrounded and dominated DNP growth. It is an essential contribution to the understanding of where we have been, as well as pointing us in the direction of the resolution of persistent, burgeoning unanswered questions and concerns. Rightfully, it does not attempt to answer all these questions but guides us toward what we need to know in order to answer them more fully and precisely. Accreditation standards have offered important guideposts for the development and standardization of programs that offer the DNP degree, while looming questions remain about what constitutes advanced practice. We do not have a viable, allowable option for the preparation of faculty with the advanced knowledge requisite to provide sophisticated and creative educational approaches that will prepare more faculty with the knowledge and skills needed to educate students at this level. Dreher articulates and clarifies these concerns using the history of the evolution of the DNP and his own significant involvement in the development and advocacy of DNP educational programs. At the same time, he is able to step back from it all offering his own reflections. He is the perfect author to make the case for ways forward while knowing that the journey is certainly infused with some uncertainties. We need this chapter to appreciate the genesis of the DNP more fully, where we stumbled and were unclear, what problems we solved and what problems we generated, what data and evidence we need in order to know how well we are doing, and what remains unanswered that is important.

I have been in nursing and nursing education for many years. I was originally a skeptic of the DNP because I became so immersed in PhD education. I remain a very strong advocate of the need for the type of theory and knowledge development that characterizes doctor of philosophy education—not just the degree in nursing. I am saddened by the now flattening enrollments given the preference and call of the DNP for so many. I bemoan our failure at the individual level to help our students from the very beginning of their professional education understand the branches of nursing knowledge. Over time I became an "acceptor" of the DNP. It felt like an inevitable tide moving over nursing and nursing education, without question. In some ways, I think it is a tide that we are still trying to navigate. I eventually realized, with some awakening awareness, that accepting was not enough if I was going to be an advocate for nursing knowledge development. When I go back to the core of nursing, why I was attracted to nursing back in the mid-1960s, growing out of my work as a volunteer and then nursing assistant working alongside hospital nurses and engaging with people in such meaningful ways, I know we need both DNP- and PhD-prepared nurses. We need them to be engaged with one another. We need them to be willing to share individually and leverage collectively the knowledge that they each bring to make the difference needed to better the lives of human beings. I call these needs, but they are also dreams and desires worth pursuing.

CHAPTER TWO

Professional and Doctor of Nursing Practice Roles in Nursing: A Theoretical and Historical Approach

H. MICHAEL DREHER AND JEANNINE URIBE

INTRODUCTION

Given the still plural and fragmented nature of the RN, it is not surprising that we still face struggles with the emerging doctor of nursing practice position and the roles associated with it. While the current roles of registered nurses are known, why do we have two degrees and one diploma (yes, there are 28 active diploma programs accredited by the Accreditation Commission on Nursing Education) that each prepare the graduate for the same professional nursing practice role and all take the same licensing exam? Shouldn't there be some role ambiguity among these degrees? One example where there is less ambiguity is in the Magnet Recognition Program® Affiliated Hospitals, where BSN-prepared RNs are hired at higher percentages according to certain guidelines. According to their May 2022 dashboard, 68% of their RNs are BSN prepared and 24% are associate prepared (American Nurses Credentialing Center, 2022). Even today, the role boundaries of the RN and APRN expand as individual state boards of nursing continue to update their scope of practice as new health practices evolve (Chapman et al., 2019; Spetz et al., 2019). How did the evolution of the work of the RN advance to a professional role (Fritter & Shimp, 2016; Yam, 2013; Zerwekh & Claborn, 2009)? The evolution of the DNP role is likely to be similar.

As one reflects on the history of nursing in the United States, one can appreciate the struggles of our still-emerging doctor of nursing practice today. The very first formal program for nursing in the United States was a 6-month training curriculum established at the Women's Hospital in Philadelphia in 1863 by physician Emmeline Horton Clevelend, MD, an 1855 alumna of the Women's Medical College of Pennsylvania, the world's first medical college for women (Robinson, 1946).[1] What was their role like? The first doctor of nursing practice degree was at the University of Kentucky College of Nursing in 2001. It did not prepare DNP clinicians but graduates educated in health systems/clinical leadership (Marion et al., 2003). What were the roles of the graduates when there were no role models?

This chapter discusses three dimensions of nursing roles. First, a discussion around unresolved issues that continue to impact the evolution of the DNP role and, in particular, role differentiation between the DNP degree and master's degree APRN practice and how the splintering education of the RN could be similar. Second, the chapter outlines some of the theoretical underpinnings of the literature on role theory that the DNP graduate will face. Last, toward a better understanding of the former two, a truncated history of American nursing and the evolution of professional roles. However, this final section of the chapter is not meant to be a comprehensive history of American nursing. Such a history has been excellently provided by Donohue (1996) in *Nursing, the Finest Art: An Illustrated History*; Reverby's (1987) *Ordered to Care: The Dilemma of American Nursing, 1850–1945*; and by Judd et al. (2009) in *A History of American Nursing: Trends and Eras*. This historical review of the history of nursing in America is included at the end of the chapter as a retrospective on where we began as a profession and how advanced we have become with the doctor of nursing practice degree.

THE EARLY EVOLUTION AND ONGOING STRUGGLES OF THE DNP ROLE

The ongoing debate on how to differentiate between the practice of the master's-prepared APRN and the DNP-prepared APRN continues. Beeber et al. (2019) write, "We know little about the role of DNP-prepared nurses in the workforce when compared to APRNs without doctoral preparation" (p. 355). Martsolf et al. (2021) similarly write, "Many employers may not know how to effectively use the advanced knowledge and skills of DNP-prepared NPs" (p. 954). This should not be discouraging. The still relatively new DNP degree and role are evolving—in some environments faster than others.

The early pronouncements about the differences between master's and DNP roles were aspirational. The American Association of Colleges of Nursing (AACN) and others stated what the DNP "will do" or "should be." In 2004, the AACN declared that "benefits of practice-focused doctoral programs [will] include … enhanced leadership skills to strengthen practice and health care delivery" (p. 8). Edwardson wrote, "The purpose of the DNP, on the other hand, is to prepare practitioners to take the knowledge created by researchers and theoretical scholars and use it in the delivery of services and advancement of policies that support high-quality health care" (2010, p. 138). Do we know if these two forecasts happened, and is there now an evidence base to support them? Will the DNP role ever be clearly differentiated from the role of the master's-prepared advanced practice nurse? The ambitious goal of 2015 by which the traditional clinical APRN (NP, CRNA, CNM, and CNS) would be transitioned to DNP entry-level practice did not occur as Cronenwett and colleagues predicted (2011). Now, after almost 20 years, the question is, "What has happened?" (McCauley et al., 2020).

Academicians aside (who developed this degree), what are DNP-educated executives and clinicians now doing in their respective practice landscapes? Are they being trapped by old views of what the CNO or NP does? Can the chief executive officer or physician-owned private practice comprehend what a DNP-educated CNO or NP can do *more* than before their new degree? Doesn't "I am a nurse practitioner (or CNO) and I have a doctor of nursing practice degree" or "I am a nurse practitioner (or CNO) and I have a master's degree" invite real confusion for them? In an attempt at greater clarity, Dreher and Montgomery (2009) have suggested using the term or acronym doctoral advanced practice nurse (DAPN). However, some serious and clarifying questions still need to be asked and answered: What should the role of the DAPN be? Now, the next aspirational deadline for the DNP for NPs by 2025 will also not be met (Idzik et al., 2021). All new CRNA students, however, will be required to enter a DNP or DANP (doctor of anesthesia practice) program by 2025. It cannot be overlooked that there were approximately 40,679 CRNAs in the United States in 2022 (U.S. Bureau of Labor Statistics, 2022), but there are over 355,000 NPs (American Association of Nurse Practitioners, 2022). Logically, it is far easier to change the entry-level educational requirement of an advanced practice nursing specialty that is almost one-ninth the size of another.

The likely disconnect from the AACN's goal of the 2015 date for the DNP to become the "standard" degree for entry level was (a) the failure to bring a broader range of stakeholders and national advanced practice nursing leaders to delineate a plan to study the practice role of the master's APN/APRN first; (b) the failure to develop adequate consensus around how another advanced degree (at great time and cost to the individual) might directly impact national health outcomes and particularly how this will be measured; and (c) promoting an ambitious goal move of "should" transition to the DNP by 2015 (Auerbach et al., 2015, p. iii) over a less demarcated "toward" instead to what some considered a premature leap. Despite tremendous growth in DNP programs, which increased from 92 in 2008 to 354 in 2018 (AACN, 2019), the American Association of Nurse Practitioners reported that 79.8% of APRNs held a master's as their highest degree and just 14% held a DNP (AANP, 2019).

The second issue that has hampered acceptance of the degree in many health sectors is a lack of understanding of how the role of the DNP clinician or executive can bring value to the organization. In a new AACN report from over 800 DNP graduates from 2005 to 2020 (Zangaro, 2023), the following findings were reported by Key Informants (we do note the low number of employer interviews conducted):

- DNP graduates have a larger and more diverse skill set and greater knowledge of policy, economics, and the business side of nursing.
- Of the 13 employers interviewed, most could not readily identify differences in the provision of direct patient care by MSN and DNP-prepared nurses.
- Academic leaders could not identify differences in clinical skills between MSN and DNP-prepared nurses. Lack of understanding among employers and other healthcare professionals about the DNP degree.
- Academic leaders and DNP graduates provided similar views on the key differences between BSN-to-DNP and MSN-to-DNP graduates.

Finally, if a more highly educated advanced practice nurse with a doctorate degree does not improve health, then why bother with the expense and effort of another degree? One important step is the creation of a minimum data set (MDS) by Covelli et al. (2022), who have developed a tool to track the outcomes of nurse practitioner DNP practice outcomes. This may be a first step toward evidence-based MS/DNP NP role differentiation if large amounts of data are collected in a standardized format and analyzed to further support the development of DNP NP practice. This chapter lays some of the groundwork with which to answer these questions in this text. Nevertheless, making definitive claims that DANP will be superior to master's ANP practice will remain elusive.

Our history has already experienced the divisiveness surrounding entry-level professional nursing practice. The American Nurses Association's (ANA's) historic 1965 position statement, which called for all RNs to be educated at the baccalaureate level, was never realized (Donley & Flaherty, 2002). There was much debate in the profession about whether this was a positive or negative step, as it might disenfranchise RNs with associate degrees and associate degree stakeholders and advocates had gained significant influence (Nelson, 2002). Even the ANA's reaffirmation of that position in 1985 (Smith, 2009) was not realized. Today, no state requires the BS except New York, which has a "BSN in Ten" initiative, that requires all associate degree nurses to get a BS degree within 10 years of graduation (Schmitz, 2022). According to the 2022 National Nurses Workforce Study by the National Council of State Boards of Nursing (NCSBN) in its new report, 47.2% of RNs identified a BSN as the degree that qualified them for their first U.S. nursing license. This percentage was 41.8% in 2020 and 39% in 2015 (2023). While the Institute of Medicine's 2011 *The Future of Nursing* report recommended increasing the percentage of nurses with a baccalaureate degree to 80% by 2020, this did not happen. However, there are now more RNs with a baccalaureate degree, largely due to the growing number of associate degree nurses completing RN/BSN degrees (National Academies of Sciences, Engineering, and Medicine, 2021).

Dr. Linda H. Aiken, a professor of nursing and sociology and the founding director of the Center for Health Outcomes and Policy Research at the University of Pennsylvania School of Nursing, has long led studies that have reported better health-related outcomes for hospitals that deliver care by BSN-prepared nurses over the care delivered by non-BSN-prepared nurses (Aiken et al., 2003, 2011, 2014; Alspach 2014; Harrison et al., 2019). Although there are increasing percentages of all RNs attaining the baccalaureate degree, the 2011 Institute of Medicine's report called for 80% BSN-prepared nurses by 2020, a goal that was not met, and the question is whether there are forces that can still undermine BSN degree education attainment. The answer is yes, and these forces are pragmatic. Just as McCauley and colleagues (2020) have identified cost as a major obstacle to attaining the post-master's DNP (and the BSN-to-DNP is more expensive; McCauley et al.), cost can also be a barrier to obtaining an associate degree. At Dreher's own college, there is a large associate degree program, an RN/BSN, master's, and a DNP program. And while a generic BS degree will soon be launched, the associate degree will remain (if downsized), as it is an access degree that can launch a graduate (often a first-generation student and/or one in financial need to attend college) into the middle class. Moreover, while many hospitals will give tuition support for master's study, our experience is that doctoral study is not included, and we have particularly sought scholarships for our DNP students to increase our graduation rates. Our view is that without a critical mass of DNP clinicians in our geographic area (New York only allows the clinical doctorate and does not permit an executive role or spin-off DNPs such as informatics or forensics, etc.), the DNP role may not be fully realized and its perceived value to the organization may be limited. This is analogous to a small department of nursing where there is only one full-time family nurse practitioner faculty (this first author was dean of a school of nursing where this was the case), there are no true peers, and some degree of isolation can occur. But again, low enrollment cannot economically support a second hire.

Whether these two-decade-old issues—the ANA position statement to require the BSN by 1965 or 1985 (there has not been a third) or to require the DNP now by 2025 (at least by the National Organization of Nurse Practitioner Faculty)—will ever be realized is yet to be seen (NONPF, 2023). One of the barriers to requiring the BSN for professional nursing practice is the lack of regulatory movement at the state level to require it (except New York). McCauley et al. (2020) mention this same barrier to the adoption of the DNP for APRN practice. But even the DNP or DNAP required for CRNA practice is an accreditor-only (not state-only) requirement. It is therefore not surprising that there is continuing controversy or concern over whether the doctorate will ever fully replace the master's degree for entry-level advanced nursing practice. Do you envision all 50 state legislatures (or even some) changing their nursing practice acts to eliminate the master's degree? That remains an interesting question. Nevertheless, the evolving role of the DAPN, the expanding boundaries of their work, the sphere of influence they will cast, and what they will do with a DNP degree that is explicitly different, are all still transforming. In other words, the history of the role of the DNP graduate is being written as you live it. The DNP degree is still young and has already had a large impact on the profession.

Challenges to differentiate the DNP from the master's degree APRN role practice may be more complex than debates and position statements around baccalaureate entry-level practice from 1965 to 1985. One has only to cite the classic randomized trial study of physician versus nurse practitioner primary care by Dr. Mary Mundinger et al. (2000). Dr. Mundinger (dean of the Columbia University School of Nursing, 1986–2010) and colleagues studied the primary care outcomes of 1,317 patients provided by 17 physicians and 7 master's-prepared nurse practitioners in four community-based primary care clinics at an urban academic medical center over the course of 1 year. Findings of this study include:

- Recruitment and retention (patients kept their first primary care appointment): higher rates of retention by the nurse practitioner group (68.2% versus 63.8%).
- Patient satisfaction of care: no significant differences.
- Health status of the study group: improvements from baseline to follow-up were equivalent in each group.
- Peak-flow measures on asthma: no significant differences.
- Hypertension: no statistically significant difference in the systolic readings, but the nursing practitioner group had a statistically smaller lower diagnostic measurement (82 mmHg vs. 85 mmHg (t test 2.09, $P = .04$)).

This study reflects positively on nurse practitioners having similar or slightly better primary care outcomes (likely to the surprise of many physicians). It is imperative that this enormous, costly DNP degree launch (possibly near a billion dollars in higher education and national healthcare resources), while attempting to elevate advanced nursing practice, differentiate itself from master's APN practice. The historical perils of the BSN degree for entry-level professional nursing should not be repeated. The pervasive dearth of DNP practice health outcome studies in the nursing and health literature is worrisome. However, one way that the DNP student and graduate can help in DNP degree differentiation (though that should not be the aim in patient care, of course) is through scholarship. DNP students are mentored by doctoral faculty, and the aim should be to produce high quality DNP projects that are publishable. Published projects (in whatever format, and there are many) will contribute to the nursing and health literature and advance the nursing discipline. DNP students or graduates should be encouraged to copublish with their mentors as long as the ethics of authorship are followed (Hein & Chinn, 2017). Science today (and nursing science is no different) is almost exclusively team-based. The days of the lone investigator are over. Collaboration is key!

Admittedly, it is not time to defend and establish a new acronym: DAPN for the doctoral advanced practice nurse and DAPRN for the practice-doctorate-educated traditional advanced practice registered nurse (APRN) and for the nurse practitioner, nurse-midwife, nurse anesthetist, or clinical nurse specialist. However, this chapter has used them for clarity to differentiate between doctoral and master's preparation and maybe other texts should too.

ROLES IN THE PROFESSION

Perhaps the seminal book on role theory in the health professions is *Role Theory: Perspectives for Health Professionals*, first published by Hardy and Conway in 1978. This chapter extends only some of the work of the contributors to this seminal text and analyzes the content that would specifically pertain to role theory for present-day DAPNs.

The term role is largely a sociological one (Biddle, 1986); however, its sociological application has universal meaning for society at both the individual and group levels and for disciplines that are accorded the status of a profession where roles and role functions are important.

Although the early classical professions were divinity, law, and medicine (Klass, 1961), a more contemporary understanding of a profession includes nursing, dentistry, engineering, architecture, social work, accountancy, and others. The profession of nursing is uniquely characterized by professional autonomy, a clearly defined, highly developed, specialized, and theoretical knowledge base, control of training, certification, and licensing for those newly entering the profession, self-governing and self-policing authority, an explicit ethical code, especially pertaining to professional ethics, and a commitment to public service (Burbules & Densmore, 1991). A more recent analysis of the word profession emphasizes that what makes the work of the professional nurse different from, for example, the work of an engineer is that there is a distinctive reliance on interpersonal skills and on ethical codes of work behavior (Dahnke & Dreher, 2016).

An interesting and perhaps historical discussion is whether nurses with associate and baccalaureate degrees are also professionals. The Institute of Medicine's 2011 *"Future of Nursing"* report called for a more highly educated nursing workforce. The recent National Academy of Medicine's (formerly the Institute of Medicine) report (2021) states that the success of the report "…will depend on leveraging the capacity and the many strengths of the current nursing workforce" (p. 61). Some, however, take the position that, while nursing is a profession, some practitioners (without a baccalaureate degree) are technically not professionals (AACN, 2000; Barter & McFarland, 2001). Liaschenko and Peter (2004) even declare that nursing is not a profession but simply "work." Melosh (1982) goes even further, asserting that "nursing is not and cannot be a profession" (p. 15). Melosh identified a key limitation in nursing's development as a profession by saying that "nurses never gained the large measure of control over their work that defines a profession" (p. 19). In addition, she writes that classical definitions of a profession maintain that "Professionals are their own bosses" (p. 15) and "if professions maintain their authority through controlling the division of labor related to their work ... then doctors' own professionalization organizes and requires nurses' subordination" (p. 19). Perhaps this last point was true in 1982 (except where military nurses could outrank their physician colleagues then and now), but in 2023, 27 states (including the District of Columbia) allow completely independent nurse practitioner practices (Ferris, 2001; NurseJournal Staff, 2023).[2] There is even an active, very reputable blog (whose authors have previously won American Journal of Nursing [AJN] Book-of-the-Year awards) that presents a very modern case for why nursing is a profession:

> Nursing is an autonomous, self-governing profession, a distinct scientific discipline with many autonomous practice features. Despite what the media may portray, nursing is not directed by physicians, even though nurses have less practical power than physicians do. In addition to extensive medical expertise, nurses have a unique, holistic patient advocacy focus, a unique scope of practice, and a unique body of knowledge, including special expertise in areas such as patient education, wound care and pain management (truthaboutnursing.org, 2015, para. 1).

By contemporary standards, at least by Melosh's definition, some nurses are indeed autonomous and classically "professional."

Dreher has graduated two master's-prepared adult-gerontological primary care nurse practitioners who have their own private practices. One is truly independent, and the other is independent but is housed with other independent NPs in a semi-group practice. This is what DNPs should do: form an independent private practice (in one of those 27 states) or semi-independent or group practices to collaborate with fellow DNP colleagues and make referrals to them when a medical plan of care is necessary. This would mean that the profession of nursing is legitimately partly professional too. This chapter, however, focuses on the roles of doctoral-educated advanced practice nursing professionals that have evolved from the emergence of professional nursing roles, but the ongoing debate about the nature of the professionalism of nursing continues. It is still a debate whether the associate degree (or diploma-prepared) RN is a professional RN by education. But the definition is mostly irrelevant, as there are highly skilled associate degree RNs who deliver excellent care. Dreher, perhaps not so humbly, was first one. Because the health of our citizenry is so important, the roles of nursing professionals are particularly critical to both the development of the profession itself and their impact on society because of the highly skilled work nurses perform.

Roles and Their Meaning for New DNP Graduates

At its most basic level, a role can be defined as "a set of goals, rights cohering in a socially recognizable whole and adopted by individuals toward achieving agreed upon common goods." A more precise sociological view would characterize roles as occurring within systems (or organizations, or relationships), and therefore a role can be considered a "set of systems states and actions of a subsystem, of an organization, including its interactions with other systems of nonsystem elements" (Kuhn, 1974, p. 298). These definitional frameworks lead us to conceptualize an operational definition of the word role for nursing. It is suggested that nursing roles are professional, socially constructed, operationalized behaviors that form the boundaries of what a professional nurse does. Only through a thorough analysis of the work of RNs and the roles they play, enact, or fulfill in the course of their professional work can one ascertain what are advanced (practice) nursing roles?

Finally, what differentiates or extends the boundaries of advanced practice to doctoral advanced (practice) nursing roles? In theory, it sounds very simple. In actuality, we believe that it is more complex. Multiple discussions have ensued in Dreher's DNP seminars in the past years about nursing roles and the nature of advanced practice nursing. For example, in the scenario of an overweight or obese patient with accompanying negative health conditions that need intervention, how does the 20-minute primary care interaction between an adult nurse practitioner and patient differ operationally from the physician-patient interaction (Dreher, 2008)? This kind of discussion is particularly germane to DAPNs, who must now identify how their roles and functions will be different and more advanced than when they had a master's degree. Again, if the skill set is the same, then nursing has a weaker argument for calling for a practice nursing doctorate. Meleis's work (1975) and that of Meleis and Trangenstein (1994) on role transitions is still very well applicable to today's doctoral advanced practice graduate, especially one who practiced previously with the master's degree. In her 2011 book, Meleis suggests that "Role insufficiency may be manifested in assuming any new roles... " (p. 2) and further indicates that there are "some losses and gains in their different roles and support systems" (p. 3). Smith Glasgow and Zoucha addressed some of the role strain among DNP students in this text's first edition (2011) and in a replication study in the second edition (Smith Glasgow et al., 2017). But we suspect there is more role strain among DNP graduates than has penetrated the nursing literature.

Sociologic Schools of Thought on Roles

There are two very prominent sociological schools of thought on roles and social interactions that serve as frameworks or even paradigms in which individuals, institutions, and systems operate. In Table 2.1, the functionalist view, as mostly attributed to the eminent sociologist Emile Durkheim (1964), and the competing symbolic interaction perspective best articulated by Mead (1934), Cooley (1964), and Blumer (1969) are summarized.

In a functionalist view, or structural-functional theory, the roles that individuals play in society evolve out of organic systems that constantly interact and are somewhat predictable. For example, in the case of the professional nurse, there is a need in society for nurses to perform certain roles (e.g., health educator, caregiver, advocate), and thus most nurses employ those roles in their daily work. DAPNs, however, are in a very different place functionally. Society does not yet know exactly what roles they will play (or be required to fill), and the new domain of this doctoral advanced practice is being created in real time, even as this text is published.

TABLE 2.1 Two Perspectives on Roles in Social Interactions

Functionalist View (Macro-Sociological Analysis)	Symbolic Interactionist View (Micro-Sociological Analysis)
Focus of perspective is on the group and its demarcation into smaller subgroups, units, and systems.	Focus of perspective is on the individual interacting and the symbolic interpretation of both verbal and nonverbal behavior and cures.
Objects and persons are stimuli that act on an individual.	Individuals construct objects on the basis of their ongoing activity. They give meaning to objects and makes decisions on the basis of their judgments.
Action is a release or response to what the situational norms demand.	Individuals decide what they wish to do and how they will do it. They take account of external and internal cues, interpreting their significance for their individual actions.
Environmental forces act to "produce" behavior.	By a process of self-indication, an individual accepts, rejects, or transforms the meaning (impact) of such forces.
Prescriptions for action, or norms, dictate appropriate behaviors. They are social facts.	Others' attitudes are the basis for individual lines of action.
An act is a unitary, bounded phenomenon; that is, it starts and stops.	An act is disclosed over time and what the end of the act will be cannot be foretold at the start.
The act (of an actor) will be followed by the response of another with or without any interpretation taking place on the part of the other.	An act is validated by the response of another.
Persons act on the basis of a generally objective reality; that is, learned responses.	Reality is defined by each actor; one defines a situation as they "see it" and acts on this perception.
People are socially molded, not forced, to perform societal functions.	Social order is maintained when people share their understanding of everyday behavior.
Group action is the expression of societal demands and shared social values.	Group action is the expression of individuals confronting their life situations.

Source: Adapted from Hardy, M., & Conway, M. (1988). *Role theory: Perspectives for health professionals.* (2nd ed.). Appleton & Lange.

We, therefore, propose that the functionalist view of the roles of the professional nurse, where a common socialization of RNs creates stability in the social system, may not theoretically or properly explain the unfolding role of a new type of advanced practice nurse. In a discussion of the roles of professionals, a symbolic interactionist view of DAPNs would indicate that their emerging roles would evolve from an ongoing examination of their meaning to a vigorous self-analysis of how satisfying, effective, or well received the exhibition of the role is. In other words, the critical feedback this new practitioner receives, processes, interprets, and reinterprets will ultimately reinforce the role being integrated and assimilated in a new domain of practice. In a study, Jackson and Stevenson (2000) describe the utility of using this critical feedback from patients (which may not be explicit) to answer this question. Similarly, Erving Goffman's (1955) original theory of "face work," which is described by Shattell (2004) as the face of the nurse interacting with the face of the patient in the simplicity or ordinariness of any basic nurse-patient interaction, is an example of how symbolic interaction theory may be highly useful in explaining how two different dyadic DAPN roles may evolve.

First, what is the new DAPN-patient role? Second, what is the new DAPN role in relation to professional clinicians in other healthcare disciplines? On an operational level, these questions are: (a) How will the individual patient perceive Dr. Jane Smith's role as a nursing primary care provider now using the title "Dr."? (b) How will fellow health profession colleagues perceive the new role of the DAPN as doctoral-prepared, not master's-prepared? Will patients have different expectations? Will colleagues have different expectations? Indeed, Goffman, in his classic sociological text *A Presentation of Self in Everyday Life* (1959), writes, "When an individual enters the presence of others, they commonly seek to acquire information about him or to bring into play information about him already possessed" (p. 1). Will this new type of doctoral advanced practice nurse use the face-to-face feedback to create solutions to any new role conflict or role strain that may occur?

Smith Glasgow and Zoucha (2011) conducted the first study on role strain in the doctorally prepared advanced practice nurse. Using a phenomenological approach from the Dutch (Utrecht) School, they developed an investigator-designed, open interview process method. They studied eight DNP- or DrNP-prepared, post-master's nursing faculty, advanced practice, or executives with a DNP program focus in nursing education ($n = 5$), advanced clinical practice ($n = 3$), and clinical research ($n = 1$). The major focus of their *current* jobs as informants was one nurse midwife, one nurse executive, three nursing faculty, three in advanced practice, and one in a dual role of nurse practitioner and nursing faculty. The demographics of the participants were seven women and one male, with a mean age of 49. One of the three themes of the study was *Context of the DNP Role*. Two comments were, "I am always introduced as a PhD nurse and then I have to explain that I do not have a PhD," and another, "I have to always explain what my role is." The nurse executive gained an expanded role at her workplace with a new DNP degree.

The second theme was *Feelings of Confidence and Empowerment in the Role as a DNP*. One participant stated "I'm a couple of years out from it and I can say that I feel it was worth it and that I'm starting to get the payoff in terms of confidence and career opportunities." Another stated, "I certainly feel more confident about standing up in front of a group of executives and senior leadership ... this is a problem, this is the solution, and this is the recommendation ... this is why I feel more confident about my role." Also, the DNP graduate in a clinical research role said, "I know how to conduct research, and I feel more confident in looking at research and my conclusions because I have had a rigorous academic exercise over and over." Another stated, "I thought it gave me a sense of empowerment to go out on my own and do things."

The last theme was *Finding My Way by Finding and Responding to Opportunity*. Comments included, "I think the hardest part for me is that I went from a position of 15 years of being on top of my game, knowing what I was doing, knowing who to contact, very autonomous, to being at the bottom and having to feel my way around. I feel like a baby learning to crawl." Another said, "We're a dynamic profession in a dynamic environment. So, who knows where we're all going to end up in the next 50 to 15 years?" The conclusions the authors draw are

> ...DNP graduates will need to differentiate their practice from the MSN in order to substantiate their value to the profession, health care community, and public, or else the forces of role strain will likely persist and perhaps worsen. Health care reform and other market forces may also drive the need for the DNP going forward as we see a growing need for innovation and evidence to improve care. (p. 225)

In a replication of their 2011 study Smith Glasgow et al. (2017) revisited role strain in the DNP-prepared practitioner, clinical executive, and educator in a replication study of eight participants, all female and white, with an older mean age of 58 (versus 47 in the 2011 study). The same phenomenological influencedly open interview process method was used. Among the sample, five were DAPRNs and three were executives. Theme changes are described in Table 2.2.

The themes do look different in the 7 years between the two studies. In that interval, there was a surging growth in DNP programs, of approximately 150 in 2010 to nearly 350 in 2017 (AACN, 2019). The progress in Theme 1 was stated by one new DNP graduate: "People sort of celebrated the fact that I had a doctorate. Other people made a big deal of it, which I found interesting." A second said, "I have become more open-minded, and I am not afraid to bring my ideas to the table." Many in this group felt more respected in their group, and their DNP advanced preparation was fundamental to this change in role perception. They described environments where they worked as supportive, and they felt valued. The nurse executives had even more clarity about their role. High-performing organizations are always seeking talented individuals with highly developed leadership skills (Wells & Hejna, 2019). And while the DAPRNs experienced acceptance and support as an "individual nurse," their environments were not necessarily prepared to create new roles for them. In the second theme, most participants expressed increased confidence in their roles. One participant felt that doors were opened by having a DNP degree. Most felt they would continue to grow and be more respected by their peers. The last theme has evolved from "Finding My Way..." in 2010 to "Finding a Settled Place..." in 2017. One participant said, "It feels good. I think I can

TABLE 2.2 Changes in Qualitative DNP Role Themes Between 2011 and 2017 Studies

2010 Study	2017 Study
Theme 1: Context of the DNP Role	Theme 1: The Changing and Evolutionary Context and Environment of the DNP Role
Theme 2: Feelings of Confidence and Empowerment in the Role as a DNP.	Theme 2: The Emerging Feeling of Confidence and Respect in the Role as a DNP
Theme 3: Finding My Way by Finding and Responding to Opportunity	Theme 3: Finding a Settled Place in the Perceived Role of the DNP

do anything." Another said, "I think people value the DNP. I think they respect it. I think that when I am at the table with physicians, I think there is a sense that the playing field is a little more level." Progress has been made toward the goal of less role strain for the still-evolving doctoral advanced practice nurse. Every environment is different, every workplace, different peers, different barriers, and even unexpected interest and support for you in your new role.

Another important concept in symbolic interaction is that of role-taking. Role-taking is a key mechanism of interaction that permits us to take another person's perspective and see what our actions might mean to the other actors with whom we interact (Schell & Kayser-Jones, 1999). One scholar suggests that the outcome of role-taking is not just the processing of the influence of the interaction on behavior but requires overt behavioral change based on the processing of those interactions (Cast, 2004). In other words, in the DAPN role, the new practitioner is likely not only to think differently but also to act differently as new face-to-face interactions with patients and colleagues are experienced. We contend that this change in perspective and change in thinking are more likely to occur as the new practitioner engages in more reflective practice. Johns and Freshwater (2005) are leading scholars supporting the practice of reflection in advanced nursing practice, and they build on and extend the classical work of Schön (1983), who coined the concepts of "reflection in action" and "reflection on action." Stew (2017) writes about how reflective practice ought to be even more mature and developed in the DNP/professional doctorate nursing graduate. With deep reflection about this new role and consideration of what it is or should be (and conversely, what it is no longer), the new practitioner is thus likely to experience ambiguity as he or she tries to "figure this new role out." Our view is that the experience of ambiguity is not detrimental but a sign of progress. As the new practitioner engages in activities that lead to more secure role delineation, we think the ambiguity will lessen. Hopefully, patients will respond differently and positively to the confidence and enhanced skill set of the DNP graduate. Over time, we predict that colleagues in the health profession will respond similarly.

A vigorous curricular focus on the concept of role is particularly important for the student pursuing a DNP degree. However, it is not likely that the expansion and ultimate role delineation of the DNP graduate will be entirely noncontroversial or always well received. There will be resistance from current master's-prepared nurse practitioners, nurse-midwives, nurse anesthetists, and clinical nurse specialists who will claim your practice is not different (or better?) than theirs. If their argument prevails, then a given institution may not compensate the doctoral graduate more highly. Thus, in supporting doctoral advanced nursing practice, we are unyielding in our plea that the necessary outcome data must be conducted and disseminated. Nevertheless, there is a bountiful amount of optimism in the profession about your future and this new degree, and as one graduate has written:

> Since attaining my doctorate, I find myself better equipped to build upon my master's-level training. I'm no longer satisfied with doing the "how to," but indeed now relish and crave the "why?" and the "why not?" As a doctoral advanced practice nurse, I am different! (Dreher & Montgomery, 2009, p. 530)

We anticipate that in your new role, you will also be different.

Emergence of Professional Roles in Nursing: Rising from the Toil of Public Health Nurses

It is with some incredulity that public health nurses are not more duly recognized for their role in the evolution of our discipline. Furthermore, while Nightingale's historic eminence still reigns over nursing, her vision for nursing was enacted very differently in the United States. In many ways, the rise of modern nursing has been accomplished despite tension between two equally dogmatic nursing subcultures: the conservative traditionalists and the elite professionalizers[3] (Melosh, 1982; Reverby, 1987). And as quarrelsome as these two camps have been over the past 100 years, progress has indeed been made, and nursing is probably more advanced here than in any other place on the globe.

THE NIGHTINGALE INFLUENCE

Florence Nightingale wrote about patients and nursing, beginning a revolution in the roles of nurses, represented up to that point by religious sisters or inmates living in the almshouses where they served. Her ideas on nursing included a reformed vision of employment for women, a profession that removed the societal attachment to the idea of womanly work and feminine intuition, and replacing the characterization of a nurse with an educated, highly moral, and stable woman to run the wards. Her nurses required both theoretical and practical training. In Deloughery's (1977) book on the nursing profession, Nightingale changed nursing to "a career and not a last resort" (p. 61) for women in need of employment. Nightingale's ideal plan separated ward service from nursing education by making student nurses' practical experiences on the hospital wards opportunities for learning with nurse instructors and physicians, rather than just providing service to the hospital.

Scientific progress in medicine, combined with the growing promotion of social reforms in many areas, helped formulate the idea that for better outcomes, physicians needed assistants to carry out their complex medical treatments. Recognizing that they were following the physician's orders, Nightingale wanted her nurses to understand the reasons for their actions, and thus promoted the idea of education. She wanted public support for nursing education, which included some medical education—a shift in thinking that was not readily accepted.

In opposition to Nightingale's educational plan for nurses were widely supported societal ideas characterizing what constituted the natural, traditional work of women and views that too much education would take away the feminine instinct that was related to delivering care. The transfer of the Nightingale tenets to hospitals in the United States altered important educational objectives, which were different from just using student nurses to fulfill the service needs of the hospital.

THE NIGHTINGALE NURSING MODEL BECOMES "AMERICANIZED"

Hospital administrators, physicians, and women in the United States studied Nightingale's ideas and brought them to hospitals that had been established since the late 18th century, staffed with employees providing care without formalized training (Rosenberg, 1987). The first nursing schools were formed by separate nursing school boards charged with planning and financing the institutions. Unfortunately, poor funding removed Nightingale's ideal of student nurses in the hospitals to learn. Instead, students became the sole hospital care providers, in effect paying for their training, which lacked public support (Rosenberg). Their education became ward service, as theoretical classroom time decreased and practical experience became the teacher. The proliferation of hospitals in the 1870s increased the need for student nurses and the growth of nursing schools, which led to the diffusion of nursing education and the graduation of a variety of levels of nurses. The reputation of nurses, as well as the quality of the care they provided, both in hospitals and in private duty positions in the home after completing training, varied.

In the late 19th and early 20th centuries, nursing leaders, including a group of women nursing superintendents, shaped nursing education and work and attempted to prescriptively require a level of consistency in nursing care, thus protecting the reputation of the schools and the work done by their graduate nurses. Although the superintendent title was mostly associated with the directors of training schools in the profession's infancy, the "nurse superintendent" was later clarified by Davis (1929) as:

> The administrator or executive head of the hospital, not the director of the training school. In some of the smaller hospitals, unfortunately, the two positions are combined. The nurse superintendent has her chief field in the nongovernmental charitable hospital of less than 100 beds. (p. 386)

This early cohort of leaders worked together to form committees to evaluate school curricula and the specialized tasks performed by nurses. They actively promoted the formation of alumni groups (and their obvious financial philanthropy) and became a formidable and interested group of active nurses. The American Society of Superintendents of Training Schools, founded in 1894, promoted leadership, higher entrance requirements for potential students, and better training schools in an effort to increase the professionalization of nursing and protect trained nurses' legitimate role in society. Renamed the National League of Nursing Education in 1912, members aimed to encourage more women to enter nursing by pushing for progressive reforms, including shorter days, a university education, and a standard curriculum (Dock & Stewart, 1938).

Many sick people stayed at home in the 1800s so that their families could take care of them due to hospitals' poor reputation. With the growth of nursing training schools, those who could afford supplementary care hired a private duty nurse to come to the home to carry out physician treatments and provide skilled nursing care to the sick individual. Demand for private duty nurses increased as female family members increasingly joined the workforce. After the turn of the 20th century, hospitals also arranged for private duty nurses to provide care within the institution, which created employment opportunities for the majority of graduate nurses (Whelan, 2005). These nurse-owned and -operated registries were formed to assist nurses with finding work while granting them the freedom to choose the job, although this type of autonomy did not add to the professional image of nurses. When caring for patients in their homes, nurses fought against the image of subservience, especially African American nurses, who had been kept in inferior positions by a white majority of nurses and society alike (Young, 2005). Following Nightingale's promotion of highly moral and educated women, nursing leaders from the first half of the 20th century promoted the ideal nurse to have "the exercise of superior intelligence, a large body of knowledge and skills, sensitiveness, and imagination" (Harmer & Henderson, 1939, p. 4). However, middle- and upper-class women did not join nursing in large numbers, leaving women of the lower socioeconomic class with a high school diploma to enter training (Dock & Stewart, 1938; Rosenberg, 1987).

The Toil Public Health Nurses and Their Contribution to Nursing
NURSING'S ROLE IN THE PUBLIC'S HEALTH

Public health nurses had specialized knowledge and skills obtained by furthering their education after hospital training and were required to be effective in the communities where they worked. Advances in medicine and science during the late 1800s, specifically the wide acceptance of the germ theory, helped change the way people thought about infections and debunked previously held moral aspects of the causes of disease (Rosen, 1993). Identifying controllable germs as the root cause of illness and disability led to a global initiative demanding that governments take responsibility by responding to public welfare needs and subsidizing improvements in community sanitation, water supplies, and other alterable situations that, if left unattended, could lead to higher morbidity and mortality rates from infectious disease. The federally funded U.S. Public Health Service (USPHS) is one example of the U.S. government's attention to the need for community services to protect the health of citizens. Although the USPHS can trace its early history back to 1798 with an act designed for the relief of sick and disabled seamen, its history was more formally established by legislation in 1889, forming the USPHS Commissioned Officer Program (Williams, 1951). At first, only physicians were admitted to the Commissioned Officer Association, with the first nurses not commissioned until July 1945 (Parascandola, 2007; U.S. Public Health Service Nursing, 2009). Nevertheless, nurses in the 20th century would serve a fundamental role in this agency.

At the turn of the 20th century, the continuing influx of immigrants from around the world and overcrowding in urban areas led to a renewal of social reforms in which nurses participated and started a new role for nurses: short-term care for and education of families in their homes. The settlement house movement, which flourished in many cities beginning in the late 1800s, interested many individuals from all walks of life who subscribed to a belief in social welfare, and who sought to help improve the lives of the poor immigrants (Wade, 1967). Their social activism was intentional and aimed at the social determinants of health by assisting immigrant families to acculturate to urban life in America by improving their employment, the sanitation of their living arrangements, and their health. Lillian Wald, Mary Brewster, and other nurses formed the world-famous Henry Street Settlement House in New York in 1893, financed by wealthy patrons who saw the value of improving the health and welfare of the urban working poor (Buhler-Wilkerson, 1991). Living in the neighborhoods they served, these nurses visited tenement homes, providing nursing care and health education to all members of the family and providing education about their capacity to care for themselves and to enhance their health. In the new role of the public health nurse, another opportunity was provided to increase the professionalism of nurses due to its requirements of higher education, specialized knowledge, and a more autonomous practice (Brainard, 1985).

During the early 1900s, public health initiatives aimed to decrease disease, but the social issues connected with disease remained. Despite great efforts by public health nurses, poverty often limits individual choices and the ability to live a healthy life. Public awareness of growing health problems created the perfect link between public health and social reforms, forging a place for nurses to address health policies caused by urbanization, poverty, and disease (Porter, 1994). In recognition of this need for more specialized training for this role, Simmons College in Boston began an 8-month course for public health nurses in 1904 (Nutting, 1904). The nurses that emerged from this program, referred to as visiting nurses, worked for two types of agencies: voluntary and official. The privately funded voluntary organizations were funded by communities and philanthropies and were run by board members who hired public health nurses. Official agencies of the federal and state governments funded public health nurse positions with tax dollars.

The National Organization of Public Health Nurses (NOPHN), started in 1912, played a role in shaping public health nursing and attempted to bring this branch of nursing to a higher professional level. The NOPHN promoted standards of education, leadership, supervision, and employment and gave advice to groups looking to employ a public health nurse. Their journal, *Public Health Nurse*, founded in 1912, was a resource for nurses and committees looking for legislation, statistics, health information, and programs. Physicians contributed to the journal, writing about communicable diseases and treatments carried out by nurses at home. Although NOPHN recommendations were available, there were only a very limited number of employable, educated public health nurses who met them. As a result, many organizations overlooked the NOPHN's minimum standards and hired unprepared nurses to public health positions, which in many cases did not have supervisors or other nurses to assist the newly hired nurses in fulfilling their job requirements (Buhler-Wilkerson, 1987). The continuing increase in the hiring of public health nurses was due to the increasing number of agencies hiring a single public health nurse, ultimately limiting the number of citizens who came into contact with this service (Giacomo, 1953).

With the continued rise of organized nursing and a growing diverse population, philanthropic organizations pushed for national policy reforms and programs that included positions for public health nurses and helped promote an increase in government support for employing nurses (Magat, 1989). These official agencies were funded at a variety of government levels and employed public health nurses to address health issues in the hope of decreasing the incidence and prevalence of disease. As public funding increased with the increased incidence of communicable diseases, public health nurses had a choice of employment in official agencies sponsored by the government at the state and federal levels or in voluntary agencies, usually run by a board of community women and men (Beckemeier, 2008).

Public health nurses working in privately funded voluntary agencies specialized in caring for the entire family at home. They routinely visited many families each day to provide nursing care and to improve public health education practices in the home. These nurses determined the needs of the families and worked in cooperation with local boards and agencies to get services delivered. There were distinct skills required by public health nurses that were not gained from private duty or hospital experience (Dock, 1906). Hospital training did not provide the education to prepare the public health nurse to work with the acute and chronic healthcare needs seen in the community. In the early 1900s, public health nurses worked autonomously, caring for patients who could not afford to seek treatment from a physician (Craig, 2003). Their role thus changed with the growing organization of public health and the interest of the federal government in providing services.

PHYSICIANS EMERGED DOMINANT OVER NURSES IN THE PUBLIC HEALTH ROLE

C. E. A. Winslow, a Yale professor, physician, and leader in public health, ranked the physician as the head of the team, but he strongly promoted nurses as integral to public health campaigns. Indeed, early on, Winslow (1911) wrote very supportively of visiting nurses, stating: "Yet it is, I think, more and more clear that the real strategic point is by the bedside of the patient and at the elbow of the convalescent or the carrier. Here the chain of infection can be broken far more surely and more economically than at any point" (Winslow, 1911, p. 909). In his view, however, physicians would still make the diagnosis or program decisions that public health nurses then carried out in the homes, schools, and workplaces in the community. Winslow pushed health education as the change factor for successful public health campaigns, giving the task to nurses to interpret and translate health information for groups, families, and individuals. Attempting to decrease the individual's exposure to communicable diseases, public health nurses broke down scientific health information into doable tasks to be carried out by mothers, workers, children, and teachers. Yet, although he respected their work and realized the necessity of their work in conjunction with public health education, his writings show his continued ambivalence about the professional role of the nurse. He described a public health nurse as "a community mother but armed with expert knowledge which few mothers can possess" (Winslow, 1923, p. 56).

Supported by administrators in the powerful, pro-medicine Rockefeller Foundation in the 1920s, physicians were formally designated as the public health team leaders in governmental agencies. Universities, medical schools, and schools of public health joined to educate physicians in bacteriology, statistics, and public health principles and administration (Winslow, 1925). Graduates took positions in health departments and were given the official title of health officer. Public health nurses in official agencies were once again viewed as being in the position of assisting physicians to carry out public health principles and programs. Under this model, public health nurses thus lost some of the autonomy of practice in the homes of their clients and responded by shifting their focus to prevention instead of treatment.

THE PUBLIC HEALTH NURSE: MORE SPECIALIZED AND MORE PROFESSIONAL?
The public health nurse of the first half of the 20th century had several unique roles described in the textbooks as translator, educator, advocate, and conservator of the public's health (Gardner, 1936). The debate heightened in the 1930s over whether their role should be further specialized into the different services provided, such as child health, maternal health, orthopedics, tuberculosis care, and others (Footner, 1998; Melosh, 1982). With significant medical advances (the first antimicrobial drugs were introduced and new surgical procedures were invented), the profession of medicine was becoming more specialized, leading to the idea that physicians needed more specialized nurses to assist them (Schulz & Johnson, 2003). However, a generalist role still worked best for most agencies to deliver community nursing care efficiently, although nurses debated this issue. Families usually had several problems among various members of the household, and to avoid duplication of services, a public health nurse generalist was able to enter the home and tackle whatever problem the family presented to her. The special tasks of public health nurses, the requirement for additional education, as well as their autonomy in the field outside of the agency, boosted the view of professionalization in nursing.

Indeed, even before the severance of the generalist nurse into the specialist, public health nursing became the first specialty in nursing (Allen, 1991; Alpi & Adams, 2007; Gardner, 1936). Various postgraduate courses educated graduate nurses in public health, sanitation, sociology, ethics, and other subjects to give them a better understanding of the problems as well as approaches to assist different immigrant and impoverished families. Seeing the need for specialized knowledge, nursing leaders promoted the idea of a university education for public health nurses, which culminated in 1949 with the Russell Sage Foundation–sponsored Brown Report calling for nurses to be educated in colleges and universities (Gebbie, 2009; Maraldo et al., 1988). However, nursing continued to be burdened with a label and reputation of "women's work," rather than work that was valued as a "profession." Furthermore, physician control over nursing continued. Group and Roberts (2001) wrote, "By the 1930's the American Medical Association (AMA) had established a set of committees on nursing that tightened its control" (p. 148), and the tensions between nursing and medicine would continue for decades.

THE FEDERAL RECLASSIFICATION OF NURSING CHANGES THE PROFESSION

The Emergence of the Recognized Professionalism of Nursing
Professionalism for nurses gained momentum just after the turn of the 20th century, with endorsements from state and federal legislation. Lusk (1997) points out in her historical study that nursing leaders pushed and promoted the professional classification of nurses based on criteria established in the literature. However, nurses' link to service sometimes placed them in the laborer category, especially students in training whose work hours were limited to 8-hour days similar to those of unionized factory workers.

Some nursing leaders fought against these limits to autonomous practice and gained the right for graduate nurses to set their own work hours (Lusk). Government institutions denied professional status to nurses, which left army nurses during World War I without rank or authority in battlefield hospitals (Donahue, 1985). Now that women held the right to vote, nurses fought the federal government's classification of nurses as "subprofessionals" in 1923 legislation (Minnigerode, 1923). However, they did not have enough influence to change the category until 1935, when Harry L. Hopkins of the federal Work Progress Administration (WPA) reclassified nurses from "skilled non-manual workers" to "Class 4 professional and technical workers" in a simple federal memo (*AJN*, 1935). Nevertheless, this historic subclassification of nurses' work negatively affected their social standing and, more importantly, the salaries they earned. Even after this important 1935 regulatory memo, the status of nurses and their work did not substantively change as the ravages of the Great Depression (1929–1940) continued and left nurses with stagnant opportunities for educational advancement (D'Antonio, 2004). However, Byers (1999) views this period as a time of emerging liberation for all women, writing: Women's roles began to change with World War II as many were forced to find employment and to assume more family responsibilities as a result of the financial devastation of the Great Depression and men being forced to serve with the Armed Forces (p. 12).

In reality, nurses used expert knowledge, indeed some of the same knowledge used by physicians and often taught to nurses by physicians, but they were not seen as colleagues of the physicians. The public health hierarchy maintained the role of the physician as the head, responsible for making the assessments and the program decisions that directed the care and education to be delivered by the nurse. Therefore, while public health nurses developed a role in a new venue outside of the hospital and changed their work from bedside treatment of illness to health promotion and education requiring specialized knowledge, their work was still viewed within the maternal role of women and not considered by society to be "professional level work." The contemporary nursing leadership held a different view and developed education programs to promote the use of scientific knowledge when addressing issues affecting the public. Two pioneers of nursing, Lavinia Lloyd Dock and Isabel M. Stewart, both wrote very provocatively (in an almost unheard language of the day by nurses) in 1938 that nursing is not:

> A subordinate or "satellite" vocation . . . nursing is as old if not older than medicine and has had an independent existence for hundreds of years. The Nightingale concept of nursing was not that of a sub-caste of medicine or a "handmaid of medicine. (pp. 365–366)

They both further stated that:

> The experience of many years in many countries tends to show that nursing flourishes best when it is directed and controlled by skilled and experienced nurses and given the largest possible measure of freedom for the exercise of its particular functions. (p. 367)

Earlier, the Rockefeller Foundation, a leader in public health research and education, wanted to evaluate the effectiveness of public health nursing education in order to have workers adequately trained in public health. Nurses effectively bridged the gap between science and home, bringing health education to families in terms they understood and in incremental steps that they could take to improve their health within their surroundings. The Committee for the Study of Nursing Education, funded by the Rockefeller Foundation in 1919, studied the education requirements for public health nurses. However, due to the requirement of nurses' training, the committee decided to study hospital training also (Winslow, 1922). Josephine Goldmark subsequently wrote the influential Goldmark Report, published in 1923 (Gebbie, 2009), which found that the long and difficult hospital training using nursing students as cheap labor for the hospitals did not attract the interest of middle-class women who were thought to be able to grasp the higher level of knowledge needed to be a public health nurse. The recommendations that came out of the report called for higher entrance standards to nursing school as well as 3 years of hospital training plus postgraduate training, which included classroom education as well as public health field work. The committee felt that these steps would encourage more middle-class women to enter nursing, thus bringing more respect to the profession. Ultimately, public health nursing became an expensive funding endeavor because their service remained limited to the poor rather than expanding health education to all levels of society (Buhler-Wilkerson, 1985). Public health nurses' numbers decreased with the draw of nurses to meet war needs; furthermore, changes in the financial arrangements to pay nurses' salaries at the public health agencies did not garner public support (Buhler-Wilkerson, 1993).

NURSING'S STATUS POST–WORLD WAR II—THE 1960S

After World War II, the specialized knowledge of the public health nurse became a basic part of nursing education, and the NOPHN blended into the ANA. In pursuing the agenda of professionalization, public health nurses attempted to bring status to all of nursing and to control their nursing work, job qualifications, and education globally. However, a shortage of educated public health nurses hampered the tremendous need to develop health programs in countries recovering from war. Many countries were building their nursing education programs and did not have established public health nursing agencies, so the leaders of the World Health Organization (WHO) endorsed the use of less trained workers in public health work (Cueto, 2007).

Post–World War II advancements in medicine and pharmaceuticals and federal funding of the Hill-Burton Act (which increased the number of hospitals) changed the U.S. healthcare system. Nurses experienced innovative programs, such as military flight nurses caring for wounded soldiers on cargo planes and in mobile surgical units close to the battles in the Korean War (Kalisch & Kalisch, 2003). The Truman administration's promotion of the community college system in conjunction with a nursing shortage ultimately made acceptable the idea of a 2-year associate degree producing a college-educated nurse. However, community colleges lacked hospital affiliations and raised educational costs through the need for the employment of additional clinical staff (Halloran, 1995). Public health nursing changed from a post-diploma specialty to a standard part of the baccalaureate nursing program. The Nurse Training Act (NTA) of 1964 helped fund nursing education; however, a smaller percentage funded baccalaureate nursing education, although the apprentice system of diploma training schools (still very prevalent but decreasing in number) and community college associate degree nursing programs received a larger share of the money. Incredulously, this inequity still persists some 40+ years later.

Dr. Linda Aiken, co-chair of the Council on Physician and Nurse Supply studied the issue of building the number of nurses and nursing faculty. The Council's report found that the majority of funding supported the shorter, two-year college programs but these ADN nurses typically did not go on to receive higher degrees thus limiting the number of future advanced practice nurses and nursing faculty. Thus, the recommendation that all states increase BSN programs (Council on Physician and Nurse Supply, 2007).

The ANA's leaders published their stance on nursing education in 1965, promoting the baccalaureate degree as the entry level for professional nurses but with support for the associate degree for technical nursing practice (ANA, 1965). The intention was to limit the scope of practice of the technical nurse and develop the leadership aspect of the baccalaureate nurse (Freund, 1990). Ultimately, an increased demand for nurses related to increased healthcare funding from the Medicare and Medicaid programs added to the persistent nursing shortage in hospitals (Lynaugh, 2007). Despite their best intentions, the nursing leadership had difficulty quantifying the intended levels of care and the lack of differentiation between roles, which seemed to blend nurses together. Today, the nursing profession is well aware of its failed efforts to ensure that all nurses have a BSN. However, Donley & Flaherty (2008) write, "If you view the 1965 statement as a call to close hospital schools of nursing and to move all nursing education inside the walls of colleges or universities, then the ANA was successful in implementing its vision" (p. 1). Notwithstanding, they further state, "If, however, you view the 1965 Position Paper as a mandate for a more educated nurse force to enhance patient care, the goal has not been achieved" (Donley & Flaherty, 2008, p. 1).

The sustained progress in medical technology and nursing's emergence as a discipline in the mid- to late-1960s again offered nurses specialized knowledge and skill in hospital settings in the newly established cardiac care units (Dreher, 2010). Small groups of specially trained nurses in these intensive observation units used the skills usually associated with physicians, which gave nurses a larger scope of practice and perhaps a boost to their professionalism (Keeling, 2004). Through skilled observation, these nurses made independent decisions to administer the needed medications based on standing orders and used the technology to save patients' lives. Keeling referred to it as "the blurry line" between medicine and nursing because these nurses gave medications to stop arrhythmias and *then* wrote the verbal orders for physicians to sign at a later time. In the 1960s, many nursing tasks involved using new machines and taking new measurements from them, although previously these functions had been limited to the realm of physicians. Physicians, however, embraced the capacity of the RNs to manage this ever-increasing technology, as they ultimately could not manage and monitor all of this technology themselves. Was this real progress toward more nursing professional autonomy? Or was it simply acquiescence by physicians that their work depended on the good functioning of nurses and nursing?

SUMMARY

In American nursing in the 1800s through the 1960s, nursing leaders gradually sought to establish higher standards for nurses, largely in response to changes in society. Woods (1996) has also recognized that the rise of professional nursing has been led primarily by nurse educators and public health nurses. Ultimately, however, those "traditionalists" and "professionalizers" (again despite their disagreement on change) did succeed in raising nursing from being simply everyday women's work to a professional career choice for women (and men to a lesser extent), giving women an economic position in the market, albeit undercompensated and still unnecessarily stereotyped.

It has been more than 150 years from the founding of the first nursing education program of six months at the Women's Hospital in Philadelphia in 1863 to a position where a doctor of nursing practice degree could replace master's entry-level degree programs for advanced practice registered nursing practice (DAPRN). Even if the DNP does not replace master's-level preparation for APRNs, it could become the "preferred preparation." It is not unlikely that the BSN and DNP may have a shared history. As McCauley et al. (2020) have outlined, while there has been enormous growth in the doctor of nursing practice programs since 2005, when eight programs were founded,[4] significant issues remain, as outlined in this chapter.

A chief one is: Why are most students seeking to become nurse practitioners choosing master's preparation? The role of what a DNP graduate should do remains an evolution, and role delineation from master's preparation seems a long way from clarity. The good news is that as DNP programs continue to be founded and current programs grow, an increase in the critical mass of DNPs will shape their impact in a variety of roles, ultimately creating an evidence base that DNPs as a whole can improve health outcomes. The roles they will acquire will gradually increase their value to their respective workplaces. It seems the DNP-prepared nurse executive may have the easiest role transition, but more research needs to be done on how each DAPN develops and matures in their role. The struggle of nurses to gain true professional status continues today as their scope of practice and their role in healthcare expand into the realm of a new doctoral degree, which may one day be required for entry into advanced practice nursing. We can only imagine how long that will take!

■ CRITICAL THINKING QUESTIONS

1. How do you think the controversy over whether nursing is truly a profession might impact the perception of the DNP graduate by other, more common doctoral-prepared healthcare professionals?
2. As you read, there have been many instances in history when nursing roles have changed but have remained constrained by internal and external forces. Can you identify any particular forces that might support or work against the proliferation of this new degree?
3. Do you agree that the role of the professional nurse is best described from a functionalist perspective, and the role of the DAPN is best described from a symbolic interactionist perspective? What about the role of the master's-prepared advanced practice nurse—is their role more structural-functional or symbolic interactionist?
4. Your new role will interact with two different populations: patients and colleagues. How do you envision your new role evolving with each one?
5. As you are most likely very early in your DNP curriculum, do you already have ideas about how you want your doctoral role to be different from your master's role?
6. As a future nursing leader, how can you use historical research for problem solving? In other words, can knowledge of the past prepare one for the future?
7. The information in this chapter points out some of the external influences that affected the nursing profession, leaving nursing leaders with their hands tied. Do you think nursing leaders are able to ascertain the external influences that are affecting nursing today? Discuss.
8. Do you think this chapter points to nurses actively promoting their professionalism or passively accepting the judgment of others? Discuss.
How will you advance your role as a DNP graduate: through active promotion, passive acceptance, or maybe somewhere in between?
9. Discuss whether nurses were handed their place in the healthcare system or whether they endeavored to develop roles for nurses in the healthcare system, placing nurses where they were most effective.
10. Discuss why you are either a conservative traditionalist or an elite professionalizer.

NOTES

1. Robinson (1946), who has written a meticulous and gripping history of nursing in *White Caps: The Story of Nursing*, indicates that five separate entities lay claim to the status of the "first nursing school or first training program for nurses," including New York Hospital (1798), the Nurse Society of Philadelphia (1828), and the New York Infirmary (1857). However, Robinson favors the authenticity of the more substantial programs established first at the Women's Hospital of Philadelphia in 1863, which was the first 6-month curriculum, and then a 12-month curriculum founded at New England Hospital in 1872.
2. We should note that this number was 23 in 2017 and has only grown by four states since the year of publication of the second edition of this book.
3. The conservative "traditionalists" and the elite "professionalizers" (Melosh, 1982; Reverby, 1987). It is Melosh's view that historians of nursing have long been preoccupied by the theme of "professionalism." Melosh suggests that they have absorbed the ideology of a nursing elite. Melosh today would likely see the early DNP advocates as elite "professionalizers" who may ultimately disenfranchise master's-prepared APNs versus "traditionalists" who opposed the DNP degree, at least at the beginning of the debate and the early launch of the degree. Traditionalists saw no need to replace the master's degree with advanced nursing practice.
4. Case Western Reserve, Columbia University, Drexel University, Rush University, Tri-College University Nursing Consortium (Concordia College; Minnesota State University, Moorhead; North Dakota State University), University of Denver, University of South Carolina, and University of Tennessee at Memphis.

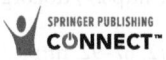 A robust set of instructor resources designed to supplement this text is located at http://connect.springerpub.com/content/book/978-0-8261-8137-4. Qualifying instructors may request access by emailing textbook@springerpub.com.

REFERENCES

Aiken, L. H., Cimiotti, J. P., Sloane, D. M., Smith, H. L., Flynn, L., & Neff, D. F. (2011). Effects of nurse staffing and nurse education on patient deaths in hospitals with different nurse work environments. *Medical Care, 49*(12), 1047–1053. https://doi.org/10.1097/MLR.0b013e3182330b6e

Aiken, L. H., Clarke, S. P., Cheung, R. B., Sloane, D. M., & Silber, J. H. (2003). Educational levels of hospital nurses and surgical patient mortality. *Journal of the American Medical Association, 290*(12), 1617–1623. https://doi.org/10.1001/jama.290.12.1617

Aiken, L. H., Sloane, D. M., Bruyneel, L., Van den Heede, K., Griffiths, P., Busse, R., Diomidous, M., Kinnunen, J., Kózka, M., Lesaffre, E., McHugh, M. D., Moreno-Casbas, M. T., Rafferty, A. M., Schwendimann, R., Scott, P. A., Tishelman, C., van Achterberg, T., Sermeus, W., & RN4CAST Consortium. (2014). Nurse staffing and education and hospital mortality in nine European countries: A retrospective observational study. *The Lancet, 383*(9931), 1824–1830. https://doi.org/10.1016/S0140-6736(13)62631-8

Allen, C. E. (1991). Holistic concepts and the professionalization of public health nursing. *Public Health Nursing, 8*(2), 74–80. https://doi.org/ 10.1111/j.1525-1446.1991.tb00649.x

Alpi, K. M., & Adams, M. G. (2007). Mapping the literature of public health and community nursing. *Journal of the Medical Library Association, 95*(1), e6–e9.

Alspach, J. G. (2014). Nurse education and patient mortality: Sorting fact from fury. *Critical Care Nurse, 34*(4) 10–12. https://doi.org/10.4037/ccn2014507. Retrieved Nurse Education and Patient Mortality: Sorting Fact From Fury | Critical Care Nurse | American Association of Critical-Care Nurses (aacnjournals.org)

American Association of Colleges of Nursing. (2000). *The baccalaureate degree in nursing as minimal preparation for professional practice.* http://www.aacn.nche.edu/Publications/positions/baccmin.htm

American Association of Colleges of Nursing. (2004). *AACN position statement on the practice doctorate in nursing March 2004.* Author.

American Association of Colleges of Nursing. (2015). *MEDICARE at 50: A look at nursing education.* http://www.aacn.nche.edu/government-affairs/ian/2015/September-2015.pdf

American Association of Colleges of Nursing. (2019). *2004–2018 Enrollment and graduations in ba-calaureate and graduate programs in nursing.* American Association of Colleges of Nursing.

American Association of Nurse Practitioners. (2016). *Safe practice environment.* https://www.aanp.org/legislation-regulation/state-legislation/state-practice-environment

American Association of Nurse Practitioners (AANP). (2019). *The state of the nurse practitioner profession: 2018.* https://bit.ly/2PmHIdt.

American Association of Nurse Practitioners. (2022). *NP Fact Sheet.* Retrieved from NP Fact Sheet (aanp.org)

American Journal of Nursing. (1935). The WPA and nursing: The nurse's status; projects; state committees [Unsigned Editorial]. *The American Journal of Nursing, 35*(12), 1154–1156. https://doi.org/10.2307/3412013

American Nurses' Association. (1965). American Nurses' Association's first position on education for nursing. *The American Journal of Nursing, 65*(12), 106–111. https://doi.org/10.2307/3419707

American Nurses Credentialing Center. (2022). Characteristics of magnet organizations. *nursingworld.org* Retrieved Characteristics of Magnet Organizations | ANCC | ANA (nursingworld.org)

Auerbach, D. I., Martsolf, G., Pearson, M. L., Taylor, E. A., Maydman, Z., Muchow, A., Spetz, J., & Lee, Y. (2015).The DNP by 2015: A study of the institutional, political, and professional issues that facilitate or impede establishing a post-baccalaureate doctor of nursing practice program. *Report by RAND Corporation sponsored by the AACN*, Retrieved The DNP by 2015 - RAND Report (aacnnursing.org)

Barter, M., & McFarland, P. L. (2001). BSN by 2010. A California initiative. *The Journal of Nursing Administration, 31*(3), 141–144. https://doi.org/10.1097/00005110-200103000-00010

Beckemeier, B. (2008). History of public health and public health nursing. In L. L. Ivanovov & C. L. Blue (Eds.), *Public Health Nursing: Leadership, Policy, & Practice* (pp. 2–26). Delmar Cengage Learning.

Beeber, A. S., Palmer, C., Waldrop, J., Lynn, M. R., & Jones, C. B. (2019). The role of Doctor of Nursing Practice-prepared nurses in practice settings. *Nursing Outlook, 67*(4), 354–364. https://doi.org/10.1016/j.outlook.2019.02.006

Biddle, B. J. (1986). Recent developments in role theory. *Annual Review of Sociology, 12*, 67–92. https://doi.org/10.1146/annurev.so.12.080186.000435

Blumer, H. (1969). *Symbolic interactionism: Perspective and method.* University of California Press.

Brainard, A. M. (1985). *The evolution of public health nursing* W. B. Saunders.

Buhler-Wilkerson, K. (1985). Public health nursing: In sickness or in health? *American Journal of Public Health, 75*(10), 1155–1161. https://doi.org/10.2105/ajph.75.10.1155

Buhler-Wilkerson, K. (1987). Left carrying the bag: Experiments in visiting nursing, 1877–1909. *Nursing Research, 36*(1), 42–47.

Buhler-Wilkerson, K. (1991). Lillian Wald: Public health pioneer. *Nursing Research, 40*(5), 316–317. https://doi.org/10.1097/00006199-199109000-00025

Buhler-Wilkerson, K. (1993). Guarded by standards and directed by strangers. Charleston, South Carolina's response to a national health care agenda, 1920–1930. *Nursing History Review: Official Journal of the American Association for the History of Nursing, 1*, 139–154.

Burbules, N., & Densmore, K., (1991). The limits of making teaching a profession. *Educational Policy, 5*(1), 44–63. https://doi.org/10.1177/0895904891005001004

Byers, B. K. (1999). *The lived experience of registered nurses, 1930–1950: A phenomenological study.* A Dissertation in Higher Education submitted to the Graduate Faculty of Texas Tech University. https://ttu-ir.tdl.org/ttu-ir/handle/2346/9563 [Restricted access for full source.]

Cast, A. (2004). Role-taking and interaction. *Social Psychology Quarterly, 67*(3), 296–309. https://doi.org/10.1177/019027250406700305

Chapman, S., Toretsky, C., & Phoenix, B. J. (2019). Enhancing psychiatric mental health nurse practitioner practice: Impact of state scope of practice regulations. *Journal of Nursing Regulation, 10*(1), 35–43. https://doi.org/10.1016/S2155-8256(19)30081-X

Cooley, C. (1964). *Human nature and social order.* Schocken Books.

Council on Physician and Nurse Supply. (2007). *New council calls for immediate increase in physician and nurse education.* http://www.physiciannursesupply.com/news-press-releases.aspx

Covelli, A. F., Buckhholz, S. W., Fowler, L. H., Beasley, S. B., & Bigley, M. B. (2022). Development of the doctor of nursing practice nurse practitioner minimum data set (DNP NP MDS). *Journal of Professional Nursing, 39,* 54–68. https://doi.org/10.1016/j.profnurs.2021.12.012

Craig, P. (2003). The development of public health nursing. In S. Cowley (Ed.), *Public health in policy and practice: A sourcebook for health visitors and community nurses* (pp. 25–43). Elsevier Science.

Cronenwett, L., Dracup, K., Grey, M., McCauley, L., Meleis, A., & Salmon, M. (2011). The doctor of nursing practice: A national workforce perspective. *Nursing Outlook, 59*(1), 9–17. https://doi.org/10.1016/j.outlook.2010.11.003

Cueto, M. (2007). *The value of health: A history of the Pan American Health Organization.* Pan American Health Organization. https://iris.paho.org/handle/10665.2/51500

Dahnke, M. D., & Dreher, H. M. (2016). *Philosophy of science for nursing practice: Concepts and applications.* (2nd ed.). Springer Publishing Company.

D'Antonio, P. (2004). Women, nursing, and baccalaureate education in 20th century America. *Journal of Nursing Scholarship, 36*(4), 379–384. https://doi.org/10.1111/j.1547-5069.2004.04067.x

Davis, M. (1929). The nurse as hospital superintendent. *The American Journal of Nursing, 29*(4), 385–387. https://doi.org/10.2307/3408499

Deloughery, G. (1977). *History and trends of professional nursing.* Mosby.

Dock, L. L. (1906). Training for visiting nursing. *The American Journal of Nursing, 7*(2), 109–111. https://doi.org/10.2307/3403716

Dock, L. L., & Stewart, I. M. (1938). *A short history of nursing from the earliest times to the present day.* G. P. Putnam's Sons, The Knickerbocker Press.

Donahue, P. (1985). *Nursing, the finest art.* Mosby.

Donohue, P. (1996). *Nursing, the finest art: An illustrated history.* (2nd ed.). Mosby.

Donley, R., & Flaherty, R. (2002). Revisiting the American Nurses Association's first position on education for nurses. *Online Journal of Issues in Nursing, 7*(2). http://www.nursingworld.org/MainMenuCategories/ANAMarketplace/ANAPeriodicals/OJIN/TableofContents/Volume72002/No2May2002/RevisingPostiononEducation.aspx

Donley, R., & Flaherty, M. J. (2008). Revisiting the American Nurses Association's first position on education for nurses: A comparative analysis of the first and second position statements on the education of nurses. *The Online Journal of Issues in Nursing, 13*(2). http://www.nursingworld.org/MainMenuCategories/ANAMarketplace/ANAPeriodicals/OJIN/TableofContents/Volume72002/No2May2002/RevisingPostiononEducation.aspx

Dreher, H. M. (2008b). Is poor weight management a failure of primary care? *Holistic Nursing Practice, 22*(6), 312–316. https://doi.org/10.1097/01.HNP.0000339342.80758.0f

Dreher, H. M., & Dahnke, M. D. (2016). What is a practice discipline? In M. D. Dahnke & H. M. Dreher's (Eds.), *Philosophy of science in a practice discipline: Concepts and application,* (2nd ed.). (pp.71–96). Springer Publishing Company.

Dreher, H. M., & Montgomery, K. A. (2009). Let's call it "doctoral" advanced practice nursing. *Journal of Continuing Education in Nursing, 40*(12), 530–531. https://doi.org/10.3928/00220124-20100525-01

Durkeim, E. (1964). *The division of labor in society.* Free Press.

Edwardson, S. (2010). Doctor of philosophy and doctor of nursing of nursing practice as complementarydegrees. *Journal of Professional Nursing, 26*(3), 137–140. https://doi.org/10.1016/j.profnurs.2009.08.004

Ferris, D. (2001). *Military intelligence.* http://www.nurseweek.com/news/features/01-06/military.html

Footner, A. (1998). Nursing specialism or nursing specialization? *Nursing Outlook, 2*(4), 219–223. https://doi.org/10.1016/S1361-3111(98)80049-6

Freund, C. M. (1990). *The unity of education, research, and practice.* American Nurses Association.

Fritter, E., & Shimp, K. (2016). What does certification in professional nursing practice mean? *Med-Surg Matters, Academy of Medical-Surgical Nurses, 25*(2), 8–10. https://go.gale.com/ps/anonymous?id=GALE%7CA452585842&sid=googleScholar&v=2.1&it=r&linkaccess=fulltext&issn=10920811&p=AONE&sw=w

Gardner, M. S. (1936). *Public health nursing.* Macmillian.

Gebbie, K. M. (2009). 20th-century reports on nursing and nursing education: What difference did they make? *Nursing Outlook, 57*(2), 84–92. https://doi.org/10.1016/j.outlook.2009.01.006

Giacomo, R. (1953). The 1953 census of nurses in public health work. *Nursing Outlook, 1*(11), 645–646.

Goffman, E. (1955). On face-work: An analysis of ritual elements in social interaction. *Psychiatry, 18*(3), 213–231. https://doi.org/10.1080/00332747.1955.11023008

Goffman, E. (1959). *The presentation of self in everyday life*. University of Edinburgh, Social Sciences Research Centre.
Group, T. M., & Roberts, J. I. (2001). *Nursing, physician control, and the medical monopoly: Historical perspectives on gendered inequality in roles, rights, and range of practice*. University Press.
Halloran, E. (1995). *A Virginia Henderson reader: Excellence in nursing*. Springer Publishing Company.
Hardy, M., & Conway, M. (1978). *Role theory: Perspectives for health professionals*. Appleton & Lange.
Hardy, M., & Conway, M. (1988). *Role theory: Perspectives for health professionals*. (2nd ed.). Appleton & Lange.
Harmer, B., & Henderson, V. (1939). *Textbook of the principles and practice of nursing*. Macmillan.
Harrison, J. M., Aiken, L. H., Sloane, D. M., Carthon, J. M. B., Merchant, R. M., Berg, R. A., & McHugh, M. D. (2019). In hospitals with more nurses who have baccalaureate degrees, better outcomes for patients after cardiac arrest. *Health Affairs, 38*(7), 1087–1094. Retrieved Health Affairs | Vol 38, No 7
Hein, L., & Chinn, P. (2017). Issues of authorship: Who and in what order? *Nurse Author and Editor, 27*(3), 1–8. https://doi.org/10.1111/nae2.34
Idzik, S., Buchholz, S. W., Kelly-Weeder, S., Finnegan, L., & Bigley, M. B. (2021). Strategies to move entry-level nurse practitioner education to the doctor of nursing practice degree by 2025. *Nurse Educator 46*(6), 336–341. https://doi.org/10.1097/NNE.0000000000001129
Institute of Medicine. (2011). *The future of nursing: Leading change, advancing health*. http://www.nationalacademies.org/hmd/Reports/2010/The-Future-of-Nursing-Leading-Change-Advancing-Health.aspx#sthash.ECAsL6ya.dpuf
Jackson, S., & Stevenson, C. (2000). What do people need psychiatric and mental health nurses for? *Journal of Advanced Nursing, 31*(2), 378–388. https://doi.org/10.1046/j.1365-2648.2000.01288.x
Johns, C., & Freshwater, D. (2005). *Transforming nursing through reflective practice*, (2nd ed.). Wiley-Blackwell.
Judd, D., Sitzman, K., & Davis, G. M. (2009). *A history of American nursing: Trends and eras*. Jones & Bartlett.
Kalisch, P. A., & Kalisch, B. J. (2003). *American nursing: A history*. (4th ed.). Lippincott Williams & Wilkins.
Keeling, A. W. (2004). Blurring the boundaries between medicine and nursing: Coronary care nursing, circa the 1960s. *Nursing History Review: Official Journal of the American Association for the History of Nursing, 12*, 139–164.
Klass, A. A. (1961). What is a profession? *Canadian Medical Association Journal, 85*, 698–701.
Kuhn, A. (1974). *The logic of social systems*. Jossey-Bass.
Liaschenko, J., & Peter, E. (2004). Nursing ethics and conceptualizations of nursing: Profession, practice and work. *Journal of Advanced Nursing, 46*(5), 488–495. https://doi.org/10.1111/j.1365-2648.2004.03011.x
Lusk, B. (1997). Professional classifications of American nurses, 1910 to 1935. *Western Journal of Nursing Research, 19*(2), 227–242. https://doi.org/10.1177/019394599701900207
Lynaugh, J. (2007). Hospitals, nurses, and education—Eternal triangle. In J. Lynaugh, H. Grace, G. Smith, R. Sena, M., & de Villabos (Eds.), *The W. K. Kellogg Foundation and the nursing profession: Shared values, shared legacy*. Sigma Theta Tau International.
Magat, R. (Ed.). (1989). *Philanthropic giving: Studies in varieties and goals*. Oxford University Press.
Maraldo, P. J., Fagin, C., & Keenan, T. (1988). Nursing and private philanthropy. *Health Affairs (Project Hope), 7*(1), 130–136.
Marion, L., Viens, D., O'Sullivan, A. L., Crabtree, K., Fontana, S., Price, M. M., & (National Organization of Nurse Practitioner Faculty [NONPF] Practice Doctorate Task Force. (2003). The practice doctorate in nursing: Future or fringe. *Topics in Advanced Practice Nursing eJournal, 3*(2), 1–8, Retrieved The Practice Doctorate in Nursing (psu.edu)
Martsolf, G. R., Komadino, A., Germack, H., Harrison, J., & Poghosyan, L. (2021). Practice environment, independence, and roles among DNP- and MSN-prepared primary care nurse practitioners. *Nursing Outlook, 69*(6), 953–960. https://doi.org/10.1016/j.outlook.2021.06.008
McCauley, L. A., Broome, M. E., Frazier, L., Hayes, R., Kurth, A., Musil, C. M., Norman, L. D., Rideout, H., & Villarruel, A. M. (2020). Doctor of nursing practice (DNP) degree in the United States: Reflecting, readjusting, and getting back on track. *Nursing Outlook, 68*(4), 494–503. https://doi.org/10.1016/j.outlook.2020.03.008
Mead, G. (1934). *Mind, self, and society*. University of Chicago Press.
Meleis, A. I. (1975). Role insufficiency and role supplementation: A conceptual framework. *Nursing Research, 24*(4), 264–271.

Meleis, A. I. (2011). Transitions from practice to evidence-based. In A. Meleis (Ed.), *Transitions theory: Middle range and situation specific theories in nursing research and practice* (pp. 1–10). Springer Publishing Company.

Meleis, A. I., & Trangenstein, P. A. (1994). Facilitating transitions: Redefinition of the nursing mission. *Nursing Outlook, 42*(6), 255–259. https://doi.org/10.1016/0029-6554(94)90045-0

Melosh, B. (1982). *The physician's hand: Work culture and conflict in American nursing*. Temple University Press.

Minnigerode, L. (1923). Report of committee on federal legislation. *American Journal of Nursing, 24*(3), 223.

Mundinger, M. O., Kane, R. l., Lenz, E. R., Totten, A. M., Tsai, W. Y., Cleary, P. D., Friedewald, W. T., Siu, A. L., & Shelanski, M. L. (2000). Primary care outcomes in patients treated by nurse practitioners or physicians: A randomized trial. *Journal of the American Medical Association, 283*(1), 59–68. https://doi.org/10.1001/jama.283.1.59

National Academy of Medicine. (2021). *The future of nursing 2020–2030: Charting a path to achieve health equity*. Retrieved Front Matter | The Future of Nursing 2020–2030: Charting a Path to Achieve Health Equity | The National Academies Press

National Council of States Boards of Nursing. (2023). *2022 National Nursing Workforce Study*, Author. Retrieved from 2022 National Nurses Workforce Study by the National Council of State Boards of Nursing

National Organization of Nurse Practitioner Faculty. (2023). *Reaffirming the Doctor of Nursing Practice Degree: Entry to Nurse Practitioner Practice by 2025*. NONPF, Retrieved NONPF (ymaws.com)

Nelson, M. A. (2002). Education for professional nursing practice: Looking backward into the future. *Online Journal of Issues in Nursing, 7*(2), 4. Education for Professional Nursing Practice: Looking Backward into the Future Retrieved | OJIN: The Online Journal of Issues in Nursing (nursingworld.org)

NurseJournal Staff. (2023). *Nurse practitioner practice authority: A state-by-state guide*. Retrieved Nurse Practitioner Practice Authority: A State-by-State Guide | NurseJournal.org

Nutting, A. (1904). A school for social workers. *The American Journal of Nursing, 4*(9), 679–681. https://doi.org/10.2307/3401566

Merriam-Webster.com. (2023). Role. Merriam-Webster.com Role Definition & Meaning - Merriam-Webster

Parascandola, J. (2007). Public health history. Commissioned Officer Association for the USPHS. https://www.coausphs.org/COA/COA/About/History.aspx

Porter, D. (1994). The history of public health and the modern state: Introduction. *Clio Medica, 26*, 1–44.

Reverby, S. (1987). *Ordered to care: The dilemma of American nursing*, 1850–1945. Cambridge University Press.

Robinson, V. (1946). *White caps: The story of nursing*. J. B. Lippincott.

Rosen, J. (1993). *A history of public health*. Johns Hopkins University Press.

Rosenberg, C. (1987). *The care of strangers: The rise of America's hospital system*. Basic Books.

Schell, E. S., & Kayser-Jones, J. (1999). The effect of role-taking ability on caregiver-resident mealtime interaction. *Applied Nursing Research, 12*(1), 38–44. https://doi.org/10.1016/s0897-1897(99)80167-0

Schmitz, K. A. (2022). *Associate degree nurse attitudes toward degree advancement when considering the "BSN in 10" in New York State*, D'Youville College, ProQuest Dissertations Publishing, 2022. 29164560.

Schön, D. (1983). *The reflective practitioner: How professionals think in action*. Basic Books.

Schulz, R., & Johnson, A. C. (2003). *Management of hospitals and health services: Strategic issues and performance*. Beard Books.

Shattell, M. (2004). Nurse-patient interaction: A review of the literature. *Journal of Clinical Nursing, 13*(6), 714–722. https://doi.org/10.1111/j.1365-2702.2004.00965.x

Smiley, R. A., Allgeyer, R. L., Shobo, L., Karen, C. L., Letourmeau, R., Zhong, E., Kaminski-Ozturk, N., & Alexander, M, (2023). The national nursing workforce study. *Journal of Nursing Regulation, 14*(1), Supplement 2, S1–S90, Retrieved The 2022 National Nursing Workforce Survey - Journal of Nursing Regulation

Smith, T. G. (2009, October 5). A policy perspective on the entry into practice issue. *Online Journal of Issues of Nursing*. Retrieved A Policy Perspective on the Entry into Practice Issue | OJIN: The Online Journal of Issues in Nursing (nursingworld.org)

Smith Glasgow, M. E., & Zoucha, R. (2011). Role strain in the doctorally prepared advance practice nurse:The experiences of doctor of nursing practice graduates in their current professional positions. In H. M. Dreher & M. E. Smith Glasgow (Eds.), *Role Development for Doctoral Advanced Nursing Practice* (pp. 213–226). Springer Publishing Company.

Smith Glasgow, M. E., Zoucha, R., & Johnson, C. (2017). Role strain in the doctorally prepared advance practice nurse: The experiences of doctor of nursing practice graduates in their current professional positions. In H. M. Dreher & M. E. Smith Glasgow (Eds.), *Role development for doctoral advanced nursing practice* (2nd ed., pp. 237–250). Springer Publishing Company.

Spetz, J., Toretsky, C., Chapman, S., Phoenix, B., & Tierney, M. (2019). Nurse practitioner and physician assistant waivers to prescribe buprenorphine and state scope of practice restrictions. *Journal of the American Medical Association, 321*(14), 1407–1408. https://doi.org/10.1001/jama.2019.0834

Stew, G. (2017). Enhancing the doctoral advanced practice nursing role with reflective practice. In H. M. Dreher & M. E. Smith Glasgow (Eds.), *Role development for doctoral advanced nursing practice* (2nd ed., pp. 429–438). Springer Publishing Company.

Truthaboutnursing.org. (2015). *Q: Are you sure nurses are autonomous? Based on what I've seen, it sure looks like physicians are calling the shots.* http://www.truthaboutnursing.org/faq/autonomy.html

U.S. Bureau of Labor Statistics. (2022). *Certified Registered Nurse Anesthetists.* Retrieved U.S. Bureau of Labor Statistics (bls.gov)

U.S. Public Health Service Nursing. (2009). *Nurse resource manual: USPHS nursing—Mission, responsibilities, and challenge.* http://phs-nurse.org/nurse-resource-manual/usphs-mission

Wade, L. C. (1967). The heritage from Chicago's early settlement houses. *Journal of the Illinois State Historical Society (1908–1984), 60*(4), 411–441.

Wells, W., & Hejna, W. (2019). Developing leadership talent in healthcare organizations. *Healthcare Financial Management, 63*(1), 66–69.

Whelan, J. C. (2005). "A necessity in the nursing world": The Chicago Nurses Professional Registry, 1913-1950. *Nursing History Review: Official Journal of the American Association for the History of Nursing, 13*, 49–75.

Williams, R. C. (1951). *The United States Public Health Service, 1798–1950.* Commissioned Officers Association of the United States Public Health Service.

Winslow, C.-E. A. (1911). The role of the visiting nurse in the campaign for public health. *American Journal of Nursing, 11*(11), 909–929.

Winslow, C.-E. A. (1922). From the report of the committee on nursing education. *American Journal of Nursing, 22*(11), 882–884. https://doi.org/10.2307/3406757

Winslow, C.-E. A. (1923). *The evolution and significance of the modern public health campaign.* Yale University Press.

Winslow, C. E. (1925). The place of public health in a university. *Science, 62*, 335–338.

Woods, C. Q. (1996). Evolution of the American Nurses Association's position on health insurance for the aged: 1933–1965. *Nursing Research, 45*(5), 304–310. https://doi.org/10.1097/00006199-199609000-00009

Yam, B. M. C. (2013). From vocation to profession: the quest for professionalization of nursing, *British Journal of Nursing, 13*(16). Retrieved from From vocation to profession: the quest for professionalization of nursing | British Journal of Nursing (magonlinelibrary.com)

Young, J. (2005). Revisiting the 1925 Johns Report on African-American nurses. *Nursing History Review: Official Journal of the American Association for the History of Nursing, 13*, 77–99.

Zangaro, G. A. (2023). The state of the doctor of nursing practice degree: A survey of DNP graduates, academic leaders and, and employers. *American Association of Colleges of Nursing,* Retrieved 2023aprn_gzangaro.pdf (ncsbn.org)

Zerwekh, J., & Claborn, J. (2009). *Nursing today: Transitions and trends* (6th ed.). Elsevier Health Sciences.

CHAPTER TWO Reflective Response

ZANE WOLF

Having inaugurated and taught in La Salle's Doctor of Nursing Practice Program, I have been sensitized to the challenges of providing the degree by many experiences since its inception. Examples include creating and revising a curriculum that meets certifying standards and establishing rigor in DNP projects. With nurse faculty, administrators, colleague faculty from other disciplines, university leaders, and doctoral students, I have discussed the role of the DNP-prepared nurse. The discussions have not been definitive or final.

Discussions with stakeholders have also highlighted the insecurities shared by students and faculty about the role of the DNP graduate. Students questioned the benefit of their education when considering skill-set development, which is not necessarily appreciated during coursework. They also contemplated whether salary increases would follow degree completion. Students wondered if their previous role as an advanced practice nurse, nurse administrator, or, more recently, baccalaureate-prepared nurse with a doctoral degree earned in tandem with nurse anesthesia-focused courses would change significantly due to the DNP.

At our university, the DNP curriculum was oriented toward the need for a clinical practice doctorate that broadened knowledge and skills in population health, ethics of care, nursing's role and participation in policy formulation, database searching, research critique, and quality outcomes in healthcare. The courses in the curriculum fostered clinical practice knowledge and leadership skills. However, the financial and personal costs of the degree continued to be concerns for students.

This chapter has helped me position my experiences as a dean, professor, and adjunct faculty in a historical context, the classic literature on roles, and the persistent role differentiation problem that has accompanied the label of *nurse as a professional role* in society. The authors have pointed out the achievement of the label professional while at the same time remarking on the lack of differentiation in role and salary for nurses with diploma, associate degree, and baccalaureate degree education at the entry level into the profession. These graduates, certified by state boards of nursing after passing the NCLEX-RN exam, are known as *professional* nurses. Going forward, the chapter substantiates the role problems of DNP graduates by interweaving historical references throughout.

The authors, while emphasizing the ambiguities of the professional role of the RN educated in diploma, associate degree, and baccalaureate degree programs, suggest that nurses earning a DNP are also in an ambiguous position due to a lack of role clarity. For example, those leaders who hire DNP-prepared nurses struggle because their advanced clinical skills may not have changed because of the DNP experience. Witness the writing of a post-baccalaureate nurse anesthetist graduate immediately after his DNP program who described his degree as a doctorate in nursing anesthesia, not a doctor of nursing practice.

Nevertheless, the intentions and hopes of faculty and administrators of DNP programs are that graduates augment their leadership skills for navigating healthcare delivery systems. Although nursing faculty's aspirations persist about the benefits of the degree, it is employers who need to decide if the broad education provided in DNP programs benefits healthcare institutions and patients. As yet, the perceived value of the DNP-prepared nurse to an organization is not secured. However, it is promising that research is focusing on the outcomes and career patterns of DNP graduates. More studies are needed on the outcomes of advanced practice nurses at the master's level as compared to DNP-prepared nurses.

The percentage of master's-prepared nurses who earn DNP degrees is lower than expected. Most nurse practitioners are prepared at the master's level, as noted in this chapter. In addition, the number of master of science in nursing programs has decreased marginally as some nursing schools have eliminated master's degree programs. The DNP curricular situation highlights the problem of role differentiation; the various types of post-baccalaureate nursing programs underscore it.

The concept of autonomy as a characteristic of a profession is emphasized in the chapter's historical antecedents. For example, the struggle that nursing has had when classified as having either professional or nonprofessional status provides a context for nursing's role fulfillment. The cases of public health and critical care nurses are highlighted from the perspective of skill development evoked during opportunities presented when they functioned in clinical settings. The clinical environment fostered innovative skill development outside of traditional roles.

One of the challenges of nursing as a professional role is explained by societal perceptions that nursing has less practical power compared to medicine. The chapter's argument was that the types of nursing programs at the entry and graduate levels complicated the role differentiation problem. Another situation for DNP nurses with a *clinical doctoral degree* has not been resolved, either. However, their nursing practice is not simply work or labor.

The hope of this chapter's authors is that DNP history is being written now in terms of its value to society, likely due to the relative newness of the degree. Already, some indicators suggest that DNP graduates advance in confidence and job opportunities. DNP graduates have earned respect for colleagues and successfully crossed boundaries as their nursing work has gradually been integrated into healthcare delivery systems. The research questions that follow will provide answers by demonstrating that DNP interventions effect institutional and patient outcomes.

CHAPTER THREE

The Evolution of Advanced Practice Nursing Roles

MARCIA R. GARDNER, BOBBIE POSMONTIER,
MICHAEL E. CONTI, AND DEBRA HANNA

Nursing, as a discipline, has struggled since the Florence Nightingale era to articulate the unique contribution of its practitioners to health and illness care. This tension comes in part from its own history and in part from its link with and historical dependence on other disciplines, including medicine, for certain types of scientific knowledge, practice skills, and, to a large degree, access to patients. Functional skills (e.g., physical examination) and functional knowledge (e.g., pharmacology, pathophysiology of disease, or psychology of illness) are shared with (some might say "borrowed" from) other health disciplines. Mastery of higher level biomedical and pharmacological knowledge, clinical reasoning, and clinical and/or diagnostic skills has emerged as a hallmark of advanced practice nursing as enacted by nurse practitioners (NPs), nurse anesthetists, nurse-midwives, and clinical nurse specialists (CNSs). Yet, at the same time, nursing has also labored to establish a distinctive knowledge and practice structure separate from these shared domains.

The scope of nursing in the United States has expanded, contracted, and reexpanded in concert with, and in response to, a variety of social, political, technological, and theoretical forces such as:

- The influx of poor immigrants into overcrowded tenements at the turn of the century, which culminated in Lillian Wald's creation of the Henry Street Settlement (Keeling, 2009)
- Congress's establishment of the Army and Navy Nursing Corps in the early 1900s (Keeling, 2009)
- The advent of World War I and the 1918 influenza epidemic (Buhler-Wilkerson, 2001; Wald, 1922)
- The Great Depression of the 1930s, the resultant closing of hospital nursing programs, and the movement of graduate nurses into hospitals (Keeling, 2009)
- The nursing shortage during World War II, which resulted in the Bolton Act that established funding for basic nursing education and postgraduate education for the preparation of certified nurse anesthetists, educators, and administrators (Spalding, 1943)

- The post-World War II development of the acute care hospital system (Fairman & Lynaugh, 1998)
- The Brown Report of 1948, funded by the Carnegie Foundation, which advocated the transition of nursing education from hospital-based diploma programs into colleges and universities and the recruitment of men and minorities (Donahue, 1996)
- Explosions in scientific, biomedical, and pharmaceutical knowledge, as well as related technologies (Keeling, 2009)
- President Johnson's "Great Society" legislation in 1964 enacting Medicare and Medicaid (Keeling, 2009)
- The growth of the third-party payment system in 1965 (Keeling, 2009)
- Economic pressures and expanding costs of healthcare and healthcare coverage (Keeling, 2009)
- The need to fill the "provider gap" in rural and underserved geographic areas (Keeling, 2009)
- Title VIII funding for advanced practice nursing education through the Health Resources and Services Administration (HRSA; American Nurses Association [ANA], n.d.)
- Creation of the National Center for Nursing Research in 1985 and the National Institute of Nursing Research (NINR) in 1993 (National Institute of Health [NIH], n.d.), providing greater opportunities for funded research and helping to document outcomes associated with advanced nursing practice, among other issues
- Publication of the Institute of Medicine's (IOM) "Future of Nursing" Report (IOM, 2011)
- Approval and implementation of the federal Affordable Care Act (ACA), beginning in 2010

In the midst of these social and scientific changes (and possibly in response to them), nursing leaders and innovators in the mid-20th century embraced a growing theoretical and practice focus on individuals and their experiences rather than on medical diagnoses and treatment (Fairman, 1999). This disciplinary and cognitive shift offered a means to recognize and consolidate nursing's distinctive knowledge and practice methods, to break away from a purely medicalized approach to patient care, and to situate nursing as an independent, collaborative healthcare discipline with a differentiated knowledge base, focus, skill set, and language—particularly differentiated from medicine. Such efforts led to the development, articulation, and scientific testing of conceptual models and related descriptive grand theories for the understanding of human responses to health and illness, such as Orem's Self-Care Framework, the Roy Adaptation Model, or Rogers's Science of Unitary Human Beings. Other crucial developments included elucidation of the generally accepted meta-paradigm for nursing practice, research, and theory construction: human/ person, environment, health, nursing, and synthesis and testing of midrange and other theories to guide practice (Baer, 1987; Fawcett & Alligood, 2005; Phillips, 1996). These efforts were integral to and important in the examination and expansion of nursing's knowledge and practice structures, including its taxonomy, processes, strategies for knowledge generation, scope of practice, and practice strategies (Blegen & Tripp-Reimer, 1997; Fawcett & Alligood, 2005; Moorhead et al.,1998; Roy, 2007). Knowledge and clinical practice set the stage for the more recent evolution and revolution in nursing advanced practice roles and scope of practice. The four advanced practice nursing roles addressed subsequently include nurse-midwife, nurse anesthetist, NP, and CNS, all of whom contributed via their own unique histories to shaping advanced practice nursing in the 21st century. We have provided a longer analysis of nurse-midwifery, as its emergence as an advanced practice role is often minimized in the broader nursing literature.

DEVELOPMENT OF THE NURSE-MIDWIFE ROLE

Although records of midwifery practice date back to 370–460 BCE at the time of Hippocrates, it was the midwives of the 18th and 19th centuries who shaped the evolution of nurse-midwives in the 21st century in the United States (McCool & Simeone, 2002). Midwifery skills among colonial midwives ranged from those formally trained in Europe to those of illiterate women who became midwives in response to community needs. In addition to assisting with childbirth, bathing women after childbirth, and cooking, most midwives also provided primary care to their communities. When the first boat of African slaves arrived from West Africa, the first granny midwives began to practice midwifery on plantations in the rural south for both White and Black women, which was based on West African tribal folklore (Graninger, 1996; Morrison & Fee, 2010). The safety and skill of midwives varied widely during the first 250 years in America because there were no educational standards. Although some were well educated, others relied on herbs and poultices (Manocchio, 2008). Most midwives were either self-taught or learned through apprenticeship from others.

Dr. William Shippen, a protégé of Dr. William Smellie in England, established the first formal educational program for midwives in Philadelphia in 1765 (Rooks, 1997). Because illiterate women could not qualify for or afford private education, and midwifery was considered beneath the stature of educated women, Dr. Shippen limited the education to men. By the end of the 18th century, colonial men traveled to England for medical training, and returned to provide obstetric care to upper-class women. Morally outraged by men providing care for women, Dr. Samuel Gregory, a graduate of Yale University, established the first formal midwifery education program for women at the Boston Female Medical College in 1848 (Rooks, 1997). The 3-month midwifery program graduated 12 midwives between 1848 and 1851 but was forced to close in 1874 due to strong opposition from the Boston Medical Society (Rooks, 1997). By the late 19th century, there had been massive immigration into the United States from southern and eastern Europe (Dawley, 2003). New immigrants were densely packed into urban areas and suffered poor working conditions, long hours in factories, and overcrowding in tenements (Keeling, 2009). High maternal-infant mortality was blamed on granny and immigrant midwives, who managed 50% of all U.S. births. Public health nursing leaders, including Carolyn Conant van Blarcom, who wrote the first obstetric nursing textbook; Lillian Wald, the founder of the Henry Street Settlement in New York City; Mary Beard, who developed prenatal care; and Mary Breckinridge, who founded the first midwifery service in America, joined with obstetricians to eliminate lay midwives in the United States (Dawley, 2005; Stone, 2000). These nursing leaders sought to combine public health nursing and midwifery to create the nurse-midwife. Dr. Fred Taussig, a Missouri physician, is credited with coining the term nurse-midwife in 1925 (Stone, 2000).

The 1920s were framed by several pivotal events, including that:

- Middle- and upper-class women embraced "twilight sleep" (a combination of morphine and scopolamine for childbirth analgesia and amnesia to decrease and forget labor pain)
- Physicians gained higher esteem (because upper- and middle-class women chose them for labor and pain management)

- Physicians became more organized politically
- Increased use of intervention methods (forceps, episiotomies, scopolamine, and morphine) was recommended for all women by obstetrician Joseph Delee (McCool & Simeone, 2002)

Despite the findings in several New York- and New Jersey-based studies, and the 1925 White House Conference on Child Health and Protection, that midwives had much better maternal-infant outcomes than obstetricians, middle- and upper-class women felt that the use of midwives should be reserved only for poor women who could not afford the prestigious care of an obstetrician (Keeling, 2009; Rooks, 1997).

The Bellevue School of Midwifery opened in 1911 to train lay midwives but was forced to close in 1935 by the New York City Commissioner of Hospitals because he considered midwifery superfluous in the current social climate as well as below current medical standards (Varney et al., 2004). In 1923, the Maternity Center Association's (MCA) Hazel Corbin, RN, and obstetrician Ralph Lobenstine, MD, sought to open a nurse-midwifery educational program in conjunction with Bellevue Hospital in New York City, but they were thwarted by the New York City commissioner, who worried that well-educated nurse-midwives would be harder to eliminate than lay midwives (Dawley, 2003; Dawley & Burst, 2005).

In 1921, Mary Breckinridge conducted a maternal-child needs assessment and lay midwifery survey in Leslie County, Kentucky, while she was studying public health nursing at Columbia University Teachers College (Dawley, 2005; Dawley & Burst, 2005). When Corbin and Lobenstin's nurse-midwifery education program failed to open in New York, Mary Breckinridge's friend and colleague Carolyn Conant van Blarcom assisted her with enrolling in an English midwifery school. After her graduation in 1925, Breckinridge returned to Hyden, Kentucky, to establish the Frontier Nursing Service (FNS). With the help of Louis Dublin, a statistician from Metropolitan Life Insurance, Breckinridge compiled statistics that showed positive outcomes among the first 10,000 births assisted by midwives and public health nurses from the FNS (Dawley, 2003; Raisler & Kennedy, 2005).

In 1923, the Preston Retreat Hospital added a midwifery course, which continued to operate despite dwindling enrollment until 1960 (Varney et al., 2004). In 1927, the FNS and MCA joined forces to draft plans for developing a nurse-midwifery educational program and to examine state laws governing midwifery practice. By 1931, the MCA opened its own home-birth service (Lobenstin Midwifery Clinic), and by 1932, it opened an educational program, the Lobenstine Midwifery School (Burst & Thompson, 2003; Dawley & Burst, 2005; Stone, 2000).

By the late 1930s, after the introduction of penicillin and sulfonamides, improved nutrition, improved sanitation, and improved housing, the maternal death rate had dropped dramatically for all women in the United States (Rooks, 1997). Changes in the U.S. healthcare system then influenced midwifery education after World War II (Dawley, 2003). In 1943, the federal government established the Emergency Maternity and Infant Care Program for the wives and children of returning servicemen who could not otherwise afford a hospital birth. In addition, the Hill-Burton Act of 1946 provided funding for the construction of hospitals. Although 9% of all U.S. citizens had health insurance in 1940, by 1950, the percentage had increased to 50%. However, despite more widespread health insurance coverage, there was a shortage of obstetricians providing hospital maternity services. In response to the shortage, there was an accelerated increase in midwifery programs from 1940 to 1950. The Medical Mission Sisters of Philadelphia designed and developed a midwifery service and educational program (Catholic Maternity Institute) in New Mexico (Barger, 2005; Dawley, 2005).

Once established, the New Mexico program provided partial funding for the education of black nurse-midwives in Tuskegee, Alabama (1941), as well as in the Flint Goodrich Hospital Nurse Midwifery Program (1942) in New Orleans. Racial tensions, however, eventually resulted in the closing of the programs in 1946 (Burst & Thompson, 2003). By 1947, the Medical Mission Sisters of Philadelphia had established the first master's in nursing program for nurse-midwives at the Catholic University of America to respond to the needs of underserved families in Washington, DC.

Despite the innovations in natural childbirth methods based on Dr. Grantly Dick Read's work developed after World War II and the increasing public dislike of "twilight sleep," 88% of women chose to deliver in hospitals (Rooks, 1997). During the 1950s, 25 university affiliated hospitals offered graduate nursing programs for maternal-child nursing to provide leaders in teaching, education, and public health. Their socialization was different from that of the nurse-midwife because they were taught to follow physician standing orders, recognize abnormal labor, and call the physician to the labor room when delivery was imminent. Midwifery was never part of these nursing programs.

In the meantime, the MCA recommended moving midwifery education into recognized universities and formulating standard admission requirements and curriculums (Burst & Thompson, 2003; Rooks, 1997). In 1955, Columbia University opened the first graduate nurse-midwifery education program with clinical training in an academic medical center. Yale University opened its own program in 1956. By 1958, three of six national midwifery education programs offered a master's degree for nurse-midwives.

In 1954, 20 nurse-midwives attended the ANA convention and formed the Committee on Organization because the National League for Nursing (NLN) and ANA would not create a special niche for nurse-midwives (Rooks, 1997). In May 1955, the Committee on Organization voted to form the American College of Nurse-Midwives (ACNM) as a separate accrediting body to develop and evaluate nurse-midwifery standards, improve nurse-midwifery education, sponsor nurse-midwifery research, and participate in the International Confederation of Midwives (Burst & Thompson, 2003).

The social changes of the 1960s were marked by counterculture activities, rejection of authority, and the enactment of Medicare and Medicaid by President Lyndon Johnson (Keeling, 2009). After Senator Robert Kennedy visited the Mississippi Delta in 1965, federal funding was established for the County Health Improvement Program for Holmes County, Mississippi, starting in 1969. In addition, the Federal Division of Nursing provided funding for nurse-midwifery education in the Department of Obstetrics and Gynecology at the University of Mississippi School of Medicine. As the requirements for admission initially included a bachelor's degree in nursing, most nurses in Mississippi could not participate. In response, the requirements were revised to allow nondegreed nurses to obtain a certificate in midwifery (Keeling, 2009).

During the 1970s, the number of infants delivered by nurse-midwives doubled, there was a shortage of physicians providing obstetric care to the poor, and the concept of using a nurse-midwife for birth moved into the middle class (McCool & Simeone, 2002). Nurse-midwifery educational programs increased from seven in 1960 to 19 in 1979, and nurse-midwifery became legal in most states. The National Health Service Corps began to offer scholarships to nurse-midwife students willing to work in underserved areas after graduation. In 1973, in response to the increased births and the shortage of physicians, the University of Mississippi began a modular curriculum for nurse-midwifery students based on self-mastery learning that could be completed in less time than traditional education. The modular program included a list of objectives for the entry-level nurse-midwife, learning materials in self-contained packages, independent and self-paced learning, and self-assessment measures by which students could decide if they were ready for testing. By 1979, the ACNM had established core competencies in nurse-midwifery, which specified the body of knowledge, skills, and behaviors expected of nurse-midwife graduates (Avery, 2005). The core competencies served as a guide for formulating curricula, accrediting nurse-midwifery programs, and setting the standards for the national certification exam.

As the three branches of military service in the United States had difficulty recruiting and retaining obstetricians, the Air Force started its own nurse-midwifery program at Andrews Air Force Base in Maryland in 1973 (Rooks, 1997). The ACNM, however, would not accredit its program. The Air Force affiliated with Georgetown University in 1975 and offered its base as a clinical site. The Army formed its own graduate nurse-midwife program in 1974 in affiliation with the University of Kentucky and offered Fort Knox as the clinical site. The Navy chose to send its personnel to already-established nurse-midwifery programs (Rooks, 1997).

By the 1980s, there were 21 accredited nurse-midwife educational programs ranging from 9- to 18-month certificate programs to two to three master's-level programs (Burst & Thompson, 2003). In 1980, the Education Program Association opened the first distance learning program for family NPs and physician assistants desiring to practice midwifery in publicly funded clinics in California. This innovation allowed students to continue to live in their own communities while rapidly completing the requirements for graduation. By 1989, the FNS had established its own distance learning program by establishing the Community-Based Nurse Midwifery Program (CNEP) to increase rural access to nurse-midwifery education. The CNEP is affiliated with the Francis Payne Bolton School of Nursing at Case Western Reserve University to offer a master's degree in nursing (Burst & Thompson, 2003).

Although the number of midwifery programs increased to 28 by 1984, enrollment dropped between 1984 and 1986, largely as a result of the malpractice crisis (Burst & Thompson, 2003; Rooks, 1997). By 1988, however, the Robert Wood Johnson Foundation had provided a grant for scholarships to educate and recruit nurse-midwifery students to work in West Virginia after graduation (Burst & Thompson, 2003). The program increased the number of nurse-midwives in West Virginia from four in 1989 to 20 in 1992. Between 1991 and 1993, federal financial support provided nurse-midwifery education in exchange for working in underserved areas. In 1991, the ACNM task force also identified barriers for nurse-midwives and established the goal of 10,000 practicing nurse-midwives by 2001. In response to a 50% decrease in practicing obstetricians and a 20% increase in births, the Florida Midwifery Resource Center established a call to action in 1993 to educate 600 additional nurse-midwives by the year 2000. By 1993, 67% to 70% of nurse-midwives were master's prepared, and 4% to 5% were doctorally prepared (Burst & Thompson, 2003; Rooks, 1997).

Between 1982 and 1997, the ACNM Division of Accreditation (now the Accreditation Commission for Midwifery Education [ACME]) only provided accreditation for nurse-midwifery programs. In 1997, however, the ACNM Division of Accreditation recognized the certified (direct entry) midwife (CM) credential. The CM was developed to provide a pathway to midwifery for those without a nursing degree. (Jefferson et al., 2021). There are only two direct-entry midwifery programs recognized by the ACNM, including the Midwifery Institute at Philadelphia University in Philadelphia, Pennsylvania, and the State University of New York (SUNY) Downstate Medical Center Midwifery Education Program in Brooklyn, New York. Graduates of these programs must meet the core competencies and may sit for the national certification exam, but only eight states and the District of Columbia currently license CMs (American College of Nurse Midwives, 2020). In 2010, the ACNM issued a position statement (Mandatory Degree Requirements for Entry into Midwifery Practice) stating that a graduate degree (minimum master's degree) is required for entry into clinical practice for both nurse-midwife and direct-entry midwifery students. The Doctor of Nursing Practice (DNP) degree, however, is not a requirement for entry into clinical practice. Nurse-midwives and certified midwives educated before 2010 without a graduate degree are permitted to retain licensure to practice. While not accredited by the Commission for Midwifery Education, Thomas Jefferson University launched the first ever Doctor of Midwifery program in 2017 that aligns with competencies outlined in the American College of Nurse-Midwives Practice Doctorate in Midwifery and is fully accredited by the Middle States Commission on Higher Education to provide professional doctoral degrees.

Certified professional midwives (CPMs) are also direct entry midwives, but they are mostly trained in the apprenticeship model (63.1%) and are certified by the North American Registry of Midwives (Jefferson et al., 2021). There are currently nine CPM educational programs in the United States that are accredited by the Midwifery Education Accreditation Council. As of 2020, there were 3,963 CPMs who were licensed in 34 states (NARM, 2020; Jefferson et al., 2021). The most recent statistics from 2017 show that CPMs attended approximately 31,000 births in the United States (MacDorman & Declercq, 2019).

In contrast, as of 2019, there were 12,218 CNMs and 102 CMs who attended 372,991 births in the United States and 38 accredited graduate CNM programs (American College of Nurse Midwives, 2019). Midwives currently practice in a variety of settings, including homes, hospitals, birth centers, and clinics. In a recent educational advance in nurse-midwifery education, Jefferson University in Philadelphia has founded the first professional doctorate in nurse-midwifery degree (DM).

■ DEVELOPMENT OF THE NURSE ANESTHETIST ROLE

The roots of the certified registered nurse anesthetist (CRNA) emerged during the American Civil War (1861–1865), when surgeons needed the assistance of Catholic sisters and Lutheran deaconesses trained as nurses to administer chloroform to wounded soldiers during surgery (Wall, 2005). Ten years after the Civil War, Dr. William Mayo of St. Mary's Hospital in Rochester, Minnesota, recognized the value of training nurse anesthetists because, unlike medical students who watched the surgery while administering anesthesia, nurses observed the patient, which resulted in reduced mortality rates (Keeling, 2007). In 1889, Dr. Mayo trained and hired nurses Edith Granham and Alice Magaw to serve as his anesthetists. By 1913, his 6-month program included theoretical education and clinical practice.

Despite the success of the Mayo Clinic training program for nurse anesthetists, other physicians began to question the authority of nurses to administer anesthesia (Keeling, 2009). Both the New York State Medical Society and the Ohio State Medical Board tried unsuccessfully to bar nurse anesthetists from practicing medicine without a license. In *Frank v. South* (1917), a landmark case, the Kentucky appellate court ruled in favor of nurse anesthetist Margaret Hatfield, stating that she was not practicing medicine because she was under the supervision of and subordinate to licensed physician Dr. Louis Frank. Later, in 1934, the Dagmar Nelson case established the precedent of nurse anesthesia practice at the California Supreme Court, stating that Neslon was practicing nursing and not medicine, as alleged by Dr. William Vane Chalmer-Francis, a California physician (Ray & Desai, 2016). During World War I, Mayo physicians and Dr. George W. Crile of the Lakeside Hospital anesthesia program in Cleveland, Ohio, advocated for nurse anesthetists to provide pain relief to wounded soldiers (Keeling, 2009). In addition, nurse anesthetist Agatha Hodgins and Dr. George Crile developed novel anesthetic techniques, including the use of nitrous oxide-oxygen combinations and scopolamine and morphine as anesthetic adjuncts.

As medicine laid claim to the specialty of anesthesiology during World War II due to scientific advances, shortages of anesthesiologists on the battlefield necessitated the training of nurse anesthetists (Keeling, 2009). In 1945, certification became a practice requirement for CRNAs (National Board of Certification and Recertification of Nurse Anesthetists, 2010). The Korean War provided yet another opportunity for the expansion of the profession. By the early 1960s, the army had established nurse anesthesia programs at Walter Reed Hospital and Letterman General Hospital. Although the number of nurse anesthesia programs decreased during the 1970s due to decreased funding, a lack of affiliation with universities, and physician opposition, by 1998, nurse anesthesia educational programs were offered at the master's level (Diers, 1991; Keeling, 2009).

Anesthesia delivery in the United States is currently accomplished by four main methods: anesthesiologists working as the sole provider, an anesthesia care team (ACT), independent CRNAs, and a variation of the ACT model where an anesthesiologist assistant works under direct supervision of the physician anesthesiologist in a one-to-one or one-to-two provider ratio. The ACT, where a physician anesthesiologist may supervise or medically direct one to four CRNAs, is the most common form of delivery. CRNAs work independently, mostly in rural areas, where they deliver approximately 70% of anesthetics in rural hospitals, and 37% of CRNAs practice in towns with fewer than 50,000 residents (Fallacaro et al., 1996; Seibert et al., 2004).

Nationally, 24 states and the Territory of Guam have enacted the "opt out," where physician anesthesiologist supervision is no longer required for Medicare and Medicaid patients (American Society of Anesthesiologists, 2023). This was intended to increase access to care for those patients who resided in primarily rural areas (Wright & Bolt, 2023). For opt-out legislation to be enacted, the Centers for Medicare and Medicaid Services (CMS) require the governor to write a letter of support delineating the following variables:

1. This policy is in the best interest of that state's constituents
2. They have consulted with the state boards of nursing and medicine
3. The law is consistent with state policy, whereas CRNAs can legally deliver anesthesia care independent of physician supervision or oversight (Feyereisen et al., 2020)

According to AANA data from 2021, about 40% of CRNAs worked for hospitals, 26% for physician anesthesia groups, 17% were independent contractors, 4% were in the military, including the Veterans Administration (VA), and 4% were the owners or partners of anesthesia groups, including ketamine clinics (AANA, 2020). The majority of CRNAs (92%) are directly engaged in clinical practice, and the remaining 8% are engaged in education or departmental/hospital administration (AANA, 2020). Military CRNAs have had a distinguished history of autonomous practice. On Navy ships, smaller military and VA hospitals, and on the battlefield, they have and continue to practice without anesthesiologist supervision as the sole provider to the U.S. military (Jenkins et al., 2006).

The current scope of practice, according to the practice guidelines, published by the AANA, includes:

- Preoperative assessment
- Development and implementation of an anesthetic plan
- Obtaining informed consent

- Anesthesia delivery (sedation, general anesthesia, regional, and neuraxial anesthesia)
- Selection and implementation of noninvasive and invasive monitoring (arterial lines, pulmonary artery [PA] catheters, central lines, and transesophageal echo [TEE])
- Airway management (natural airway, endotracheal intubations, laryngeal mask airway [LMA] placement and implementation of alternative airway techniques, fiber-optic intubations [FOI], needle cricothyrotomy)
- Facilitation of emergence from anesthesia; transfer to the postanesthesia care unit (PACU); and PACU management
- Conducting a postanesthesia evaluation.
- Chronic and acute pain management, including interventional pain management
- The ability to function as a member of emergency response teams (providing cardiopulmonary support)
- Ordering, evaluating, and interpreting diagnostic and point of care (POC) testing
- Use and supervision of the use of fluoroscopy and ultrasound for diagnosis and care delivery (AANA, 2020)

Nursing boards and the facilities where CRNAs practice determine the scope of practice for CRNAs in accordance with their bylaws.

Nurse anesthesia has, since its inception, had to continuously and diligently prove its important contribution to the delivery of anesthetic care within the matrix of the U.S. healthcare system. Two important studies examined the effect of the anesthesia provider on mortality rates (Canadian Coordinating Office for Health Technology Assessment, 2004). First, Pine et al. (2003) examined risk-adjusted mortality rates for the following provider models: anesthesiologists as sole providers, CRNAs as sole providers, and the ACT model. Medicare patients undergoing eight surgical procedures were the focus of the study. Results indicate that there was no statistically significant difference between provider types. Similar results were found among the sole CRNA provider, anesthesiologists, and ACT personnel (Pine et al., 2003), meaning anesthesia care outcomes were equivalent regardless of provider type. Second, Jordan et al. (2001) found no statistical difference in adverse outcomes between type of provider and preoperative physical status, patient age, surgical procedure, or method of anesthesia in a study that reviewed 223 closed claims studies from 1989 to 1997. In 2010, Dulisse and Cromwell's retrospective study of Medicare data from 1999 to 2005 reported no adverse outcomes when CRNAs are not supervised by a physician. This study, published in *Health Affairs*, was important in that it was not biased, and the authors recommended that the Centers for Medicare and Medicaid Services allow CRNAs to practice without physician supervision in every state. Although only two studies have been cited, it is important to note that CRNAs, who now almost universally have a master's degree and by 2022 will have a practice doctorate, DNP, or doctor of nurse anesthesia practice (DNAP), have a long history of providing quality, cost-effective patient care with positive patient outcomes (Hoyem et al., 2019).

Development of the NP Role

The NP's role has been prominent in terms of controversies, visibility in public and social policy, and scope of practice considerations, particularly concerning the role's uniqueness and overlap with medical practice. The history of the NP movement can be seen as another exemplar the development of advanced practice nursing. NP practice moved beyond the range of extended healthcare services, including education, direct care, chronic illness management, and community services, that public health nurses had been providing since the 1920s. Formal NP practice was "birthed" in 1965 through the joining of primary care pediatrics and public health/family-community nursing. This was the vision of Dr. Henry Silver, a pediatrician associated with the University of Colorado School of Medicine, and Dr. Loretta Ford from the University of Colorado School of Nursing. The NP role emerged at a time when pediatric medicine was struggling to extend care to underserved populations due to a shortage of healthcare professionals. At the same time, nursing was also struggling to expand its scope beyond hospital care to develop autonomous practice, fully embed nursing education in higher education, and professionalize as a workforce (Bullough, 1976; Ford, 1975; Richmond, 1965).

The new breed of pediatric care providers in the original University of Colorado program were baccalaureate-prepared clinicians with: (a) advanced clinical and diagnostic skills and knowledge; (b) the ability to monitor child health, growth, and development; and (c) the ability to provide guidance to families, manage minor acute health problems in pediatric primary care, and function within healthcare teams—particularly for medically underserved populations. The program involved four months of university-based education, followed by clinical training in underserved rural community/primary care pediatric settings. Dr. Ford subsequently argued strongly for embedding NP education fully within a graduate nursing education framework; both Ford and Silver were instrumental in communicating the effectiveness of this pediatric NP model and in ensuring its replication (Ford, 1975; Mason et al., 2000; Silver et al., 1968).

A comparable pediatric NP program for the care of children from underserved urban families developed soon after at the Massachusetts General Hospital in Boston. In addition, other academic medical care settings also developed NP programs that would similarly extend the skills of public health nurses, address access to care for urban underserved children, and serve the needs of children in underserved rural areas (Murphy, 1990).

In the following decade, NP certificate training programs began to proliferate across the country. Most of these had a particular emphasis on pediatrics and/or family health and on extending primary care to underserved urban and rural children and families in a time of expanding healthcare needs and growing recognition of disparities in access to care (Davidson et al., 1975; Mason et al., 2000). Most required a short-term commitment (less than 1 year), and not all required a bachelor's degree for entry (Mason et al., 2000). The scope of NP practice expanded to include family planning and women's health within 10 years after Ford and Silver's innovation (Lewis, 2000) and continues to expand in response to current healthcare needs nationally and globally.

Federal funding through Title VIII of the Nurse Training Act (American Association of Colleges of Nursing, 2009) provided opportunities for the expansion of NP use in family-focused primary care, in women's health, and then in other populations. In addition, regional programs funded by the federal Title X family planning initiative prepared NPs, therefore significantly expanding the NP workforce in women's health (Bednash et al., 2009; Manisoff, 1981). By 1978, the IOM had taken the stand that state regulations should be revised to accommodate an increased scope of practice and prescription authority for NPs, albeit under physician supervision (Mason et al., 2000). As the advanced nursing role began to fully take hold, university-based schools of nursing began to integrate NP education and training at the graduate level. Title VIII funding was essential in supporting nurses' completion of these programs (AACN, 2009), thus expanding the advanced practice nursing workforce. The scope of practice expanded beyond family and pediatric foci, and beyond primary care to include adult health as well as highly specialized and/or system-focused practice (e.g., oncology, cardiology, and psychiatric specialties).

Coincidentally, a variety of forces created opportunities for the expansion of the NP role. There were regulatory changes for medical education, including pass-through funding adjustments and state-level regulatory restrictions for physician residency training (hours permitted on duty). There was also a growing body of evidence supporting the cost and treatment outcome effectiveness of NPs, as well as a growing and better educated NP workforce. Along with other forces, these recognized improvements created opportunities for greater inclusion of NP scope and practice into high-acuity patient care. As fewer physician residents were able/available to provide acute patient care coverage, additional opportunities for NP employment developed (American Academy of Pediatrics Committee on Hospital Care, 1999; American Academy of Pediatrics Committee on Pediatric Workforce, 2013). Adult, pediatric, and neonatal acute care NP education was introduced and solidified as nurse clinicians were poised to fill gaps in the acute care system (Hinch et al., 2005). In the 1990s, the National Council of State Boards of Nursing (NCSBN); American Academy of Nurse Practitioners Certification Board; the American Nurses Credentialing Center; the National Certification Board for Pediatric Nurse Practitioners and Nurses, now the Pediatric Nursing Certification Board (PNCB); and the National Certification Corporation (NCC) began to jointly consider a cohesive approach to the regulation of NP practice (NCSBN, 1998). In 2018, the National Organization of Nurse Practitioner Faculties (NONPF) established its definitive policy statement, committing to the DNP as the entry-level credential for NP practice (NONPF, 2018). At this time, NP preparation continues to reside mostly at the master's level. However, there is increasing movement in colleges and universities toward the BS to DNP pathway for entry into advanced practice registered nurse (APRN) practice (Idzik et al., 2021). In alignment with the American Association of Colleges of Nursing's approval of *The Essentials: Core Competencies for Professional Nursing* (2021), which established a new model of professional nursing education at entry-level practice and advanced levels, NONPF developed a set of revised, detailed *NP Role Core Competencies* in 2022. The document establishes specific shared competencies and subcompetenciesas outcomes of nurse practitioner education and specifically indicates that these core outcomes will be evaluated at the "clinical doctoral level" (NONPF, 2022).

The NP movement, particularly in its overlap with medicine's functions, created and continues to create controversies both within and outside of its own discipline. The IOM's landmark report, *The Future of Nursing: Leading Change, Advancing Health* (IOM, 2011), called for nurses to practice to the full scope of their skills and the full extent of their education as equal partners in both designing and providing healthcare services. Great strides have been made toward this goal. According to Stanley (2012), the consensus model for APRN regulation demonstrated the evolving leadership roles that advanced practice nurses (APNs) must have in the redesign of the U.S. healthcare system. In 2016, the U.S. Department of Veterans Affairs (VA) amended its regulations to provide for full practice authority for NPs, CNS, and CNMs, although not for CRNAs (U.S. Department of Veterans Affairs, 2016). By 2022, 26 states plus the District of Columbia had a version of independent practice authority by statute and/or regulation (AANP, 2022). NPs continue to press for legislative initiatives promoting full practice authority on the federal and local levels. Educational preparation, qualifications for practice, role functions, and differentiation from other providers (e.g., physicians, physician assistants, and CNSs) are among the areas continuing to need clarification for legislation, regulation, and reimbursement. NP practice has expanded beyond health profession shortage areas into the mainstream of primary and acute care. Furthermore, NP clinicians, through their lobbying efforts, have made inroads in reimbursement for the provision of healthcare services, such as the formal ability to order durable medical equipment for their patients, the inclusion of NPs in the first year of the Merit-Based Incentive Payment System (MIPS), and ensuring that NP-led patient-centered medical homes are eligible to receive incentive payments for the management of patients with chronic disease, all part of the sustainable growth rate repeal for Medicare Part B. The American Medical Association (AMA), American College of Physicians, and the American Academy of Pediatrics (AAP), among others, have periodically attempted to limit NP scope of practice, particularly related to autonomous practice, through lobbying efforts as well as the creation of policies and standards for physician supervision of nonphysician providers (AMA, n.d.; Buppert, 2005; Hedger, 2009). The Federal Trade Commission (FTC), in a landmark report, Policy Perspectives: Competition and Regulation of Advanced Practice Nurses (2014), encouraged state legislatures to look closely at state regulations for NP practice and notes that

> Mandatory physician supervision and collaborative practice agreement requirements are likely to impede competition among health care providers and restrict APRNs' ability to practice independently, leading to decreased access to health care services, higher health care costs, reduced quality of care, and less innovation in health care delivery. (FTC, 2014, p. 38)

According to the FTC report, APRNs provide safe and effective care within the scope of their training, certification, and licensure. The report notes that, in addition, significant shortages of primary care practitioners can be alleviated by reducing undue regulatory burdens.

DEVELOPMENT OF THE CNS ROLE

Development, Evolution, and Renewal of the Clinical Nurse Specialist (1900–2020s)

Like the other three categories of advanced practice nurses, clinical nurse specialists (CNSs) are in an elite group. CNSs are experts in their clinical specialty who hold either a graduate or a doctoral degree and are nationally certified in their specialty. In most states, their licenses reflect clinical nurse specialists' advanced practice status. The National Association of Clinical Nurse Specialists (NACNS) lists 44 competencies of CNSs in three spheres of impact: direct patient care, nurses and nursing, and organizational/systems (NACNS, 2019). This recent model of CNS practice differs from the original 1986 American Nurses Association *Role of the Clinical Nurse Specialist* document, which defined the scope and standards of practice for CNSs with five subroles. Yet the new model does not eliminate those subroles—it builds upon them. Recent depictions of CNS practice show the breadth, depth, and creativity that experienced clinical nurse specialists contribute to today's healthcare system.

Many agencies expect clinical nurse specialists to act as clinical educators, clinical consultants, evidence-based practice researchers, and engage in administrative duties to monitor and consistently improve patient care quality and safety. Yes—clinical nurse specialists are capable of all that and more. Clinical nurse specialists guide healthcare teams to solve complex patient problems. They nurture, guide, and develop nursing staff. Most of all, clinical nurse specialists work within organizational systems as collaborative, savvy leaders capable of leading systemwide changes that result in cost-effective, high-quality patient care.

In September 2022, the president of the NACNS told members there are 88,000 working clinical nurse specialists in the United States. So why is the public largely unaware of this advanced practice role? The short answer is that nearly 80% of working CNSs were downsized from the U.S. national healthcare system between 1990 and 1995, thus CNSs were sparsely present for three decades. The rebirth of clinical nurse specialists in the U.S. healthcare system is the result of several forces. To get to the heart of the story, it's important to start from the beginning.

Historical Evolution of the Clinical Nurse Specialist Role

Katherine DeWitt (1900) wrote about specialist nurses—a trend she had observed and that she thought would continue—in the first issue of the *American Journal of Nursing*. By 1900, professional nurses worked in specialized areas such as anesthesia, obstetrics, pediatrics, and public health. And yet, in 1900, the professionalization of nursing was still in flux. Licensure, which was discussed as one way to protect the public from unsafe, uneducated, self-proclaimed nurses, was still a goal that would take nearly 30 more years to achieve in some states. Combining specialization with ideas of an "expanded" or "advanced" scope of nursing practice came later, decades after licensure for minimum safe professional nursing practice was achieved.

Nurse scholar and theorist Dr. Hildegard Peplau (1909–1999) envisioned and advocated for the clinical nurse specialist role. In the late 1940s, Peplau taught her ideas about advanced nursing practice to graduate students studying psychiatric nursing at Columbia University. In the mid-1950s, Peplau started the first graduate program for psychiatric clinical nurse specialists at Rutgers University in New Jersey. Over time, Peplau's grasp of what clinical nurse specialists could contribute to healthcare deepened. In 1965, Peplau wrote an article called "Specialization in Professional Nursing" in a journal edited by Martha Rogers, *Nursing Science*. That article, which established her deep grasp of specialization, was reprinted in full in *Clinical Nurse Specialist* in 2003.

During the 1960s and 1970s, advances in diagnostic and monitoring technology, pharmaceutical agents, and ventilatory support helped critical care emerge as a new healthcare specialty for cardiac, neurological, pediatric, and other patient populations. As new specialties arose, specialty-based professional organizations began to meet specialist nurses' professional needs. Specialization raised questions about the nature, scope, and standards of general nursing practice and about specialist nursing. In 1979–1980, Peplau came out of retirement to work with an ANA task force charged with defining the nature and scope of nursing practice and specialization in nursing. That work led to the ANA's 1980 Social Policy Statement (SPS).

CNS Role Formally Delineated, but Controversy Ensues (1980–1990)

According to the Social Policy Statement (1980), nurses who pursued specialization did so by becoming experts in their clinical specialty, first through "intense personal studies," and then by obtaining additional formal education beyond a baccalaureate degree. Upon graduation from their master's or doctoral degrees, specialists were expected to become certified to validate mastery of their specialty-based knowledge. In 1980, a doctoral degree for nurses meant a research doctorate, usually a PhD or an EdD. The DNP practice doctorate would come two decades later.

Some scholars believe that Peplau left her mark in the original SPS in Section III. "Specialization in Nursing Practice," pages 21–29. After defining what specialization in nursing practice was and why it had occurred, the SPS document claimed that nursing specialization was "clearly established." That claim was followed by four subsections: 1) Criteria for Specialists in Nursing Practice, 2) Roles and Functions of Specialists in Nursing Practice, 3) Need for Specialists in Nursing Practice, and 4) Areas of Specialization.

An SPS draft version was circulated at the June 1980 ANA convention in Houston, Texas, so nurses could provide comments (Hobbs, 2009). The concise definition of nursing, as *"the diagnosis and treatment of human responses to actual or potential health problems"* (ANA, 1980, p. 9) led to protests mainly by nurse practitioners. According to Hobbs (2009), nurse practitioners were upset by language that placed a boundary on their role. Nurse practitioners diagnosed and treated diseases, not only symptoms of or human responses to diseases. However, the definition still left nurses with a single scope of practice for all nurses. The scope of advanced nursing practice was left undefined.

In 1980, the SPS referred only to "specialists," not specifically to clinical nurse specialists, as registered nurses who, through supervised study at the graduate level (master's or doctorate) have become experts "in the defined area of knowledge and practice in a selected clinical area of nursing" (ANA, 1980, p. 1). However, the SPS reference applied to nurse practitioners, certified nurse midwives, and certified nurse anesthetists as well. Six years after the SPS was ratified, the ANA published *The Role of the Clinical Nurse Specialist* (1986), a scope and standards document. By then, CNSs were viewed as advanced practice nurses who kept patient care quality high. In fact, the 1986 ANA document specified five functional CNS subroles: 1) expert clinician, 2) clinical educator, 3) clinical consultant, 4) clinical researcher, and 5) administrator to oversee policies, procedures, and quality of care. CNSs were experts at managing complex patient care situations, and they analyzed and changed organizational systems to improve patient care quality. Their efforts to problem-solve and tailor care for complex patients, nurture professional nurse development, undertake projects, evaluate programs, and initiate and support large organizational changes made clinical nurse specialists unique clinical nurse leaders.

An important point made in the 1986 CNS Role document was that a "clinical nurse specialist's expertise is derived from combining graduate study with clinical experience" (ANA, 1986, p. 1). Requirements to become a clinical nurse specialist included well-developed clinical expertise, an earned graduate degree, and certification in the nurse's specialty clinical area (ANA, 1986). These three elements were meant to show that the path to becoming a CNS was rigorous and trustworthy. The public could feel safe whenever a CNS intervened. Although CNS role criteria were established between 1980 and 1986, title protection for the CNS role was not yet well-established nationwide. That meant that in some states, nurses could call themselves clinical nurse specialists without having the proper education, certification, or clinical expertise. Title protection for legitimate clinical nurse specialists became a larger issue in the early 2000s.

Clinical Nurse Specialists Downsized From the U.S. Healthcare System (1990–1996)

During the 1980s, healthcare economics changed to a dramatic degree. In his 1980 inaugural address, President Ronald Reagan promised to reduce healthcare spending. Throughout the 1980s, strategies such as capitated payments by insurers, diagnostic related groups, and managed competition were used to reduce national healthcare costs. CNSs were told to reduce patients' length of hospital stay, and to have nurses "work smarter, not harder." CNSs created critical pathways and reduced the average length of hospital stays. Those efforts were not enough.

Reductions in third-party reimbursement during the late 1980s led healthcare agencies nationwide to the edge of insolvency. Mergers between small and large institutions that began in the early 1990s prompted a downsizing of the nursing workforce. First, vacant staff nurse positions were eliminated, and staff nurse workloads increased beyond reason. Job freezes were instituted. Nurses with graduate degrees who worked in leadership, management, or supervisory positions lost their jobs. By 1995, some nurse managers concurrently supervised as many as four or five units. The phrase "span of control" began to appear in nursing literature. Early 1990s downsizing decimated the clinical nurse specialist work force. According to Hamric et al. (2009), "By 1996, of the 61,601 Clinical Nurse Specialists in the United States, only 23% were practicing in CNS-specific positions (USDHHS, 1996)." That means that although 14,168 working CNSs remained, 47,433, or 77% of all CNSs, had lost their positions. CNSs were master's-prepared, nationally certified, highly experienced clinical experts whose job it was to keep patient care quality high. Removing CNSs and so many others from the nursing workforce might have saved money in the short term, but by 1998, the quality of care nationwide was quite low. Downsizing, poor staffing, work speed-ups, and other "cost-saving" strategies had led to an estimated 98,000 preventable fatal errors (Kohn et al., 2000).

In 1995, the revised Social Policy Statement addressed nurse practitioners' concerns. Specialization was redefined. Advanced practice nursing roles (clinical nurse specialist, nurse practitioner, nurse midwife, and nurse anesthetist) were discussed in general, inclusive terms so that no role overshadowed any other advanced practice role. A single scope of practice endured.

A year later, the American Association of Colleges of Nursing (AACN) released the *Essentials of Master's Education for Advanced Practice Nursing* (1996). That document specified that all advanced practice nurses must have a baccalaureate and a graduate degree with three substantive advanced practice courses in pathophysiology, physical assessment, and pharmacology, and 500 clinical practice hours in each advanced practice role. If graduate students wanted to become nurse practitioners and clinical nurse specialists, they were required to complete 500 clinical hours for each advanced practice role.

Unification of Advanced Practice Roles: The LACE Initiative (2004–2008)

When the SPS was revised in 1995, specialization was tied to four APRN roles: CNS, nurse practitioner, certified nurse midwife, and nurse anesthetist. CNS jobs had disappeared, and so few working CNSs were left in 1996. By 2000, as the number of CNS graduate programs declined due to low student enrollments, nurse practitioner programs prospered.

Mundinger and colleagues (2000) proposed the Doctor of Nursing Practice degree, originally aimed at expanding nurse practitioners' education. Their logic was that NPs needed more education to independently provide high-quality primary care. From 2000 to 2004, members discussed the DNP degree at the American Association of Colleges of Nursing (AACN) annual meetings for Deans. In 2004, AACN members approved a resolution to make the DNP practice doctorate a requirement for entry to advanced practice nursing by 2015 (Cronenwett et al., 2011). The DNP requirement and the 2003 AACN proposal for a new master's-prepared generalist role called clinical nurse leader affected CNSs directly. In 2004, when the AACN released its DNP position statement, only nurses in any of the four advanced practice nursing roles were expected to have a DNP degree by 2015, not clinical nurse leaders.

In 2004, APRN representatives from many professional specialty organizations began to engage in regular consensus building meetings. Their conversations focused on shared expectations for educational preparation for advanced practice, certification, and licensure. The committee's consensus model of advanced practice nursing became known colloquially as the "LACE initiative" (Goudreau, 2009). The acronym LACE stands for licensure, accreditation, certification, and education. Each advanced practice nurse today must obtain proper advanced practice licensure, national certification, and graduate education through accredited programs (also see the Unification of APRN Education, Regulation, and Practice section of this chapter).

Consensus model talks had been underway for 2 years when, in 2006, an APRN Task Force of the National Council of State Boards of Nursing (NCSBN) released a vision statement recommending that clinical nurse specialists no longer be considered advanced practice nurses (Goudreau, 2009). APRN leaders responded to the NCSBN's direct threat to the clinical nurse specialist role by forming a smaller "joint dialogue" group. One unsolved licensure problem in 2006 was that all registered nurses shared one scope of practice. That generalist scope did not cover advanced practice nursing. A second scope of advanced practice was developed by the joint dialogue group that could be tied to licensure (Goudreau, 2009).

Title protection for APRNs was also discussed during the LACE consensus meetings. Without title protection, nurses who were not properly credentialed could call themselves clinical nurse specialists without being able to safely fulfill the role. As of September 2022, most states and U.S. territories have title protection laws for clinical nurse specialists.

In December 2009, an NACNS task force issued a statement called *Core Practice Doctorate: Clinical Nurse Specialist Competencies*. It affirmed a practice doctorate for clinical nurse specialists and aligned DNP competencies into three spheres of influence. In 2015, NACNS members approved 2030 as the year when all CNSs will be required to have a DNP or doctoral degree (Anonymous, 2015).

The Institute of Medicine Quality of Health Care America Project (1998–2008)

The recent resurgence in the 2020s of the clinical nurse specialist role is the legacy gift that individual CNSs from the 20% who kept their jobs in 1996 gave to all of us, their future colleagues. They collaborated, negotiated, and met daunting challenges with energy and intelligence these past three decades. However, the Institute of Medicine's 10-year Quality of Health Care America project also aided in the transition from the 1990s downsizing, when the CNS role was almost extinct, to the CNS role rebirth in 2020.

By 1998, Congress had become aware of the decline in healthcare quality that had followed the nursing workforce reduction. The Institute of Medicine initiated the Quality of Health Care America project in June 1998 with the charge to improve patient care quality in the next 10 years (1998–2008; Kohn et al., 2000, p. 205). The committee's work led to several key reports: *To Err Is Human* (2000); *Crossing the Quality Chasm* (2001), *Keeping Patients Safe* (2004), and others. Those reports recommended changes to improve healthcare quality. In 2010, Congress changed healthcare financing when it passed the Affordable Care Act. With that law in place, fee-for-service reimbursement was replaced with pay-for-performance, which depends on patient satisfaction and patient care quality. If patient satisfaction is low or if patients suffer adverse events, care will not be reimbursed, and agencies can be fined.

Affordable Care Act provisions became fully effective in 2014. The need to improve patient care quality driven by the new law inspired healthcare administrators to seek out one group of advanced practice nurses with a record for consistently improving care: clinical nurse specialists. Between 2019 and 2022, the CNS work force grew from 70,000 to 88,000. Healthcare agencies are hiring clinical nurse specialists again. Students now see the clinical nurse specialist role as a viable advanced practice role. It was a long, complicated journey. CNSs helped define an APRN scope of practice, clarified their own role competencies and outcomes, and became an integral part of the U.S. healthcare system again.

UNIFICATION OF APRN EDUCATION, REGULATION, AND PRACTICE

Professional and regulatory organizations continued to move toward a cohesive approach relative to the preparation of advanced practice nurses for entry into practice and toward a unified vision of the scope of advanced practice nursing in general. Lewis (2000) notes that, in 1992, both the ANA and the NCSBN took similar positions regarding the need for advanced practice nursing education (with advanced practice nursing defined as NP, nurse anesthetist, nurse-midwife, and CNS) to be situated only at the graduate level and made an initial effort to create a regulatory model (NCSBN, 1998). As nursing professional organizations began to take similar positions regarding advanced nursing practice and advanced nursing education, the transition of certificate programs preparing advanced practice nurse clinicians to formal graduate-level programs accelerated.

In the 1990s, the AACN convened a national group representing multiple organizations and specialty stakeholders for the development of consensus guidelines for advanced practice nursing education at the graduate (master's) level: The Essentials of Master's Education for Advanced Practice Nursing (AACN, 1996). This document recognized only four types of clinicians providing direct, advanced patient care as advanced practice nurses: nurse-midwives, nurse anesthetists, NPs, and CNSs. It specified clearly that education for advanced nursing roles should occur at the master's level. The National Task Force for Quality Nurse Practitioner Education, comprised of representatives from a variety of organizations, including the AACN, the National Organization of Nurse Practitioner Faculties (NONPF), NP certifying bodies, and a variety of other stakeholder organizations, promulgated targeted educational guidelines for NP preparation. The NONPF established a set of specialty-specific educational guidelines outlining competencies for NP education in both general and specialty areas of practice (NONPF, 2002, 2003, 2004, 2022). In 2008, the National Task Force produced the consensus document, Criteria for Evaluation of Nurse Practitioner Programs. Nurse anesthetist, nurse-midwife, and CNS education are, in addition, more specifically guided by the respective specialty accrediting organizations. Educational "landmarks" are critical, because they demonstrate the evolution of a cohesive view of advanced nursing practice on the part of those involved in preparing advanced clinicians for practice.

CONSENSUS MODEL AND LACE

Advanced practice nursing has continued to grow toward a unified licensure and practice model through the collaboration of a variety of advanced practice nursing stakeholder organizations, including the NCSBN, the APRN Consensus Workgroup, and representatives from multiple professional nursing organizations, building on a framework established in the 1990s. The Consensus Model for Advanced Practice Registered Nurses (APRN Consensus Workgroup and NCBSN APRN Advisory Committee, 2008), created through this collaboration, prescribed the regulatory strategy for APRNs, identified the same four direct care providers as APRNs, and specified that other nurses prepared at the graduate level, whose scope is not direct care, do not fall under the definition of the APRN as stated in the model. A proposed timeline for implementation of the model has been developed; as it is implemented and state regulations are amended, the title "advanced practice registered nurse" will be restricted. The model specifies that APRNs are licensed and practice in one of the following clinical roles: certified nurse practitioner (CNP), certified nurse-midwife (CNM), certified nurse anesthetist, or certified CNS. Education for practice will occur within six population foci (adult-geriatric, pediatric, neonatal, women's/gender-related health, psychiatric-mental health, or family/individual life span), with certification and licensing within the respective population focus as well. Specialization will involve an additional layer of certification, via professional organizations, beyond the population focus (e.g., adult-gerontology population focus, specialty of oncology; APRN Consensus Workgroup and NCBSN APRN Advisory Committee, 2008; Partin, 2009; Stanley et al., 2009). It is important to note the definition of the CNS as an APRN with relevant licensing and regulatory expectations, because the title CNS is not currently universally restricted, nor are there license/certification requirements across all states for the CNS role.

The model gives a clear definition of advanced practice nursing and outlines recommendations for uniform regulation of APRN practice through LACE: "licensure, accreditation [of APRN educational programs], certification, and education" (APRN Consensus Workgroup and NCBSN APRN Advisory Committee, 2008, p. 7). The characteristics of APRNs as outlined in the consensus statement, are that they are clinicians:

1. Who have completed an accredited graduate-level education program preparing them for one of the four recognized APRN roles
2. Who have passed a national certification examination that measures APRN role and population-focused competencies and who maintain continued competence as evidenced by recertification in the role and population through the national certification program
3. Who have acquired advanced clinical knowledge and skills preparing them to provide direct care to patients, as well as a component of indirect care; however, the defining factor for all [sic] APRNs is that a significant component of their education and practice focuses on the direct care of individuals
4. Whose practice builds on the competencies of RNs by demonstrating a greater depth and breadth of knowledge, a greater synthesis of data, increased complexity of skills and interventions, and greater role autonomy
5. Who are educationally prepared to assume responsibility and accountability for health promotion and/or maintenance, as well as the assessment, diagnosis, and management of patient problems, which includes the use and prescription of pharmacologic and nonpharmacologic interventions
6. Who have clinical experience of sufficient depth and breadth to reflect the intended license
7. Who have obtained a license to practice as an APRN in one of the four APRN roles: CRNA, CNM, CNS, or CNP (APRN Consensus Workgroup and NCBSN APRN Advisory Committee, 2008, pp. 7–8)

UNIQUENESS OF APRN "PRACTICE"

Contemporary views of advanced nursing practice are grounded in the intersection of medical knowledge and skills with nursing's meta-paradigm and knowledge base. The unique contribution that APRNs can make in the current healthcare system can be conceptualized as emerging from a distinctive blend of biomedical and nursing perspectives, skills, and knowledge sets. One crucial challenge for contemporary and future advanced nursing practice is to fully elucidate and articulate the mechanisms by which this fusion occurs (resulting in excellent, cost-effective patient outcomes). Our discipline's appreciation of holism incorporates an understanding of persons as integrated, continually interacting with their environment, and engaged in the creation of meaning, and our disciplinary attention to the influences of life transitions and health conditions on individuals, families, and communities forms a matrix of underpinnings for advanced nursing practice. Holism, patient/client centeredness, respect for individual autonomy, respectful communication with active listening, focused preventive care, health education, and integration of services, all of which are combined with clinical knowledge and expertise, are potentially some of the essential components of APRN effectiveness that grow from the nursing meta-paradigm (Donnelly, 2003; Erikson, 2007; Neill, 1999).

Despite an evolving, but sparse, evidence base for the uniqueness of APRN practice, many of these disciplinary dimensions of practice still need to be systematically examined. For example, Charlton et al. (2008) reported the findings of their integrative review of NP communication styles. Their review suggested that NPs' patient-centered communication styles, which they termed "biopsychosocial," compared with "biomedical" styles (2008, p. 383), influenced patient satisfaction, adherence, and health indicators, and were consistent with a specialized model of APRN effectiveness based on nursing's disciplinary perspective. Dunphy and Winland-Brown (2006) proposed a model of APRN practice: The Circle of Caring, which accounts for and formalizes the overlapping multidisciplinary perspectives integrated in APRN practice from the standpoint of contextualized understanding in a scientific caring framework. Dunphy and Winland-Brown state that "caring is suggested as one way to bridge the gulf between holistic nursing theories and biomedical nursing praxis" (2006, p. 288). Table 3.1 offers other perspectives by summarizing a variety of studies that examined the influence of a nursing-disciplinary perspective as the underpinning for effective patient care by NPs. This literature continues to be somewhat sparse.

APRN PRACTICE OUTCOMES

Compelling evidence of the effectiveness of APRN-managed care has been in the literature since the 1970s (Lenz et al., 2004). Studies have looked at a variety of patient outcomes for APRN-provided care, primarily in comparison to that from doctors. Patient satisfaction with, and quality outcomes of, APRN care have been extensively studied in the United States during the past three decades, and more recently in Canada, Britain, and European countries that have adopted advanced practice/NP roles. Satisfaction with the quality of NP-provided care in primary care, emergency departments, and specialty care settings has consistently been found to be high, while researchers acknowledge that various methods, definitions, instruments, data sets, and time frames have been used in the measurement of these outcomes. However, across multiple studies and reviews, findings consistently documented the quality of, and patient satisfaction with,

TABLE 3.1 Sample of Studies Examining the Influence of Disciplinary Underpinnings on NP Practice Outcomes

Authors	Design	Related Findings
Benkert et al. (2009)	Descriptive-correlational	African American subjects with moderate cultural mistrust of European Americans; high satisfaction/moderate trust of NPs.
Benkert et al. (2002)	Descriptive	Low-income African American subjects with significantly higher trust scores for NPs vs. MDs; no significant difference in mistrust or satisfaction between providers; significant higher trust scores for clinicians in nurse-managed vs. jointly managed clinics.
Castro (2009)	Descriptive-correlational	Latina (female) subjects seen at least once by an NP clinician; all NP clinicians had cultural proficiency, competence, or awareness; no clinicians had cultural incompetence; a higher NP cultural competence score is correlated with higher patient satisfaction scores, and higher time spent with the provider is correlated with higher satisfaction.
Donohue (2003)	Descriptive, naturalistic	Middle-aged female subjects described resources expected and received from NP encounters; resources included services, information, support, time, respect, reassurance, affirmation, reinforcement, and trust.
Green and Davis (2005)	Predictive modeling	Predictors of patient satisfaction and relationships among NP demographic characteristics, components of Caring Behaviors Inventory, patient satisfaction measures, all NPs with high CBI scores, no differences between male and female; no significant relationships among CBI components and satisfaction.
Hayes (2007)	Descriptive-mixed method	Patients aged 18–86 years receiving NP care; 86% female; high satisfaction with NP communication and style of interaction; high recall of instructions; intention to adhere to treatment plan very likely; themes connected with intention to follow treatment plan: trust, expertise, and concern for one's own health.
Kinchin (2022)	Descriptive	Degree of NP incorporation of shared decision making and holistic approaches in their practice. Most common holistic strategies are listening, communication with patients, expertise, solicitation of patient input, and exploration of the effects of medical conditions on patient life.
Kotzer (2005)	Descriptive survey	Advanced practice nurses in tertiary pediatric settings: 59% in the NP role; 21% in the combined CNS/NP role. Primary job functions: education/guidance/counseling, care coordination, and direct care.
Kozlowski et al. (2015)	Pre-experimental single group pre/post	PNPs in primary care using the evidence-based COPE model decreased anxiety symptoms and improved anxiety measures in children aged 8–13 years.

(continued)

TABLE 3.1 Sample of Studies Examining the Influence of Disciplinary Underpinnings on NP Practice Outcomes (*continued*)

Authors	Design	Related Findings
O'Reilly et al. (2020)	Instrument validation	Generated psychometrics of the Patient Enablement and Satisfaction Survey for evaluation of APN care. Findings were a three-factor outcome: satisfaction, quality, and enablement.
Roots and McDonald (2014)	Descriptive, qualitative, case study	NPs added to rural Canadian fee-for-service practices; extended access and appointment times; emphasis on team approach; increased satisfaction; increased connection to community services for patients.
Sawatsky et al. (2013)	Randomized trial	NP-directed care after cardiac surgery is more likely to result in a higher rating of functional status, fewer reported symptoms, and higher satisfaction with the amount and quality of services received.
Van Leuven and Prion (2007)	Descriptive, naturalistic	Interviews of NPs for perspectives on health promotion activities in practice; health promotion viewed as implicit in the nursing role; differentiates NPs from MDs; valued by NPs; obstacles; time, patient care needs, limitations of scope of practice, patient scheduling, practice model (HMO vs. other practice).

CBI, Caring Behaviors Inventory; CNS, clinical nurse specialist; COPE, creativity, optimism, planning, and expert information; HMO, health maintenance organization; NP, nurse practitioner; PNP, PhD in nursing program.

APRN-provided care to be equivalent to or higher than physician-provided care (Carter & Chochinov, 2007; Cooper et al., 2002; Dierick-van Daele et al., 2009; Horrocks et al., 2002; Jennings et al., 2009; Kleinpell et al., 2008; Knudtson 2000; Roblin et al., 2004). For example, Mundinger and associates' large randomized controlled trial of NP-provided primary care, compared with physician-provided care with a 2-year follow-up demonstrated no significant differences in patient satisfaction, utilization of services, self-reported health status, or physiological measures related to diabetes, hypertension, and asthma outcomes (Lenz et al., 2004; Mundinger et al., 2000). Significantly improved access to care and improved health outcomes have been documented in states where NPs have full, unrestricted practice authority (Oliver et al., 2014; Yang et al., 2021). Full scope of practice has also been associated with positive NP-administration relationships, professional visibility, and support for independent practice (Poghosyan et al., 2022). Aiken et al. (2021) found higher quality of care and safety in acute settings with higher ratios of nurse practitioners to the number of hospital beds, along with other positive findings.

In another large randomized controlled trial of 2,957 low-income, low-risk women, Jackson et al. (2003) found that birth outcomes of women receiving nurse-midwife collaborative care were equivalent to those of women receiving traditional physician care, but women receiving nurse-midwife care had lower operative intervention, lower use of epidural anesthesia, more spontaneous vaginal deliveries, and less use of medical resources. Pine et al.'s (2003) and Jordan et al.'s (2001) studies of anesthesia morbidity and mortality, noted earlier, demonstrated in a similar fashion the effectiveness, safety, and quality of nurse anesthetist–delivered care. Both the historical and recent literature document the effectiveness of APN-provided care across multiple, diverse populations and in diverse settings.

APRN CURRENT AND FUTURE OUTCOMES

Providers and researchers need to broaden their focus on quality to include a thorough evaluation of how APRN-provided care affects the entire healthcare system, including primary, acute, and specialty care, and especially to change policies about the full scope of autonomous, fully independent APRN practice. There is evidence, evolving over several decades, that nurse anesthetist–provided care has resulted in high-quality patient outcomes that are at least equivalent to those achieved by physicians (AANA, 2020). In addition, CNM-provided maternity care in the United States has resulted in excellent neonatal and maternal outcomes, including the physical health of mothers and infants and satisfaction with care, among others (Davidson, 2002; Oakley et al., 1996; Wilson, 1989). Overall, NP-directed care has achieved excellent outcomes, including care quality, cost-effectiveness, length of stay, and equivalence to physician-provided care (Lenz et al., 2004). However, all of these findings should be considered in the context of a changing healthcare system and rapidly changing population demographics.

The primary care needs of the population are expanding in an era of significant health reform, and many more primary care providers will be required to fill these needs. The management of chronic illness is a growing APRN focus as the burden of chronic illness grows in our society. This is magnified by an increasingly aged population, by evolutionary technologies that extend life across the developmental continuum, and by healthcare reform that further pressures the economic bottom line while additionally emphasizing chronic care management, medical homes, and primary care access (Blumenthal et al., 2015; Kocher et al., 2010). APRNs are increasingly responsible for caseloads of chronically ill clients who have complex social, behavioral, mental health, and medical needs in primary, acute, and long-term care. The evidence of the quality and effectiveness of APRN-provided care in the past five decades is strong. The evidence foundation for outcomes of care as provided by NPs, CNMs, CRNAs, and CNSs, including their impact on client health in the short- and long-term, utilization of services, cost, access, quality, and other factors, should and will continue to grow in the now-transformed healthcare system of the 21st century and beyond.

SUMMARY: FROM SILOS TO COMMON VISION

On March 23, 2010, President Barack Obama signed into law the Patient Protection and Affordable Care Act (ACA), the first overhaul of the American healthcare system since Lyndon Johnson signed Medicare and Medicaid into law on July 30, 1965. The ACA's planned focus on better access to and affordability of health insurance, health services integration and coordination, expanded use of electronic health records, expansion of primary care services, and redefinition of healthcare team member roles, especially those of NPs (Kocher et al., 2010), helped to solidify the importance of advanced practice nurse providers in improving the health of American citizens. Despite political controversies and state-level discrepancies related to its implementation, this historic legislation has indeed helped millions of Americans access health insurance and thus healthcare services, and has promoted the expansion of primary care and chronic care management services (Blumenthal et al., 2015); APNs will continue to be needed to provide these crucial services (National Academies of Sciences, Engineering, and Medicine, 2021). During the past two decades, significant changes that mesh with healthcare reform have occurred. Advanced practice nursing has matured into a powerful force ready to determine its own future. Once separated by practice into separate professional silos, 100,000 APRNs (nurse-midwives, nurse anesthetists, NPs, and CNSs) stand ready to join forces under a uniform umbrella to push the profession forward through a common vision (Pearson, 2010).

APRNs have continued to fight for 100% insurance parity with physicians, universal coverage, and expansion of APRN practice to increase access to care, especially for the underinsured and underserved (Advance for Nurse Practitioners, 2010; Pearson, 2010). The National Council of State Boards of Nursing has created model language for an APRN compact, defined as multistate licensure allowing APRNs with licensure in one compact state to practice in other compact states. The compact will be implemented after seven states have approved it; currently, Utah, North Dakota, and Delaware have such legislation (NCSBN, 2020). APRNs have continued to decrease barriers to practice and have won the ability to receive Medicaid reimbursement for healthcare services. Progressive legislation has resulted in the authority for APRNs to write prescriptions for services for disabled individuals, including ordering placards, prescribing home healthcare services, performing physical exams for drivers and students, signing death certificates, writing "do not resuscitate" (DNR) orders, and becoming empaneled and recognized as primary care providers. APRNs have won the ability to write for Schedule II through Schedule V controlled substances, and have their names printed on prescription labels.

Historically, APRNs have held their ground in their struggles with Boards of Medicine across the United States to reduce medicine's influence, resulting in regulation, supervision requirements, and authority over advanced nursing practice (Pearson, 2010). APRNs have lobbied for regulatory changes in language from "physician supervision" to "collaboration" or "independent practice" and have removed mandatory APRN-to-physician ratios. Increasingly, state legislatures are removing barriers to independent NP practice. During the most acute period of the COVID-19 pandemic, between 2020 and 2021, through gubernatorial executive orders, states, such as New York, removed APRN scope of practice restrictions as well as state-specific licensure requirements (New York State Association of Counties, 2021). The temporary relaxation of these restrictions permitted qualified providers to cross state lines and expand the respective healthcare workforce when states experienced COVID-19 crises related to the pandemic, to provide telehealth services broadly, and more specifically allowed APRNs to function independently across their full scope of practice. Despite the beneficial outcomes of these changes, such executive orders expired and restrictions on practice returned as the prevalence of COVID-19 morbidity began to drop.

APRNs have also increased their numbers in leadership positions on state boards of nursing. In several states, advanced practice nurses have won the protection of the title of APRN (Advance for Nurse Practitioners, 2010; Pearson, 2010). In addition, they have increased their involvement in the business of state legislatures and the federal government. Four NPs have been elected to powerful positions as state representatives. In several states, APRNs have become major players in malpractice reform and have been integrally involved in state Medicaid legislation. As the profession has matured, APRNs have hired their own professional lobbyists and formed political action committees. In *Kentucky Association Health Plans, Inc. v. Miller*, Kentucky Commissioner of Insurance (2003), the United States Supreme Court upheld the any-willing provider law, where insurers must open their networks to any provider recognized by the state, including APRNs.

In addition to promoting external changes, APRNs have also focused inwardly to improve the quality of practice. APRNs are reexamining the essential degree for entry-level advanced nursing practice and moving toward unification through the Consensus Model for Advanced Practice Registered Nurses (Advance for Nurse Practitioners, 2010;

Pearson, 2010). In addition, APRNs are moving toward uniform regulation of practice through licensing, accreditation, certification, and education. As the nation experiences dynamic changes in its healthcare system, APRNs—both master's-level and now including those doctorally prepared—stand ready to move the profession forward to provide the highest quality, universally accessible healthcare.

CRITICAL THINKING QUESTIONS

1. How have social, professional, and economic changes from the 1950s to the present influenced the APRN scope of practice?
2. How can historical factors in the evolution of the APRN shape the role and practice of future APRNs?
3. How is APRN practice different from generalist and medical practice? What accounts for its outcome in terms of patient satisfaction and health status?
4. APRN practice, particularly NP and CNM practice, may be conceptualized as built on a social justice foundation—to increase access to care for underserved and/or economically vulnerable populations. Current APRN practice has expanded beyond these boundaries, and many APRNs provide health services to clients who have access to adequate healthcare services and who have adequate financial resources. How does this fit with nursing's values? How does this fit with the argument that APRNs should provide lower-cost care than physicians and care that is more accessible?
5. What factors will influence the full implementation of the consensus model for APRN practice? How? What are the barriers to fully autonomous APRN practice?
6. What strategies could be used to increase physician support for autonomous APRN practice?
7. What are the advantages and disadvantages of the APRN movement toward the consensus model for APRNs and uniform regulation of practice through licensing, accreditation, certification, and education?
8. What are the factors of APRN practice that make it uniquely different from medical practice? How do they enhance or weaken the profession?
9. What are the theoretical factors that set APRNs apart from the discipline of medicine? How does this theory base influence research and practice?
10. What impact will the move to entry-level APRN practice at the DNP level have on healthcare access, quality, and cost?

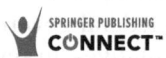

A robust set of instructor resources designed to supplement this text is located at http://connect.springerpub.com/content/book/978-0-8261-8137-4. Qualifying instructors may request access by emailing textbook@springerpub.com.

REFERENCES

AANA. (2020). *Scope of nurse anesthesia practice*. https://www.aana.com/wp-content/uploads/2023/01/scope-of-nurse-anesthesia-practice.pdf

Advance for Nurse Practitioners. (2010). *Annual legislative updates 2000–2010*. http://nurse-practitioners.advanceweb.com/Editorial/Search/SearchResult.aspx?KW= annual+legislative +update

Aiken, L. H., Sloane, D. M., Brom, H. M., Todd, B. A., Barnes, H. Cimiotti, J. P., Cunningham, R. S. & McHugh, M. D. (2021). Value of nurse practitioner inpatient hospital staffing. *Medical Care, 59*(10), 857–863. https://doi.org/10.1097/MLR.0000000000001628

AMA. (n.d.). *AMA successfully fights scope of practice expansions that threaten patient safety.* https://www.ama-assn.org/practice-management/scope-practice/ama-successfully-fights-scope-practice-expansions-threaten

American Academy of Pediatrics Committee on Hospital Care. (1999). Role of the nurse practitioner and physician assistant in the care of hospitalized children. *Pediatrics, 103,* 1050–1052. http://www.pediatrics.org/cgi/content/full/103/5/1050

American Academy of Pediatrics Committee on Pediatric Workforce. (2013). Scope of practice issues in the delivery of pediatric healthcare. *Pediatrics, 131*(6), 1211–1216. https://doi.org/10.1542/peds.2013-0943

American Association of Colleges of Nursing. (1996). *The essentials of master's education for advanced practice nursing.* https://www.aacnnursing.org/Portals/0/PDFs/Publications/MastersEssentials11.pdf

American Association of Colleges of Nursing. (2004). *AACN position statement on the practice doctorate in nursing.* Author. https://www.aacnnursing.org/portals/42/news/position-statements/dnp.pdf

American Association of Colleges of Nursing. (2009). *Title VIII nursing workforce development programs achieving success: Student recipients report the benefits.* https://www.apna.org/wp-content/uploads/2021/03/Title_VIII_Nursing_Workforce_Development_Programs_Brochure.pdf

American Association of Nurse Anesthetists. (n.d.). *Quality of care in anesthesia.* http://www.aana.com/qualityofcare.aspx

American Association of Nurse Practitioners. (2022). *State practice environment.* https://www.aanp.org/advocacy/state/state-practice-environment

American College of Nurse-Midwives. (2010). *Accreditation commission for midwifery education.* https://www.midwife.org/acme---accreditation-information

American College of Nurse-Midwives. (2019). *Fact sheet: essential facts about midwives.* https://www.midwife.org/acnm/files/cclibraryfiles/filename/000000007531/EssentialFactsAboutMidwives-UPDATED.pdf#:~:text=Standards%20for%20education%20and%20certification%20in%20midwifery%20are,ACME-accredited%20midwifery%20education%20programs%20in%20the%20United%20States.5

American College of Nurse Midwives (2022). *Fact sheet: Essential facts about midwives.* https://www.midwife.org/acnm/files/cclibraryfiles/filename/000000008273/EssentialFactsAboutMidwives_Final_2022.pdf

American Nurses Association. (n.d.). *Funding for nursing workforce development.* http://nursingworld.org/DocumentVault/GOVA/Federal/Federal-Issues/Nursing WorkforceDevelopment.html

American Nurses Association. (1980). *Nursing's social policy statement.* Author.

American Nurses Association. (1986). *The role of the clinical nurse specialist. ANA,* Author.

American Society of Anesthesiologists. (2023). *Opt-Outs.* https://www.asahq.org/advocacy-and-asapac/advocacy-topics/opt-outs

Anonymous. (2015). Clinical nurse specialists should have a doctor's degree. *Nursing Matters, 4,* 6. https://doi.org/10.14303/irjpp.2015.0121

APRN Consensus Workgroup and NCBSN APRN Advisory Committee. (2008). *Consensus model for advanced practice registered nurses.* https://www.ncsbn.org/public-files/Consensus_Model_Report.pdf

Avery, M. D. (2005). The history and evolution of the core competencies for basic midwifery practice. *Journal of Midwifery & Women's Health, 50*(2), 102–107. https://doi.org/10.1016/j.jmwh.2004.12.006

Baer, E. D. (1987). 'A cooperative venture' in pursuit of professional status: A research journal for nursing. *Nursing Research, 36*(1), 18–25.

Barger, M. K. (2005). Midwifery practice: Where have we been and where are we going? *Journal of Midwifery & Women's Health, 50*(2), 87–90. https://doi.org/10.1016/j.jmwh.2004.12.013

Bednash, G., Worthington, S., & Wysocki, S. (2009). Nurse practitioner education: Keeping the academic pipeline open to meet family planning needs in the United States. *Contraception, 80*(5), 409–411. https://doi.org/10.1016/j.contraception.2009.07.010

Benkert, R., Barkauskas, V., Pohl, J., Corser, W., Tanner, C., & Wells, M. (2002). Patient satisfaction outcomes in nurse-managed centers. *Outcomes Management, 6*(4), 174–181.

Benkert, R., Hollie, B., Nordstrom, C. K., Wickson, B., & Bins-Emerick, L. (2009). Trust, mistrust, racial identity and patient satisfaction in urban African American primary care patients of nurse practitioners. *Journal of Nursing Scholarship, 41*(2), 211–219. https://doi.org/10.1111/j.1547-5069.2009.01273.x

Blegen, M. A., & Tripp-Reimer, T. (1997). Implications of nursing taxonomies for middle range theory development. *Advances in Nursing Science, 19*(3), 37–49. https://doi.org/10.1097/00012272-199703000-00005

Blumenthal, D., Abrams, M., & Nuzum, R. (2015). The affordable care act at 5 years. *New England Journal of Medicine, 372*(25), 2451–2458. http://www.nejm.org/doi/full/10.1056/NEJMhpr1503614?af=R&rss=currentIssue&

Buhler-Wilkerson, K. (2001). *No place like home: A history of nursing and home care in the United States*. Johns Hopkins University Press.

Bullough, B. (1976). Influences on role expansion. *American Journal of Nursing, 76*(9), 1476–1481.

Buppert, C. (2005). Scope of practice. *Journal for Nurse Practitioners, 1*(1), 11–13. https://doi.org/10.2307/3424083

Burst, H., & Thompson, J. (2003). Genealogic origins of nurse midwifery education programs in the United States, Brief report. *Journal of Midwifery & Women's Health, 48*(6), 464–472. https://doi.org/10.1016/j.jmwh.2003.09.004

Canadian Coordinating Office for Health Technology Assessment. (2004). Surgical anesthesia delivered by nonphysicians, No. 37 [Report]. http://www.cadth.ca/media/pdf/273_No37_surgicalanesthesia_preassess_e.pdf

Carter, A. J. E., & Chochinov, A. H. (2007). A systematic review of the impact of nurse practitioners on cost, quality of care, satisfaction and wait times in the emergency department. *Canadian Journal of Emergency Medical Care, 9*(4), 286–295. https://doi.org/10.1017/s1481803500015189

Castro, A., & Ruiz, E. (2009). The effects of nurse practitioner cultural competence on Latina patient satisfaction. *Journal of the American Academy of Nurse Practitioners, 21*(5), 278–286. https://doi.org/10.1111/j.1745-7599.2009.00406.x

Charlton, C. R., Dearing, K. S., Berry, J. A., & Johnson, M. J. (2008). Nurse practitioners' communication styles and their impact on patient outcomes: An integrated literature review. *Journal of the American Academy of Nurse Practitioners, 20*(7), 382–388. https://doi.org/10.1111/j.1745-7599.2008.00336.x

Cooper, M. A., Lindsay, G. M., Kinn, S., & Swann, I. J. (2002). Evaluating emergency nurse practitioner services: A randomized controlled trial. *Journal of Advanced Nursing, 40*(6), 721–730. https://doi.org/10.1046/j.1365-2648.2002.02431.x

Davidson, M. H., Burns, C. E., St. Geme, J. W., Cadman, S. G., Newman, C. G., & Bullough, B. (1975). A short term intensive training program for pediatric nurse practitioners. *Journal of Pediatrics, 87*(2), 315–320. https://doi.org/10.1016/s0022-3476(75)80609-3

Davidson, M. R. (2002). Outcomes of high risk women cared for by certified nurse midwives. *Journal of Midwifery & Women's Health, 47*(1), 46–49. https://doi.org/10.1016/s1526-9523(01)00217-3

Dawley, K. (2003). Origins of nurse-midwifery in the United States and its expansion in the 1940s. *Journal of Midwifery & Womens Health, 48*(2), 86–95. https://doi.org/10.1016/s1526-9523(03)00002-3

Dawley, K. (2005). Doubling back over roads once traveled: Creating a national organization for nurse-midwifery. *Journal of Midwifery & Women's Health, 50*(2), 71–82. https://doi.org/10.1016/j.jmwh.2004.12.002

Dawley, K., & Burst, H. V. (2005). The American College of Nurse-Midwives and its antecedents: A historic time line. *Journal of Midwifery & Women's Health, 50*(1), 16–22. https://doi.org/10.1016/j.jmwh.2004.09.011

DeWitt, K. (1900). Specialties in Nursing. *American Journal of Nursing, 1*(1): 10–14.

Dierick-van Daele, A. T. M., Metsemakers, J. F. M., Derckx, E. W. C. C., Spreeuwenberg, C., & Vrijhoef, H. J. M. (2009). Nurse practitioners substituting for general practitioners: Randomized controlled trial. *Journal of Advanced Nursing, 65*(2), 391–401. https://doi.org/10.1111/j.1365-2648.2008.04888.x

Diers, D. (1991). Nurse-midwives and nurse anesthetists: The cutting edge in specialist practice. In L. H. Aiken & C. M. Fagin (Eds.), *Charting nursing's future: Agenda for the '90s* (pp. 159–180). J. B. Lippincott.

Donahue, P. (1996). *Nursing, the finest art: An illustrated history* (2nd ed.). Mosby.

Donnelly, G. (2003). Clinical expertise in advanced practice nursing: A Canadian perspective. *Nurse Education Today, 23*(3), 168–173. https://doi.org/10.1016/s0260-6917(02)00236-8

Donohue, R. K. (2003). Nurse practitioner–client interaction as resource exchange in a women's health clinic: An exploratory study. *Journal of Clinical Nursing, 12*(5), 717–725. https://doi.org/10.1046/j.1365-2702.2003.00790.x

Dulisse, B., & Cromwell, J. (2010). No harm found when nurse anesthetists work without supervision by physicians. *Health Affairs, 29*(8), 1469–1475. https://doi.org/10.1377/hlthaff.2008.0966

Dunphy, L. M., & Winland-Brown, J. E. (2006). The circle of caring: A transformative model of advanced practice nursing. In W. K. Cody (Ed.), *Philosophical and theoretical perspectives for advanced nursing practice* (4th ed.). Jones & Bartlett.

Erikson, H. L. (2007). Philosophy and theory of holism. *Nursing Clinics of North America*, 42(2), 139–163. https://doi.org/10.1016/j.cnur.2007.03.001

Fairman, J. (1999). Thinking about patients: Nursing science in the 1950's. *Reflections*, 23(3), 30–32.

Fairman, J., & Lynaugh, J. (1998). *Critical care nursing: A history.* University of Pennsylvania Press.

Fallacaro, M., Obst, T., Funn, I., & Chu, M. (1996). The national distribution of certified registered nurse anesthetists across metropolitan and nonmetropolitan settings. *Journal of the American Association of Nurse Anesthetists*, 64(3), 237–242.

Fawcett, J., & Alligood, M. R. (2005). Influences on advancement of nursing knowledge. *Nursing Science Quarterly*, 18(3), 227–232. https://doi.org/10.1177/0894318405277523

Federal Trade Commission. (2014). *Policy perspectives: Competition and regulation of advanced practice nurses.* https://www.ftc.gov/reports/policy-perspectives-competition-regulation-advanced-practice-nurses

Feyereisen, S. L., Puro, N. & McConnell, W. (2020). Addressing provider shortages in rural America: The role of the state opt-out policy adoptions in promoting hospital anesthesia provision. *The Journal of Rural Health.* 37(4). 684–691. https://doi-org.une.idm.oclc.org/10.1111/jrh.12487

Ford, L. (1975). An interview with Dr. Loretta Ford. *Nurse Practitioner*, 1(1), 9–12.

Frank vs. South. (1917). 175 Ky 416, 427–428; 194 SW 375, 380.

Goudreau, K. A. (2009). What clinical nurse specialist need to know about the consensus model for advanced nursing practice. *Clinical Nurse Specialist*, 53(2), 50–51.

Graninger, E. (1996). Granny-midwives: Matriarchs of birth in the African-American community 1600–1940. *Birth Gazette*, 13(1), 9–13.

Green, A., & Davis, S. (2005). Toward a predictive model of patient satisfaction with nurse practitioner care. *Journal of the American Academy of Nurse Practitioners*, 17(4), 139–148. https://doi.org/10.1111/j.1041-2972.2005.0022.x

Hamric, A. B., Spross, J. A., Hanson, C. M. (2009). *Advanced practice nursing: An integrative approach*, (4th ed.). W.B. Saunders.

Hayes, E. (2007). Nurse practitioners and managed care: Patient satisfaction and intention to adhere to nurse practitioner plan of care. *Journal of the American Academy of Nurse Practitioners*, 19(8), 418–426. https://doi.org/10.1111/j.1745-7599.2007.00245.x

Hedger, B. (2009). ACP urges doctors and NPs to work together. *American Medical News.* http://www.ama-assn.org/amednews/2009/03/02/prsa0302.htm

Hinch, B., Murphy, M., & Lauer, M. K. (2005). Preparing students for evolving nurse practitioner roles in healthcare. *MEDSURG Nursing*, 14(4), 240–246.

Hobbs, J. L. (2009). Defining Nursing Practice: The Social Policy Statement 1980-1983. *Advances in Nursing Science*, 32(1), 3–18. https://doi.org/10.1097/01.ANS.0000346283.29730.d1

Horrocks, S., Anderson, E., & Salisbury, C. (2002). Systematic review of whether nurse practitioners working in primary care can provide equivalent care to doctors. *British Medical Journal*, 324(7341), 819–823. https://doi.org/10.1136/bmj.324.7341.819

Hoyem, R. L., Quraishi, J. A., Jordan, L., Wiltse Nicely, K. L. (2019). Advocacy, research and anesthesia practice models: key studies of safety and cost-effectiveness. *Policy, Politics & Nursing Practice.* 20(4). https://doi-org.une.idm.oclc.org/10.1177/1527154419874410

Idzik, S., Buchholz, S. W., Kelly-Weeder, S., Finnegan, L. & Bigley, M. (2021). Strategies to move entry-level nurse practitioner education to the Doctor of Nursing Practice Degree by 2025. *Nurse Educator*, 46(6), 336–341. https://doi.org/10.1097/NNE.0000000000001129

Institute of Medicine. (2000). *To err is human: Building a safer health system.* National Academies Press.

Institute of Medicine. (2001). *Crossing the quality chasm: A new health system for the 21st century.* National Academy Press.

Institute of Medicine. (2004). *Keeping patients safe: Transforming the work environment of nurses.* National Academies Press.

Institute of Medicine. (2011). *The future of nursing: Leading change, advancing health.* National Academies Press.

Jackson, D. J., Lang, J. M., Swartz, W. H., Ganiats, T. G., Fullerton, J., Ecker, J., & Nguyen, U. (2003). Outcomes, safety, and resource utilization in a collaborative care birth center program compared with traditional physician-based perinatal care. *American Journal of Public Health*, 93(6), 999–1006.

Jefferson, K., Bouchard, M. E., Summers, L. (2021). The regulation of professional midwifery in the United States. *Journal of Nursing Regulation 11*(4), 26–38. https://doi.org/10.1016/S2155-8256(20)30174-5

Jenkins, C. L., Elliott, A. R., & Harris, J. R. (2006). Identifying ethical issues of the department of the army civilian and army nurse corps certified nurse anesthetists. *Military Medicine, 171*(8), 762. https://doi.org/10.7205/milmed.171.8.762

Jennings, N., Lee, G., Chao, K., & Keating, S. (2009). A survey of patient satisfaction in a metropolitan emergency department: Comparing nurse practitioners and emergency physicians. *International Journal of Nursing Practice, 15*(3), 213–218. https://doi.org/10.1111/j.1440-172X.2009.01746.x

Jordan, L. M., Kremer, M., Crawforth, K., & Shott, S. (2001). Data driven practice improvement: The AANA foundation closed malpractice claims study. *AANA Journal, 69*(4), 304–311.

Keeling, A. (2007). *Nursing and the privilege of prescription, 1893–2000*. The Ohio State University Press.

Keeling, A. (2009). A brief history of advanced practice nursing in the United States. In A. Hamric, J. Spross, & C. Hanson (Eds.), *Advanced practice nursing: An integrative approach* (4th ed.). Elsevier.

Kentucky Association of Health Plans, Inc. vs. Miller. (2003). 538 U.S.329.

Kinchin, E.(2022). Holistic nurse practitioner care including promotion of shared decision-making. *Holistic Nursing, 40*(4), 326–335. https://doi.org/10.1177/08980101211062704

Kleinpell, R. M., Ely, E. W., & Grabenkort, R. (2008). Nurse practitioners and physician assistants in the intensive care unit: An evidence-based review. *Critical Care Medicine, 36*(10), 2888–2897. https://doi.org/10.1097/CCM.0b013e318186ba8c

Knudtson, N. (2000). Patient satisfaction with nurse practitioner service in a rural setting. *Journal of the American Academy of Nurse Practitioners, 12*(10), 405–412. https://doi.org/10.1111/j.1745-7599.2000.tb00146.x

Kocher, R., Emmanuel, E. J., & DeParle, N. M. (2010). The affordable care act and the future of clinical medicine. *Annals of Internal Medicine, 153*(8), 536–540. https://doi.org/10.7326/0003-4819-153-8-201010190-00274

Kotzer, A. M. (2005). Characteristics and role functions of advanced practice nurses in a tertiary pediatric setting. *Journal for Specialists in Pediatric Nursing, 10*(1), 20–28. https://doi.org/10.1111/j.1088-145x.2005.00004.x

Kozlowski, J. L., Lusk, P., & Melnyk, B. M. (2015). Pediatric nurse practitioner management of child anxiety in a rural primary care clinic with the evidence-based cope program. *Journal of Pediatric Health Care, 29*(3), 274–282. https://doi.org/10.1016/j.pedhc.2015.01.009

Lenz, E. R., Mundinger, M. O. N., Kane, R. L., Hopkins, S. C., & Lin, S. X. (2004). Primary care outcomes in patients treated by nurse practitioners or physicians: Two-year follow-up. *Medical Care Research & Review, 61*(3), 332–351. https://doi.org/10.1177/1077558704266821

Lewis, J. A. (2000). Advanced practice in maternal/child nursing: History, current status, and thoughts about the future. *The American Journal of Maternal/Child Nursing, 25*(6), 327–330. https://doi.org/10.1097/00005721-200011000-00010

Manisoff, M. (1981). The nurse practitioner in family planning clinics. *Family Planning Perspectives, 13*(1), 19–22.

Manocchio, R. T. (2008). Tending communities, crossing cultures: Midwives in 19th-century California. *Journal of Midwifery & Women's Health, 53*(1), 75–81 https://doi.org/10.1016/j.jmwh.2007.03.006.

Mason, D. J., Vaccaro, K., & Fessler, M. B. (2000). Early views of nurse practitioners: A Medline search. *Clinical Excellence for Nurse Practitioners, 4*(3), 175–183.

McCool, W. F., & Simeone, S. A. (2002). Birth in the United States: An overview of trends past and present. *Nursing Clinics of North America, 37*(4), 735–746. https://doi.org/10.1016/s0029-6465(02)00020-8

MacDorman, M. F., & Declercq, E. (2019). Trends and state variations in out-of-hospital births in the United States, 2004–2017. *Birth. 46*(2), 279–288. https://doi.org/10.1111/birt.12411

Moorhead, S., Head, B., Johnson, M., & Maas, M. (1998). The nursing outcomes taxonomy: Development and coding. *Journal of Nursing Care Quality, 12*(6), 56–63. https://doi.org/10.1097/00001786-199808000-00010

Morrison, S. M., & Fee, E. (2010). Nothing to work with but cleanliness: The training of African American traditional midwives in the South. *American Journal of Public Health, 100*(2), 238–239. https://doi.org/10.2105/AJPH.2009.182873

Mundinger, M. O., Cook, S. S., Lenz. E. R. Piacientini, K., Auerhahn & C., & Smith, J. (2000). Assuring access and quality in advanced practice nursing: A challenge to nurse educators. *Journal of Professional Nursing, 16*(6), 322–329. https://doi.org/10.1053/jpnu.2000.18177

Mundinger, M. O., Kane, R. L., Lenz, E. R., Totten, A. M., Tsai, W. Y., Cleary, P. D., Friedewald, W. T., Siu, A. L., & Shelanski, M. L. (2000). Primary care outcomes in patients treated by nurse practitioners or physicians: A randomized trial. *Journal of the American Medical Association, 283*(1), 59–68. https://doi.org/10.1001/jama.283.1.59

Murphy, M. A. (1990). A brief history of pediatric nurse practitioners and NAPNAP 1964–1990. *Journal of Pediatric Health Care, 4*(6), 332–337. https://doi.org/10.1016/0891-5245(90)90084-j

National Academies of Sciences, Engineering, and Medicine. (2021). *The Future of nursing 2020–2030: Charting a path to achieve health equity.* The National Academies Press. https://www.ncbi.nlm.nih.gov/books/NBK573922/

National Association of Clinical Nurse Specialists. (2019, December). *Core Practice Doctorate Clinical Nurse Specialist (CNS) Competencies.* Author.

National Association of Clinical Nurse Specialists. (2019, November). *Statement on Clinical Nurse Specialist Practice & Education,* (3rd ed.). NACNS author.

National Board of Certification and Recertification of Nurse Anesthetists. (2010). *Certification.* http://www.nbcrna.com/certification.html

National Council of State Boards of Nursing. (1998). *Using nurse practitioner certification for state nursing regulation: A historical perspective.* Author.

National Council of State Boards of Nursing. (2020). *APRN compact.* https://www.ncsbn.org/compacts/aprn-compact.page

National Institutes of Health. (n.d.). *Important events in the National Institute of Nursing Research history.* https://www.ninr.nih.gov/aboutninr/history#.VwJ82-a9-t4

National Organization of Nurse Practitioner Faculties. (2002). *Nurse practitioner primary care competencies in specialty care areas: Adult, family, gerontological, pediatric, and women's health.* https://cdn.ymaws.com/www.nonpf.org/resource/resmgr/competencies/primarycarecomps02.pdf

National Organization of Nurse Practitioner Faculties. (2003). *Psychiatric-mental health nurse practitioner competencies: National panel for psychiatric mental health NP competencies.* Author.

National Organization of Nurse Practitioner Faculties. (2004). *Acute care nurse practitioner competencies: Faculties national panel for acute care nurse practitioner competencies.* Author.

National Organization of Nurse Practitioner Faculties. (2018). *The doctor of nursing practice degree: Entry to nurse practitioner practice by 2025.* https://www.nonpf.org/news/400012/NONPF-DNP-Statement-May-2018.htm

National Organization of Nurse Practitioner Faculties. (2022). *NONPF's NP role core competencies.* https://www.nonpf.org/page/NP_Role_Core_Competencies

National Task Force on Quality Nurse Practitioner Education. (2008). *Criteria for evaluation of nurse practitioner programs.* AACN. http://www.aacn.nche.edu/education/pdf/evalcriteria2008.pdf

Neill, K. M. (1999). A holistic interdisciplinary health care research model. *Holistic Nursing Practice, 13*(2), 54–60. https://doi.org/10.1097/00004650-199901000-00009

New York State Association of Counties. (2021). *Executive orders.* https://www.nysac.org/content.asp?contentid=264

Oakley, D., Murray, M. E., Murtland, T., Hayashi, R., Anderson, H. F., & Mays, F. (1996). Comparison of outcomes of maternity care by obstetricians and certified nurse midwives. *Obstetrics & Gynecology, 88*(5), 832–829. https://doi.org/10.1016/0029-7844(96)00278-5

Oliver, G., Pennington, L. Revelle, S. & Rantz, M. (2014). Impact of nurse practitioners on health outcomes of Medicare and Medicaid patients. *Nursing Outlook, 62*(6), 440–447. https://doi.org/10.1016/j.outlook.2014.07.004

O'Reilly, D., Brady, A., Bryant-Lukosius, D., Varley, J., Daly, L., Cotter. P., Elliot, N., Lehane, E., Fleming, S., Savage, E., Hegarty, J. & Drennan, J. (2020). Patient-reported experiences of consulttoin with an advanced nurse practitioner: Factor structure and reliability analysis of the patient enablement and satisfaction survey. *Journal of Advanced Nursing, 77*(10), 4279–4289. https://doi.org/10.1111/jan.15026

Partin, B. (2009). Consensus model for APRN regulation. *The Nurse Practitioner, 34*(6), 8. https://doi.org/10.1097/01.NPR.0000352281.51487.f3

Pearson, L. (2010). *The Pearson report 2010.* http://www.pearsonreport.com

Peplau, H. (2003/1965) Specialization in Professional Nursing. *Clinical Nurse Specialist, 17*(1), 3–14. https://doi.org/10.1097/00002800-200301000-00002 [Reprinted from the original that appeared in *Nursing Science*, 1965]

Phillips, J. R. (1996). What constitutes nursing science? *Nursing Science Quarterly, 9*(2), 48–49. https://doi.org/10.1177/089431849600900202

Pine, M., Holt, K. D., & Lou, Y. B. (2003). Surgical mortality and type of anesthesia provider. *AANA Journal*, *71*(2), 109–116.

Poghosyan, L, Stein, J. H., Liu, J., Spetz, J., Osakwe, Z. T., & Martsolf, G. (2022). State-level scope of practice regulations for nurse practitioners impact work environments: Six state investigation. *Research in Nursing and Health*, *45*(5), 516–524. https://doi.org/10.1002/nur.22253

Raisler, J., & Kennedy, H. (2005). Midwifery care of poor and vulnerable women, 1925–2003. *Journal of Midwifery & Women's Health*, *50*(2), 113–121. https://doi.org/10.1016/j.jmwh.2004.12.010

Ray, W.T. & Desai, S. P. (2016). The history of the nurse anesthesia profession. *Journal of Clinical Anesthesia*, *30*, 51–58. https://doi.org/10.1016/j.jclinane.2015.11.005

Richmond, J. B. (1965). Gaps in the nation's services for children. *Bulletin of the New York Academy of Medicine*, *41*(12), 1237–1247.

Roblin, D. W., Becker, E. R., Adams, E. K., Howard, D. H., & Roberts, M. H. (2004). Patient satisfaction with primary care: Does type of practitioner matter? *Medical Care*, *42*(6), 579–590. https://doi.org/10.1097/01.mlr.0000128005.27364.72

Rooks, J. (1997). *Midwifery and childbirth in America*. Temple University Press.

Roots, A., & McDonald, R. (2014). Outcomes associated with nurse practitioners in collaborative practice in rural settings in Canada: A mixed methods study. *Human Resources for Health*, *12*(69). https://doi.org/10.1186/1478-4491-12-69

Roy, C. (2007). Advances in nursing knowledge and the challenge for transforming practice. In C. Roy & D. A. Jones (Eds.), *Nursing knowledge development and clinical practice* (pp. 3–37). Springer Publishing Company.

Sawatsky, J. A., Christie, S., & Singal, R. K. (2013). Exploring outcomes of a nurse practitioner managed cardiac surgery follow up intervention: A randomized trial. *Journal of Advanced Nursing*, *69*(9), 2076–2087. https://doi.org/10.1111/jan.12075

Seibert, E. M., Alexander, J., & Lupien, A. E. (2004). Rural nurse anesthesia: a pilot study. *AANA Journal*, *72*(3), 181–191.

Silver, H. K., Ford, L. R., & Day, H. C. (1968). The pediatric nurse practitioner program: Expanding the role of the nurse to provide increased health care for children. *Journal of the American Medical Association*, *204*(4), 298–302. https://doi.org/10.1001/jama.1968.03140170014003

Spalding, E. (1943). The Bolton act provides federal funding for postgraduate programs. *American Journal of Nursing*, *43*, 833. https://doi.org/10.2307/3456437

Stanley, J. M. (2012). Impact of new regulatory standards on advanced practice registered nursing: The APRN Consensus Model and LACE. *Nursing Clinics of North America*, *27*(2), 241–250. https://doi.org/10.1016/j.cnur.2012.02.001

Stanley, J. M., Werner, K. E., & Apple, K. (2009). Positioning advanced practice registered nurses for healthcare reform: Consensus on APRN regulation. *Journal of Professional Nursing*, *25*(6), 340–348 https://doi.org/10.1016/j.profnurs.2009.10.001.

Stone, S. E. (2000). The evolving scope of nurse-midwifery practice in the United States. *Journal of Midwifery & Women's Health*, *45*(6), 522–531. https://doi.org/10.1016/s1526-9523(00)00084-2

U.S. Department of Veterans Affairs. (2016). *VA grants full practice authority to advance practice registered nurses*. https://www.va.gov/opa/pressrel/pressrelease.cfm?id=2847

Van Leuven, K., & Prion, S. (2007). Health promotion in care directed by nurse practitioners. *Journal for Nurse Practitioners*, *3*(7), 456–461. https://doi.org/10.1016/j.nurpra.2007.04.024

Varney, H., Kriebs, J., & Gegor, C. (2004). *Varney's midwifery*, (4th ed.). Jones & Bartlett.

Wald, L. (1922). The origin and development of the Henry Street Settlement Text for Broadcasting. [Reel #25 Lillian Wald Papers]. In *The Westinghouse Electric Manufacturing Co. (Producer)*. The New York Public Library.

Wall, B. M. (2005). *Unlikely entrepreneurs: Catholic sisters and the hospital marketplace, 1863–1925*. The Ohio State University Press.

Wilson, B. (1989). Delivery outcomes of low risk births: Comparison of certified nurse midwives and obstetricians. *Journal of the American Academy of Nurse Practitioners*, *1*(1), 9–13.

Yang, B. K., Johangen, M. E. Trinkoff, A. M., Idzik, S. R., Wince. J., & Tomlinson, C. (2021). State nurse practitioner practice regulations and U.S. health care delivery outcomes: A systematic review. *Medical Care Research and Review*, *78*(3), 183–196. Jones & Bartlett.

CHAPTER THREE

Reflective Response 1

DANA PEARLMAN

In 2021, the American College of Nurse-Midwives published a Truth and Reconciliation Resolution speaking to the harm done to midwifery by nurse-midwives. It is imperative that nursing more broadly recognize that "[n]ursing's participation in the campaign to eliminate the midwife served neither the interests of pregnant women nor the goals of the nursing profession" (Dawley, 2000). If advanced practice registered nurses (APRNs) value evidence-based practice to improve outcomes, the time has come to fully embrace midwifery, not solely nurse-midwives, and implement change.

Nurse-midwife is hyphenated, but nurse anesthetist, clinical nurse specialist, and nurse practitioner are not. Why is that? The word "nurse" in the title nurse-midwife is not an adjective. Nurse is a noun in this context, representing an individual educated in the two disciplines of nursing and midwifery. "Nurse-midwifery" is, therefore, an incorrect conceptualization of the profession of midwifery being modified by nursing; the correct terminology would be nursing and midwifery. In truth, it is easier to say nurse-midwife, which flows similarly to how nurses talk about being a nurse educator, nurse scientist, or nurse entrepreneur, where nursing deeply informs our work as educators, scientists, or entrepreneurs, but nursing is not the sole avenue to becoming an educator, scientist, or entrepreneur.

Uniform midwifery education program accreditation with defined core competencies and national certification for nurse-midwives long predates the LACE working group and consensus model for advanced practice nursing. However, APRN legislation that recognizes that nurse-midwives may be educated outside of schools of nursing and hold graduate degrees other than nursing degrees has benefited nurse-midwives regulated by boards of nursing. Despite the care taken in the LACE discussions, most nurse-midwives in the United States are educated in colleges of nursing, where nursing and midwifery education is often referred to as a "specialty" of nursing rather than a professional role that an RN with graduate education in midwifery may claim.

The American College of Nurse-Midwives is recognized as an influential midwifery association worldwide, but because certified nurse-midwives (CNMs) are licensed as APRNs rather than as midwives in 44 states, U.S. midwifery does not meet the International Confederation of Midwives' (ICM) criteria for midwifery self-regulation. The American College of Nurse-Midwives (ACNM) developed a white paper in 2011 outlining the ideal regulating body for CNMs as boards of midwifery, in compliance with the ICM. When a board of midwifery is not feasible and CNMs are regulated by boards of nursing, the ACNM recommended that the boards regulate the direct entry equivalent to CNMs, certified midwives (CMs) as well.

The United States now has three nationally recognized midwifery credentials: the CNM, the CM, and the certified professional midwife (CPM). Midwifery looks at education, regulation, and association as the pillars of a strong profession. For CPMs, the accrediting agency for education programs is the Midwifery Education Accreditation Council (MEAC), the national certifying body is the North American Registry of

Midwives (NARM), and the professional association is the National Association of Certified Professional Midwives (NACPM). The professional association for CNMs and CMs is the ACNM. The Accreditation Commission for Midwifery Education (ACME) accredits programs leading to eligibility for CM or CNM credentials. Both CNMs and CMs take the same exam given by the American Midwifery Certification Board (AMCB) to earn their respective national certifications. The ACNM publishes standard-setting documents for the practice of midwifery by CNMs and CMs. These include standards of practice, a code of ethics, competencies for basic midwifery practice, and competencies for master's and doctoral education in midwifery.

The ACNM launched the CM credential in 1994. The first CMs educated in an accredited program to identical core competencies, standards, scope, and code of ethics, side-by-side with nurse-midwife students, were nationally certified and state licensed in 1997. CMs are now recognized for licensure in 10 states and the District of Columbia. Unfortunately, CMs face the same hurdles for full practice authority that APRNs do, though they often need to overcome lingering bias and tropes stemming from the campaign to eliminate the midwife as well as resistance from both medicine and nursing. Thankfully, this appears to be evolving as Colorado, the District of Columbia, and Maryland have moved to license CMs with parity to CNMs, and several other state affiliates of ACNM are seeking to expand access and diversify the midwifery workforce through the expansion of the CM credential. However, it is difficult for individuals to invest in accredited education within a regionally accredited college or university when professional licensure and recognition are absent, fraught, or, in some cases, hostile.

The United States has the worst maternal mortality among other wealthy nations and unconscionable health disparities among black, brown, and indigenous people. Tens of thousands of qualified applicants have been turned away from entry into nursing because of a bottleneck in clinical education. The future of midwifery in the United States is a both/and scenario: nurses can continue to advance their education in midwifery and be recognized as APRNs, while other educational pathways to midwifery simultaneously expand to increase the midwifery workforce through accredited education, national certification, and full-practice authority consistent with educational competencies. Our National Provider Identification already recognizes CNMs and CMs as advanced practice midwives and CPMs as midwives. Adding midwives to the Social Security Act would be one way to rapidly increase access to midwifery jobs and equitable reimbursement.

The United States adopted the sequential educational model of nurse-midwifery from Great Britain. In the 1980s, Great Britain shifted away from sequential education in nursing followed by midwifery for registered midwives (RMs). Now RMs in the United Kingdom enter midwifery programs directly. Most countries around the world educate nurses AND midwives with separate roles and regulations. Many second-degree nurse-midwife students today attend accelerated nursing programs at great expense, primarily to practice the ACNM Core Competencies, have legal access to hospitals, and have the ability to serve all who seek midwifery care. Nursing and midwifery can cooperate and promote a *both/and* solution, meaning that we work to promote evidence-based care and improve outcomes through *both* nursing *and* midwifery. If we follow the evidence, the United States can finally create the opportunity to enter the profession of midwifery directly, while precious seats in nursing programs can be saved for the expansion of the nursing workforce, and both professions can grow and flourish.

The path to both/and requires a paradigm shift in the nursing conceptualization of midwives. Careful use of the language describing midwifery as a respected sibling rather than an offspring of nursing can help. This distinction is as important as the distinction between medicine and nursing. All three professions have overlapping skills, while midwifery and nursing share whole-person paradigms, but the practices are not the same. When midwives are caring for families during the perinatal cycle, attending births, caring for newborns, providing contraception, and providing primary care services, they are practicing midwifery. Nursing is one entry point to midwifery, but it need not be the only entry point. Just as nurses are no longer holding the velvet box with a thermometer for the physician, fundamental healthcare skills can be taught to students entering a range of professions. Aspiring midwives emerge not only from nursing, but also from social work, physical therapy, law, public health, or their own birth and life experiences. The future of the maternity care workforce demands mutual respect and reconciling the harm done in the 19th and 20th centuries to midwifery. Nursing can and must restore midwives, not only nurse-midwives, to health.

REFERENCE

Dawley, K. (2000). The campaign to eliminate the midwife. *American Journal of Nursing, 100*(10), 50–56.

CHAPTER THREE Reflective Response 2

MICHAEL NEFT

▪ RECENT WORK EFFORTS AND ON-GOING ISSUES IN THE CRNA ROLE

Conti emphasizes the clinical role of the CRNA since its genesis during the Civil War. Since then, certified registered nurse anesthetists (CRNAs) have given anesthesia everywhere from harsh battle conditions for the military to high-tech hospitals. They have given anesthesia for cutting-edge procedures like awake craniotomies, transcatheter aortic valve replacements (TAVR), and hyperthermic intraperitoneal chemoperfusion (HIPEC). As noted in the preceding chapter, studies have documented the safety and economy of nurse anesthesia care. Hoyden et al. (2019) note that while the idea of doing further studies to document the efficacy and cost-effectiveness of nurse anesthesia has been considered, mortality and morbidity rates are so low in anesthesia that the idea has been all but abandoned. I often tell my students that they can do anything they want when they graduate. There are many different patient populations who need anesthesia care, as well as different venues in which to provide it: hospitals, doctor's offices, free-standing surgery or gastroenterology centers, as well as the military or mission trips.

There is an ongoing discussion within the profession about what type of practice a CRNA should strive to be part of. Some practitioners discover that independent practice, in which they make all of their own clinical decisions without anesthesiologist supervision or direction, is the best fit for them. Others do not mind working in a more team-oriented practice, though sometimes they may be over-supervised to the point of domination and intimidation, as is commonly encountered in some of the "team practices" in anesthesia. When these methods of control are used, it is no longer a team practice but a dictatorship. CRNAs are taught to think critically and independently, being able to develop a care plan, justify it, implement it, and constantly reevaluate its efficacy, adjusting it as needed. In strongly supervised practices, this ability is stifled. Our education and nursing background, which instill in us the capacity to think and act independently, make CRNAs a positive alternative for anesthesia care.

While other advanced practice nursing (APN) groups have supported the American Association of Colleges of Nursing's (AACN) movement toward clinical doctorates for all APNs in theory, only nurse anesthesia has done so in practice. All nurse anesthesia programs are now taught within a doctoral framework. This demonstrates the anesthesia profession's commitment to doctoral education as the basis for entry into practice. A CRNA educated at the DNP level learns not only the clinical skills that are important for their careers but also how to assess and solve problems. These skills create practitioners who can tackle educational, clinical, and administrative problems important to the running of their departments as soon as they graduate. While the number of DNP programs in other APN areas has continued to rise, it is taking longer for BSN-DNP enrollment to increase. Many APN-MSN programs still exist, but their graduates do not have a terminal clinical degree. They may have to return to school for the "add-on" DNP degree (McCauley et al., 2020). According to McCauley and colleagues, the intent of the DNP degree was to produce doctorally prepared clinicians at the bedside. However, it seems that those in other APN fields who return to school for the DNP after being an MSN-prepared APN are moving into administrative or education positions. Often, when many do earn their NP credentials, they move into education or administrative positions and do not ever practice as an NP.

For CRNAs to practice to their full scope, as highly educated problem-solvers and to move their profession forward, the reins of some practice patterns must be loosened. Hoyden et al. (2019) note that political influences in the anesthesia community trump evidence when considering the scope of practice for CRNAs. In their integrative review, Vitale and Lyons (2021) found that the leadership in some healthcare organizations does not want to implement a CRNA-heavy anesthesia department because it will upset the medical staff, namely surgeons and anesthesiologists. They also found that CRNAs in more rural practices tend to have wider scopes of practice, and states where CRNAs practice more toward their full scope have higher numbers of CRNAs.

Patient care suffers when advanced practice nurses, such as CRNAs, are not permitted to work within their full scope of practice. CRNAs provide safe care, and when allowed to practice to the full extent of their education, they can provide much-needed anesthesia services in all settings, expanding care access for patients, especially those in vulnerable populations.

With the problem-solving skills learned in their DNP programs, CRNAs can lead interprofessional teams whose goal is to solve or manage ongoing problems in healthcare (Bowie et al., 2019). Service equity, burnout, patient safety, and care efficiency are all areas that require constant management and monitoring. CRNAs can help tackle these issues as they face them in their daily practice. A prime example is the oversight of the consolidation of the healthcare system/hospital services. An anesthesia department in one facility may close, change case mix, or be completely absorbed by another provider group, health system, or hospital. CRNAs can be key members of groups that plan those mergers, not only because of their clinical knowledge but also because of the insight and skills they gain in their DNP education. Not only do they know their clinical jobs best, but they also know what resources need to be in place for them to be effectively executed.

The diversification of the nurse anesthesia profession is an ongoing process in which many CRNAs play a role. The Diversity in Nurse Anesthesia Mentorship Program (DNAMP; Gould, 2020) organization actively seeks out minority nurses and student nurses to mentor and help guide them into nurse anesthesia programs. It is also "committed to dismantling inequities and disparities among underrepresented, racially diverse, marginalized nurse anesthesia and faculty workforces" (pp. 177–178). This organization was established in 2007 by Wallena Gould, Ed.D., CRNA. One of its primary roles is to assist minority critical-care nurses and nursing students in understanding the application process for nurse anesthesia programs and being able to anticipate all aspects of it. It does this through educational offerings several times per year. The programs take place over a weekend at a university-based nurse anesthesia program. Lectures, group/panel discussions, and role play are the chief educational tools. Additionally, the participants spend time in the simulation lab with CRNAs who teach skills such as airway management and subarachnoid block placement. CRNAs from both the DNAMP and local CRNA faculty and students take part in presenting these workshops. It empowers nurses and students from underserved backgrounds by giving them the skills to navigate the difficult process of applying to and interviewing for admission to nurse anesthesia programs and to have the best possible experience as students.

What I Think the Future of CRNA Practice Should Look Like

CRNAs need to be able to practice to the full scope of their education. This will improve access to care by having more independent anesthesia practitioners available. In that light, we should be able to provide care outside the operating room, such as chronic pain management, supervision clinics specializing in preoperative patient optimization, and being able to serve as true leaders in anesthesia departments, that is, being able to make autonomous decisions affecting CRNA management and practice, not only executing the decisions of physician leaders. The CRNA practice faces ongoing challenges. The physician community is obstructionist in allowing us to practice within our full scope of care. It says this is because of concerns for patient safety, without any empirical evidence. If we are not allowed to practice to our full scope, patient care is jeopardized by those who implement and enforce those restrictions. Our education prepares us not only as expert clinicians but as engaged, autonomous practitioners whose nursing backgrounds give them a unique perspective on and approach to patient care. We need to be part of the discussion and solution for any problems involving the anesthesia department or its patients. Often, CRNAs are busy with patient care, and their physician counterparts are the ones making decisions about their futures. If our practice, including our DNP skill set, received its due respect, we would be at those discussions. While the future is bright for CRNAs where there is a need for our skills, both clinical and quality oriented, the path forward is turbulent.

REFERENCES

Bowie, B., DeSoscio, J., & Swanson, K. M. (2019). The DNP degree: Are we producing the graduates we intended? *The Journal of Nursing Administration, 49*(5), 280–285. https://doi.org/10.1097/NNA.0000000000000751

Gould, W. (2021). Historical underpinning to diversifying nurse anesthesia programs: A model of success. *Teaching and Learning in Nursing, 16*(2), 175–180. https://doi.org/10.1016/j.teln.2020.11.004

Hoyden, P., Quraishi, J., Jordan, L., & Nicely, K. (2019). Advocacy, research, and anesthesia practice models: Key studies of safety and cost-effectiveness. *Policy, Politics, and Nursing Practice, 20*(4), 193–204. https://doi.org/10.1177/1527154419874410

McCauley, L., Broome, M., Frazier, L., Hayes, R., Kurth, A., Musil, C., Norman, L., Rideout, K., & Villarruel, A. (2020). Doctor of nursing practice (DNP) degree in the United States: Reflecting, readjusting, and getting back on track. *Nursing Outlook, 68*(4), 494–503. https://doi.org/10.1016/j.outlook.2020.03.008

Vitale, C., & Lyons, K. (2021). The state of nurse anesthetists practice and policy: An integrative review. *AANA Journal, 89*(5), 403–412.

CHAPTER THREE Reflective Response 3

KSENIA ZUKOWSKY

■ A PERSONAL JOURNEY AS A PIONEERING NEONATAL NURSE PRACTITIONER

From a very early age, as I recall, I always wanted to be a nurse. Anytime that I think of my active childhood play memories, nursing play kits and dolls were a part of my active play. I traveled from the suburbs of South Jersey to a small hospital in Philadelphia, Pennsylvania, to volunteer my time as a candy striper during the summer following my freshman year of high school. In 1975, I graduated from the University of Pennsylvania Presbyterian School of Nursing, University of Pennsylvania Medical Center, diploma program in Philadelphia.

I was subsequently hired for my first professional nursing position at St. Christopher's Hospital for Children (SCHC) in Philadelphia, which I held from 1975 through 1986. At SCHC, I held a few accomplished roles, including being a nurse in the NICU, assistant NICU nurse manager, and eventually NICU nurse manager.

Responding to the nursing profession's call to elevate the RN's level of education from a nursing diploma to a bachelor's of science in nursing, I returned to the classroom in 1980, enrolling in LaSalle University's bachelor of science in nursing (BSN) program. Over the course of five years, I completed the in-person evening BSN program while maintaining my full-time position at SCHC, graduating in 1985.

After obtaining my BSN, I kept my education momentum going and was accepted to the University of Pennsylvania's School of Nursing (UPENNSON) master's of science in nursing (MSN) Perinatal/Neonatal program in 1985. At that time, my concentration preferences were either perinatal/neonatal clinical nurse specialist (CNS) or pediatric nurse practitioner. As an expert neonatal nurse and NICU nurse manager, initially I chose perinatal/neonatal CNS with a minor in nursing administration.

My aspiring graduate choices would be altered. When I met with the chair of the Perinatal/Neonatal and Women's Health program at UPENNSON during my admission interview for the MSN program, she advised me that I would be the perfect candidate for the new Neonatal Nurse Practitioner (NNP) program. After that interview, my new graduate concentration was solidified.

Completing the Neonatal Nurse Practitioner MSN program was a near-false start. In the early 1980s, the Philadelphia/Southern New Jersey/Delaware Valley region did not recognize the Neonatal Nurse Practitioner role. Additionally, upon further investigation and discussion with my interprofessional colleagues, among whom were neonatologists, they were unsure of how to utilize the NNP role in a NICU. Obtaining a clinical site and preceptor to meet my neonatal clinical competencies during clinical rotations as a graduate student almost did not happen.

Finally, after many inquiries and engaging the full support of the UPENNSON faculty and two regional neonatologists, my clinical experiences were successfully completed, and I graduated from the UPENNSON with my Neonatal Nurse Practitioner Master of Science in Nursing degree in August of 1987.

Securing an advanced practice nursing NNP position in the Philadelphia/Southern New Jersey/Delaware Valley region in 1987 proved to be quite challenging, as the role was still so new and the profession was still navigating what specific role the NNP would play in the interprofessional neonatal healthcare team. There was very little opportunity for the role to be developed in Philadelphia and New Jersey. The two neonatologists who precepted me during my graduate studies expressed support and wanted to have the neonatal nurse practitioner role established in their NICU, yet the emphasis on the priority of neonatal medical fellowships and pediatric residency education outweighed the opportunity for integrating an advanced practice nursing role into the neonatal team.

Following my MSN graduation and after no luck securing an advanced practice nursing position in the Philadelphia/Southern New Jersey region, I interviewed for an NNP position in Fairfax, Virginia. The NNP position was offered to me, but I wanted to stay in this region. I had family members who were dependent on my support, and moving out of the area would have been a hardship. In the fall of 1987, the chair of Perinatal/Neonatal Nursing at the UPENNSON called and offered me a position as a clinical expert. My role was to set up all clinical sites for the NNP program for the School of Nursing and to teach neonatal content to the perinatal/neonatal students.

I eagerly accepted and stayed in this role for 7 years. Additionally, during that time, I acquired a clinical NNP position, first at a level II NICU and subsequently at a level III NICU, both in Philadelphia. In both instances, I was the first in-house advanced practice nurse and NNP hired by the organizations.

Continuing with my role at the University of Pennsylvania's graduate nursing program, I was able to meet with and integrate NNP students at several academic and community NICUs in the Delaware Valley region. Graduate nursing students were placed in New Jersey, Delaware, Philadelphia, and the surrounding suburban community hospitals. These neonatal NP students were initially precepted by the neonatal attendings and then, over time, by the advanced practice nursing graduates. Over the next several years, graduates from other NNP programs would join the NICU teams in the region. Interprofessional teams of physicians and advanced practice nurses were established. Precepting NNP students was welcomed and, in some cases, used as a means to add NNPs to the established NNP teams by hiring them post-graduation. Neonatologists who agreed to precept NNP students often hired the NNPs after graduating and obtaining passing board scores. This allowed for a win-win, as the NNP knew the NICU team and vice versa.

Though the successful amalgamation of the NNP student role and NNP professional role was being attained in many NICUs in the Delaware Valley, competition with residency-based programs in the Philadelphia region remained an intense issue. Though advanced practice nursing has been shown to have a significant impact on patient care, some physician teams equate the NNP role with a perpetual resident position. Through the sheer determination of many practicing NNPs in neonatal integrative healthcare teams, some of that mindset dissipated. This was more of an issue in the late 1980s through the 1990s, yet it is still present in our current time.

After obtaining substantial professional experience and being part of the initiation of the neonatal nurse practitioner across neonatal integrative healthcare teams, I continued my graduate education by attaining my PhD from New York University, Steinhardt School of Education, Division of Nursing. I lived in southern New Jersey and commuted to New York City several times a week for in-person classes at NYU, which became a routine that continued for several years. Simultaneously, I practiced clinically in a level III NICU in Philadelphia as an NNP and continued teaching at the University of Pennsylvania for several of those years, until I was nearing the dissertation phase of my doctoral program.

After finishing my PhD in 2002 and practicing as an NNP in a level III NICU, I was approached by my clinical neonatal director and the chair of the Department of Nursing at Thomas Jefferson University (TJU) to develop a graduate nursing program. The Department of Nursing evolved into the School of Nursing, then the College of Nursing, and the chair became the dean of the TJU School of Nursing. The NNP MSN graduate program was written and approved by the Pennsylvania State Board of Nursing and the TJU board, and students started to enroll in the program. I joined the academic nursing department at Thomas Jefferson University as the NNP coordinator/program director. In that role, I continued teaching NNP students and integrating them into clinical sites in the Delaware Valley. Leading this program brought many opportunities to my professional career, including holding board member and treasurer positions on the Philadelphia Perinatal Society as well as a board member position for *Advances in Neonatal Care*, the journal for the National Association of Neonatal Nurses (NANN). As a former National Faculty for Neonatal Resuscitation Program (NRP) (1986–1990), my interaction with this interprofessional education program remained current as a teacher and a learner of the program from 1990–2019 through my active NNP full-time/part-time status.

In time, I interviewed and was given the opportunity to be the associate dean for Graduate Programs (2012–2016) and senior associate dean for Academic Programs (2016–2018). Throughout my tenure in these leadership roles, the doctor of nursing practice was developed at the Jefferson School/College of Nursing for both nurse practitioner and nurse anesthesia programs. Enrollment in graduate nursing programs increased across all program specialties. As responsibilities in academics increased, my clinical practice went to a part-time status and was completed on weekends. Though remaining current and experienced for many years at this part-time status, I am now the chair of Graduate Programs at Jefferson College of Nursing. While holding these leadership roles, there have been several new programs and courses that have been developed, and I have assisted with or led the development and implementation processes. In summary, do I consider myself a pioneer in the neonatal nurse practitioner and educator role? With humility, I will say I do not, but I am honored that there are those who say I am.

CHAPTER THREE

Reflective Response 4

MARY T. BOUCHAUD

In reading Chapter 3, specifically the section on the history of the advanced practice role of the clinical nurse specialist (CNS), I could not help but look back on how and why I became a registered nurse, my educational journey, my clinical practice, and my sustainability in academia.

The decision to be a nurse was easy; going about becoming one and being accepted in my career has been a life-long challenge. My entry into the profession began in August 1976, when I was accepted into the first 2-year ADN program in the state of New Jersey and into a 3-year, 36-month hospital-based diploma program affiliated with a community college. Because the clinical rotations were 3 days a week for 3-month blocks, I chose the hospital-based program. It wasn't long after graduating, passing the 2-day nursing state boards, and beginning my career at the University of Pennsylvania that I was informed I did it all wrong; to be considered a legitimate member of the healthcare team, to be "heard," I should have gotten my bachelor's degree in nursing. So eventually I *had* to go back to school for my BSN—notice I did not say I *wanted* to get my degree. Every university/college of nursing I investigated said the same thing: "As far as we are concerned, your nursing education does not exist. You will need to either repeat all your nursing courses or take challenging CLEP [College-Level Examination Program®] exams in those courses and pass with an 88% or better." I finally found a university that accepted my college courses and offered 13 challenging exams and three CLEP exams for my nursing courses. Once I paid for and passed all those exams, I was required to take 45 credits in non-nursing courses to earn a BSN degree at their college. During this time, I continued working full time, gaining nursing and leadership experience but still being unable to make changes.

I settled on two areas of practice: community/public health and adult rehabilitation/traumatic brain injury. My colleagues encouraged me to sit for the rehab certification exam and directed me to a prep course. On the first day of the 3-day course, the attendees were informed that a major university was offering a federally funded MSN degree in the clinical nurse specialist track (CNS) of adult rehabilitation and traumatic brain injury. The degree was also in community health nursing. I sat for the certification exam, passed, and completed the MSN program. I have been a licensed CNS in the state of New Jersey with prescriptive authority in adult rehabilitation and traumatic brain injury since 1994 and a certified rehabilitation registered nurse (CRRN) since 1992. But again, my dilemma with being *accepted* for the nursing education decisions I made continued. Dr. Hanna's discussion in Chapter 3 regarding the five roles of the CNS and "title protection" in particular felt biographical, as I can personally and professionally attest to the realities of her cited NCSBN's recommendation "that clinical nurse specialists no longer be considered advanced practice nurses" (Goudreau, 2009).

In my clinical career as a licensed CNS, in the role of expert clinician and consultant, I created the first and only pediatric rehab homecare agency in the state of New

Jersey. In the role of expert clinician and administrator, I was hired as an allied professional services (APS) supervisor in a home care agency to build teams and promote collaboration between the rehab and nursing teams. In all five roles, with an emphasis on expert clinician and clinical researcher, I acquired a $100,000 grant from the Multiple Sclerosis Society to create a home companion program designed to eventually serve as a national template for all Visiting Nurses Associations (VNAs) across the United States. I also acquired a Welfare-To-Work grant and developed a career ladder program for community residents who had been on welfare and now were required to go to work.

In academia, in the role of clinical educator and clinical researcher, 21 years ago I developed a correctional health rotation for senior-level nursing students in an accelerated 1-year BSN program and conducted a 15-year research study related to student experiences in prison. In the role of expert clinician, clinical educator, and consultant, I led a team of faculty and community members to redesign and reimagine the undergraduate BSN curriculum at a major healthcare university. Over a span of 15 years in these roles, I also conducted multiple innovative interprofessional collaborative and community efforts between BSN, radiography, nuclear medicine, biological and laboratory sciences, physical therapy, occupational therapy, and medical students. Although I know these and many other accomplishments came about as a result of my roles as an advanced practice nurse, a CNS, and a registered nurse, they were noticed only as a part of the employment environment and "duties as assigned." Hanna's discussion on the previous NCSBN's vision statement "recommending clinical nurse specialists no longer be considered advanced practice nurses" serves as an explanation as to why my CNS work, though appreciated, was not seen as that of a licensed advanced practice nurse.

I did and still do take the five roles of a CNS very seriously; however, when I began my nursing education journey, I found colleagues and administrators telling me, "You should have gone to school to be a nurse practitioner." The lack of respect through the years for my CNS education, licensure, and practice despite my demonstrated contributions to what Hanna refers to as "complex patient care situations" in both clinical practice and my 24 years of academia has been unsettling. The fact that hospital-based nurses who lack the educational training and licensure can continue to publicly and professionally promote themselves as CNSs because there is still no title protection (in all states) has forced me to refer to myself as a "real" clinical nurse specialist. Yet no nurse can legally identify themselves as a nurse practitioner (NP) unless they receive the educational preparation and pass a national board certification exam. This lack of title protection continues to aggravate me, especially in academia, where I see the valued investment and support of NP programs while CNS programs are no longer offered. The irony is that clinical preceptors are guiding students while claiming to be clinical nurse specialists in the fields of practice where they are working.

Reflecting on my career and on Dr. Hanna's presentation in this chapter solidified my convictions that if given the chance to do it all over again, I would become a registered nurse by starting in a hospital-based program, then pursue my MSN and PhD and become a CNS and a certified rehab registered nurse. With all the education, experience, and knowledge I have today, I would still choose CNS over becoming an NP because my commitment to patient care, patient education, and the preparation of future generations of registered nurses transcends the singular role of diagnosing and prescribing. The five roles of the CNS consistently provide me with opportunities to exercise my professional and clinical expertise, to be accepted and heard, and not only to contribute to change but also be the change agent. Academia is an ideal environment to buoy the fulfillment of all aspects of my nursing expertise as a CNS and a CRRN.

CHAPTER FOUR

What Is Evidence?

MICHAEL D. DAHNKE

"Evidence" does not seem an especially esoteric term. It seems one that most people would assume they have a clear understanding of. Most would affirm that it is associated with knowledge claims, with what we claim to know. It is mostly heard in the contexts of science and the law. Scientists use evidence to prove (or disprove) scientific claims, hypotheses, or theories. Lawyers use evidence to prove the guilt of defendants or to raise doubts regarding the possible guilt of a defendant. But the relationship between evidence and knowledge may not be entirely clear or simple. Evidence implicates certain logical functions. This is because evidence is associated not simply with knowledge but with the discovery or production of knowledge and knowledge typically of matters often not directly before us, beyond our direct sensory perception. In this way, the study of evidence further implicates certain logical functions but also problems or puzzles that may further complicate and modify our understanding of evidence. In what follows, I hope to enlighten the concept of evidence through an examination of its meaning and use and the logical questions it raises.

WHAT ARE THE CLASSIC THEORIES OF EVIDENCE?

As with any sufficiently complex, abstract concept, there exist numerous competing theories of evidence, none of which boasts uncritical acceptance amongst those who study such things. There are some general similarities we can glean from such theories in general. And some of the differences can alert us to the more uncertain and questionable aspects of the concept. As this text in general and this chapter, in particular, is not intended as a complete philosophical investigation into the concept of evidence or an attempt at yet another hopefully adequate and justified theory of evidence, I will forego any in-depth critique of these theories and include them only to the extent that they illuminate the general thinking and problems of the concept toward the goal of enlightening, rather than obscuring the concept.

In his critique of major theories of evidence, Julian Reiss (2015) identifies four criteria for a good theory of evidence. The first two are that a good theory should be both a theory of support and warrant. These criteria point to a fundamental ambiguity in our use of the word evidence, or sometimes "proof." Often when we say that we have evidence for X being true, we mean that we have a piece of evidence that is a sign that X is true but may not by itself establish that X is true. In other words, supporting evidence. So, a good theory should explain how evidence functions in this way. Alternatively, sometimes we use "evidence" to refer to a body of evidence that establishes or warrants the truth of X or warrants our inference that X is indeed true. In other words, "warranting evidence." Thus, a good theory of evidence should also explain this function of evidence. Reiss (2015) explains the distinction with the example of a crime scene in which two different sets of fingerprints are found. Each set of prints provides support for the belief that the owner of the fingerprints committed the crime. However, with two (at least two) alternative accounts of the crime, neither set of prints is sufficient warrant to believe that either suspect definitely committed the crime. Although support and warrant are related, they are distinct. Support is more fundamental and a necessary condition for warrant, and it is possible to have support absent warrant. And both are necessary elements of a complete theory of evidence: "A theory of evidence that didn't tell us about support would be impracticable; a theory that didn't tell us about warrant would not be useful" (Reiss, 2015, p. 36). The third criterion is that a good theory should apply to nonideal cases. "A practicable theory must be able to count as evidence that which has been produced under the conditions in which typical scientists find themselves …" (Reiss, 2015, p. 36). Science is often conducted in nonideal circumstances, lacking complete control over conditions and variables or lacking complete background knowledge. A theory of evidence that only enlightened ideal cases would not be very practical. It is one thing for a theory to make sense in a merely theoretical manner. But if it only applies to theoretically ideal or perfect cases, then it has limited application for actual scientific activities. Last, a theory of evidence should be descriptively adequate. By "descriptively adequate," Reiss (2015) means consistent with the practical activity and evidentiary assessments of actual scientists: "it should … regard as evidence what practicing scientists regard as evidence and confer assessments on hypotheses roughly in line with practice" (Reiss, 2015, p. 36). In Reiss's (2015) criteria we see an emphasis on avoiding a theory-practice gap. From this perspective, theory should not simply describe the conceptual reality of an idea, but it should align closely with the use-value of that concept in the real world. Let us now review a few of the classic theories of evidence.

If we look to the beginning of the scientific revolution, with the work of Francis Bacon (2019), we see a decidedly simple approach to evidence through conceptualization and implementation of inductive reasoning. To hypothesize on the cause of heat, Bacon (2019) merely created a list of items that contained heat (fire, the sun, living bodies) and a contrasting list of items that lacked heat (ice, the cold ground, etc.). From these two lists, he abstracted what was common in the first list and what was lacking in the second. The problem here is that this method lacks practical selectivity. Each list could continue indefinitely, if not infinitely, before we know that we have an adequate sample to abstract from. Despite this problem, Bacon's conclusion, that heat is motion, is surprisingly consistent with our current understanding of heat. Applying Reiss's (2015) criteria, this theory of evidence appears to function generally as a theory of support but is left wanting in terms of a theory of warrant. The perceived connection between the indicated evidence and the conclusion leaves open the possibility of various logical connections beyond the assumed one.

In the 19th century British philosopher John Stuart Mill, although known more for his work in ethics and political philosophy, seemingly built upon Bacon's insights on evidence in an attempt to better understand and provide a logical foundation for inductive reasoning in his *A System of Logic: Ratiocinative and Inductive* (2015). In this work, Mill formulated what he called "methods of experimental inquiry" and what are now commonly referred to as "Mill's methods." These are essentially inductive inferential techniques that provide analytical clarity to the various types of inferences to be made in the course of experimental science. These include the method of agreement, the method of difference, the joint method of agreement and difference, the method of residues, and the method of concomitant variation. These "methods" are techniques for assuring the quality of inductive inferences, particularly in terms of causation. In doing so, they similarly formulate several distinct and discrete functions of evidence. The first three methods are reflective of Bacon's approach, but they are developed with greater sophistication beyond mere enumeration and are extended with the addition of the last two methods.

According to the method of agreement, in investigating different instances of a particular effect, when we find one antecedent event, action, condition, or circumstance (what Mill simply calls an "antecedent") in common among these different instances, then we can infer that this common element is the causal factor that results in the effect under investigation. The fact that this antecedent is present or precedes all instances of this phenomenon is evidence of its causal nature. In investigating the cause of a disease like acquired immune deficiency syndrome, for example, we discover that all persons suffering from this disease test positive for the human immunodeficiency virus. From this, we might infer that HIV is likely the cause of AIDS.

The method of difference identifies a distinction between cases in which the effect to be studied occurs and when it does not. If the cases in which it does occur have a preceding factor or event in common that is lacking from cases in which it does not occur, that points to this element missing in the latter cases as a causal factor in the former cases. If one finds a broken window in one's house but all other windows intact and beneath the broken window is found a baseball, it is reasonable to infer that a baseball in flight was the cause of the broken window, as no baseballs are found near the intact windows. Copi et al. (2014) provide a historical example, exhibiting questionable research ethics as well, from the determination of yellow fever as transmitted by mosquitos. A room was divided with a mosquito-proof screen. On one side were two volunteers and no mosquitoes. On the other fifteen yellow fever-infected mosquitoes were released with one volunteer. The mosquito-side volunteer soon developed yellow fever while the others did not.

The joint method of agreement and difference, as it sounds, combines the first two methods. The fact that this is included as a distinct method makes clear that Mill understands the limitations of inductive reasoning, that neither the agreement nor the difference method proves causality, but both together provide stronger reasoning (though still not absolute proof) than either by itself.

The method of residues relies upon knowledge of certain preceding or existing causes to infer a newly understood cause. In a complex event or effect in which we know the causes of some parts of the event but not some other particular part, we can look to the antecedent events to discount the known causes. Whatever is left in the antecedent event (the residue) is the cause of this other part of the event. A simple example is that of calculating the cargo of a truck by weighing the loaded truck and subtracting the weight of the truck when empty (Copi et al., 2014). The discovery of the planet Neptune presents a real-world example of this method. When the movement of the planet Uranus did not meet the expected movement based upon calculations that functioned for all other planets, it was inferred that the discrepancy was caused by an undiscovered planet, which turned out to be Neptune (Copi et al., 2014).

The first four methods are eliminative, meaning that the inference involves the total elimination of some particular factor or factors. However, experience has demonstrated that the world is not always so neat and clean. Factors involved are not always wholly eliminated. This is where the method of concomitant variation is useful. In this method, it is observed that the increase of a particular factor is accompanied by the concomitant increase or decrease of some other factor. Mill (2017) provides the example of heat and its effects on physical matter. Since heat cannot be entirely removed from a body of matter, the first four methods are impracticable. But what we can observe is that an increase in heat is accompanied by the expansion of bodies, while contraction of bodies accompanies a decrease in heat, leading to the conclusion that heat causes expansion in bodies.

Though conceptually and theoretically a significant step forward from Bacon's induction, Mill's view of induction and evidence also has some severe limitations. First, Mill seems to oversimplify the type of situations we might be investigating from a scientific point of view, assuming that cases can easily be compared in reference to a single similarity or difference. The method also ignores the role of assumptions and preexisting knowledge in the testing and development of scientific knowledge. In the yellow fever case, for example, mosquitoes as a possible cause is not something happened upon by chance or through a mere arbitrary selection (Copi et al., 2014). There is a reason someone thought to test mosquitoes. That reasoning seems elided in this method. In terms of Reiss's (2015) criteria, this raises questions of the third and fourth: non ideal practicality and descriptive adequacy.

In the 20th century, philosophers attempted to address the latter problem with Mill's methods as well as the selectivity problem of Bacon's method through development of hypothetico-deductivism, an approach to understanding evidence and its function in the scientific process put forth by the logical positivist school of philosophy (Hempel, 2000). We begin with a phenomenon to be explained. A hypothesis meant to explain it is put forth based on antecedent knowledge and inferences. This hypothesis is tested by logically deducing what would and would not follow if that hypothesis were true. Evidence then are those predictions that either affirm or fail to affirm the given hypothesis. Suppose that you pick up your television remote, point it at the television, press the power button, and nothing happens. Anyone with experience with modern electronics knows that there are several possible problems here but only a few of which a layman will likely be able to address. This background knowledge helps to formulate our next steps forward. One possibility is that the batteries in the remote control are dead. This model of remote control has no indicator for power in the batteries outside of the device itself functioning or not. So, you formulate the hypothesis that the TV did not turn on because the remote-control batteries are dead. If this hypothesis is true, then, also due to background knowledge, there are a couple of predictions that you can make. One is that if you remove the batteries and place them in another device that takes the same type and number of batteries, then you would expect that device also not to turn on. The inability of this new device to turn on is evidence in favor of the hypothesis. Alternatively, you could put a set of fresh batteries in the remote control and expect, if your hypothesis is true, that the remote control will now turn on the TV. However, if these predictions do not bear out, then your hypothesis may not be true. You may need then to explore and test other hypotheses, such as whether the television is plugged in or whether there is a power outage in your area. Despite the attempts by logical positivists to ground induction with greater certainty, this method has the limitations of all other forms of induction. But it has another limitation in terms of elimination of hypotheses. It is assumed that a failed test is deductive proof against a hypothesis. However, even this is not so clear or certain. If you test the batteries by placing fresh ones in the remote control and find that the device still does not function, there is a possibility that those fresh batteries are faulty. Thus, it could still be true that the problem you are having is one of dead batteries, despite this apparent evidence dismissing that hypothesis. The other test seems more certain in a practical sense. If you place your presumed dead batteries in another device, and that device works, that appears to be strong evidence against your dead battery hypothesis. However, there is still some small room for error.

The alternative device may require less power, and there may be just enough power left in those batteries to power the alternative device but not the remote control. And while strictly speaking, it may not be true that the batteries are "dead" (i.e., wholly drained of power), it may still be true that the remote control failed to turn on the television due to a lack of sufficient power in the batteries. These types of problems point to once again an issue with Reiss's (2015) third criterion.

The Bayesian theory of evidence utilizes the probability formula known as Bayes' theorem to formulate data as knowledge (Howson & Urbach, 2006; Reiss, 2015). According to the Bayesian theory, if there is greater probability that a hypothesis is true, given a particular fact or datum than absent that fact, then that fact is evidence. Consider the hypothesis that a high-fat diet leads to an increase in serum cholesterol. There is a greater probability that this is true when we have instances of persons with high serum cholesterol who have maintained a diet high in fat. Thus, those instances of persons in which a high-fat diet and high serum cholesterol correlate would count as evidence. According to Reiss's (2015) evaluation, the Bayesian theory of evidence provides a criterion of relevance and functions as a theory of support but not one of warrant. In other words, it allows us to determine which facts can be scientifically claimed more likely to be true but are "not in [themselves] a good reason to infer it" (p. 38).

None of these classic theories of evidence faultlessly explains how evidence functions in a scientific context. Thus, this is a question that philosophers of science are still examining and developing new theories for, though these theories are mostly refinements, emendations, and combinations of the above classic theories, including Reiss's (2015) own a posteriori hypothetico-deductivism. Let us now explore a more pointed question on the essence of evidence.

IS EVIDENCE KNOWLEDGE?

My initial impulse is to provide a stereotypically frustrating philosophical answer of "yes and no" to this question. Unfortunately, in the short term, this is as accurate an answer as I can muster. So, let us explore the "yes" and the "no" of it more fully.

Let us consider examples of evidence. Anyone who has watched a crime procedural or read an Agatha Christie story is familiar with various types of evidence related to criminal investigation. The most classic of these is the fingerprint. Fingerprints are of course the patterned, oily remnants of a person's fingers that remain after touching an object. But is that truly what a fingerprint is? In one sense, yes. But these fingerprints are typically invisible to the naked eye. And for that reason, they are, by themselves, useless to the investigative process. Alternatively, what we might mean by "fingerprints" are the lifted (and reversed) images taken by investigators and made to be visible and useful for investigative purposes. The term "fingerprint" might be used to apply to either of these, yet, of course, there is an essential relationship between the two. The former can exist (but an existence left unknown) without the latter, but the latter cannot exist without the former. Despite (or perhaps due to) the usefulness of the latter, there is a certain artifice to it which includes a reflection (reinforced by the mirror-reversal) of nature, of reality, of the former type of fingerprint. What I mean by "artifice" is that the fingerprint that is conceptualized as evidence is a lifted creation of human activity. It is separate, though essentially related to, the natural fingerprint that exists on an object.

Let us consider a scientific example. Pharmaceutical company Anciana is developing a new medication to treat rheumatoid arthritis. The new medication is now in Phase III. A double-blind study is performed on a screened selection of patients suffering from rheumatoid arthritis comparing the new medication with existing medications. As part of this trial, a battery of information will be collected from each patient in a regular, systematic manner. Such information could include vital measurements such as blood pressure and heart rate. It could include blood tests to determine elimination rate. It could include self-reporting of adverse events. This information is collected as data and could qualify as evidence. This information refers back to the reality of what occurs in the study but, as evidence, it exists abstractly as raw data.

A nursing researcher is investigating the effect of caffeine-reduction on the quality of sleep of persons with HIV (Dreher, 2000). The researcher gathers a group of 80 self-selected, qualified subjects who meet the study criteria. At the beginning of the study, each subject completes a Caffeine Intake Survey to estimate individual daily intake of caffeine. The subjects were then to maintain a Caffeine Tracking Diary to record all caffeine intake and a Compliance Form to determine the adherence to abstinence for the experimental group. These and other data gathered through the course of this study will function as evidence. Again, the evidence is the abstract information that refers back to the natural events that occur, rather than the natural events themselves.

But does the evidence indicated in these three examples qualify as knowledge? From a certain perspective, yes, but from a low level of what we mean by knowledge.

WHAT DO WE MEAN BY "KNOWLEDGE"?

The classic understanding of knowledge is the Platonic definition of "justified true belief." Granted, this is not a perfect definition. It famously fails Gettier's (1963) challenges. However, I will ignore that problem here for three reasons. Despite the failure of Gettier's challenges, it is still the most widely referred to definition of knowledge. Those challenges are, arguably, of a limited and artificial sort. And this definition and Gettier's challenges have been analyzed, investigated, and studied in countless books, journal articles, and conference proceedings. This is not the place to further that already voluminous discourse.

I present here merely a brief analysis of the Platonic definition to ensure collective understanding. First, knowledge refers to a belief. This means that knowledge is an internal, cognitive state, a state of affirming a proposition about the world. In this sense, if we take the forms of data above strictly, they cannot qualify as knowledge. As data that exist external to our minds, they cannot themselves be knowledge. However, our apprehension of them may instead qualify as knowledge. Second, knowledge is belief that is true. This aspect seems quite intuitive. If we claim to know something that is false, it seems mistaken to consider that as knowledge. If I believe that Jupiter has twelve moons and that turns out to be false, that false belief can in no way be considered a form of knowledge. And third, knowledge must be a true belief that is justified. If I merely guess, absent any research or presumed expertise, that Jupiter has eighty moons and I happen to be right about that, that still does not qualify as knowledge. If I believe that Jupiter has eighty moons based upon competent research and it is true that Jupiter has eighty moons, then that would qualify as knowledge.

The fingerprint could qualify as a form of knowledge but of a particularly limited type, thus, the "no" of the frustrating philosophical answer. Our apprehension of the lifted fingerprint manifests in the cognitive state of belief that the pattern of a particular finger was found on a particular object. If that belief is true and justified, it can be conceived as a knowledge claim. But I call this a limited type of knowledge because that knowledge is highly specific and far from our practical goal. We are after knowledge that is broader and of greater use: Who committed this crime? The fingerprint then can become evidence (supporting evidence) that a particular person was present at the crime scene. This brings us closer to what we are after.

The data retrieved from the patients in the pharmaceutical study or the sleep and caffeine study will work similarly. As data, it qualifies as particularized bits of knowledge, assuming belief, truth, and justification. But each datum by itself is not very useful knowledge. What it points to in its function as evidence provides more useful knowledge.

Of course, my analysis here of the scientific examples suffers from oversimplification on several levels, not least of which is that evidence from a single study may not be sufficient to truly point to a belief (true or not) that is justified. Science is a fallibilistic and self-correcting enterprise and experiments and studies require replication to better ensure actual or accepted knowledge. Thus, with such caveats in mind, we can say that what we call evidence can qualify as knowledge, but of a limited form and without the ultimate use-value that we typically are pursuing.

THE LOGIC OF EVIDENCE

So, yes, evidence is or can be knowledge but not typically of the form we wish to attain. Rather, it points to, or eventually or potentially points to, that knowledge we wish to attain. The fingerprint points to the presence of a person who may be the criminal. Data from the pharmaceutical study points to (or not) the efficacy and safety of the new medication. Data from the sleep-caffeine study point to the truth of the relationship between caffeine intake and sleep quality for persons with HIV. This is where logic enters the picture. Any piece of evidence is most fundamentally a fact about the world. But not just a fact, it must be an observable fact. The fingerprint as an invisible remnant of a person's fingers is not evidence. Once the technology is developed to make that fingerprint visible, then it becomes evidence (potentially). But evidence is further not just an *observable* fact but an *observed* fact. There are many observable facts about the world, but not all of them are observed. The latent fingerprint is observable, but it cannot exist as evidence until it is lifted and becomes observed. Further, evidence is only evidence within a logical context in which it functions to provide reasons for belief. In the context of science, we are typically attempting to verify a hypothesis. As far as evidence is knowledge, it is direct knowledge of observations or self-reporting. They are facts as such. But as such, they exist as evidence only due to their inferential relationship to the knowledge we aim to obtain. This inferential relationship is one of induction or inductive reasoning.

WHAT ARE INDUCTIVE REASONING AND THE PROBLEM OF INDUCTION?

"Generalization," wrote philosopher Hans Reichenbach, "is the origin of science" (1951, p. 5). Any law or hypothesis invariably takes the form of a generalization. Science, qua science, is not interested in the facts surrounding instances or individuals. What is meaningful, scientifically, is that which we can claim about reality in a general sense. One can record that water boiled at 100°C at sea level on a given date and time, but this fact by itself lacks any scientific meaning. To claim that water, *in general*, boils at 100°C at sea level is at once a broader, bolder, and more scientifically meaningful claim. Generalization is a form of inductive reasoning. Inductive reasoning is an ampliative form of reasoning, meaning that the conclusion of an inference adds to the information contained within the premises. In deductive reasoning, there is no information in the conclusion that is not also in the premises. This is why deductive reasoning can achieve logical validity or "proof" in the mathematical sense. Because inductive reasoning, including generalizations, is ampliative, logical validity or proof is impossible to achieve. Regarding scientific investigation, the information-adding conclusion would be the hypothesis and the premises would be the observations, facts, pieces of evidence. A classic example of inductive reasoning involves the color of swans:

1. Every swan that has been observed has been white.
2. Therefore, all swans are white.

Here, the observational facts include the indication of the color of swans observed. Since it is likely not possible to directly document the color of every swan in the world, an inductive inference is employed to infer from those swans observed to all swans. Fittingly, this simple example also provides an initial illustration of the problem of induction. For centuries, this conclusion was believed based upon this type of reasoning. Then, in the late 17th century, black swans were discovered, inspiring what is now known as "the black swan problem," the occurrence of an unprecedented and unexpected event. In greater depth, the problem of induction involves the question as to whether there is truly any logical connection between the premises and the conclusion, whether we are ever rationally justified in inferring a general conclusion from specific premises or whether we can infer the future from knowledge of the past. Eighteenth-century Scottish philosopher David Hume famously examined this problem and concluded that such inferences were based more in psychological expectations than in logical justification. We believe that the sun will rise tomorrow. But our only foundation for such a belief is that it has risen every day of our lives and every day of recorded history. And no matter how many times it has risen in the past, that is no guarantee that it will rise again tomorrow. Psychologically, we associate disparate events together and begin to expect them to be conjoined in what we identify as causal relationships or natural uniformities. Our conceptualization of this pattern is based in habit or custom, argued Hume, rather than in actual logic. British philosopher Bertrand Russell (2013) more dramatically illustrates this problem with the story of a chicken who is fed every morning by the farmer. Eventually, the chicken associates the sight of the farmer with food. And for a long time that association is reinforced until one day the chicken sees the farmer and instead of receiving food, the farmer wrings its neck. The meaning here is twofold. First, the story dramatizes the "black swan problem." The past association of two elements does not in itself guarantee a continued association of such. Second, and a little more deeply, Russell is implying, following Hume, that in our acceptance of inductive conclusions we are not employing our higher cognitive functions but rather acting in a manner no different from many nonrational animals, no different than a chicken associating a farmer with food or a dog associating the sound of a can opener with food. Our inductive associations may be more complex and may cover a wider range of subject areas (than mostly food), but fundamentally, they function in the same manner. Thus, what we call inductive reasoning is less high cognition and closer to the types of nonrational associations that we are not surprised nonhuman animals make.

In defense of the power and centrality of inductive reasoning in science, a group of twentieth-century philosophers known as logical positivists (and later, logical empiricists) developed the principle of verifiability, which reduced all meaning to empirical generalizations. This, in a sense, elevates evidence even further than the place it holds in most scientific and nonscientific discourse. Empirical evidence becomes a measure not only of what can be known in a general sense, but of what is meaningful at all. In the words of logical positivist Rudolf Carnap (1967), "One can know that a statement is meaningful even before one knows whether it is true or false" (p. 325). Essentially, the fact that the statement (which may or may not express a hypothesis) is based upon empirical observations such as the color of particular swans observed or fingerprints found or even self-reported sleep quality[1] means that it is meaningful, even before its truth as a generalization has been established. The primary critical targets of the logical positivists with this restrictive approach to meaningfulness were metaphysical philosophy, like that of Hegel, Heidegger, or F. H. Bradley (Ayer, 2000; Carnap, 1959, 1967). They claimed that this type of metaphysical philosophy was not merely bad or mistaken philosophy but meaningless blather. The positivists were not only attempting to establish the logical function of evidence in the context of scientific investigation but attempting to expand that to meaning in general to eliminate studies and claims they believed to be meaningless but were nonetheless being taken seriously by some scholars. Eventually, the rather strict and narrow views of the logical positivists morphed into the somewhat looser views of the logical empiricists, both of which eventually suffered greatly under the powerful critique of works such as W. V. O Quine's (1951) "Two Dogmas of Empiricism." Quine argued that the severe and restrictive view of empiricism held by both the positivists and the empiricists could not sustain the weight it placed upon itself.

Eventually, inductive inferences came to be understood as probabilistic inferences. From the observation of individual instances, we cannot infer a definite conclusion but only a probabilistic one. This conceptualization in reality lacks complete justification, but pragmatically, it nods to the undeniable use-value of inductive reasoning. Even lessening the strength of our conclusions to that of probability does not adequately answer Hume's critique. However, even Hume admitted that in everyday life one could not wholly abjure and renounce the use of inductive logic. The probabilistic theorem is a compromise that allows us to intellectually retain induction as a valuable tool but not allow it the assumed, quasi-deductive, authority it held prior to Hume.

This problem brings a degree of uncertainty to any scientific hypothesis. We can only hold any scientific hypothesis in a provisional or even defeasible manner. Even when, after sufficient testing, hypothesis moves to theory, it is still held as provisional and defeasible. No amount of evidence will change this in a logical sense, only in a psychological sense.

We tend to have greater confidence in a theory that exists for greater time without being disproven. For this reason, philosopher Karl Popper flipped the logical focus and treatment of scientific evidence from induction to deduction. For Popper (2002), the logical focus of scientific activity was not using evidence to *prove* hypotheses or theories true. Such an endeavor, it has been shown, is logically impossible. We can only provide more and more affirming evidence. But no amount or even variety of affirming evidence will prove, in the strict mathematical sense of that word, a general scientific claim true. Popper (2002) argued that a more logically appropriate approach was to employ deductive reasoning toward disproving a theory or hypothesis. The central question then is no longer, "Can we prove this hypothesis true?" but "Has this hypothesis been disproven?" And with the proper counterevidence, a theory could be deductively disproven through application of a modus tollens form of argument. If my hypothesis is that reduction in caffeine intake by persons with HIV will improve sleep, and one person with HIV who has reduced caffeine intake credibly reports no improvement in sleep, then my hypothesis has been disproven. This has been called falsificationism or the falsifiability thesis. The point is not that a hypothesis is proven false but that it can possibly or theoretically be proven false. This then also replaces the logical positivists standard for meaningfulness as well as a demarcation between scientific and nonscientific claims. As the ability to provide instances of empirical evidence provided a standard of meaning for general claims for the positivists, the possibility of a statement being disproven by hypothetical counterevidence became a standard for meaningfulness according to Popper. This led him to discount certain theorists like Marx, Freud, and Adler as engaging in nonscientific speculation rather than meaningful scientific research (Popper, 2000). The claims made by these thinkers, along with astrologers and theologians are nonfalsifiable claims, according to Popper, in that the "theory" is malleable enough to adjust to (i.e., explain away) any apparently disconfirming evidence. Thus, as a theory, it is designed or engineered to never be proven wrong. A proper theory or hypothesis must be structured so that it is possible to prove it wrong, if it is indeed wrong. Such theories are bolder and take a risk. Good science then requires not just sound reasoning and careful observation but boldness and risk-taking as well. The scientist unwilling to take a risk will not make the discoveries that the risk-taking scientist is more likely to make.

Critics of Popper, such as Hungarian philosopher Imre Lakatos (1970), note that the deductive method that Popper describes does not accurately reflect how science is in fact done. Typically, one counterinstance or a single piece of counterevidence does not wholly refute a hypothesis or theory. Because science is acknowledged as both logically and methodologically imperfect, one simple instance of counterevidence cannot always be accepted as an accurate representation of reality as contrary to the hypothesis in question. In other words, the supposed counterevidence could be a fluke of some kind. So, once again, replication is built into the scientific method to protect against such problems. Also, as noted by Lakatos (1970), scientists tend toward conservatism in relation to changing or rejecting theories. This conservatism does not necessarily imply dogmatism, but instead a presumption that what has worked in the past will continue to work. One simple counterinstance is not enough, psychologically, to convince most scientists to abandon a theory or hypothesis with some history of success. How many counterinstances are enough to justify abandoning a theory is not a question that can be given a specific answer. But after enough contrary evidence arises that it can no longer be dismissed or provisionally set aside, then serious reflection on the propriety of the hypothesis or theory must be considered. However, some of Popper's insights can still be retained. His description may not reflect the reality of scientific investigation in all its specifics, but the general approach of maintaining a theory or hypothesis until it is disproven through counterevidence does seem an accurate, though general, descriptive reflection of science, as well as a reasonable, within limitations, normative understanding of science.

WHAT IS GOOD EVIDENCE?

Doubtless, the concept of "good evidence" is highly contextual. The specific nature of a particular scientific claim or hypothesis will dictate to a great extent the quality of evidence that is needed to support or warrant it. However, at the same time a few general points can be made on ensuring or pursuing quality evidence that is more likely to justify belief in a claim. Let us consider a few of these.

The first point to note is one that has been partially addressed above, what can be called "the asymmetry between verification and falsification" (Horwich, 2011, loc. 192). Evidence against a hypothesis can theoretically refute the hypothesis in a deductively definitive manner, whereas evidence affirming a hypothesis can only add more and more confirmation of the hypothesis but never prove it. This is of course due to the distinction between deductive and inductive logic indicated above. However, also as noted above, this is not exactly how science works in practice. A single piece of disconfirming evidence will often or typically not refute, by itself, a hypothesis. That one piece of evidence may be enough to refute the hypothesis if other background knowledge already places its truth in question. However, for a hypothesis that conforms to background knowledge and that has already been confirmed by other evidence, a single disconfirming instance will not be enough to dismiss the hypothesis by itself. This single instance could be a fluke or an error of artifice. But in general, disconfirming evidence has a stronger effect than confirming evidence.

Second, the predictions of a hypothesis or theory are often indicated as forms of evidence. This is key to hypothetico-deductivism, for example. But not all predictions are equal in terms of quality of evidence. The prediction of an expected, mundane event does not present very strong evidence. But predictions that are surprising, unexpected, even risky, present stronger evidence. This mirrors, of course, Popper's (2000) norm regarding the boldness of good theories. Bold theories take risks. Therefore, the predictions they make are risky, surprising, unexpected. These bolder, stronger theories themselves need stronger evidence and are made stronger by unexpected evidence that pays off.

A hypothesis or theory is better supported or warranted by a diverse range of evidence than a narrow and repetitive set of data (Horwich, 2011). This relates back to the prior standard of boldness and risk in that a hypothesis supported by more diverse evidence is both less likely a fluke and more likely to be true given that it is tested or supported from a variety of angles. It then likely applies also to a broader, more meaningful circumstance. If we test a new medicine among a narrow range of people, its breadth and efficacy are less established than were we to study a broad and diverse group of people. If Galileo's experiments regarding motion had only ever been conducted on cannonballs, the conclusions would not be as broad, meaningful, or justified as when conducted on various types of matter.

Supporting, possibly even warranting, evidence can be found for even false theories and hypotheses. Consider discarded theories in the history of science like phlogiston, geocentrism, or miasma. These theories were not complete contrivances. There existed reasons, that is, evidence, for believing each of them. In some cases there was arguably even warrant to believe them and at the time greater warrant even than to believe their presumably more accurate contemporary counterparts. The existence of phlogiston, the undetectable, theoretical substance believed in the 18th century to be that which allows substances to burn, was supported by the fact that substances such as wood weighed less after burning than before and that phlogisticated (phlogiston-rich) air (in reality, deoxygenated air) suffocated animals (Grant, 2006). However, proponents of the theory ran into a problem because phlogiston was also used to explain the phenomenon of rusting metal. It was believed that metal rusted due to loss of phlogiston. Yet it was discovered that unlike wood ash and wood, the rust of metal weighs more (though less dense, has more mass) than the metal itself. This would seem to contradict the theory. If scientists were to respond strictly as the positivists or Popper would hold, then the phlogiston theory should be discarded immediately. However, proponents of the theory attempted to retain it by adjusting some details. To explain the rust phenomenon, it was proposed that phlogiston actually had *negative* weight or mass. So, the fact that rust was explained by loss of phlogiston was retained because the loss of a substance with negative mass would presumably increase rather than decrease mass. There are of course a number of problems with this explanation. The first and most obvious is that it is inconsistent with the observation of burning. If phlogiston is still to explain burning as well as rust, it must be recognized that loss of phlogiston through burning results in less mass or weight. Now, it seems that phlogiston sometimes has positive mass and sometimes negative mass. This attempt to preserve the theory merely seems to have created more problems or puzzles. Either we have a profound and untenable inconsistency in the theory, or we must explain how a particular substance can have at different times a negative mass or a positive mass. But even before that, we must explain what it means to have a negative mass and how that occurs. And this bumps up against Popper's (2000) later formulated falsifiability principle. Rather than accepting disconfirming evidence, proponents of the theory were willing to twist the theory until it conformed to this new evidence. Yet, as indicated previously, Imre Lakatos (1970) maintains that this happens in even "good" science. Scientists, as a matter of prudence and consistency, retain a sense of conservatism to avoid throwing out theories and hypotheses overly rashly. And they will even adjust a theory to fit new evidence before discarding it. However, even for Lakatos, there must be a limit. There must be a point at which holding onto a hypothesis or theory in the face of contrary evidence surpasses reasonable prudence and becomes irrational dogmatism, although there likely can be no wholly objective determination for such a point.

The geocentric theory, the theory that the sun and the other planets revolve around the earth, has much common-sense evidence to back it up. To the casual observer, it appears that the sun is revolving around the earth. It rises in the east and sets in the west. Even for the astronomical observer in the past, it seemed patently true that other celestial bodies are similarly revolving around the earth. That is a lot of evidence in favor of geocentrism. When more careful calculations began to be made, however, seemingly contrary evidence began to arise. The planets did not move completely as one would expect given the theory. At times, they appeared to stop and move backwards. Even more than phlogiston, geocentrism is remembered as a symbol of unreasonable retention of an idea in the face of contrary evidence. Although it is often seen as more representative of religious dogmatism, there is a good deal of scientific conservatism involved in the retention of this theory as well. To preserve this theory, the concept of epicycles, intraorbital movements of planets, was introduced. This would allow the observations (of planet motion) to align with the theory or model of planets revolving around the earth. As these observations and measurements became more precise, more epicycles became necessary. Interestingly, even Copernicus's heliocentric model required the use of epicycles, even more epicycles than the preceding geocentric systems, to match observations with the theory. It was not until Kepler proposed elliptical rather than circular orbits for the heliocentric theory that epicycles could be eliminated. Finally, observations matched the theory without the use of artificial, unobserved constructs.

Well into the 19th century the germ theory of disease and the miasma theory, that disease was caused by wafting fumes from rotting garbage and corpses, were in competition with one another. The miasma theory was even the motivation for the inception of public sanitation programs. The fact that these programs resulted in lower rates of infectious diseases then presented evidence in favor of this mistaken theory. The interesting thing here is that this incorrect theory led to one of the most important modern advances in public health and the results of that change then appeared to confirm that this theory was true. Among many other important lessons, we can see from a study of evidence in these three examples that science is a continuous, fallibilistic, self-correcting process. Due to the logical processes as well as the abstraction we often find with evidence (recall the earlier fingerprint analysis), there is a great deal of uncertainty in applying evidence to hypotheses and producing knowledge. However, no matter how uncertain, one other thing we have learned from the history of science and scientific research is that the only remedy for the errors of science is further and better science.

A CONTEMPORARY CASE: IS VAERS EVIDENCE?

During the COVID-19 pandemic the VAERS (Vaccine Adverse Event Reporting System) system, which has been in place since 1990, became more widely known to the general public. At the same time, it became a source of contentious debate and dispute in the public realm. VAERS is a passive reporting system, managed jointly by the Centers for Disease Control and the U.S. Food and Drug Administration, intended to function as an early warning system for adverse events or side effects related to new vaccines. Following the introduction of the various COVID-19 vaccines, the system began receiving reports of adverse events associated with those vaccines. And the system also began receiving unprecedented attention from the mainstream press and the general public. Reports of adverse events in the media became commonplace, and references to these reports in public discourse surrounding the safety and efficacy of these new vaccines became unavoidable. Without a doubt, in public discourse, whether in traditional media or other forms of discourse and dissemination of ideas and information, the data from VAERS was treated as evidence (U.S. Department of Health and Human Services, n.d.).

However, there are severe problems with treating the data from VAERS in this manner. To begin with, VAERS is a passive reporting system open to anyone. It is not exclusive to experts, nor does inclusion of data require vetting of reporters or the data. So, the data, even qua data, is mired in uncertainty and potential unreliability. Second, the purpose of VAERS is not to determine, establish, or assert a causal relationship between reported adverse events and particular vaccines. Its purpose is merely to record and document data and detect patterns in that data. Third, the data that VAERS collects is just that, data. Data requires a certain conceptualization or reconceptualization to be transformed into evidence. As it sits in a databank, it is merely raw data. This data can be collected and analyzed and transformed into evidence in the context of a study with the goal of knowledge production. The problem was that during the pandemic, as part of the contentious public discourse surrounding COVID-19 vaccines, VAERS data was treated, by mostly non-healthcare professionals, as evidence meant to establish or verify certain preexisting beliefs about the vaccines. But given that this raw data is highly uncertain, and it is not intended to function as evidence in itself, any such inferences made will be highly suspect and not warrantable to the standards of modern medical science. This takes us to the last section of this chapter (U.S. Department of Health and Human Services, n.d.).

WHAT IS EVIDENCE-BASED MEDICINE/PRACTICE?

First, a note on terminology. Is there a difference between "evidence-based medicine" (EBM) and "evidence-based practice" (EBP)? There seems some dispute about this in the literature. Indeed, related terminology is not exhausted by this pair. One can also find "evidence-based clinical practice," "evidence-based healthcare," and even "evidence-based medicine and healthcare" (Puljak, 2022). Some have attempted to identify a distinction between these terms, sometimes focusing on the inclusion or not of the term "practice," but of course, even the term evidence-based medicine implies practice (Puljak, 2022). Thus, a clear and tenable distinction between these terms is difficult to maintain. I only see two significant points of difference. "Evidence-based medicine" appears to be the most common term and term most associated with the development of the concept. Second, "evidence-based medicine" carries an exclusionary risk, with the term "medicine" possibly implying the sole domain of physicians; whereas "practice" or "healthcare" implies domains more inclusive of nursing, medicine, and all other forms of healthcare. Since my focus here is on the first, "evidence-based," part of the term, "evidence-based medicine" has a history more grounded in the literature, and most of the literature that I will refer to uses the "medicine" term, that will be my focus as well. But I will use broader, more inclusive language where I can.

The term "evidence-based medicine" seems curious. One would think that all medicine, all healthcare practice, is "evidence-based." And on some level that is true. Even before Paracelsus threw the works of Galen and Avicenna into the flames, symbolically rejecting the dogmatism of his predecessors and contemporaries, medicine was based on some appeal to evidence, even more so in modern medicine prior to the 1990s when the term "evidence-based medicine" was coined. The movement to which the term "evidence-based medicine" refers conceptualizes evidence and its relation to practice in a specific manner.

The term "evidence-based medicine" was introduced in the early 1990s as a normative concept and a "new paradigm" (Evidence-Based Medicine Working Group, 1992; Howick, 2011). As a normative concept, the point of "evidence-based medicine" (and by extension the later variations) is not merely to describe an approach to practicing medicine but to establish standards that should be met to practice medicine (and later healthcare more generally) in what is held to be the best or most effective manner. One of the most common definitions explicates EBM as "the conscientious, explicit, and judicious use of current best evidence in making decisions about the care of individual patients ... integrating individual clinical expertise with the best available external clinical evidence from systematic research" (Sackett et al., 1996, p. 71). Elsewhere, Sackett (1997) defines it more succinctly as "integrating clinical expertise with the best available external clinical evidence from systematic research" (p. 3). The normativity is clear from these definitions by inclusion of the valuations of conscientiousness, judiciousness, and best evidence. The point of evidence-based medicine, then, is not simply to include evidence but to include the "best" evidence in a methodologically sound manner.

As a "new paradigm," the claim is that EBM represents a fundamental shift in the concept and practice of medicine. This is claimed to be not merely a slight change or gradual evolution in the way medicine is practiced but a complete upheaval in the understanding and practice of medicine. The appeal to new paradigms and paradigm shifts is often overused. I will leave it to the individual reader to judge whether evidence-based medicine (and by extension, evidence-based practice, evidence-based healthcare, etc.) does in fact represent a paradigm shift. To the extent that it might, that shift is found primarily in the conceptualization of evidence and its relation to practice. This is presumed to be a shift even from the previous 100 years of modern medicine. Despite the infusion of modern science, until the introduction of EBM, modern medicine and healthcare practice still made authoritative appeal to intuition, unsystematic observation and clinical experience, tradition, and pathophysiological rationale, that is, assumptions based on the underlying mechanisms of health and illness (Evidence-Based Medicine Working Group, 1992; Howick, 2011; Sackett, 1997). Even though this period of medicine and medical research saw tremendous advances in knowledge and practice, "EBM practitioners unearthed dozens of examples where comparative clinical studies revealed that treatments adopted based on mechanistic reasoning or lower-quality comparative clinical studies were harmful (even fatal) or useless" (Howick, 2011, p. 20). However, certain resistant diseases, like cancer, infectious diseases, and new major killers like cardiovascular disease, diabetes, and obesity proved by the 1990s to be too much of a challenge for the old intellectual and practice regime (Howick, 2011). A transition to a higher epistemic standard seemed necessary to make any headway with these troublesome conditions.

EBM recognizes a hierarchy in evidence. The top of that hierarchy is the random-controlled trial as the "gold standard" with comparative clinical studies and expert clinical judgment beneath in terms of quality and reliability (Howick, 2011). This does not mean, though, that the randomized controlled study is the only acceptable form of evidence. The phrase "best evidence" in the above definition is a relative term. In the hierarchy, the random controlled trial is explicitly the "best," but is not practicable in every practice context. Thus, at times the "best" evidence may be that produced by a "lesser" method (Sackett et al., 1996).

EBM proponents have argued that relying on "lower" forms of evidence when "higher" forms are possible has led to harm such as the use of antiarrhythmic drugs following heart attack, which was based upon "mechanistic reasoning" (Howick, 2011). At the same time, however, too strict an adherence to the hierarchy of evidence can result in unreasonable demands, particularly regarding "successful interventions for otherwise fatal conditions" (Sackett et al., 1996, p. 72). Howick (2011) provides as a comical example a satirical, fictional study employing a randomized clinical trial to determine the efficacy of parachutes.

The above points are sometimes presented as criticisms of the EBM/EBP movement, but that is unfair as proponents recognize also the relative value of lower forms of evidence and the value of individual clinical experience and expertise (Howick, 2011; Sackett et al., 1996; Sackett, 1997; Straus & McAlister, 2000). Thus, we see also in the definitions above a balance between external research and clinical expertise. There is no requirement for a practitioner to slavishly follow external research and abandon their own judgment and unique expertise: "Without clinical expertise, practice risks becoming tyrannized by evidence … Without current best evidence, practice risks becoming rapidly out of date, to the detriment of patients" (Sackett et al., 1996, p. 72).

Other criticisms of EBM include that it ignores or dismisses clinical experience and intuition, but according to proponents, EBM does in fact validate these sources of knowledge (Howick, 2011; Straus & McAlister, 2000). But such sources are conceptualized in their proper capacity or context, as "role models, teachers, and intuitive diagnostic agents but not for providing evidence that therapy works" (Howick, 2011, p. 21). Others complain that this is an impractical, ivory tower approach to medicine and healthcare (Sackett et al., 1996; Straus & McAlister, 2000). Yet, Sackett et al. (1996) maintain that much documented employment of the approach refutes this. Some fear that EBM is or will become merely an excuse to cut costs rather than an attempt to improve patient care, but that would not necessarily be borne out by actual EBM-recommended therapies (Sackett et al., 1996).

Whether EBM represents a new paradigm or simply a development of previous trends in scientific medicine remains a point of discussion for philosophers and historians of medicine. Either way, it brings with it both strengths and limitations. It can provide better assurance for both researchers and clinicians regarding the effectiveness of new treatments. However, critics may also be correct that it is not always the best or preferred route for selecting treatment options.

CONCLUSION

Evidence is doubtless a central concept in the study and practice of science. It is not conceptually identical with knowledge but has a complex relationship with knowledge, the production or verification of which is of course the primary goal of science. Having a sound and meaningful concept of evidence can better ensure this production of knowledge. Erroneous conceptualizations of evidence lead to errors in knowledge production.

Given the uncertain and provisional nature of science at its best, we need to then guard against those preventable errors when we can. In science, we will never attain absolute knowledge, but we can still remove the uncertainties that are within our power to remove.

CRITICAL THINKING QUESTIONS

1. What, according to Reiss (2015), makes a good theory of evidence?
2. Are these sensible criteria?
3. Which theory of evidence seems the best model for the essence of evidence itself?
4. How do the limitations of inductive reasoning place limits on knowledge production in science?
5. What makes evidence good evidence?
6. What qualifies VAERS as evidence or disqualifies it as nonevidence?
7. What is the value of evidence-based practice? What are its shortcomings?

NOTE

1. In regard to this self-reporting, what is empirically observed is the self-reporting rather than what was reported.

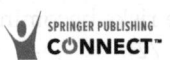

A robust set of instructor resources designed to supplement this text is located at http://connect.springerpub.com/content/book/978-0-8261-8137-4. Qualifying instructors may request access by emailing textbook@springerpub.com.

REFERENCES

Ayer, A. J. (2000). The elimination of metaphysics. In J. McErlean (Ed.), *Philosophies of science: From foundations to contemporary issues* (pp. 28–34). Wadsworth Publishing.
Bacon, F. (2019). *Novum Organum*. Anodos Books.
Carnap, R. (1959). The elimination of metaphysics through logical analysis of language. In A. J. Ayer (Ed.), *Logical positivism* (pp. 60–81). Greenwood Press.
Carnap, R. (1967). *The logical structure of the world: Pseudoproblems in philosophy* (R.A. George, Trans.) University of California Press.
Copi, I. M., Cohen, C., & MacMahon, K. (2014). *Introduction to logic* (14th ed.). Pearson Education Unlimited. https://dorshon.com/wp-content/uploads/2018/03/Introduction-to-Logic.pdf
Dreher, H. M. (2000). *The effect of caffeine reduction on sleep and well-being in persons with HIV* [Doctoral dissertation, Widener University].
Evidence-Based Medicine Working Group. (1992). Evidence-based medicine. A new approach to teaching the practice of medicine. *Journal of the American Medical Association, 268*(17), 2420–2425. https://doi.org/10.1001/jama.1992.03490170092032
Gettier, E. (1963). Is justified true belief knowledge? *Analysis, 23*(6), 121–123. https://doi.org/10.2307/3326922
Grant, J. (2006). *Discarded science: Ideas that seemed good at the time*. AAPPL Artists' and Photographers' Press Ltd.
Hempel, C. G. (2000). The role of induction in scientific inquiry. In T. Schick (Ed.), *Readings in the philosophy of science: From positivism to postmodernism* (pp. 41–49). Mayfield Publishing.
Horwich, P. (2011). *Probability and evidence*. Cambridge University Press. https://www.amazon.com/Probability-Evidence-Cambridge-Philosophy-Classics-ebook/dp/B01GG093GO/ref=sr_1_1?crid=2RES1M4CLKC52&keywords=paul+horwich+probability+and+evidence&qid=1673364742&sprefix=paul+horwich+probability+and+evidence%2Caps%2C123&sr=8-1

Howick, J. (2011). *The philosophy of evidence-based medicine.* BMJ Publishing Group.
Howson, C., & Urbach, P. (2006). *Scientific reasoning: The Bayesian approach.* Open Court.
Lakatos, I. (1970). Falsification and the methodology of scientific research programmes. In I. Lakatos & A. Musgraves (Eds.), *Criticism and the growth of knowledge* (pp. 91–196). Cambridge University Press.
Mill, J. S. (2017). *A system of logic: Ratiocinative and inductive.* Library of Alexandria.
Popper, K. (2000). Science: Conjectures and refutation. In T. Schick, Jr. (Ed.), *Readings in the philosophy of science: From positivism to postmodernism* (pp. 9–13). Mayfield Publishing.
Popper, K. (2002). *The logic of scientific discovery.* Routledge.
Puljak, L. (2022). The difference between evidence-based medicine, evidence-based (clinical) practice, and evidence-base health care. *Journal of Clinical Epidemiology, 142,* 311–312. https://doi.org/10.1016/j.jclinepi.2021.11.015
Quine, W. V. O. (1951). Main trends in recent philosophy: Two dogmas of empiricism. *The Philosophical Review, 60*(1), 20–43. https://doi.org/10.2307/2181906
Reichenbach, H. (1951). *The rise of scientific philosophy.* Routledge.
Reiss, J. (2015). *Causation, evidence, and inference.* Taylor & Francis.
Russell, B. (2013). *The problems of philosophy.* Martino Publishing.
Sackett, D. L. (1997). Evidence-based medicine. *Seminars in Perinatology, 21*(1), 3–5. https://doi.org/10.1016/s0146-0005(97)80013-4
Sackett, D. L., Rosenberg, W. M. C., Muir Gray, J. A., Haynes, R. B., & Richardson, W. S. (1996). Evidence based medicine: What it is and what it isn't. *BMJ, 312,* 71–2.
Straus, S. E., & McAlister, F. A. (2000). Evidence-based medicine: A commentary on common criticisms. *Canadian Medical Association Journal, 163*(7), 837–841.
U.S. Department of Health and Human Services. (n.d.). *VAERS: Vaccine Adverse Event Reporting System.* U.S. Department of Health and Human Services. https://vaers.hhs.gov/index.html

CHAPTER FOUR

Reflective Response

GRAHAM J. MCDOUGALL, JR.

Professor Michael Dahnke, PhD, has written a comprehensive essay on Evidence. The various sections cover theories, what is knowledge, the relationship of evidence to knowledge, logic of evidence, inductive reasoning, what is good evidence, a contemporary case of evidence, and a conclusion.

My research programs consist of more than 25 funded and unfunded studies conducted over 30 years. This reflective essay emphasizes three purposes related to the phenomenon chosen to guide my program of research. First, the concept of metamemory, next the various funded studies completed over 30 years, and finally, the quality of the evidence generated by these studies.

METAMEMORY

Metamemory refers to knowledge, beliefs, and feelings, specifically about memory, including the ability to monitor one's memory processes. This concept was first tested with older adults in 1978. The scientific understanding of memory self-appraisals and the cognitive changes that precede the onset of dementia has implications for the diagnosis and clinical care of individuals in the earliest stages of neurodegenerative decline. The subjective perception of memory loss or memory complaints is very common in older adults, though there is no straightforward relationship between cognitive complaints and performance as assessed with conventional neuropsychological instruments. Deficits in memory performance are often nonspecific predictors of cognitive decline and may portend a future diagnosis of mild cognitive impairment. Therefore, the cognitive complaints of older adults are an important area of clinical research. The three skills often associated with metamemory that are often evaluated are awareness, diagnosis, and monitoring.

THE STUDIES AND SCIENTIFIC EVIDENCE

The studies followed the National Institutes of Health (NIH) guidelines to support the highest quality science, meet public accountability, and maintain social responsibility in the conduct of science. These goals were accomplished by including a scientific premise, scientific rigor, the consideration of relevant biological variables, such as sex, and the authentication of key biological and/or chemical resources. When these criteria are met, other researchers are highly likely to replicate a study for confirmation of the findings.

The scientific premise emphasized the soundness of the scientific foundation of the project, such as concepts, previous work, and data (when relevant). This aspect was fully developed by providing sufficient justification for the project. This component was established by citing appropriate work and/or preliminary data as well as appropriately identifed strengths and weaknesses in prior work in the field. The goal emphasized how a study proposed to fill a significant gap in the field, and, if not, an explanation was offered why this was not possible.

Scientific rigor was ensured by adhering to the application of scientific methods that support robust and unbiased design, analysis, interpretation, and reporting of results, and sufficient information for the study to be assessed and reproduced. For example, in each study that was reviewed, determining group size was implemented a priori, analyzing anticipated results, methods to reduce bias were implemented, in clinical trials, ensuring independent and blinded measurements, improving precision and reducing variability. Other measures operationalized were focused on including or excluding research subjects, and managing missing data.

Biological variables, specifically sex, were stated in all studies, as were all biological variables, relevant to the research, such as sex, age, source, weight, or genetic strain when the question required this information. The relevant biological variables were controlled or factored into the study design when appropriate.

In my study designs, enough subjects were provided to inform the presence or absence of sex differences. Statistically powered comparisons between sexes were a strong consideration in the studies. If sex differences were known not to exist, a strong justification should be provided if the application proposes to study one sex. If sex differences are known, experiments should be designed with appropriate group sizes to detect sex differences.

The studies were quantitative in nature and were guided by answerable research questions (Figure 4.1). They were designed to be hierarchical and included descriptive, correlational, predictive, and interventional questions. Rigor was maintained regardless of the study designs; they were planned with internal validity. This was accomplished by using reliable and valid instruments that had previous history in the literature on cognitive aging. External validity was possible with one funded study that recruited a random sample.

QUALITY OF THE EVIDENCE GENERATED BY THE STUDIES

The findings and knowledge generated leading to the evidence from the studies were published in peer-reviewed scientific journals. The journals chosen represented a combination of general nursing and interdisciplinary aging research–based journals, such as *Multivariate Behavioral Research, Nursing Research, Western Journal Nursing Research,* or nursing and interdisciplinary journals focused on a population of older adults, such as *The Gerontologist, Geriatric Nursing,* or *Aging and Mental Health*. Other clinical journals often published my research to emphasize the translation nature of studies to clinical populations, such as *HIV/AIDS Research and Treatment*.

In each funded study the major findings that answered the research questions were often the first manuscript published; however, in a multiyear project, such as a randomized clinical trial, these findings were not available until the completion of the study. To maintain relevance as a tenured research professor, unique aspects of the study were published before the study was completed. An example might include unique methods for the recruitment procedures for minority populations. Other examples where an early set of findings might be published included in *Ethnicity and Disease* and the *International Journal of Geriatric Psychiatry*.

140 ■ I: HISTORICAL AND THEORETICAL FOUNDATIONS FOR ROLE DELINEATION

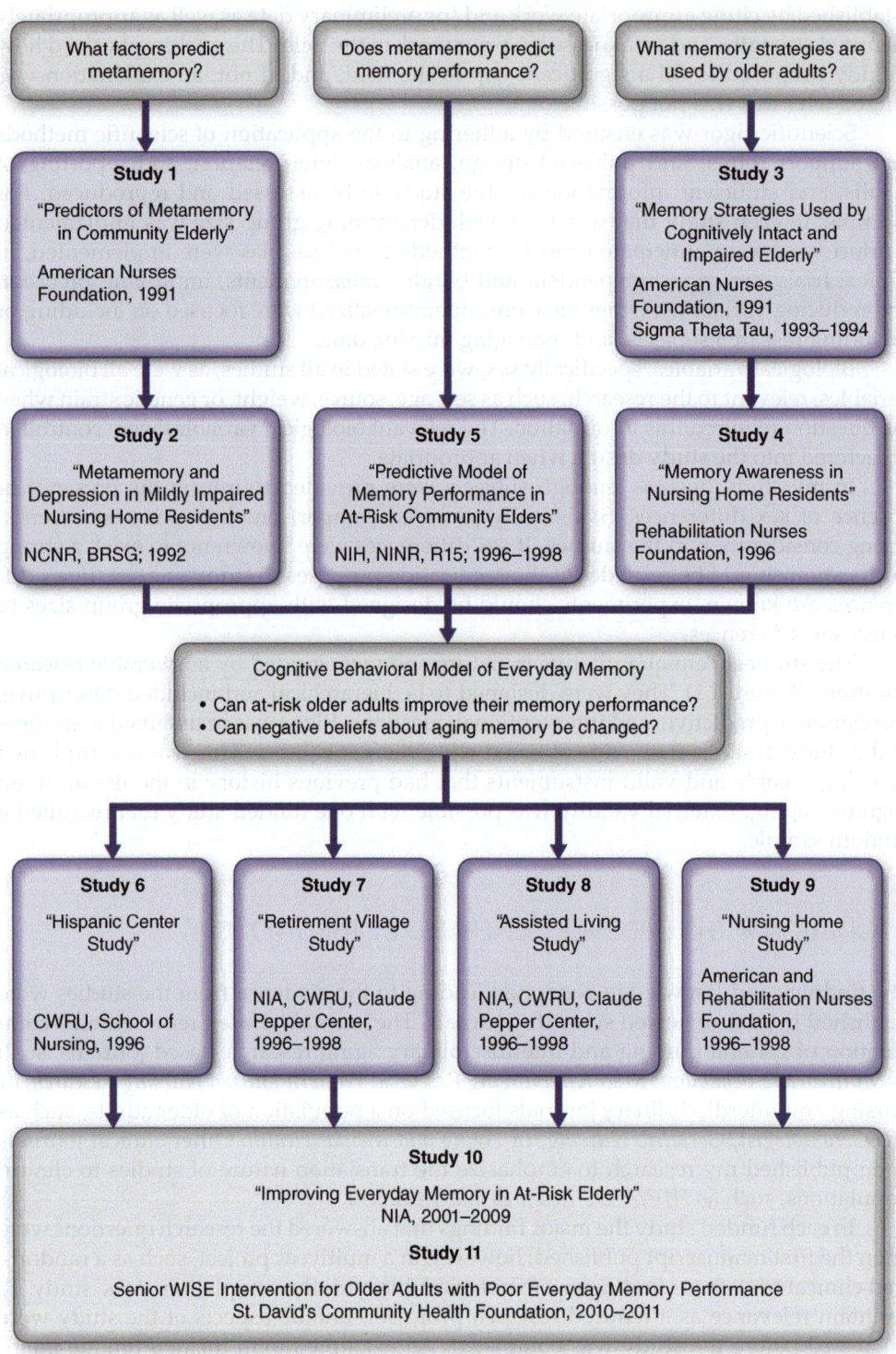

FIGURE 4.1 Funded Programmatic Studies

Finally, the evidence is supported in the scientific community as a product of other scientists citing an individual's research. As a research scientist, our work appears in the National Library of Medicine database and can be searched on PubMed.

In addition, Google Scholar is another user-friendly mechanism to recognize an individual's scientific publications. This interactive site is connected to your university email address. In addition, statistical rankings are continuously updated to this database to determine the reach of your influence.

https://scholar.google.com/citations?user=N01dFRQAAAAJ&hl=en

CHAPTER FIVE

Engaging in Evidence-Based Practice to Maximize Healthcare Outcomes by the Advanced Practice Registered Nurse

CINDY ZELLEFROW AND BERNADETTE MELNYK

On October 25, 2004, the member schools affiliated with the American Association of Colleges of Nursing (AACN) voted to endorse the doctor of nursing practice (DNP). Their vision was to produce leaders in both advanced practice and nursing leadership with advanced competency in evidence-based practice (EBP), quality improvement (QI), leadership, health policy, and informatics (AACN, 2022b). When prepared in the manner initially intended by the AACN, DNP-prepared nurses are well positioned to lead the rapid translation of evidence into practice so that we may address the quality and safety issues that continue to plague healthcare (Melnyk, 2016). In doing so, we increase our chances of meeting the Quintuple Aim in Healthcare: improved patient experience, including quality and safety; better population health outcomes; lower costs; high level of clinician well-being; and enhanced health equity (Itchhaporia, 2021; Nundy et al., 2022).

This chapter discusses why EBP is essential to advanced practice nursing and how it has evolved since it became a cornerstone of clinical practice. It describes, what EBP is, what it is not, how it interfaces with research, evidence-based QI (EBQI; Sherman et al., 2004), and the application of implementation strategies based on implementation science (a new opportunity for DNPs to further their impact). In addition, the chapter highlights what it takes to integrate EBP into organizations, the frameworks and models that help guide and structure the work of EBP or EBQI, and how to plan for sustainability. Finally, opportunities for DNP-prepared advanced practice registered nurses (APRNs) considering the evolution of EBP are discussed.

■ WHY EBP?

Although the United States spends more on healthcare than any other country, our outcomes remain among the worst in the world (The Commonwealth Fund, 2021; see Table 5.1).

TABLE 5.1 2021 Comparison of Healthcare System Performance Rankings in High-Income Countries

	AUS	CAN	FRA	GER	NETH	NZ	NOR	SWE	SWIZ	UK	US
OVERALL RANKING	3	10	8	5	2	6	1	7	9	4	11
Access to Care	8	9	7	3	1	5	2	6	10	4	11
Care Process	6	4	10	9	3	1	8	11	7	5	2
Administrative Efficiency	2	7	6	9	8	3	1	5	10	4	11
Equity	1	10	7	2	5	9	8	6	3	4	11
Health Care Outcomes	1	10	6	7	4	8	2	5	3	9	11

Source: Eric C. Schneider et al., *Mirror, Mirror 2021 — Reflecting Poorly: Health Care in the U.S. Compared to Other High-Income Countries* (Commonwealth Fund, Aug. 2021). https://doi.org/10.26099/01DV-H208.

A strong body of research, including a recent scoping review (Connor et al., 2023), has provided quality evidence that EBP benefits patients, clinicians, organizations, and the communities they serve. It has become a key component of accreditation (The Joint Commission, 2023), reimbursement (Centers for Medicaid and Medicare Services, 2021), and education (AACN, 2021). Many professional organizations endorse EBP as a critical strategy and competency to provide patient-centered, safe, and quality care (AACN, 2021; American Association of Nurse Anesthesiology [AANA], 2022; American Association for Nurse Practitioners [AANP], 2022; National Association of Nurse Practitioner Faculties [NONPF], 2022; American Nurses Association [ANA], 2022).

So why all the hype? EBP has a widespread positive impact, including:

1. Better outcomes for all: A scoping review of 636 articles concluded that EBP improves patient and healthcare system outcomes (Connor et al., 2023). In all, 792 outcomes were measured at least 20 times across the body of literature, with 90% reporting improvement. Outcomes most often reported included reduced length of stay, mortality, and readmissions, as well as increases in patient compliance/adherence. Infection prevention, behavioral healthcare, pain management, transitional care, diabetes management, pediatric care, nutrition management, rehabilitation, and geriatrics care all showed positive outcomes from EBP.

2. Better patient experience: According to the literature, patient satisfaction improves when patients receive evidence-based care (Beeber et al., 2019; Berryman, 2021; Williams, 2022).

3. Lower costs: Healthcare has become big business, needing to generate revenue to keep the business healthy and the doors open. With limited resources and a limit to the number of patients an APRN can see in a day, APRNs must find other ways to optimize revenue. EBP and EBQI are the perfect mechanisms by which to do so. Engaging in EBP and EBQI allows APRNs to optimize efficiency and maximize reimbursement. Several opportunities to increase revenue include increasing Medicare reimbursement and capturing return on investment (ROI) and value of investment (VOI) for all EBP and EBQI initiatives.

- *Increasing Medicare payments.* In 2015, Congress passed the Medicare Access and CHIP Reauthorization Act (MACRA). This legislation transitioned the Medicare payment structure from a fee-for-service to a quality-based reimbursement (Primary

Care Collaborative, n.d.). In addition, in 2019, Medicare Part B payments became tied to quality reporting, resource use, and meaningful use of the Health Electronic Record. Engaging in EBP and EBQI is integral to identifying best practices to be implemented and monitored using quality improvement methodology to maximize reimbursement while getting credit for engaging in quality improvement in the primary care setting.

- *Capturing ROI and VOI:* When evaluating the success of an EBP or EBQI initiative, it is important to capture two important measures of success: the clinical outcomes and fiscal savings. ROI is a performance measure that reflects an initiative's efficiency and profitability (Birken, 2022). The Connor et al. (2023) scoping review reported that ROI was reported in only 19% of the 636 articles included, with a positive return on investment noted 94% of the time.

When engaged in EBP and EBQI, ROI may come in the form of actual cost savings (i.e., you eliminate equipment that is not supported by the evidence, such as incentive spirometers, bed alarms, etc., saving money) or cost avoidance (i.e., implementing interventions, such as a nurse-driven indwelling urinary catheter removal protocol to *prevent* catheter-associated urinary tract infections of residents in a rehabilitation hospital).

The benefits of providing evidence-based care may not directly produce outcomes that can be captured in dollars and cents. VOI reflects the nonmonetary rewards of implementing evidence-based practices. For example, implementing mental health support services to address the rising rates of depression and anxiety in healthcare workers would be an example of an evidence-based initiative that does not necessarily reflect a direct cost reduction. This sort of initiative may, in fact, create a cost increase initially to get the program up and running. However, research suggests increasing utilization of mental health support services by clinicians results in a healthier workforce, resulting in positive monetary outcomes downstream, such as decreased absenteeism and increased retention as well as reduced preventable medical errors (Melnyk et al., 2021). This is an excellent example of the value of an investment. Although these outcomes may not be immediately quantified monetarily, they are every bit as important in reflecting the success of an EBP or EBQI initiative.

When clinicians engage in EBP and EBQI, every initiative's implementation plan should always include a business plan to capture the ROI, potential cost savings through cost avoidance, and VOI. Doing so will justify the investment of resources necessary to engage in EBP and EBQI. (See Box 5.1: EBP LIVE for a real-life example of implementing an EBQI initiative to impact outcomes for adolescents who screened positive for depression in a primary care practice.)

4. *Improved clinician experience:* Research suggests that when nurses engage in EBP, job satisfaction, retention, intent to stay, and group cohesion increase (Beeber et al., 2019; Kim et al., 2017; Melnyk et al., 2010, 2021).

5. *Enhances the value brought to organizations:* According to research, DNP-prepared APRNs bring additional value to organizations (Chipps et al., 2018; Kesten et al., 2022). A study by Beeber et al. (2019) on the role of doctor of nursing practice-prepared nurses in practice settings suggested that employers recognized DNP-prepared APRNs as an asset to their organizations. Employers reported advanced competency in EBP and a sound understanding of accessing and utilizing data as two attributes that have positively impacted patient-, clinician-, and system-level outcomes.

6. *Decreases your exposure to litigation:* There is a second "ROI" in EBP; risk of ignoring. When clinicians are not aware of or ignore EBPs, they increase their personal

> **BOX 5.1 EBP Live: Improving Outcomes for Adolescents Screening Positive for Depression in a Primary Care Office**
>
> Upon employment in an APRN-led primary care practice, a pediatric psych/mental health practitioner (PMHPNP) discovered quality issues around referrals for adolescents who screened positive for depression using the PHQ-9. She discovered psych/mental health referrals were not consistently made for adolescents screening positive for mild or moderate depression despite automatic prompts built into the electronic medical record.
>
> Taking an EBQI approach, the PMHPNP took the following steps:
>
> - Established baseline using the QI data on referral rates and wait times for first appointments
> - Discovered, appraised, and synthesized the evidence around best practices for referrals to psych/mental health services for adolescents screening positive for mild and moderate depression
> - Reviewed the current referral processes and structures for process/structure issues
> - Engaged key stakeholders to gain insight regarding attitudes and barriers to making referrals
> - Amended the referral process based on staff feedback
> - Educated staff on modifications to the screening and referral process
> - Created an implementation plan and rolled out the practice change
>
> As a result of this EBQ initiative, referral rates for adolescents who screened positive for mild depression went up by 62%. Wait times from referral to initial appointment dropped from an average of 15 weeks to 1 week and 1 day. The practice captured increased revenue of $41,000/year.

and professional exposure to litigation. In an ever-changing healthcare environment, APRNs must remain current to ensure they provide clients with the best available care. Engaging in EBP helps clinicians remain current with changes in recommendations and policies around such topics as wellness, disease prevention, treatments, and management, practice guidelines, and legislative policy. Engaging in EBP also means engaging in shared decision-making to bring patients and key stakeholders into conversations as collaborating partners. People are much less likely to sue someone they like and respect. Bringing an evidence-based practice approach to decision-making builds positive relationships with key stakeholders that can lessen exposure to litigation.

Despite all the positive outcomes from EBP, studies of APRNs and chief nursing officers indicate a disconnect in understanding that EBP is the way to achieve quality and safety (Melnyk et al., 2012b, 2016; Zolot, 2016). Findings from a recent study of chief nurse executives and chief nurse officers indicate that the majority invest little of their budgets in implementation of EBP in their healthcare systems (Melnyk et al., 2023).

Studies on APRN engagement are also a source for concern. The literature suggests that APRNs are sometimes challenged to fully engage in EBP due to barriers created by the nature of their educational preparation, the responsibility of their roles, and the environments and contexts in which they practice (Melnyk et al., 2018; Serra et al., 2022; Ylimaki et al., 2022). A scoping review by Clarke et al. (2021) reports that APRNs' implementation of EBP has been low and findings from a national study indicated that

APRNs only felt competent in meeting one of the 24 EBP competencies (Melnyk et al., 2014). APRNs who are DNP-prepared are well-positioned to mentor and lead EBP in a wide variety of practice sites, increasing the chances of shifting our society from a focus on sick care to a focus on prevention and wellness.

EBP: ITS DEFINITION, CLARIFICATION, AND EVOLUTION

Evidence-based practice is an approach to problem-solving that brings together the best evidence (external and internal), clinical expertise, and preferences and values (notice we did not say "patient preferences and values" as EBP has evolved to have application well beyond patient care; Melnyk & Fineout-Overholt, 2023). EBP is not something else to do, but rather a way of being, a way of thinking, a way of doing EVERYTHING. It means approaching every aspect of being an APRN with curiosity and wonder. Academicians strive to raise clinicians who ARE evidence-based rather than those who DO evidence-based practice. The goal is to skill DNP-prepared APRNS in a way that creates advanced competency in EBP (Melnyk et al., 2014), meaning you have the advanced knowledge, skills, and attitudes needed to engage in, mentor, and, most important, lead EBP in your professional circles, committees, collaboratives, practice sites, and professional organizations. Before you can mentor and lead EBP, you must understand what it is, what it is not, and how it has evolved.

EBP, Research, and EBQI Defined

Despite much discussion, confusion still exists between EBP, research, and quality improvement. The following comments are examples of such confusion heard in conversations and presentations and read in correspondents and publications. NOTE: Responses are provided to clarify the difference between EBP and research.

Comment: "Our **evidence-based research** looked at...."
Response: There is no such thing as "evidence-based research," for if we have the evidence, there is no knowledge gap for research to fill.
Comment: "**The sample size in our EBP initiative** was small."
Response: Sample size is not a concern in EBP; it is only a concern in quantitative research.
Comment: "We **did not reach statistical significance**."
Response: Statistical significance, reported as a significant *p*-value, is a concern in research as it is a statistic that reflects the probability that an outcome was the result of the intervention being tested and not something that happened by chance. NOTE: Most healthcare organizations report quality improvement metrics using raw numbers and percentages versus statistics as *p*-values, Cronbach alphas, and confidence intervals.

There must be clarity about the differences between EBP, research, and EBQI so we can utilize the proper models, knowledge, and skills to address problems taking an EBP approach.

RESEARCH

Research is defined as a detailed study of a subject to discover new information or reach a new understanding (Cambridge Dictionary, 2023). Research addresses the question, **"What should we do?"** In the case of quantitative research, it starts with an identified gap in knowledge, an idea about what to try, a hypothesis about what will happen, and a structured, systematic approach to implementing the intervention in question, measuring the impact, analyzing the data, and reporting the outcomes so recommendations can be made. It is often framed around theories and theoretical frameworks to help the researcher connect their ideas to existing knowledge since they are generating new knowledge to fill a knowledge gap that can be used externally (generalized). Research may be done by individuals or in teams. Those who are the leaders of a research study are called the "principal investigator" or "PI." Typically, these leaders are either PhD-prepared or have advanced education and experience in conducting research.

Researchers may apply for grant funding through various avenues to fund their work. Otherwise, it may be accomplished through paid positions for nurse scientists who are part of the organization's infrastructure dedicated to engaging in research to address organizational concerns and priorities, made possible thanks to leaders who are willing to allocate resources to allow this work to happen.

EBP

Most experts define EBP as a problem-solving approach that brings together the best evidence with clinical expertise and patient preferences and values to address clinical issues (Cullen & Adams, 2010; Melnyk & Fineout-Overholt, 2005, 2023). EBP addresses the question, *"Are we doing the best thing based upon a body of quality evidence?"* It starts with wondering about an issue, problem, or practice, heads to discovery, critical appraisal, and synthesis of evidence that exposes best practices based on the literature. Recommendations are then made based on the body of evidence. Once identified, recommendations are implemented, measured, evaluated, hardwired for sustainability, and results are disseminated. Honoring the preferences and values of end users through shared decision-making is also a cornerstone of EBP.

The work of EBP is structured using models of various types: organizational change models, EBP project process models, implementation models based on implementation science, and change theory models. In real-world settings, it is typically done in teams led by an EBP mentor. The advancing research and clinical practice through close collaboration (ARCC) model was the first EBP model to establish that a critical mass of EBP mentors in a healthcare system results in greater EBP implementation and competency by clinicians as well as improved healthcare system and patient outcomes (Melnyk et al., 2017, 2021b; see Figure 5.1 for the ARCC model [Melnyk & Fineout-Overholt, 2023]). Anyone can be a member of an EBP team, regardless of educational preparation, as long as they have an EBP mentor to teach, guide, and support the team through the process. According to the ARCC model, those with advanced EBP education typically take on the role of mentor. Those who have advanced EBP education and hold positions that have budgetary oversight lead EBP by allocating the resources needed to build infrastructure to create and support a culture that promotes evidence-based decision-making at all levels. DNP-prepared APRNs are well positioned to take on these roles.

Historically, little to no funding has been available or allocated in healthcare systems for EBP. Research indicates nursing leaders have a disconnect around the impact of EBP on quality improvement (Caramanica & Spiva, 2018; Melnyk et al., 2016). A recent national study with chief nursing officers and chief nursing executives revealed that little of nursing budgets are allocated to EBP (Melnyk et al., 2023). However, the healthcare systems of those chief nurses who invested more of their budgets in EBP had better patient and nurse outcomes. As a result, this work is often done on a voluntary basis by clinicians who are passionate about it. However, as of late, more funding has been made

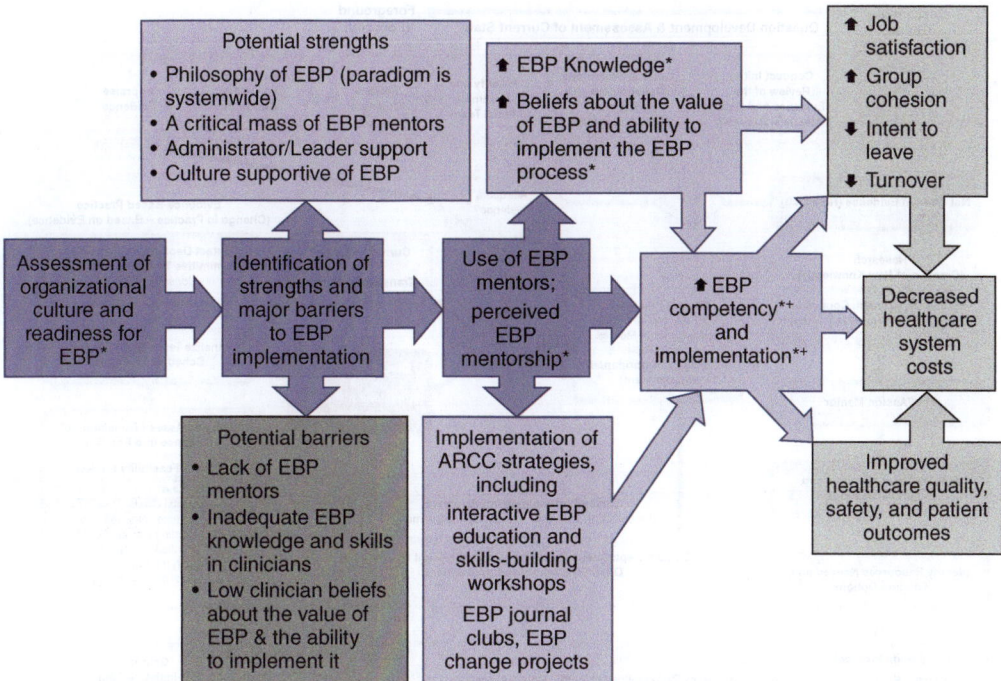

FIGURE 5.1   The Advancing Research and Clinical Through Close Collaboration (ARCC) Model, 2023

*Scale developed

+Based on the EBP paradigm and using the EBP process

Source: Melnyk, B.M., & Fineout-Overholt, E. (2005). *Evidence-based practice in nursing and healthcare: A guide to best practice* (1st ed.), Williams & Wilkins. Revised 2017, Revised 2021.

possible through grants, visionary leaders who have allocated the necessary resources or shifted the work to organizational committees.

EVIDENCE-BASED QUALITY IMPROVEMENT (EBQI)

The Centers for Medicaid and Medicare Services (CMS) defines quality improvement as a systematic process that seeks to standardize processes and structures, cut down on variation, achieve predictable results, and improve outcomes for all (CMS, 2021). Quality improvement answers the question, *"Are we doing the best thing the best way every time?"* It starts with identifying a clinical issue (based on benchmarks and internal data), explores the processes, structures, and environments where care is provided, and identifies why outcomes are not what they should be. However, not all quality improvement is evidence-based, and leaders often do not base their decisions in solving problems on the best evidence. In 2004, Sherman et al. introduced the concept of evidence-based quality improvement (EBQI), bringing forth the notion that interventions, processes, and structures being improved upon should be based on best evidence versus tradition or an idea conceived during brainstorming (Melnyk et al., 2015; Melnyk & Fineout-Overholt, 2023; Sherman et al., 2004).

QI frameworks and models most often used include the Institute for Healthcare Improvement (IHI)'s Model for Improvement (Langley et al., 2009); Lean and Six Sigma Quality Improvement are typically led by quality improvement specialists who are employees of the organization.

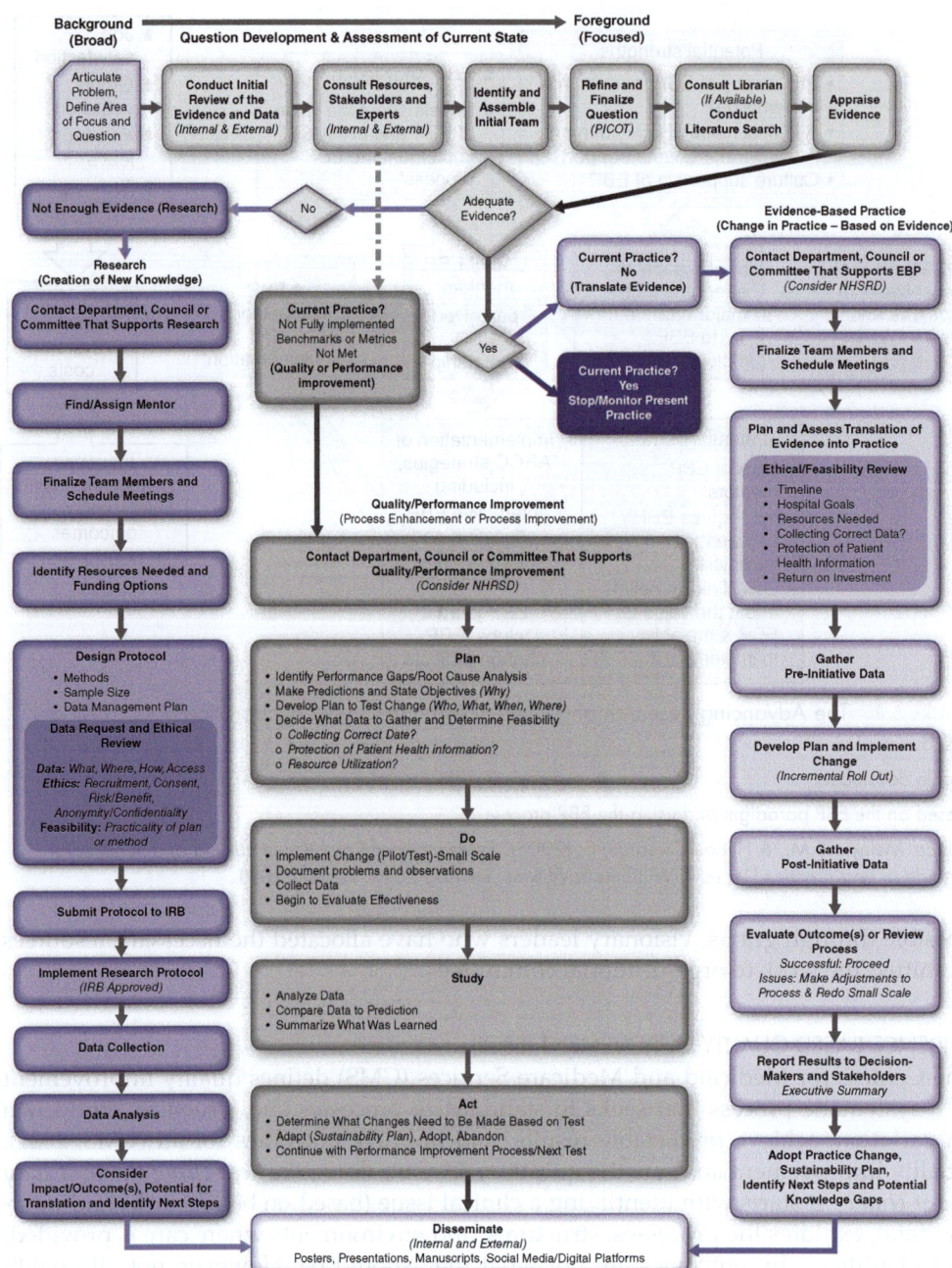

FIGURE 5.2 The Clinical Inquiry Process Diagram
Source: Brown, R. E. (2023). *The clinical inquiry process diagram (Version 4)*. https://scholarscompass.vcu.edu/libraries_pubs/78

The resources needed to engage in EBQI are part of the operational budget, as engaging in QI is driven by regulations, accreditation, reimbursement, and finances. Quality improvement is typically done in teams led by quality improvement specialists who may have advanced education in quality improvement and may or may not be certified as quality specialists. See Figure 5.2 for more details about how EBP, research, and QI interplay and deciding which approach to take (Brown, 2023).

The Evolution of EBP

When the Patient Protection and Affordable Care Act (ACA) was fully implemented in 2014, its goals were to change the dynamics of healthcare accessibility, quality, and affordability. No longer was reimbursement based on quantity; it became about quality (CMS, 2023; Levin et al., 2022). This created an uptick in interest in EBP as clinicians, providers, reimbursing bodies, and accreditors alike sought improved quality, safety, and better outcomes for all.

When something moves from theory into real-life settings, we discover nuances, weaknesses, and glitches that were not seen when it existed in the pages of a book or in theory. This prompts changes to the original theory, model, process, structure, intervention, etc. Such was the case with EBP. Prior to the full implementation of the ACA in 2014, EBP existed in the vision of the pioneers of EBP, textbooks, and academia. The healthcare organizations that were engaging in EBP were often doing so in the context of academic-practice partnerships or as a result of relationships with EBP pioneers such as Bernadette Melnyk and Ellen Fineout-Overholt (the ARCC model), Iowa Model Collaborative (Marita Titler and Laura Cullen-Leads), Robin Newhouse and Deborah Dang (Johns Hopkins model of evidence-based practice), and Kathleen Stephens (the star model). After the implementation of the ACA, healthcare systems began seeking out experts in EBP to help them integrate EBP into decision-making to improve quality and safety.

As internationally recognized leaders in EBP integration and education, we at the Helene Fuld Health Trust National Institute for Evidence-Based Practice in Nursing and Healthcare (Fuld National Institute for EBP) have been privileged to bring EBP to healthcare and education across the world. As such, we have been part of the evolution of EBP, including such things as changes in the way people think about the connection between EBP, research, and EBQI, the definition and language of EBP, the birth of EBQI, the importance of implementation science, and hardwiring EBPs for sustainability.

THE CONNECTION AND INTERSECTION OF EBP, RESEARCH, AND QI

In the early days of EBP, people thought EBP, research, and quality improvement were three concepts that were related but separate. Now, we have a better understanding how these methodologies are interrelated. For example, if not for research, there would be no EBP, and EBP gives us hope that the 15-year (Kahn et al., 2021) to 17-year research publication-to-implementation gap will lessen. QI metrics provide internal evidence to support that there are issues that may be addressed, but QI is most often done by QI specialists who may or may not be nurses and are often not trained in EBP so tend to engage in QI separately from EBP and research.

In 2014, Dr. Lynn Gallagher-Ford created the EBP, research, innovation, and QI alignment model, suggesting that instead of inquiry around EBP, research, and QI being independent of one another, all inquiry begins with the EBP process. If sufficient evidence is available and supports change, recommendations are implemented based on the evidence, and EBQI methodologies are utilized to measure, evaluate, and hardwire for sustainability. If there is insufficient evidence to support change, we engage in research to fill the knowledge gap, implement it, and apply QI methodologies to measure and evaluate the change. On those occasions when we need to take action to prevent harm while research is being conducted, we innovate and measure and evaluate the outcomes of our innovation using QI methodology. This approach showcases the importance of approaching inquiry with wonder and letting the evidence guide your journey. See Figure 5.3 (O'Leary et al., 2022).

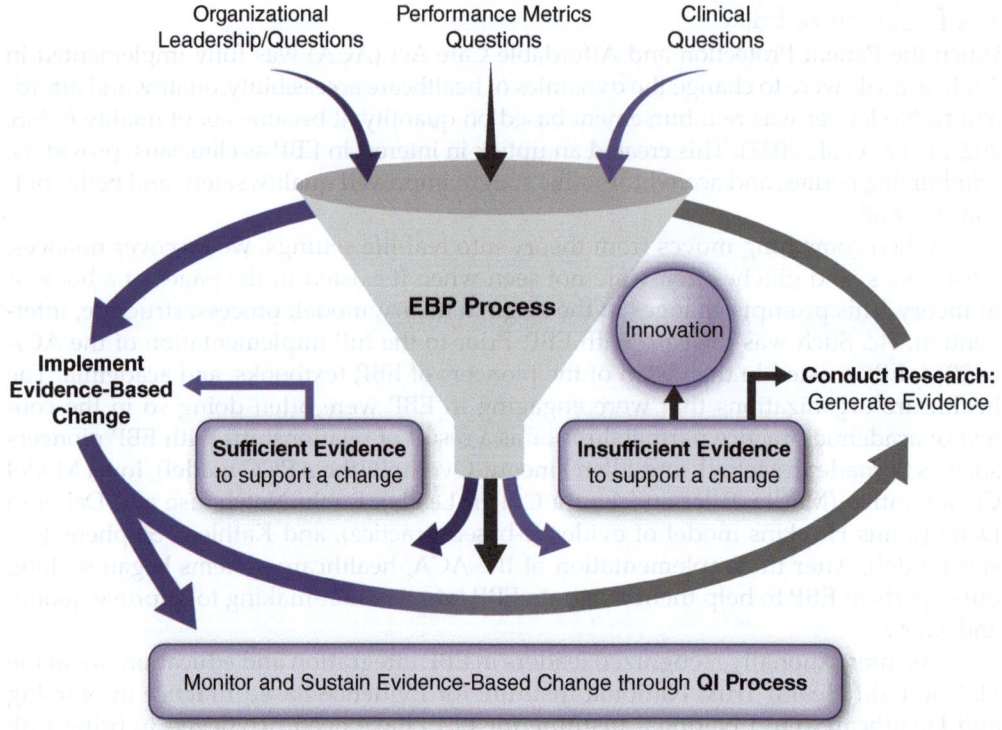

FIGURE 5.3 The EBP, Research, Innovation, and QI Alignment Model
Source: Copyright © 2014 Lynn Gallagher-Ford, PhD, RN, NE-BC, FAAN 2014.

THE BIRTH OF EBQI

As mentioned above, QI does not always start with confirming the "thing" one is trying to improve upon is evidence-based to begin with. Many times, the "thing" one is trying to improve upon is a policy, solution, intervention, process, etc., arrived at through brainstorming, leveraging of power and/or hierarchy, a presentation seen at a conference, or inquiry about how similar organizations are addressing the issue. This sets everyone up to do less-than-best-practice effectively and efficiently, resulting in poorer outcomes. With a heightened commitment to attaining optimal outcomes for all, it occurred to EBP proponents that QI must be applied to best practices, for anything less than beginning with best practices based on evidence will prevent us from realizing optimum outcomes regardless of how efficient or effective our implementation is. This gave birth to the term "evidence-based quality improvement" (EBQI; Sherman et al., 2004).

Like any new concept, many definitions and approaches have emerged. A scoping review of 170 articles by Hempel et al. (2022) went to the literature to find the most widely adopted approaches to evidence-based quality improvement (EBQI). The literature suggests EBQI is a strategy to enhance QI initiative impacts by systematically incorporating evidence-based practices and methods into the QI process. Keeping in line with all three components of EBP (best evidence, clinical expertise, and end-user preferences and values), it encourages collaboration with practice to engage their expertise and gain their perspective. Healthcare organizations stand a much better chance to move quality indicators in a positive direction when they engage in EBQI.

IMPLEMENTATION SCIENCE

Clinicians are becoming more comfortable with the first part of the EBP process; identifying clinical issues, creating a searchable question, searching for, critically appraising, synthesizing, and making recommendations based on the evidence. The real challenge begins when it is time to implement change into complex healthcare systems. Without effective implementation, best practices never get infused into routine work, and healthcare systems lose the time, energy, and resources that were invested to address the many issues facing healthcare. These challenges have sparked the creation of implementation science.

According to Eccles and Mittman (2006), implementation science is the scientific study of methods to promote the systematic uptake of evidence-based practices and research findings into practice to improve quality and safety and maximize outcomes. Understanding which implementation models are most effective in different situations can expedite the uptake of best practices, positively impacting outcomes. Doctoral-prepare APRNs are well positioned to lead the application of implementation strategies based on implementation science to realize practice improvements that positively affect patient, clinician, and organizational outcomes, while further demonstrating their worth to practice.

EVOLUTION OF THE DEFINITION OF EBP

Early EBP models focused on providing a structured process to walk clinicians through the steps of EBP as they applied it to patient care issues. However, in recent years, EBP has become an approach to decision-making in all areas, from bedside to chairside to tableside. Since EBP is no longer just about decision-making in patient care, the definition of EBP is evolving. Whereas early definitions focused on the integration of best evidence from *research*, we now understand other kinds of literature, such as the various types of literature reviews, policy and position papers, clinical practice guidelines, EBP and EBQI project manuscripts, and expert opinions also add value to a body of evidence when they are appraised as quality work. Likewise, current definitions speak to integrating "patient preferences and values." However, as EBP is becoming a decision-making process in all realms, it lends itself to integrating "end-user preferences and value."

EVOLUTION OF THE LANGUAGE OF EBP

Words matter. They define concepts, communicate ideas, give direction and context, and convey sentiments. As EBP is evolving, the language around it must also evolve to reflect our deeper understanding of EBP and the evolution of its processes, reach, and impact.

- *From "patient preferences and values" to "end-user preferences and values":* The definition of EBP holds an opportunity for evolution of the language of EBP. Early definitions focused on integrating "patient preferences and values" into decision-making. However, as EBP has been integrated into clinical practice and across healthcare organizations, it has become an approach to problem solving in all aspects of healthcare; from bedside to chairside (e.g., in clinic visits and consultations) to tableside (i.e., in administrative meetings at all levels). As a result, the definition has evolved from considering patient preferences and values to "end-user" preferences and values.

- *From "EBP project" to "EBP initiative":* Another opportunity for language evolution is a shift from the words *"EBP project"* to **"EBP initiative."** Although similar, both words bring their own unique nuances. In the context of the business world, Indeed, a global leader in pay-for-performance recruitment and career guidance, describes "initiatives" as comprehensive and a means to reach strategic and long-term goals. They go on to describe them as being transformative and a way to bring about positive change in an organization. In contrast, they describe "projects" as a temporary endeavor done to meet a unique and specific goal (Indeed, 2022). Historically, we have referred to the work of EBP as an *"EBP project,"* often leaving the impression that once it is done, it is done, and clinicians revert to doing things the way they have always done them (practice based on tradition). This has created yet another barrier to hardwiring change for sustainability. Using the term *"EBP initiatives"* allows us to change that dynamic.

- *From "PICO(T) question" to "searchable question in PICO(T) format"*: Another opportunity for the evolution of the language around EBP is using the term "PICO(T) question." The term "PICO(T) question" implies that this is a question to be answered. In fact, clinicians and academicians alike will sometimes make comments like "I found literature to answer my PICO(T) question" rather than "I found literature that addresses my clinical inquiry." The PICO(T) question is not a question to be answered, but rather a search strategy that helps identify the key words that lay the foundation for an effective, efficient, quality search of the electronic databases to identify literature that may become part of your body of evidence. DNP faculty sometimes ask students to change their PICO(T) question because the initiative does not align with the original PICO(T) question. It is important to note that the original PICO(T) question will not always align with the final initiative. This is the perfect example of what happens when clinicians allow *the* literature to guide the work. Clinicians begin searching using key words identified through creation of their original PICO(T) question, but once they get into the electronic databases and begin discovering literature, they sometimes discover other terms and/or interventions and solutions they never even knew about. That is the ultimate expression of an evidence-based practice initiative where the evidence has truly guided decision-making.

Once a PICO(T) question is used, it becomes part of the story of that initiative. You may add additional terms, expand your search strategy, or create new PICO(T) questions that address other aspects of an initiative (i.e., PICO(T) questions that allow you to search for the "What," "How," "Who," "When," and/or "Where"), but once you use your original PICO(T) question, it should never be changed. It is part of the story of your EBP journey.

Evolving the language from *"PICO(T) question"* to **"searchable question in PICO(T) format"** clarifies the one and ONLY job of the PICO(T) question: to serve as a search strategy.

BUILDING AN EBP ORGANIZATION: WHAT DOES IT TAKE?

Now that this chapter has covered what EBP is, what it is not, why it is important, how it has evolved and the opportunities DNP-prepared APRNs have to rise and be the leaders they are prepared to be, it is essential to understand what it takes to make EBP part of the DNA of an organization.

Creating an EBP Culture

Peter Drucker's famous quote, "Culture eats strategy for breakfast" attests to the vital role culture plays in the success of an organization. DNP-prepared APRNs are positioned

BOX 5.2 Tools to Assess Organizational Readiness for EBP

Organizational Readiness for EBP Assessment Tool	Citation
1. Context Assessment Instrument (CAI)	McCormack, B., McCarthy, G., Wright, J., Slater, P., & Coffey, A. (2009). Development and testing of the Context Assessment Index (CAI). *Worldviews on Evidence-Based Nursing, 6*(1), 27–35. https://doi.org/10.1111/j.1741-6787.2008.00130.x
2. Alberta Context Tool (ACT)	Estabrooks, C. A., Squires, J. E., Cummings, G. G., Birdsell, J., & Norton, P. G. (2009). Development and assessment of the Alberta Context Tool. *BMC Health Services Research, 9*(1). 234. https://doi.org/10.1186/1472-6963-9-234
3. Organizational Readiness to Change Assessment (ORCA)	Helfrich, C. D., Li, Y. F., Sharp, N. D., & Sales, A. E. (2009). Organizational Readiness to Change Assessment (ORCA): Development of an instrument based on the Promoting Action on Research in Health Services (PARIHS) framework. *Implementation Science, 4*(38). https://doi.org/10.1186/1748-5908-4-38
4. Organizational Culture & Readiness for System-wide Integration of Evidence-Based Practice Survey (OCRSIEP)	Melnyk, B. M., Fineout-Overholt, E., Giggleman, M., & Cruz, R. (2010). Correlates among cognitive beliefs, EBP implementation, organizational culture, cohesion, and job satisfaction in evidence-based practice mentors from a community hospital system. *Nursing Outlook, 58*(6), 301–308. https://doi.org/10.1016/j.outlook.2010.06.002

to build organizational cultures that promote EBP. Key components to creating an EBP culture include the following.

ASSESS THE ORGANIZATION OR PRACTICE SITE FOR EBP READINESS

Before we can move forward and create an EBP culture, we must first assess where we are in the process and what we already have as described in the ARCC model. Several valid and reliable tools exist to assess organizational readiness for EBP (see Box 5.2).

MITIGATE BARRIERS AND LEVERAGE FACILITATORS OF EBP

EBP is the way to meeting the Quintuple Aim in Healthcare (Nundy et al., 2022). However, it does not happen easily. Healthcare organizations are complex systems with many moving pieces and parts, people, personalities, policies, and places where work gets done. This can lead to facilitators of EBP to leverage and barriers to overcome. The most common barriers reported include deficits in EBP knowledge and skills, lack of time, workload, fear of resistance to change, and lack of leadership support (Crawford et al., 2023; Melnyk et al., 2018). It is important to identify both the barriers and the facilitators, so leadership and the EBP team can strategize how to best leverage the facilitators and mitigate the barriers to bring best practices to the forefront.

CREATE A SHARED MENTAL MODEL

In real-world settings, EBP is typically not done by individuals, but rather by teams; ideally interprofessional teams. Creating a shared mental model helps facilitate effective

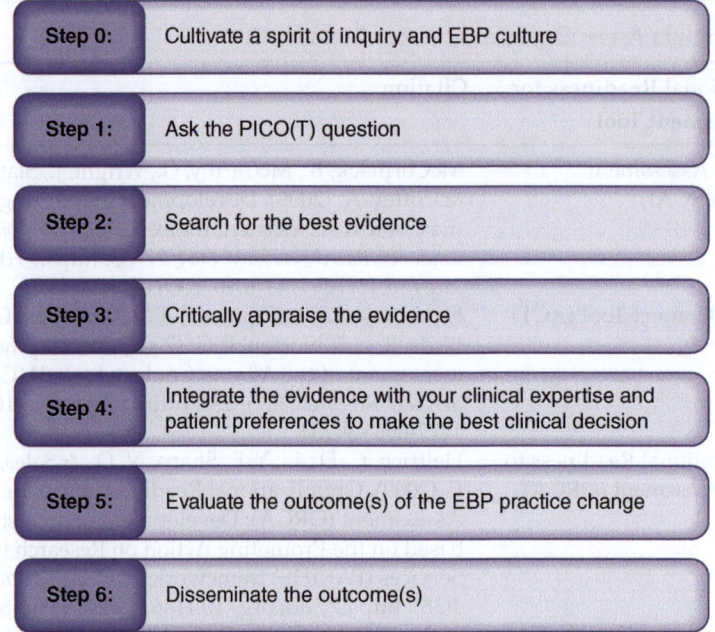

FIGURE 5.4 The Seven Steps of EBP

Source: Melnyk, B. M., & Fineout-Overholt, E. (2023). *Evidence-based practice in nursing and healthcare: A guide to best practice* (5th ed.), Wolters Kluwer.

teamwork by putting everyone on the same page (McComb & Simpson, 2014). A shared mental model allows everyone to understand the vision, goals, and expectations, as well as the processes and structures that will be used to move the work forward expeditiously through effective collaboration. In EBP, creating a shared mental model includes such things as having a shared vision and mission that explicitly call out EBP, an understanding of the organization's strategic plan and priorities, identifying common goals and processes, and agreeing on common models/frameworks, resources, and tools to be used for each phase of the seven-step EBP process (see Figure 5.4; Melnyk & Fineout-Overholt, 2023).

ADOPT MODELS/STRUCTURES TO SUPPORT AND GUIDE THE WORK

Just as one needs a blueprint to build a house, clinicians need models and frameworks of various types to structure the work of EBP. Several different types of models are needed to structure the work at all phases. These include:

- *System-wide organizational EBP models:* Over the years, research has strongly suggested that having an organizational culture and infrastructure that supports EBP is vital to successful engagement in EBP, resulting in improved outcomes for all. The ARCC model, created by Drs. Bernadette Melnyk and Ellen Fineout-Overholt in 2005, with revisions made in 2017 and 2021, is the only EBP model that outlines the process for creating and sustaining evidence-based organizations (Melnyk & Fineout-Overholt, 2005). The ARCC model begins by conducting an organizational assessment to discover what is already in place so leadership understands what is in place and what additional infrastructure and resources are needed. Barriers and facilitators are identified to create awareness, allowing organizational leaders and EBP teams to create strategies to mitigate barriers and leverage facilitators. Next,

EBP education and skill building is provided to create a critical mass of EBP mentors needed to mentor EBP teams through EBP and EBQI. Last, EBP implementation occurs that leads to improvements in healthcare and patient outcomes (see Figure 5.1).

Numerous research studies have tested the effectiveness of the ARCC model in a variety of practice sites across the continuum (Fineout-Overholt et al., 2004; Gorsuch et al., 2020; Levin et al., 2011; Melnyk et al., 2012, 2017, 2021; Underhill et al., 2015). Research demonstrated many positive outcomes, including increased EBP competency, EBP implementation, job satisfaction, group cohesion, quality, safety, and patient outcomes, as well as decreased intent to leave, turnover and healthcare costs when the ARCC model is used to integrate EBP into organizations.

The PARiHS model is an EBP implementation model that also acknowledges the importance of systemwide organizational characteristics, including the use of facilitators to help guide those engaging in EBP (Kitson et al., 1998; Rycroft-Malone, 2004).

- *EBP project process models:* EBP project process models guide us through the steps of engaging in an EBP initiative from start to finish. Some of the more widely used EBP project process models include the Iowa model/Iowa model-revised (Buckwalter et al., 2017; Titler et al., 2001), Johns Hopkins nursing evidence-based practice model (JHNEBP; Dang et al., 2022; Newhouse et al., 2007), ACE (Academic Center for Evidence-Based Practice) star model of knowledge transformation (Kring, 2008; Stevens, 2004), Promoting Action on Research Implementation in Health Services (PARiHS) framework (Rycroft-Malone, 2004), and the Stetler model (Ciliska et al., 2011; Stetler, 2001). Each has its own unique nuances, so organizations should explore each and decide which model will be used to engage in EBP across the enterprise.

- *Implementation frameworks based on implementation science:* Of all the steps of EBP, implementation is often where things fall apart. Discovering what best practice is based on the evidence is only part of EBP. Optimal outcomes can only be realized when best practices are successfully implemented and hardwired for sustainability. Planning for implementation from the very beginning can help set the stage for successful implementation. Utilizing implementation strategies and frameworks based on implementation science can dramatically increase the uptake and sustainability of EBPs (McNett et al., 2021; Tucker et al., 2021).

There are a number of different implementation models, frameworks, and theories available, over 30 of which have been tested using implementation science. Identifying and choosing an implementation framework or model based on implementation science that aligns with the organization's resources, processes, and structures is key to successful implementation.

- *Change theories:* Change is hard, and healthcare is laden with practices that have been based on tradition, some for more than 100 years. Humans find comfort in things that are familiar to them. That is part of why implementation is so challenging. Change theories help us understand how change happens, the phases people go through, behaviors, attitudes, and emotions we might expect along the way, and what it takes to reach a place where change is not only adopted but sustained. Some of the more familiar change theories and models include Rogers' diffusion of innovation (2003), Kotter's eight steps for leading change (Kotter, 2023), and Lewin's change model (Hussain et al., 2018). Being able to anticipate the ebb and flow of creating change within an organization allows teams to identify strategies to help them push through the tough times and leverage the good times.

- *EBP competencies:* One thing needed to effectively create an EBP organization are frontline clinicians who have entry-level competency in EBP and experienced clinicians with advanced competency in EBP to mentor and lead the work. In 2014, Melnyk et al. conducted a national two-phase Delphi study to identify EBP competencies for all professional nurses and for advanced practice nurses. The study resulted in a set of 24 EBP competencies; 13 for all practicing nurses plus an additional 11 for advanced practice nurses and others who sit in positions where they are expected to mentor and lead EBP. The EBP competencies provide a tool to measure EBP competency for all employees coming into the organization, assess the need for professional development around EBP, and measure the impact of EBP education programs. This knowledge can help organizations make decisions about where to invest resources to elevate integration of and engagement in EBP.

BUILD THE CRITICAL COMPONENTS OF AN EBP CULTURE

There are six critical components to building an EBP culture. They include:

- *A philosophy, mission, and vision that demonstrate commitment to EBP:* Having an organizational philosophy, mission, and vision that reflect and call out EBP is essential. Making EBP a visible part of the mission and vision sets the expectation and lays the foundation for integrating EBP into your strategic plan.
- *A spirit of inquiry:* EBP can only exist in an organization or practice where inquiry is not merely allowed but encouraged and expected. Healthcare professionals must be curious as they review and analyze guidelines, practices, policies, procedures, and processes to be sure they are created and updated using an EBP approach.
- *EBP mentors:* EBP mentors are vital to successful integration of EBP into practice. Prepared with advanced EBP competency, they guide EBP teams through the EBP process, helping to keep them on track, pointing them toward needed resources, and giving them the courage to keep moving forward. Building a critical mass of EBP mentors within an organization is vital for developing EBP competency and supporting consistent implementation (Melnyk et al., 2021; Treiger & Kurland, 2021).
- *Administrative role modeling and support*: Organizational leaders at all levels and in all practice settings are critical to building an EBP culture. Caramanica et al. (2022) established EBP nurse manager leadership competencies to support clinicians in EBP using a Delphi approach. These competencies were divided into three categories: leading EBP, building infrastructure for EBP, and promoting EBP. Leaders must not only "talk the talk" but put action behind their words by allocating resources to EBP, building infrastructure within the organization that supports EBP, and publicly navigating and mitigating barriers to EBP implementation.
- *Infrastructure*: To make EBP a reality, leadership must create the organizational infrastructure necessary to support the integration of EBP across the enterprise. Key elements are building EBP into job descriptions and clinical ladders, allocating resources, and creating processes to make them available. Having resources that cannot be accessed undermines EBP. For example, one organization had a medical library at the main hub of the organization, but employees at regional sites could not access the medical library while at work due to firewalls. Things like dedicated time and access to resources such as EBP mentors, data, and electronic databases are essential to EBP engagement. Leveraging academic-practice partnerships is one way to access resources such as EBP mentors and access to electronic databases that may not be readily available within the healthcare organization. Engaging in

these partnerships is a win/win for both academic institutions and the practice sites. Academic institutions benefit as they have clinical sites for students to earn required clinical hours, potential sites to engage in research, and can keep apprised of current practices and trends. In turn, healthcare organizations can gain access to resources necessary for engaging in EBP that they may not otherwise have access to.

- *Work in interprofessional teams:* Just like the African proverb "it takes a village," it takes a team to provide high-quality, safe healthcare and create healthy environments in which to do it. EBP is the perfect shared competency for it is a standard of care in healthcare professions across the continuum and all specialties. When interprofessional teams come together, the unique perspective brought by each professional creates a rich lens to address the needs of patients and practice issues alike. DNP-prepared APRNs are well-positioned to create and lead interprofessional teams engaging in EBP.

OPPORTUNITY AWAITS

As we have seen, EBP is the way to better, safer, higher quality care and experiences for patients, their support systems, clinicians, providers, the organizations they work in and the communities they serve. When we engage in EBP, outcomes, work environments, costs, and satisfaction improve. The literature suggests that APRNs have struggled to figure out how to engage in EBP with the lack of development of APRN competencies around research, EBP and QI, the demands of their role, and the environments they work in (Clarke et al., 2021; Serra et al., 2021). APRNs are the perfect leaders of EBP in various settings across healthcare. They have unique insight and understanding of how care is provided, the environments in which it is provided, and the members of the healthcare team who work together to provide optimum care. APRNs know how to coordinate and collaborate, bringing a commitment to providing safe, quality, person-centered care, and the best patient experience so we can achieve the best possible outcomes.

Opportunity waits for there has never been a greater need or a more critical time for APRNs to become DNP-prepared than today as our healthcare system faces the monumental task of navigating the many challenges facing healthcare post-pandemic. Opportunities abound for DNP-prepared APRNs to advocate for the enhancement and permanent integration of new models for care that were leveraged during the COVID-19 pandemic, lobby to move emergency health policy and regulatory statutes passed during the pandemic that elevated APRN scope of practice and increased billable services to permanent policy (Poghosyan et al., 2022; Snyder & Kerns, 2021; Stucky et al., 2021), and address issues around healthcare equity and accessibility that became glaring during the healthcare emergency caused by COVID-19 (Kleinpell et al., 2022). DNP-prepared APRNs have the knowledge and skills to bring EBP to their organizations. In doing so, they are part of changing healthcare across the continuum for the better.

Evidence-based practice is not something else to do. It is a way of thinking, a way of being, a way of doing everything as you grow and become an evidence-based clinician. To do so, it is necessary to deepen your knowledge, skills, and attitudes around EBP and then make it the norm—that is, the way you approach practice.

DNP-prepared APRNs can change the way we approach healthcare through EBP, EBQI, and engaging implementation strategies based on implementation science. Be the change and let the evidence guide your journey. The time is now.

■ CRITICAL THINKING QUESTIONS

1. Describe some of the challenges and opportunities involved in developing, implementing, and sustaining EBP in practice settings.
2. Describe the interface between EBP, EBQI, and research.
3. Explain how a PICO(T) question serves as the basis for a comprehensive search strategy and guides the work of EBP.
4. What are the key components to creating an EBP culture in your organization?

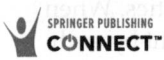

A robust set of instructor resources designed to supplement this text is located at http://connect.springerpub.com/content/book/978-0-8261-8137-4. Qualifying instructors may request access by emailing textbook@springerpub.com.

■ REFERENCES

American Association of Colleges of Nursing. (2021). *The Essentials: Core competencies for professional nursing education.* https://www.aacnnursing.org/Essentials

American Association of Colleges of Nursing. (2022a). *DNP fact sheet.* https://www.aacnnursing.org/News-Information/Fact-Sheets/DNP-Fact-Sheet

American Association of Colleges of Nursing. (2022b). *State of the DNP summary report in 2022.* https://www.aacnnursing.org/Portals/42/News/Surveys-Data/State-of-the-DNP-Summary-Report-June-2022.pdf

American Association of Nurse Anesthesiology. (2022). *Evidence-based practice.* https://www.aana.com/practice/evidence-based-practice

American Association of Nurse Practitioners. (2022). *Standards of practice for nurse practitioners.* https://www.aanp.org/advocacy/advocacy-resource/position-statements/standards-of-practice-for-nurse-practitioners

Bauer, M. S., & Kirchner, J. (2020). Implementation science: What is it and why should I care? *Psychiatry Research, 283,* 112376. https://doi.org/10.1016/j.psychres.2019.04.025

Beeber, A. S., Palmer, C., Waldrop, J., Lynn, M. R., & Jones, C. B. (2019). The role of doctor of nursing practice-prepared nurses in practice settings. *Nursing Outlook, 67*(4), 354–364. https://doi.org/10.1016/j.outlook.2019.02.006

Berryman, J. (2021). Use of EBP as a problem-solving approach to improve patient satisfaction while overcoming the COVID pandemic barriers. *Worldviews on Evidence-Based Nursing, 18*(6), 389–391. https://doi.org/10.1111/wvn.12541

Birken, E. (2022). Return on investment. *Forbes Advisor.* https://www.forbes.com/advisor/investing/roi-return-on-investment

Brown, R. E. (2023). *The clinical inquiry process diagram (Version 4).* https://scholarscompass.vcu.edu/libraries_pubs/78

Buckwalter, K. C., Cullen, L., Hanrahan, K., Kleiber, C., McCarthy, A. M., Rakel, B., Steelman, V., Tripp, R. T., & Tucker, S. (2017). Iowa model of evidence-based practice: Revisions and validation. *Worldviews on Evidence-Based Nursing, 14*(3), 175–182. https://doi.org/10.1111/wvn.12223

Cambridge Dictionary. (2023). *Research.* https://dictionary.cambridge.org/us/dictionary/english/research

Caramanica, L., Gallagher-Ford, L., Idelman, L., Mindrila, D., Richter, S., & Thomas, B. K. (2022). Establishment of nurse manager leadership competencies to support clinicians in evidence-based practice. *JONA: The Journal of Nursing Administration, 52*(1), 27–34. https://doi.org/10.1097/NNA.0000000000001099

Caramanica, L., & Spiva, L. (2018). Exploring nurse manager's support of evidence-based practice: Clinical nurse perceptions. *JONA: The Journal of Nursing Administration, 48*(5), 272–278. https://doi.org/10.1097/NNA.0000000000000612

Centers for Medicaid and Medicare Services. (2021). *Quality measurement and quality improvement.* https://www.cms.gov/Medicare/Quality-Initiatives-Patient-Assessment-Instruments/MMS/Quality-Measure-and-Quality-Improvement-#:~:text=Quality%20improvement%20is%20the%20framework,%2C%20healthcare%20systems%2C%20and%20organizations.

Chipps, E., Tussing, T., Labardee, R., Nash, M., & Brown, K. (2018). Examining the roles and competencies of nurse leaders, educators, and clinicians with a doctor of nursing practice at an academic medical center. *Journal of Doctoral Nursing Practice, 11*(2), 119–125. https://doi-org/10.1891/2380-9418.11.2.119

Ciliska D., DiCenso, A., Melynk, B. M., Fineout-Overholt, E., Stettler, C. B., Cullen, L., & Dang, D. (2011) Models to guide implementation of evidence-based practice. In B. M. Melnyk & E. Fineout-Overholt (Eds.), *Evidence-based practice in nursing and healthcare: A guide to best practice* (2nd ed., pp. 241–275). Wolters-Kluwer.

Clarke, V., Lehane, E., Mulcahy, H., & Cotter, P. (2021). Nurse practitioners' implementation of evidence-based practice into routine care: A scoping review. *Worldviews on Evidence-Based Nursing, 18*(3), 180–189. https://doi.org/10.1111/wvn.12510

Crawford, C. L., Rondinelli, J., Zuniga, S., Valdez, R. M., Tze, P. L., & Titler, M. G. (2023). Barriers and facilitators influencing EBP readiness: Building organizational and nurse capacity. *Worldviews on Evidence-Based Nursing, 20*(1), 27–36. https://doi.org/10.1111/wvn.12618

Cullen, L., & Adams, S. (2010). What is evidence-based practice? *Journal of Perianesthesia Nursing, 25*(3), 171–173. https://doi.org/10.1016/j.jopan.2010.03.004

Dang, D., Dearholt, S., Bissett, K., Ascenzi, J., & Whalen, M. (2022). *Johns Hopkins evidence-based practice for nurses and healthcare professionals: model and guidelines* (4th ed.). Sigma Theta Tau International

Eccles, M. P., & Mittman, B. S. (2006). Welcome to implementation science. *Implementation Science. 1*(1). https://doi.org/10.1186/1748-5908-1-1

Fineout-Overholt, E., Levin, R. F., & Melnyk, B. M. (2004). Strategies for advancing evidence-based practice in clinical settings. *Journal of the New York State Nurses Association, 35*(2), 28–32.

Gorsuch, C. (ret) P. F., Gallagher-Ford, L., Koshy Thomas, B., Melnyk, B. M., & Connor, L. (2020). Impact of a formal educational skill-building program based on the ARCC Model to enhance evidence-based practice competency in nurse teams. *Worldviews on Evidence-Based Nursing, 17*(4), 258–268. https://doi.org/10.1111/wvn.12463

Hempel, S., Bolshakova, M., Turner, B. J., Dinalo, J., Rose, D., Motala, A., Fu, N., Clemesha, C. G., Rubenstein, L., & Stockdale, S. (2022). Evidence-based quality improvement: A scoping review of the literature. *Journal of General Internal Medicine, 37*(16), 4257–4267. https://doi.org/10.1007/s11606-022-07602-5

Hussain, S. T., Lei, S., Akram, T., Haider, M. J., Hussain, S. H., & Ali, M. (2018). Kurt Lewin's change model: A critical review of the role of leadership an employee involvement in organizational change. *Journal of Innovation & Knowledge, 3*(3). https://doi.org/10.1016/j.jik.2016.07.002

Indeed editorial team. (2022, July 22). *What is the difference between "initiatives" vs "projects"?* https://ca.indeed.com/career-advice/career-development/initiatives-vs-projects

Itchhaporia D. (2021). The evolution of the quintuple aim: Health equity, health outcomes, and the economy. *Journal of the American College of Cardiology, 78*(22), 2262–2264. https://doi.org/10.1016/j.jacc.2021.10.018

Langley, G. L., Moen, R., Nolan, K. M., Nolan, T. W., Norman, C. L., & Provost, L. P. (2009). *The improvement guide: A practical approach to enhancing organizational performance* (2nd ed.). Jossey-Bass Publishers.

Levine, D. M., Chalasani, R., Linder, J. A., & Landon, B. E. (2022). Association of the patient protection and affordable care act with ambulatory quality, patient experience, utilization, and cost, 2014-2016. *JAMA Network Open, 5*(6). https://doi.org/10.1001/jamanetworkopen.2022.18167

Kitson, A., Harvey, G., & McCormack, B. (1998). Enabling the implementation of evidence-based practice: A conceptual framework. *BMJ Quality & Safety, 7*, 149–158. https://doi.org/10.1136/qshc.7.3.149

Lewis, C., Horstman, C., & Ramsey, C., (2019, August 5). Evidence-based strategies for improving primary care in the U.S. *The Commonwealth Fund: Improving Healthcare Quality.* https://www.commonwealthfund.org/blog/2022/evidence-based-strategies-strengthening-primary-care-us

Kesten, K. S., Moran, K., Beebe, S. L., Conrad, D., Burson, R., Corrigan, C., Manderscheid, A., & Pohl, E. (2022). Drivers for seeking the doctor of nursing practice degree and competencies acquired as reported by nurses in practice. *Journal of the American Association of Nurse Practitioners, 34*(1), 70–78. https://doi.org/10.1097/JXX.0000000000000593

Kim, S. C., Ecoff, L., Brown, C. E., Gallo, A.-M., Stichler, J. F., & Davidson, J. E. (2017). Benefits of a regional evidence-based practice fellowship program: A test of the ARCC model. *Worldviews on Evidence-Based Nursing, 14*(2), 90–98. https://doi.org/10.1111/wvn.12199

Kotter. (2023). *The 8 steps for leading change.* https://www.kotterinc.com/methodology/8-steps

Kring, D. L. (2008). Clinical nurse specialist practice domains and evidence-based practice competencies: A matrix of influence. *Clinical Nurse Specialist*, 22(4), 179–183. https://doi.org/10.1097/01.NUR.0000311706.38404

Levin, R. F., Fineout-Overholt, E., Melnyk, B. M., Barnes, M., & Vetter, M. J. (2011). Fostering evidence-based practice to improve nurse and cost outcomes in a community health setting: A pilot test of the advancing research and clinical practice through close collaboration model. *Nursing Administration Quarterly*, 35(1), 21–33. https://doi.org/10.1097/NAQ.0b013e31820320ff

Mazurek Melnyk, B. (2016). The doctor of nursing practice degree = evidence-based practice expert. *Worldviews on Evidence-Based Nursing*, 13(3), 183–184. https://doi.org/10.1111/wvn.12164

McCauley, L. A., Broome, M. E., Frazier, L., Hayes, R., Kurth, A., Musil, C. M., Norman, L. D., Rideout, K. H., & Villarruel, A. M. (2020). Doctor of Nursing Practice (DNP) degree in the United States: Reflecting, readjusting, and getting back on track. *Nursing Outlook*, 68(4), 494–503. https://doi.org/10.1016/j.outlook.2020.03.008

McComb, S., & Simpson, V. (2014). The concept of shared mental models in healthcare collaboration. *Journal of Advanced Nursing*, 70(7), 1479–1488. https://doi.org/10.1111/jan.12307

McNett, M., Masciola, R., Sievert, D., & Tucker, S. (2021). Advancing evidence-based practice through implementation science: Critical contributions of doctor of nursing practice- and doctor of philosophy-prepared nurses. *Worldviews on Evidence-Based Nursing*, 18(2), 93–101. https://doi.org/10.1111/wvn.12496

Melnyk, B. M. (2012a). Achieving a high-reliability organization through implementation of the ARCC model for systemwide sustainability of evidence-based practice. *Nursing Administration Quarterly*, 36(2), 127–135. https://doi.org/10.1097/NAQ.0b013e318249fb6a

Melnyk, B.M., Buck, J., & Gallagher-Ford, L. (2015). Transforming quality improvement into evidence-based quality improvement: A key solution to improve healthcare outcomes. [Ed.] *Worldviews on Evidence-based Nursing*, 12(5), 251–252. https://doi.org/10.1111/wvn.12112

Melnyk, B. M., & Fineout-Overholt, E. (2005). *Evidence-based practice in nursing and healthcare: A guide to best practice* (1st ed.) Williams & Wilkins.

Melnyk, B., M., & Fineout-Overholt, E. (2023). *Evidence-based practice in nursing and healthcare: A guide to best practice* (5th ed.) Wolters Kluwer.

Melnyk, B. M., Fineout-Overholt, E., Gallagher-Ford, L., & Kaplan, L. (2012b). The state of evidence-based practice in US nurses: Critical implications for nurse leaders and educators. *The Journal of Nursing Administration*, 42(9), 410–417. http://www.jstor.org/stable/26822475

Melnyk, B. M., Fineout, O. E., Giggleman, M., & Choy, K. (2017). A test of the ARCC© model improves implementation of evidence-based practice, healthcare culture, and patient outcomes. *Worldviews on Evidence-Based Nursing*, 14(1), 5–9. https://doi.org/10.1111/wvn.12188

Melnyk, B. M., Fineout-Overholt, E., Giggleman, M., & Cruz, R. (2010). Correlates among cognitive beliefs, EBP implementation, organizational culture, cohesion, and job satisfaction in evidence-based practice mentors from a community hospital system. *Nursing Outlook*, 58(6), 301–308. https://doi.org/10.1016/j.outlook.2010.06.002

Melnyk, B. M., Gallagher-Ford, L., Thomas, B. K., Troseth, M., Wyngarden, K., & Szalacha, L. (2016). A study of chief nurse executives indicates low prioritization of evidence-based practice and shortcomings in hospital performance metrics across the united states. *Worldviews on Evidence-Based Nursing*, 13(1), 6–14. https://doi.org/10.1111/wvn.12133

Melnyk, B. M., Gallagher-Ford, L., Long, L. E., & Fineout-Overholt, E. (2014). The establishment of evidence-based practice competencies for practicing registered nurses and advanced practice nurses in real-world clinical settings: Proficiencies to improve healthcare quality, reliability, patient outcomes, and costs. *Worldviews on Evidence-Based Nursing*, 11(1), 5–15. https://doi.org/10.1111/wvn.12021

Melnyk, B. M., Gallagher, F. L., Zellefrow, C., Tucker, S., Thomas, B., Sinnott, L. T., & Tan, A. (2018a). The first U.S. study on nurses' evidence-based practice competencies indicates major deficits that threaten healthcare quality, safety, and patient outcomes. *Worldviews on Evidence-Based Nursing*, 15(1), 16–25. https://doi.org/10.1111/wvn.12269

Melnyk, B. M., Hsieh, A. P., Messinger, J., Thomas, B., Connor, L., & Gallagher-Ford, L. (2003). Budgetary investment in evidence-based practice by chief nurses and stronger EBP cultures associated with less nursing turnover and better patient outcomes. *Worldviews on Evidence-based Nursing*, 20(2), 162–171. https://doi.org/10.1111/wvn.12645

Melnyk, B. M., Orsolini, L., Tan, A., Arslanian-Engoren, C., Melkus, G. D., Dunbar-Jacob, J., Rice, V. H., Millan, A., Dunbar, S. B., Braun, L. T., Wilbur, J., Chyun, D. A., Gawlik, K., & Lewis, L. M. (2018b). A national study links nurses' physical and mental health to medical errors and perceived worksite wellness. *Journal of Occupational & Environmental Medicine, 60*(2), 126–131. https://doi.org/10.1097/JOM.0000000000001198

Melnyk, B. M., Tan, A., Hsieh, A. P., Gawlik, K., Arslanian-Engoren, C., Braun, L. T., Dunbar, S., Dunbar-Jacob, J., Lewis, L. M., Millan, A., Orsolini, L., Robbins, L. B., Russell, C. L., Tucker, S., & Wilbur, J. (2021a). Critical care nurses' physical and mental health, worksite wellness support, and medical errors. *American Journal of Critical Care, 30*(3), 176–184. https://doi.org/10.4037/ajcc2021301

Melnyk, B. M., Tan, A., Hsieh, A. P., & Gallagher, F. L. (2021b). Evidence-based practice culture and mentorship predict EBP implementation, nurse job satisfaction, and intent to stay: Support for the ARCC© model. *Worldviews on Evidence-Based Nursing, 18*(4), 272–281. https://doi.org/doi-org/10.1111/wvn.12524

National Organization of Nurse Practitioner Faculties. (2022). *National Organization of Nurse Practitioner Faculties' nurse practitioner role core competencies.* https://www.nonpf.org/page/NP_Role_Core_Competencies

Newhouse, R. P. (2010). Instruments to assess organizational readiness for evidence-based practice. *JONA: The Journal of Nursing Administration, 40*(10), 404–407. https://doi.org/10.1097/NNA.0b013e3181f2ea08

Newhouse, R. P., Dearholt, S. L., Poe, S. S., Pugh, L. C., & White, K. M. (2007). *Johns hopkins nursing: evidence-based practice model and guidelines.* Sigma Theta Tau International.

Nundy, S., Cooper, L. A., & Mate, K. S. (2022). The quintuple aim for health care improvement: A new imperative to advance health equity. *JAMA: Journal of the American Medical Association, 327*(6), 521–522. https://doi-org/10.1001/jama.2021.25181

Sherman, S. E, Chapman, A., Garcia, D., & Braslow, J. T. (2004). Performance improvement: Improving recognition of depression in primary care: A study of evidence-based quality improvement. *Joint Commission Journal on Quality & Safety, 30*(2), 80–88. https://doi.org/10.1016/s1549-3741(04)30009-2

O'Leary, C., King, T. S., Gallagher-Ford, L., & Kue, J. (2022). Use of a framework to integrate research, evidence-based practice, and quality improvement. *Nurse Leader, 20*(6), 589–593. https://doi.org/10.1016/j.mnl.2022.04.008

Oncology Nursing Society. (2023). *Evidence-based practice learning library.* https://www.ons.org/learning-libraries/evidence-based-practice

Poghosyan, L., Pulcini, J., Chan, G. K., Dunphy, L., Martsolf, G. R., Greco, K., Todd, B. A., Brown, S. C., Fitzgerald, M., McMenamin, A. L., & Solari-Twadell, P. A. (2022). State responses to COVID-19: Potential benefits of continuing full practice authority for primary care nurse practitioners. *Nursing Outlook, 70*(1), 28–35. https://doi.org/10.1016/j.outlook.2021.07.012

Ranji, S. (2016). *Measuring and responding to deaths from medical errors.* Agency for Healthcare Quality and Research Patient Safety Network. https://psnet.ahrq.gov/perspective/measuring-and-responding-deaths-medical-errors

Rogers, E. M. (2003). *Diffusion of Innovations* (5th ed). Free Press (a division of Simon & Schuster, Inc.)

Serra, B. M. A., Benito, A. L., Pla, C. M., & Ferro, G. T. (2022). Delphi survey on the application of advanced practice nursing competencies: Strong points and unfinished business in cancer care. *Journal of Nursing Management (John Wiley & Sons, Inc.), 30*(8), 4339–4353. https://doi.org/10.1111/jonm.13843

Snyder, E. F., & Kerns, L. (2021). Telehealth billing for nurse practitioners during COVID-19: Policy updates. *Journal for Nurse Practitioners, 17*(3), 258–263. https://doi.org/10.1016/j.nurpra.2020.11.015

Stucky, C. H., Brown, W. J., & Stucky, M. G. (2021). COVID-19: An unprecedented opportunity for nurse practitioners to reform healthcare and advocate for permanent full practice authority. *Nursing Forum, 56*(1), 222–227. https://doi.org/10.1111/nuf.12515

Taylor, C., Mulligan, K., & McGraw, C. (2021). Barriers and enablers to the implementation of evidence-based practice in pressure ulcer prevention and management in an integrated community care setting: A qualitative study informed by the theoretical domains framework. *Health & Social Care in the Community, 29*(3), 766–779. https://doi.org/10.1111/hsc.13322

The Joint Commission. (2023). *Implement standards to improve care.* https://www.jointcommission.org/what-we-offer/accreditation/health-care-settings/hospital/learn/our-standards#a617b731bd4346e4aa4b83a1cb8074bf_2e3b11e92bd9402b97e35a609e98d63b

Titler, M. G., Kleiber, C., Steelman, V. J., Rakel, B. A., Budreau, G., Everett, L. Q., Buckwalter, K. C., Tripp-Reimer, T., & Goode, C. J. (2001). The iowa model of evidence-based practice to promote quality care. *Critical Care Nursing Clinics of North America, 13*(4), 497–509.

Treiger, T. M., & Kurland, M. (2021). The power of mentoring: Leveraging evidence-based practice. *Professional Case Management, 26*(5), 264–266. https://doi.org/10.1097/NCM.0000000000000524

Underhill, M., Roper, K., Siefert, M. L., Boucher, J., & Berry, D. (2015). Evidence-based practice beliefs and implementation before and after an initiative to promote evidence-based nursing in an ambulatory oncology setting. *Worldviews on Evidence-Based Nursing, 12*(2), 70–78. https://doi.org/10.1111/wvn.12080

Tucker, S., McNett, M., Mazurek Melnyk, B., Hanrahan, K., Hunter, S. C., Kim, B., Cullen, L., & Kitson, A. (2021). Implementation science: Application of evidence-based practice models to improve healthcare quality. *Worldviews on Evidence-Based Nursing, 18*(2), 76–84. https://doi.org/10.1111/wvn.12495

Williams, K. (2022). Sleep protocol—use of Evidence-Based Practice (EBP) to improve patient outcomes and patient satisfaction while hospitalized. *Worldviews on Evidence-Based Nursing, 19*(5), 423–425. https://doi.org/10.1111/wvn.12562

Ylimäki, S., Oikarinen, A., Kääriäinen, M., Holopainen, A., Oikarainen, A., Pölkki, T., Meriläinen, M., Lukkarila, P., Taam-Ukkonen, M., & Tuomikoski, A.-M. (2022). Advanced practice nurses' experiences of evidence-based practice: A qualitative study. *Nordic Journal of Nursing Research, 42*(4), 227–235. https://doi.org/10.1177/20571585221097658

Zolot, J. (2016). Evidence-based care is highly valued but underused by many nurse executives. *American Journal of Nursing, 116*(6), 18. https://doi.org/10.1097/01.NAJ.0000484219.14929.0e

CHAPTER FIVE Reflective Response

JENNIFER DEBERG

As a health sciences librarian regularly working with DNP-educated practitioners in support of EBP and contributing to the EBP education of DNP students, I was delighted to be asked to reflect on this chapter. It includes a useful overview of the value of EBP, a thorough description of the differences between EBP, QI, and research, and a summary of available models. Throughout the chapter, references are consistent and plentiful, indicating that the authors practice the skills discussed.

My favorite theme of this chapter is that EBP is a mindset, not merely a competency to be achieved. One is never done with EBP. Being curious, thinking critically, and investing the energy to discover are attributes that are essential for an individual to engage in EBP. The spirit of inquiry is the perfect phrase to capture this idea. And what a joy it is to watch DNP students (or any clinician, for that matter) figure out how to capitalize on this spirit by adding knowledge, skills, and experience to improve patient care. However, I would point out that the foundation for EBP is not something that can be taught, regardless of how hard educators may try. This is one reason that arming DNP students with the skills to implement EBP is not always successful.

A more pervasive problem acknowledged in this chapter is that organizations sometimes fail to embrace EBP. The ARCC model, as well as several other models described, provide guidance for working with, rather than against, complex systems. Continuous improvement, investment in staff innovation, and dedication to reflective practices are prerequisites for a culture of EBP at the organizational level. Though the authors provide compelling evidence for how EBP improves outcomes, it is a sad truth that healthcare institutions often do not prioritize resources for EBP. There is a desperate need for solutions to these issues. My perspective is somewhat grim, as I routinely watch clinical libraries close in staggering numbers. A recent study revealed a 32% reduction in hospital libraries from 2007 to 2017 (Harrow et al., 2019). Even in hospitals with electronic library subscriptions, there is not always funding to employ a librarian to educate clinicians on the very resources that are essential for EBP. Further evidence of institutional failure to commit to EBP can be easily observed, as clinicians everywhere struggle to find time for bedside care, documentation, communication, education (etc!). How can there be room for EBP without enough staff to allow dedicated time and effort?

Another message from this chapter may be that DNP-prepared practitioners have a responsibility to lead healthcare organizations in EBP. Though I believe in this potential, I do not view it as an obligation. Expecting newly trained practitioners of any discipline to transform our flawed system seems unfair. The most dedicated EBP curriculum can produce a practitioner who is well equipped but unable to succeed due to an unsupportive culture, a lack of resources, or the absence of necessary commitment. Years of EBP learning can be rapidly undone. Most students I observe seem to be more likely to overestimate their knowledge, relying too much on their intuition, due to time constraints, high expectations, and external pressures. I suspect that for many

DNP students, the spirit of inquiry has been diminished by working in an environment that does not feed it.

With regard to the changing definitions and language used for EBP discussed here, a few points should be considered. The authors recommend that "end user preferences" replace "patient values and preferences." Though I find this wording imprecise, I am more concerned that removing "patient" could be harmful. The patient is and should be at the center, even if systems/processes are what most needs attention. Our society is in the midst of redefining cultural competency and striving to better understand how bias operates. I do not feel the time is right. We need more focus on the patient, not less. If this wording were to be modified, there are other terms that seem more appropriate, such as recipients of healthcare, individuals/families receiving care, or patients/caregivers. Another proposed language change is from "PICO(T) question" to "searchable question in PICO (T) format." I would argue against PICO altogether. There is an absence of evidence that using PICO to structure the search for evidence is effective. Furthermore, there are many inquiries that cannot fit into the PICO framework. Although I value how PICO may help the clinician/student determine appropriate search terms and inclusion criteria for the body of literature, this method is far too restrictive. When I have the freedom to do so, I coach students/clinicians to develop a focused question with a clearly identified purpose and defined context. The question is the foundation for search terms, though it is not identical to the search strategy.

Finally, I would like to comment more specifically about how to better prepare DNP students and newly trained DNP clinicians for EBP. It is important to reflect that it is quite early in the development of the DNP degree. From my experiences in contributing to EBP education in a well-established DNP program, the learning outcomes are different for each graduate, which is unsurprising given that students come from a variety of backgrounds, with differing levels of expertise, motivation, and personal obligations. Most students nearing graduation do not seem to have a complete skillset to function as EBP leaders. I am not alarmed by this, as we are still figuring out both what and how to incorporate EBP content throughout the program. In my role as an instruction librarian, I often need to challenge the notion that technologically savvy digital natives already know what they need to know about searching, organizing, and appraising information. Incorporating objective EBP measurement at the start and completion of a DNP program is one suggestion. Teaching and modeling cognitive flexibility is also important, as are building habits for the continual pursuit of learning. Creating teaching partnerships with librarians, statisticians, information technologists, and faculty from other disciplines may enrich the value and meaning of EBP education. Fortunately, DNP educators seem to be continually learning about what is needed to support clinical skills in addition to those in leadership, information literacy, implementation science, informatics, and scholarship. DNP educators need to remain adaptive and collaborative, making necessary changes to meet the demands placed on graduates. More specific standards for curricula will likely aid in this process, as additional knowledge and evidence are being generated.

REFERENCE

Harrow, A., Marks, L. A., Schneider, D., Lyubechansky, A., Aaronson, E., Kysh, L., & Harrington, M. (2019). Hospital library closures and consolidations: A case series. *Journal of the Medical Library Association, 107*(2), 129–136. https://doi.org/10.5195/jmla.2019.520

SECTION TWO

Primary and Secondary Contemporary Roles for Doctoral Advanced Nursing Practice

CHAPTER SIX

The Role of the Practitioner

DIANE C. SEIBERT

INTRODUCTION

Nursing is a highly diverse and complex profession, with multiple academic levels to enter the profession, including an associate degree, a baccalaureate degree, an accelerated baccalaureate, or master's-level entry, all of which prepare the student to sit for the national nursing certification exam and receive an RN license. After earning the RN license, there are literally hundreds of ways for nurses to contribute to human or population or global health; they can earn specialty certificates, obtain advanced clinical or research degrees, or use their nursing perspective to inform and shape other professions such as law, politics, and business. This chapter explores issues unique to nurses who have elected to return to graduate school to obtain a graduate degree as an advanced practice registered nurse (APRN) to expand their clinical knowledge and expertise.

APRN EDUCATION

There are four types of APRN roles; the certified registered nurse anesthetist (CRNA), the certified nurse midwife (CNM), the clinical nurse specialist (CNS), and the nurse practitioner (NP), all of which are licensed to provide patient care outside or above the normal scope of nursing practice in the United States. Currently, there are two academic paths to becoming an APRN: a master's degree in nursing (MSN) and a clinical doctoral degree, specifically the doctor of nursing practice (DNP) degree. Unlike the research doctorate (most commonly a doctor of philosophy [PhD]) which is focused on creating new knowledge (research), the DNP is a clinical provider, focused on applying current knowledge to practice.

Just as educational preparation for RNs has evolved steadily from diploma to baccalaureate, with an associate degree added along the way, academic requirements for APRNs have been equally fluid, evolving from an apprenticeship, to a certificate, to an MSN, and now the DNP. It's particularly challenging to regulate APRN practice because the roles and practice environments are so diverse. Each APRN specialty has an organization responsible for creating educational standards (American Association of Nurse Anesthetists [AANA], American College of Nurse Midwives [ACNM], National Association of Clinical Nurse Specialists [NACNS], and National Organization of Nurse

Practitioner Faculties [NONPF]), and two APRN communities (CNM and CRNA) have created accreditation standards and accrediting bodies as well.

In the early 2000s, the American Association of Colleges of Nursing (AACN), the "national voice" for academic nursing, began a campaign to shift the "terminal degree" for APRNs to the doctoral degree. This urgency was in response to several contextual issues: the 2020 Institute of Medicine report "To Err Is Human" (IOM, 2000); a need to better prepare APRNS for practice in an increasingly complex healthcare system; and to address the "credit creep" in APRN education (AACN, 2004). The AACN laid out its vision for the future of nursing education (AACN, 2004), declaring that APRNs should enter the profession with a practice doctorate.

Two major white papers on the nursing workforce published since 2004 have reinforced the need for doctoral education in nursing (IOM, 2011; NAM, 2020). The 2011 Institute of Medicine paper titled *The Future of Nursing: Leading Change, Advancing Health,* called on the nursing profession to

> include opportunities for seamless transition to higher degree programs—from licensed practical nurse (LPN)/licensed vocational nurse (LVN) degrees, to the associate's degree in nursing (ADN) and bachelors of science in nursing (BSN), to masters of science in nursing (MSN), and to the PhD and doctor of nursing practice (DNP).

Most recently, in 2021, the National Academy of Medicine report *The Future of Nursing 2020–2030: Charting a Path to Achieve Health Equity* (National Academies of Science, Engineering, and Medicine, 2021) lauded the 500% increase in the number of doctorally educated nurses, but expressed concern about the lack of growth in the number of nurses completing research-focused degrees. So, the importance of a doctoral terminal degree in nursing is still front and center.

The first document describing the key educational components of a clinical doctorate was published by the AACN in 2006 as a companion document to the AACN Baccalaureate Essentials and AACN Master's Essentials. The "Essentials of Doctoral Education for Advanced Nursing Practice" listed the educational competencies felt to be critical to preparing APRNs to be safe and effective clinicians as well as effective healthcare system leaders. The 2006 Essentials contained eight competency areas, two of which focused on developing clinical expertise (scientific underpinnings for practice and advanced nursing practice) and the remaining six focused on systems change, including organizational and systems leadership, clinical scholarship and analytical methods for evidence-based practice, information systems/technology, healthcare policy, interprofessional collaboration, and clinical prevention and population health.

A decade later, the AACN established an AACN Essentials Task Force, composed of a diverse set of nursing professionals representing nursing education, nursing practice and healthcare system executives to create an entirely new framework for nursing education at the baccalaureate and graduate (master's and doctorate) levels. After many iterations and listening sessions, the AACN endorsed a set of Essentials that is a completely different model compared to previous versions that includes competency-based language (AACN, 2021a, 2021b). The 2021 Essentials divides nursing into levels: level one guides prelicensure students and level two identifies competencies that nurses being educated at the graduate level are expected to attain, regardless of degree. Both levels of students are expected to achieve competencies in the same domain areas, but entry to practice and graduate-level students must demonstrate competency at different levels. The 10 domains are: Knowledge for Nursing Practice; Person-Centered Care; Population Health; Scholarship for Nursing Practice; Quality and Safety; Interprofessional Partnerships: Systems-Based Practice; Informatics and Healthcare

Technologies; Professionalism and Personal, Professional, and Leadership Development. The essentials also contain 8 cross-cutting concepts that are woven into the 10 domains where appropriate. These concepts include Clinical Judgment; Communication; Compassionate Care; Diversity, Equity, and Inclusion; Ethics; Evidence-Based Practice; Health Policy; and Social Determinants of Health (AACN, 2021a, 2021b). All APRNs graduating after 2022, regardless of degree level, will be expected to be competent in these 10 domains and 8 concepts.

The Value of Doctoral Education for APRNs

AACN is very interested in assessing the value of these educational changes. To get the data they need to support these important (and impactful changes), they have commissioned two large studies to evaluate the effectiveness and impact of the practice doctorate in nursing. The first was a Rand study commissioned by the AACN in 2015 called "The DNP by 2015; A Study of the Institutional, Political, and Professional Issues that Facilitate or Impede Establishing a Post-Baccalaureate Doctor of Nursing Practice Program." The second, called "The Doctor of Nursing Practice Education in 2022," was awarded to IMPAQ, who conducted a 1-year study between February 2021 and February 2022.

In 2015, the Rand team used surveys and qualitative interviews to identify how many schools had adopted the DNP (quantitative data from AANP annual survey), and then conducted interviews with 29 deans/program directors to identify barriers or facilitators to launching the DNP at their institution. At that time, there was strong interest in a post-master's DNP (PM-DNP) from currently practicing APRNs but the demand for the DNP degree was less pronounced for nurses entering an APRN role and MSN was still the primary pathway to the APRN. They speculated that until the market dried up for the PM-DNP, two paths to the DNP would exist: the MSN to DNP and the BSN to DNP. Interestingly they noted that "autonomous" nursing schools were more likely to have transitioned to the BSN entry, speculating that this might be due to fewer institutional barriers. In terms of value of the DNP, participants almost universally agreed that the added content in the DNP was important, but noted that a significant factor driving adoption would be a requirement for the doctoral degree by certifying and accrediting bodies. As for employers, in 2015 they were relatively unaware of the practice doctorate, so hiring had not changed. In summary, the most pressing concerns included market demand, institutional barriers, state policy and regulatory structures, university system constraints, and resource and financial factors (Auerbach et al., 2015).

The 2022 study provided an update on the status of the practice doctorate. Like the Rand team, the IMPAQ team used a mixed-methods approach to conduct their assessment, completing five discrete studies in 1 year: (a) a scoping review of literature published on the DNP since 2015; (b) a curriculum analysis of 50 DNP programs; (c) interviews with 42 DNP graduates, employers, and academic leaders; (d) analysis of AACN survey data; and (e) a survey of over 800 DNP graduates.

The scoping review revealed several interesting findings, including the quality of the literature, individual practice differences, impact of the DNP project, and the "value" of the additional content. In terms of the literature quality, since 2015 over 50 articles on the topic of DNP education have been published and were available for review. They reported that most of the variability in the skills of DNP graduates is related to the knowledge and skills RNs brought with them to school, and that many DNP graduates were working as direct care providers, and may not be recognized for their skills, and are likely not fully using their DNP education. The DNP project was an important topic of discussion in the literature and revealed that there was agreement that the overall goal of the DNP project is to improve patient outcomes and effect practice change, but that there was significant variability in terms of how the DNP project was implemented. Many articles concluded by saying that APRNS with practice doctorates have the potential to improve patient and system-level outcomes significantly through leadership, influence on health policy, translation of evidence, and interdisciplinary collaboration.

The curriculum analysis was conducted at 50 DNP programs accredited by the Commission on Collegiate Nursing Education (CCNE). The research team assessed educational pathways and DNP program options at each school, explored how faculty secured clinical placements and/or clinical site partnerships, compared credit hours and assessed DNP project requirements. They found that most schools offered both BSN-to-DNP and MSN-to-DNP tracks, most of the DNP programs regardless of entry level (BSN or MSN) were educating nurse practitioners, with a much smaller percentage offering CRNA or CNS specialties. In terms of clinical placements, approximately one-third of the schools required students to find their own placements, one-third secured all placements for students, and one-third "split the difference," asking students to secure some but not all of their clinical placements, and most programs did not maintain clinical site partnerships for students. Most BSN to DNP programs were 74 credit hours, and MSN to DNP programs were 38 credits in length, although the hours varied depending on the number of transfer credits that might be accepted. Every program required students to complete a DNP project, the vast majority of which were focused on practice change and/or quality improvement (QI), but there was significant variability between programs regarding where the project was implemented, whether a project could be focused on policy change, whether students were permitted to conduct a secondary data analysis and whether or not group projects were allowed. Most programs required students to obtain 500 direct patient care hours and dedicate the remaining 500 hours to the DNP project.

The IMPAQ team interviewed 14 DNP graduates, 13 employers, and 15 faculty leading a DNP program to explore how these key stakeholders viewed the "value" of DNP graduates in the workforce. Most people across all three groups reported that DNP graduates were more prepared to manage system change because they had acquired a larger and more diverse skill set related to how healthcare organizations worked, including better preparation in the areas of policy, economics, and the "business" side of healthcare. When it came to direct patient care, however, faculty and employers couldn't identify any differences in the care provided by MSN- versus DNP-prepared nurses, possibly because both are required to obtain the same level of practice competencies. Neither graduates nor employers fully understood the unique set of skills DNP graduates possess, they couldn't clearly identify what roles DNPs should fill, and they weren't clear if the goal of the DNP was to produce expert clinicians, healthcare leaders, or both. Graduates felt that post-master's students were more mature, had years of clinical experience, and were therefore better positioned for leadership positions compared to graduates who entered DNP programs at the baccalaureate level. There were many additional themes and comments made by these three stakeholder groups in the report.

AACN survey data between 2005 to 2020 was used to assess growth in the overall number of DNP programs, student enrollment, student demographics, and DNP program tracks and concentrations. The data was clear regarding the increase in the overall number of programs and students enrolled. Each year since 2005 the number of DNP programs has increased. In 2005, only 13 schools had DNP programs and by 2020, 384 nursing schools reported having active DNP programs. The number of students enrolled in DNP programs has increased exponentially as well, rising steadily from 6,599 in 2010 to 35,755 in 2020 and more qualified applicants are being denied admissions because programs are at capacity. Most DNP students are female, although this demographic is changing as well, declining to 86% in 2020. The percentage of nonwhite students has risen steadily as well, increasing from 13% in 2006 to 37% in 2020, a trend that seems likely to continue. Although the total number of programs offering a BSN-to-DNP has increased, the MSN-to-DNP has not disappeared, but it is declining; in 2020, 57% of students were working toward a BSN-to-DNP track compared to 43% transitioning from MSN-to-DNP. Most DNP students (78%) are interested in becoming NPs, but the number of nurses interested in the CRNA is growing rapidly as well (currently 20%). The numbers of students enrolling in CNS and CNM programs remain small at around 2% overall.

The final component of the study was the results of a survey that asked 875 DNP-prepared nurses questions regarding their degree satisfaction, salary, role preparation, and employment experiences. Demographics revealed that most respondents were white (87%), from the South (47%), were NPs (33%), over 45 years old (50%); more than half (56%) were full-time, 43% were part-time; one third attended fully online programs, 9% attended fully in-person programs and the rest attended programs with a heavy virtual component. Overall, they were highly satisfied with their DNP preparation. In terms of their roles, 28% were administrators, 23% were nurse executives, 14% were faculty in a nursing program, and 13% held other positions. NPs reported being better prepared for clinical roles and less prepared for administrative, QI, policy/advocacy, or scholarship activities and nurse executives were less likely to report that their clinical skills had improved. PM-DNP graduates were significantly more likely to report being involved in scholarship activities and reported more policy/advocacy and QI skill than BSN-DNP respondents. Older respondents (>age 55) were significantly more satisfied with their decision to obtain a DNP than those younger than 35, and felt at least as well prepared for various DNP roles with a few exceptions; older respondents felt more prepared to design and conduct QI projects and research. BSN-to-DNP graduates were significantly more likely to report increased preparation for clinical practice after graduation, likely for two reasons: they were baccalaureate prepared when they started their DNP program, so had much less clinical skills than their PM-DNP colleagues (many of whom may already have been certified as APRNs) and BSN-to-DNP programs were more likely to offer APRN certification to prepare BSN nurses for clinical practice. Respondents who were not NPs (administrators, executives, faculty members) reported feeling like their employers and colleagues respected and valued their additional degree and they reported feeling a sense of goal attainment and career fulfillment. CNMs were the least likely to report that obtaining a DNP had a positive impact on their responsibilities or the respect they felt from colleagues, and CRNAs were less likely than NPs to report career fulfillment or that their employer valued them differently.

APRN LEGISLATION

One more thing to discuss before discussing how each of the APRN communities is addressing the practice doctorate is how RN and APRN practice is regulated and legislated. The purpose of regulation is to protect the public by ensuring that only safe, competent providers receive a license. Over the decades, each state developed state practice acts and only states had the authority to issue professional licenses. Established in 1896, the American Nurses Association (ANA) transitioned steadily over the years from representing nursing to regulating nursing practice. In 1978, recognizing the inherent conflict of interest, the ANA established the National Council of State Boards of Nursing (NCSBN) to create a separation between regulation and representation of professional nurses. The NCSBN, is responsible for ensuring that licensed nurses practicing in the

United States provide safe and competent nursing care. In 1995, the NCSBN recognized that the state-run, state-controlled, state-limited licensing model existing in the United States at the time was creating significant inefficiencies; for example, nurses were unable to cross state lines to assist during a natural or man-made disaster. A 1995 Pew Commission paper titled "Reforming Health Care Workforce Regulation: Policy Considerations for the 21st Century" reported that single-state licensure was expensive, restrictive, and did not significantly improve care outcomes, so in 1997 the NCSBN proposed a licensure model called the Nursing License Compact (NLC) in which states would retain regulatory authority, nurses could practice across state lines if the states could agree on a set of uniform rules and policies. At the time this book went to press, 39 states/territories have fully adopted the NLC, 6 have partially implemented, 3 are in the implementation phase, and 7 are pending legislation (Milian, 2022; NCSBN, 2022a).

Regulation of APRN Practice

Regulating APRN practice, regardless of degree level, is challenging because it does not remain within the boundaries of RN practice. In addition, many other laws and regulations influence APRN practice, including Medicare/Medicaid regulations, other boards (some states have a Board of Midwifery), and public health laws. In some states, the CNS role is not described in their Nurse Practice Act, so the practice of CNSs licensed in those states must remain at the RN level.

Rescinding or revising outdated, restrictive laws, policies, and regulations has been a decades-long effort by the APRN community. Some policies (prescriptive practice, supervision, independent practice) have had to be changed at the state level, requiring a state-by-state effort, while others (Medicare reimbursement rates, signing death certificates, permission to order durable medical equipment) have to be (and are still being) dealt with at the federal level.

The NCSBN has been involved in regulating APRN practice as well. Shortly after the launch of the NCL, the NCSBN attempted to apply a similar regulatory model to APRN practice in an effort to increase uniformity in APRN practice and education. The initial attempt foundered over issues of confidentiality and reporting, but a few years later NCSBN reconvened APRN stakeholders to explore the acceptability of a third-party review option, which was ultimately adopted (NCSBN, 2022b). The model called "The Consensus Model for APRN Regulation: Licensure, Accreditation, Certification & Education (APRN Consensus Model)" aligns licensure, accreditation, certification, and education (LACE) for APRNs (Nursing World, 2022). The model describes how APRN practice is regulated, legislates APRN titles, and defines APRN specialties to include the four roles (CRNA, CNM, NP, and CNS) and six population foci (family/individual across the lifespan, adult-gerontology, pediatrics, neonatal, psych/mental health, and women's health/gender-related) that each APRN specialty must adhere to. Regardless of degree (master's or doctoral) all APRNs are *educated, certified,* and *licensed* in a role and one or more population foci, and specialization **beyond** that role is via certification and not licensure (AACN, 2022a, 2022b).

■ THE CURRENT STATUS OF APRN EDUCATION BY APRN ROLE

The nursing profession clearly wants APRNs to be educated at the doctoral level, but transitioning from the master's to a doctoral entry level comes at a cost to both the individual seeking the degree and to those involved in educating and certifying those individuals. Each APRN specialty has its own governing body that determines the level of graduate degree required to sit for the certification exam, and when a doctoral degree would be required to enter practice in that specialty. A brief review of each APRN specialty is provided below, including the current status of transition to the doctoral degree, and includes a description of certification, licensure, and subspecialty practice within that specialty. A graphical representation of the APRN roles, populations, and current status regarding the degree required to enter practice is shown in Figure 6.1.

Certified Nurse Midwife (CNM)

The CNM role dates back to 1925, making it the oldest of the four APRN roles. Despite their long presence in the nursing community, CNMs have faced significant, persistent, and ongoing challenges from organized medicine and despite a national shortage of obstetric providers, and many women struggle to find safe and competent obstetric care. According to the U.S. Bureau of Labor Statistics, in May 2021 7,750 CNMs were employed (BLS, 2022), and the American Midwifery Certification Board reports that 13,640 CNMs were nationally certified in May 2022 (AMCB, 2022).

The CNM community has a certifying body, the American Midwifery Certification Board (AMCB), an accrediting agency, the Accreditation Commission for Midwifery Education (ACME), and a professional association, The American College of Nurse-Midwives (ACNM), which sets standards for midwifery education and practice and represents American CNMs on the national stage. Thirty-nine midwifery programs are accredited in the United States, and the number of qualified applicants, matriculants, and graduates has gradually increased since 2014 (https://www.midwifeschooling.com/accredited-nurse-midwife-programs).

DEGREE REQUIREMENTS

Nurses interested in midwifery practice can choose from three educational paths all accredited by ACME: a postgraduate certificate, a master's degree, and a doctoral

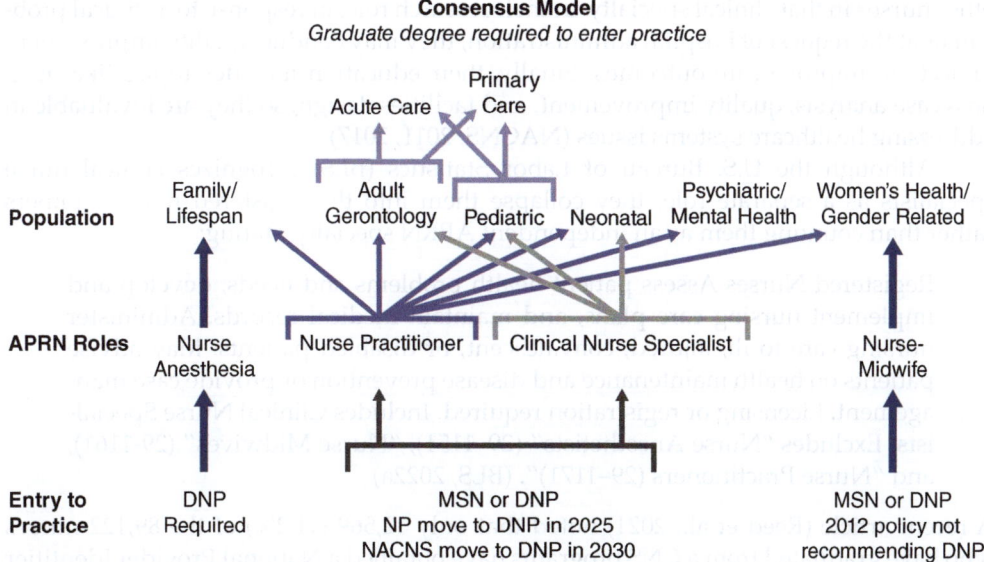

FIGURE 6.1 Consensus Model and Graduate Degree Required to Enter Practice by APRN Specialty

degree. The ACNM does not endorse the DNP degree for entry into midwifery practice, stating in its 2012 Position Paper that "It is the position of the American College of Nurse-Midwives (ACNM) that The Doctor of Nursing Practice (DNP) may be one option for some nurse-midwifery programs, but should not be a requirement for entry into midwifery practice."

ROLE AND POPULATION
The CNM is one of the four APRN roles and the population foci is "women's health/gender related." The ACNM website describes the CNM scope of practice thus: "As a certified nurse-midwife (CNM), you will be qualified to manage prenatal, delivery, and postpartum care. You will also be able to provide most of the primary care, family planning and gynecological needs of women throughout the lifespan" (https://www.midwife.org/nurses).

CERTIFICATION
All CNM graduates must pass a national certification exam administered by the American Midwifery Certification Board (AMCB).

SPECIALTY AREAS (NONCERTIFIED)
There are several women's health specialty areas that CNMs may focus their practice in, such as menopause, breast health, or infertility, but these additional certifications are optional.

Clinical Nurse Specialist (CNS)
Clinical nurse specialists are different from the other three APRN specialties in that they split their time roughly between three distinct areas: they are clinical experts, they apply evidence to improve care outcomes, and they are prepared to address problems in healthcare systems. CNSs often work in high volume, high acuity inpatient care settings. In direct care roles they commonly serve as consultants, teaching or mentoring other nurses in that clinical specialty. In their research role, in response to a clinical problem or at the request of hospital administration, they may conduct quality improvement projects to improve care outcomes. Finally, their education includes topics like business case analysis, quality improvement, and facilities design, so they are invaluable in addressing healthcare systems issues (NACNS, 2011, 2017).

Although the U.S. Bureau of Labor Statistics (BLS) recognizes clinical nurse specialists as a separate role, they collapse them into the registered nurse numbers rather than counting them as an independent APRN specialty, stating:

> Registered Nurses Assess patient health problems and needs, develop and implement nursing care plans, and maintain medical records. Administer nursing care to ill, injured, convalescent, or disabled patients. May advise patients on health maintenance and disease prevention or provide case management. Licensing or registration required. Includes Clinical Nurse Specialists. Excludes "Nurse Anesthetists" (29–1151), "Nurse Midwives" (29-1161), and "Nurse Practitioners (29–1171)". (BLS, 2022a)

A recent article (Reed et al., 2021) noted that only 12,569 (11.2%) of the 89,122 nurses who have graduated from a CNS programs have obtained a National Provider Identifier

(NPI) number which allows organizations like the BLS to count and categorize the healthcare workforce, helping to demonstrate the value of individual roles. The fact that so few CNSs have obtained the free NPI number makes it difficult to identify CNSs in the healthcare system and challenging to create policy that supports their practice.

ROLE AND POPULATION

The CNS is one of the four APRN roles, and the population foci can be adult-gerontology (acute or primary Care), pediatrics (acute or primary care), or women's health/gender related. CNSs spend approximately 35% of their time providing or supporting others in the provision of direct patient care; 20% teaching (academia or inpatient staff); 20% providing consultation services, and 14% leading evidence-based practice projects (NACNS, 2017).

DEGREE REQUIREMENTS

There are two degree options for nurses interested in obtaining a CNS, a master's or a doctoral degree, but a 2015 Position Paper clearly articulates the goal of the NACNS to adopt the doctor of nursing practice (DNP) degree as entry into practice by 2030. In their position paper they stated:

> While NACNS has consistently supported both masters and DNP preparation for entry into the CNS role, considering the complex needs of patients and the future direction of nursing practice, we believe that DNP preparation for practice in the CNS role will better position the CNS to meet the demands of an evolving healthcare system. Consistent with the strategic recommendations proposed to facilitate health care transformation, NACNS believes it is imperative to increase the number of doctorally-prepared Advanced Practice Registered Nurses (APRNs), which will increase the number of doctorally prepared nurses overall (IOM Future of Nursing, 2010; Educating Nurses: A Call for Radical Transformation, 2009). As a result, NACNS endorses the DNP degree as an important opportunity for CNS education and supports the need to increase doctoral preparation for nursing practice (IOM, 2010).

ACCREDITATION

The CNS community does not have a stand-alone accrediting body. The NACNS makes recommendations for CNS practice, but they are not an accrediting body.

CERTIFICATION

Two organizations offer certification exams for CNSs: the American Nurses Credentialing Center (ANCC), which offers one exam, the Adult-Gerontology CNS (AGCNS-BC), and the American Association of Critical-Care Nurses (AACN), which offers four exams: Acute Care CNS - Adult (ACCNS-A), the Acute Care CNS - Pediatrics (ACCNS-P), the Acute Care CNS - Neonatal (ACCNS-N), and the Acute/Critical Care CNS (CCNS).

SPECIALTY AREAS (NONCERTIFIED)

CNS practice is perhaps one of the most diverse of the APRN roles, with CNSs practicing in virtually every clinical setting, typically in inpatient settings. They can be found in maternal child, pediatrics, oncology, transplant, orthopedics, intensive care, cardiac care, etc.

Certified Nurse Anesthetist (or Nurse Anesthesiology; CRNA)

The certified registered nurse anesthetist (CRNA) is the oldest and second largest APRN role. As of May 2021, 43,950 CRNAs were licensed to practice in the United States (BLS, 2022b).

ROLE AND POPULATION

The CRNA is one of the four APRN roles and the population foci is "family/lifespan." According to the AANA website (https://www.aana.com/membership/become-a-crna), "CRNAs provide anesthetics to patients in every practice setting, and for every type of surgery or procedure. They are the sole anesthesia providers in nearly all rural hospitals, and the main provider of anesthesia to the men and women serving in the U.S. Armed Forces."

ACCREDITATION

Every CRNA program is accredited by the Council on Accreditation of Nurse Anesthesia Educational Programs (COA), and the COA publishes accreditation standards for their community as well.

DEGREE REQUIREMENTS

The COA published a position statement announcing three changes to the Accreditation Standards for schools offering CRNA programs (https://www.coacrna.org/about-coa/position-statements):

> A4: The governing body appoints a CRNA as program administrator with leadership responsibilities and authority for the administration of the program. The CRNA administrator must be qualified by experience and have an earned graduate degree from an institution of higher education accredited by a nationally recognized accrediting agency
> A5: The governing body appoints a CRNA, qualified by graduate degree, education, and experiences to assist the CRNA program administrator and, if required, assume leadership responsibilities. This individual must have an earned graduate degree from an institution of higher education accredited by a nationally recognized accrediting agency.
> C2: The faculty designs a curriculum that awards a master's or higher-level degree to graduate students who successfully complete graduation requirements.*
> *The COA will not consider any new master's degree programs for accreditation beyond 2015. All accredited programs must offer a doctoral degree for entry into practice by January 1, 2022. On January 1, 2022 and thereafter, all students matriculating into an accredited program must be enrolled in a doctoral program.

In addition to the DNP, the COA accredits three other practice doctorates for CRNA programs: the doctor of nursing practice (DrNP), the doctor of nurse anesthesia practice (DNAP), and the doctor of nurse anesthesia practice and management (DMPNA).

CERTIFICATION

All CRNA graduates must pass a national certification exam administered by the National Board of Certification and Recertification for Nurse Anesthetists (NBCRNA).

SPECIALTY AREAS (NONCERTIFIED)

Several CRNA specialty areas are available, such as pain, pediatric, obstetric, cardiovascular, plastic, dental, neurosurgical, and military, some of which are offered through the fellowship model.

Nurse Practitioner (NP)

The NP role is the newest and largest of the APRN specialties. The first NP program was developed in 1965 and the demand for NP programs and graduates has been growing ever since (Dellabella, 2015). The American Association of Nurse Practitioners reports that over 355,000 NPs are currently certified to practice in the United States.

Despite being the youngest of the APRN roles, NPs are the largest and most diverse of the APRN communities (Black, 2022), with over 355,000 licensed NPs practicing in the United States as of April 2022.

This was a 9% increase over 2021, which was partially attributed to the COVID-19 global pandemic. Interestingly, the COVID-19 pandemic created a situation eerily similar to the changes in healthcare that occurred during the First and Second World Wars. The nursing profession was again on the "front lines" and healthcare regulations were changing rapidly and in unexpected ways to increase access to care. Despite the publication of a book highly critical of NP practice in December 2021, as COVID-19 cases and deaths were peaking, legislative restrictions on NP practice were being waived (at least temporarily) through the Coronavirus Aid, Relief and Economic Security (CARES) Act. The CARES Act, passed in March 2020 temporarily (and later permanently), authorized NPs to certify/recertify home healthcare services for Medicare patients, ensuring that vital resources were accessible during the pandemic, increasing access to care in many states.

ROLE AND POPULATION

The NP is one of the four APRN roles and there are NP programs preparing graduates in the each of the six population foci: family/individual across lifespan, pediatrics, women's health/gender related, adult-gerontology, neonatal, and psychiatric/mental health. The scope of practice for NPs is based on the needs of the patient and not the setting in which the care is provided. The American Association of Nurse Practitioners (AANP) describes the NP scope of practice thus:

> As licensed, independent practitioners, NPs practice autonomously and in coordination with health care professionals and other individuals. NPs provide a wide range of health care services, including the diagnosis and management of acute, chronic and complex health problems; health promotion; disease prevention; health education; and counseling to individuals, families, groups and communities. They may also serve as health care researchers, interdisciplinary consultants and patient advocates. (www.aanp.org/advocacy/advocacy-resource/position-statements/scope-of-practice-for-nurse-practitioners#:~:text=NPs%20provide%20a%20wide%20range,%2C%20families%2C%20groups%20and%20communities)

ACCREDITATION

The National Organization of Nurse Practitioner Faculties (NONPF) organizes a committee called the National Task Force (NTF) that regularly updates NP practice standards to maintain currency and relevance with other national nursing standards and evolutions in clinical practice. Nursing programs that offering NP specialties are assessed for compliance with the NTF accreditation standards during routine accreditation visits by the Commission on Collegiate Nursing Education (CCNE) or the National League for Nursing (NLN), Accreditation Commission for Education in Nursing (ACEN) but there is no stand-alone NP accrediting body

DEGREE REQUIREMENTS
On April 20, 2018, the NONPF voted to require that all entry-level (NP) education be moved to the DNP degree by 2025.

CERTIFICATION
Several certification bodies produce certification examinations for different NP specialties: the American Association of Nurse Practitioners Certification Board (AANP-CB), the American Nurses Credentialing Center (ANCC), the National Certification Corporation (NCC), the Pediatric Nursing Certification Board (PNCB), and the American Association of Critical Care Nurses (AACN).

CERTIFICATIONS AVAILABLE FOR NPS
- Adult-Gerontology Primary Care (A-GNP) is offered by the AANPCB and ANCC
- Adult-Gerontology Acute Care (ACNPC-AG or AGACNP-BC) is offered by the AACN and ANCC
- Family (FNP-C or FNP-BC) is offered by the AANPCB and ANCC
- Women's Health (WHNP-BC) is offered by the NCC
- Neonatal (NNP-BC) is offered by the NCC
- Pediatric Primary Care (CPNP-PC) is offered by the PNCB
- Pediatric Acute Care (CPNP-AC) is offered by the PNCB
- Psychiatric-Mental Health (PMHNP-BC) is offered by the ANCC

SPECIALTY CERTIFICATIONS AVAILABLE AFTER INITIAL CERTIFICATION
- Emergency (ENP-BC) is offered by the AANPCB

SPECIALTY AREAS (NONCERTIFIED)
- Military
- Oncology
- Cardiology
- Wound Care
- Dermatology
- Neurology
- Diabetes
- Ophthalmology
- Infectious Disease and HIV
- Endocrine
- Gerontology
- Otolaryngology
- Pain Management
- Pulmonary and Sleep

- Orthopedics
- Convenient and Urgent Care
- Gastroenterology
- Obesity
- Urology
- School Nursing
- Occupational and Environmental Health
- Health Informatics

CONCLUSION

There is good evidence that APRNs are safe, cost effective, and valuable members of the healthcare system. The evidence that earning a practice doctorate is worth the additional time and money is still emerging. After the AACN DNP Essentials was published in 2006, the number of nursing programs offering the DNP increased. In 2022, the AACN reported that in 1 year (between 2000 and 2001), the number of nurses enrolling in and graduating from DNP programs increased significantly (AACN, 2022a, 2022b). Data is not yet available about the value of the DNP because most of these DNPs are still early in their career and perhaps focusing on honing their clinical skills. They have not yet risen to positions of leadership in which they can demonstrate their ability to apply evidence to improve practice or lead organizational change (McCauley et al., 2020). As reported in *The state of Doctor of Nursing Practice Education in 2022* published by the AACN in June 2022 (AACN, 2022a, 2022b), DNP graduates were largely satisfied with their degree. APRNs felt better prepared for their clinical roles and less prepared for leadership, while administrators felt the opposite. Post-master's DNP graduates were more involved in scholarship and policy than BSN-DNP respondents, and DNPs who were not APRNs (administrators, executives, faculty members) felt more respected and valued by their employers and colleagues. CNMs and CRNAs were less likely to report that the DNP changed much about their practice or the respect they received from colleagues or their employers. That said, in their conclusions, many of the authors who wrote the articles reviewed during the scoping review commented that they believed DNP-prepared APRNs have the potential to improve patient and system-level outcomes significantly through leadership, influence on health policy, translation of evidence, and interdisciplinary collaboration. It will be interesting to see how these young BSN-prepared nurses who enter their APRN careers with a DNP shape healthcare. Once they solidify their clinical skills, how will they use their DNP degree to assess evidence to improve healthcare systems?

CRITICAL THINKING QUESTIONS

1. What strengths do preparation as a DNP bring to the advanced practice role? In what ways do you think advanced practice will change once the majority of NPs are prepared at the DNP level?
2. What is the role of teachers of various educational backgrounds in the education of the DNP practitioner? Should the majority of DNP educators be practicing clinicians? Explain.

3. Do you anticipate that outcomes should be different from MS-prepared practitioners? What outcomes can be expected from DNP-prepared practitioners?
4. Do you think that attaining competency as an advanced practice nurse is necessary before becoming a change agent? How will DNP student practitioners gain the skills to become change agents in clinical practice if they cannot practice in advanced roles until they complete their DNP education?
5. Should DNP students be encouraged to develop original scholarly work through the scholarship of application? Would this approach better prepare advanced practice nurses with the skills to demonstrate enhanced patient outcomes resulting from their care? In what way?
6. Should NPs and MDs take the same certification exams? What are the advantages and drawbacks of this approach to determining competencies?
7. Are the new AACN's Essentials relevant and futuristic enough to provide guidance in the development of the practitioner going forward? Should an essentials document be futuristic?
8. Should ethics be added as an essential? Discuss ways to incorporate ethics appropriately throughout the curriculum.
9. Should PhD and DNP students be educated together? Are there areas where each should be educated separately? What areas should be shared?
10. What level of rigor should exist in a DNP program? Should it be similar to the PhD program?

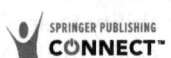

A robust set of instructor resources designed to supplement this text is located at http://connect.springerpub.com/content/book/978-0-8261-8137-4. Qualifying instructors may request access by emailing textbook@springerpub.com.

REFERENCES

American Association of Colleges of Nursing (AACN). (2004). *AACN position statement on the practice doctorate in nursing.* https://www.aacnnursing.org/Portals/42/News/Position-Statements/DNP.pdf

American Association of Colleges of Nursing (AACN). (2021a). *The essentials: Core competencies for professional nursing education; Executive Summary.* https://www.aacnnursing.org/Portals/42/AcademicNursing/pdf/Essentials-Executive-Summary.pdf

American Association of Colleges of Nursing (AACN). (2021b). *Understanding the re-envisioned essentials: A roadmap for the transformation of nursing education.* https://www.aacnnursing.org/Portals/42/AcademicNursing/pdf/Roadmap-to-New-Essentials.pdf

American Association of Colleges of Nursing (AACN). (2022a). *The state of Doctor of Nursing Practice education in 2022.* https://www.aacnnursing.org/Portals/42/News/Surveys-Data/State-of-the-DNP-Summary-Report-June-2022.pdf

American Association of Colleges of Nursing (AACN). (2022b). *DNP Fact Sheet.* AACN Fact Sheet - DNP (aacnnursing.org)

Auerbach, D. I., Martsolf, G. R., Pearson, M. L., Taylor, E. A., Zaydman, M., Muchow, A. N., Spetz, J., & Lee, Y. (2015). The DNP by 2015: A study of the institutional, political, and professional issues that facilitate or impede establishing a post-baccalaureate doctor of nursing practice program. *Rand Health Quarterly, 5*(1), 3.

American Nurses Association (ANA). *Historical Review.* https://www.nursingworld.org/~48de64/globalassets/docs/ana/historical-review2016.pdf

American Midwifery Certification Board. (2022). *Number of Certified Nurse-Midwives (CNM) / Certified Midwives (CM) by State.* https://www.amcbmidwife.org/docs/default-source/reports/number-of-cnm-cm-by-state---february-2019-present607d50819fd7410f84b748c059e9a2d9.pdf?sfvrsn=cce5f80_6

Black, B. (2022). *Nurse practitioner, no. 1 ranked health care job, reports increase in numbers, american association of nurse practitioners.* https://www.aanp.org/news-feed/nurse-practitioner-no-1-ranked-health-care-job-reports-increase-in-numbers

BLS. (2022). *U.S. Bureau of Labor Statistics.* https://www.bls.gov/oes/current/oes291151.htm

Dellabella, H. (2015). *50 years of the nurse practitioner profession.* Clinical Advisor. https://www.clinicaladvisor.com/home/web-exclusives/50-years-of-the-nurse-practitioner-profession

Hawkins, R., & Nezat, G. (2009). Doctoral education: Which degree to pursue? *AANA Journal, 77*(2), 92–6.

Institute of Medicine. (2000). *To err is human: Building a safer health system.* The National Academies Press. https://doi.org/10.17226/9728.

Institute of Medicine. (2011). *The future of nursing: Leading change, advancing health.* The National Academies Press.

Institute of Medicine of the National Academies. (2010). *The future of nursing leading change, Advancing Health.* https://nap.nationalacademies.org/resource/12956/Future-of-Nursing-2010-Report-Brief.pdf

McCauley, L. A., Broome, M. E., Frazier, L., Hayes, R., Kurth, A., Musil, C. M., Norman, L. D., Rideout, K. H., & Villarruel, A. M. (2020). Doctor of Nursing Practice (DNP) degree in the United States: Reflecting, readjusting, and getting back on track. *Nursing Outlook. 68*(4), 494–503. https://doi.org/10.1016/j.outlook.2020.03.008. PMID: 32561157; PMCID: PMC7161484.

Milian, J. (2022). *A brief history of the Nurse Licensure Compact.* Ascend: A magazine by thentia. https://ascend.thentia.com/united-states/a-brief-history-of-the-nurse-licensure-compact

National Academy of Medicine. (2020). *The future of nursing 2020–2030.* https://nam.edu/publications/the-future-of-nursing-2020-2030/

National Academies of Sciences, Engineering, and Medicine. (2021). *The future of nursing 2020–2030: Charting a path to achieve health equity.* The National Academies Press. https://doi.org/10.17226/25982.

National Council of State Boards of Nursing. (2022a). *Nurse Licensure Compact (NLC).* https://www.ncsbn.org/compacts/nurse-licensure-compact.page

National Council of State Boards of Nursing. (2022b). *Historical actions on APRNs.* https://www.ncsbn.org/nursing-regulation/practice/aprn/aprn-consensus/history-of-aprn.page

Nursing World Org. (2022). *Consensus model for APRN regulation FAQs.* https://www.nursingworld.org/certification/aprn-consensus-model/faq-consensus-model-for-aprn-regulation

National Association of Clinical Nurse Specialists (NACNS). (2011). *Criteria for the evaluation of clinical nurse specialist master's, practice doctorate, and post-graduate certificate educational programs.* https://nacns.org/wp-content/uploads/2016/11/CNSEducationCriteria.pdf

National Association of Clinical Nurse Specialists (NACNS). (2017). *2017 CNS week fact sheet.* http://nacns.org/wp-content/uploads/2017/07/CNS-Week-Fact-Sheet-2017.pdf

Reed, S. M., Arbet, J., & Staubli, L. (2021). Clinical nurse specialists in the united states registered with a national provider identifier. *Clinical Nurse Specialist CNS, 35*(3), 119–128. https://doi.org/10.1097/NUR.0000000000000592

U.S. Bureau of Labor Statistics (BLS). (2022a). *Registered nurses.* https://www.bls.gov/ors/factsheet/pdf/registered-nurses.pdf

U.S. Bureau of Labor Statistics (BLS). (2022b). *Nurse anesthetists 29-1151.* https://www.bls.gov/Oes/current/oes291151.htm

CHAPTER SIX — Reflective Response

KYMBERLEE MONTGOMERY

"It is not the strongest of the species that survives, nor the most intelligent, but the one most responsive to *change.*"

—Charles Darwin

Change! Change: alter, variate, modify, to make or become different; not always easy to accept, but always needed to improve. Our world and everything in it operates in a state of constant **change** and healthcare is no exception. We are just emerging from an unprecedented COVID-19 global pandemic that has further stressed an already battered and broken healthcare system, further exposing a nation in a state of "health" chaos, grappling with rapidly deteriorating care-related issues around the nursing shortage and burnout, healthcare disparities/inequalities, and systemic racism, to name only a few. As an expert nurse administrator, advanced practice nurse, educator, and scholar, I have witnessed **"change"** in our complex healthcare system and the nursing profession for over 35 years. As a women's health nurse practitioner with a doctor of nursing practice degree (DNP), I hope to inspire advanced practice registered nurses (APRN) to uncover the hidden gems in this chapter and thoughtfully reflect on how to be a catalyst for continuous, positive **change** through innovational leadership, practice, and engagement.

In Chapter 6, *The Role of the Practitioner,* the author presents a comprehensive and thoughtful discussion of the evolution and multifaceted **changes** in education, legislation, and practice regulation of APRNs, as well as an exploration of the literature regarding nursing doctoral degree options and value, with specific focus on the DNP. Additionally, the author correctly posits that after the emergence of the first APRNs in the 1960s, coupled with the educational advancement opportunities for doctoral preparation, the uncertainty and confusion on how to operationalize the skillset of the DNP-prepared practitioner to benefit nurses, their employers, and society continues to exist. The published data targeted on outcomes attributed to DNP practitioners versus non-DNP-prepared nurses and healthcare professionals remains sparse (AACN, 2022).

The American Association of Colleges of Nursing (AACN, 2004) describes the DNP as a clinically focused doctorate that prepares nurses to become leaders, innovators, **change** agents, and research translators, at the highest level of nursing practice, to improve patient outcomes and translate research into practice as the leaders in advanced clinical practice. The current curricula include competencies in evidence-based practice, quality improvement, critical thinking, systems leadership, organizational management, health policy, business and finance, and much more. The APRN DNP skill set uniquely qualifies nurses to make significant impact in all realms of healthcare through service as flexible leaders, health policy **change** agents, independent healthcare providers, executives, and entrepreneurs (National Academy of Sciences, 2021).

The COVID-19 pandemic clearly demonstrated the importance of nurses within the healthcare system and now is the time DNP-prepared APRNs can lead our nation through yet another necessary **change,** redeveloping and rebuilding the healthcare system. From leading interprofessional healthcare organizations, hospital boards, national advisory councils for creation or adaptation of health policy and serving as officials in all levels of government, the DNP equips APRNs with the skills to affect quality. Who better than practitioners in the trenches understand the depth and breadth of the real issues, nursing shortages, national supply chain issues, quality indicators, organizational financial stressors impacting patient care, and has the advanced skills to make **changes**? Isn't this why we put our blood, sweat, and tears into obtaining the DNP? Are we satisfied to be experts in patient care and sit idly by while our healthcare system continues its downward spiral and cost cutting seems to be the only answer? The author and I agree we must not and are not sitting idle. We know anecdotally that many doctorally prepared nurses are running hospitals, health systems, and clinics. They are deans and directors of higher educational programs ensuring high quality education of the nurses of the future, and they are the clinicians striving to improve patient care and processes. The author of Chapter 5 highlights that there is a dearth of data regarding the current activities of DNP-prepared APRNs and that the full potential of APRNs with a DNP is not fully known. We have a range of experience in nursing, from novice (BSN to DNP) to expert nurses (post-master's DNP) entering the workforce, each eager to make **change,** each ready to "pivot" and adapt quickly as needed, and all enthusiastic to be of value. How will employers and stakeholders know the value of the DNP if we don't collect and document their efforts and success?

If organized nursing does not lead this effort, then data on the past, present, and future incredible outcomes influenced by DNPs will remain scarce and the participation in **changes** made through hard work, high level skill sets, and dedication will go unnoticed.

Another astute point made by the author of Chapter 6 is the resemblance of the changes in healthcare during the COVID-19 pandemic to those in past world wars regarding access to care. The author discusses ways in which the nursing profession was front and center making sure that critical resources were readily available in times of greatest need. Waivers in legislative restrictions in APRN practice were critical to providing the access to care and the necessary care needed, which included home service, telehealth, and telephone triage. Although many waivers have become permanent, some states continue to impose restrictive scope-of-practice laws that limit the capacity of the nursing workforce even though the pandemic has ended, thus ending access to care for some (Martin et al., 2023).

The COVID-19 pandemic, one of the most significant public health emergencies in over a century, is finally coming to an end, but the crisis has uncovered serious issues of health disparities and inequities that have been seething well under the surface, or possibly in some cases ignored (Moore & Hart, 2021). Nursing as a profession is rooted in holism, which encompasses diversity, equality, and equity. To lead in the development of effective strategies in improving health for all, attention to the needs of the most underserved individuals, neighborhoods, and communities and the crucial importance of advancing health equity is paramount (National Academy of Sciences, 2021). "DNP graduates should be prepared to provide direct care in communities, conduct scholarship to validate effect, and address public health issues on a personal and policy level" (Moore & Hart, 2021). Additionally, DNP prepared APRNs possessing both strong leadership and clinical skills are poised to bridge the complicated gap between healthcare systems and community needs. For example, designing impactful ways in which private insurers, governmental payers, policy makers, hospitals, health organizations, and social services agencies can incorporate health equity into their fundamental goals and missions to help give all individuals the opportunity to attain better health and well-being fits right into the expertise of the DNP (National Academy of Sciences, 2021). Conversely, DNP-prepared APRNs can assist these stakeholders to elevate nursing in all sectors of healthcare to improve health outcomes.

Another example of the power of DNP skills is developing, leading, and participating in community needed outreach clinics such as COVID-19 testing and vaccination efforts, diabetes screening and testing mobile units, and opioid educational programs, etc. Assessing, developing, leading, evaluating, and improving through **change** is the specialty of the DNP and *is* nursing taking a rightful seat at the table! Not all DNPs will have the ability to affect **change** at this level; however, staying informed, engaged, and active in professional organizations and policy development will indeed move crucial missions forward.

In summary, it is imperative that a national database is developed to keep track of the accomplishments of the DNP-prepared APRN to promote this degree for the future of the nursing profession. Nursing is the largest workforce in the United States, thus the changes we can make as leaders and practitioners is without boundary! It will continue to take convincing (and at times proof) of our stakeholders, organizational systems, our interprofessional healthcare partners, our patients, and in some cases, even our own nursing colleagues to move this degree forward and properly give it the respect it deserves. As DNP-prepared APRNs we need to never lose sight of the notion that **change** to improve is always necessary. Our community, our patients, our health systems are counting on us. I challenge you to reflect on how far nursing has come, what we have accomplished, and to "continue to be the **change** you wish to see in the world" (Gandhi).

REFERENCES

American Association of Colleges of Nursing (AACN). (2022). *The state of doctor of nursing practice education in 2022. Updated 2022.* https://www.aacnnursing.org/Portals/42/News/Surveys-Data/State-of-the-DNP-Summary-Report-June-2022.pdf

American Association of Colleges of Nursing. (2004). *AACN position statement on the practice doctorate in nursing.* https://www.aacnnursing.org/Portals/42/News/Position-Statements/DNP.pdf

Martin, B., Buck, M., & Zhong, E. (2023). Evaluating the impact of executive orders lifting restrictions on advanced practice registered nurses during the COVID-19 pandemic. *Journal of Nursing Regulation 14*(1), 50–58. https://doi.org/10.1016/S2155-8256(23)00068-6.

Moore, K., Hart, A.M. (2021). Critical juncture: The doctor of nursing practice and COVID-19. *Journal of the American Association of Nurse Practitioners, 33*(2), 97–99. https://journals.lww.com/jaanp/Fulltext/2021/02000/Critical_juncture__The_doctor_of_nursing_practice.2.aspx

National Academies of Sciences, Engineering, and Medicine. (2021). *The future of nursing 2020-2030: Charting a path to achieve health equity.* The National Academies Press. https://doi.org/10.17226/25982.

CHAPTER SEVEN

The Role of the Clinical Executive

BARBARA WADSWORTH, TUKEA L. TALBERT, AND
MARY ELLEN SMITH GLASGOW

■ THE CLINICAL NURSE EXECUTIVE OVERVIEW

The significant role of the clinical nurse executive in leading healthcare organizations has been examined in recent years. The nurse executive is foundational to ensuring the voice and value of nursing are considered at an organizational level to create a culture of safety, quality, and equity and to improve the health and well-being of those under their leadership. Despite time pressures and a myriad of responsibilities, nurse executives are challenged at the same time to assess personal strengths and development opportunities to master the skills required to lead healthcare organizations into the future (Boston-Fleischhauer, 2020; Morse & Warshawsky, 2021). The American Association of Colleges of Nursing (AACN) has been instrumental in shaping nurse executive education. Early on and throughout the COVID-19 pandemic, nurse executives led their organizations with a focus on advocacy, transparency, and innovation to provide leadership to manage resources, to provide clinical care in a time of uncertainty, and to care for the care team, assuring their wellness throughout the multiple waves and significant challenges with workforce, supply chain issues, crisis standards, magnified emphasis on health inequities and the disproportionate impact of COVID-19 on black and Indigenous people of color (BIPOC), and the need for rapid decision making with unprecedented visitor restrictions.

The AACN in its position statement (2004) puts forth that the transformation in the healthcare delivery system will require clinicians to design, evaluate, and constantly improve the context in which care is delivered. The AACN strongly believes that nurses with doctoral preparation that encompasses clinical, organizational, economic, and leadership skills are most likely capable of critiquing scientific findings and subsequently developing programs of care that significantly impact healthcare and that are economically feasible. The AACN adopted the doctor of nursing practice (DNP) position statement in October 2004 calling for a transformational change in the education necessary for professional nurses who will practice at an advanced level of nursing practice (see *The Essentials of Doctoral Education for Advanced Nursing Practice*, AACN, 2006), and has continued to serve as a steady guide to nurse educators and leaders. In 2018, the AACN formed the Essentials Revision Taskforce and encouraged taskforce members to reenvision the Essentials in alignment with the future workforce needs of nurses entering the profession and for those entering advanced nursing practice The Essentials Taskforce, composed of 35 nursing leaders from academia and practice, represented a unique and powerful collaboration in the framing of educational standards (Giddens et al., 2022). Based on the recent AACN report, *The State of Doctor of Nursing Practice Education in 2022*, DNP graduates reported they are using evidence-based practices to change systems and policies in their organization, which is having a positive impact on patient and system outcomes (AACN, 2022). The majority of the employers surveyed responded that whether a DNP is required or even desired depends on the position/ job description. Academic employers reported that they require a doctoral degree for faculty positions, with some requiring a DNP specifically, and employers in hospitals or hospital systems reported that a DNP is usually only required for leadership and executive positions. A finding regarding nursing executive DNP preparation that requires more dialogue and discussion is that "Nurse executives were, on average, 22 percentage points less likely than NPs [nurse practitioners] to believe that their preparation to work in a clinical setting improved as a result of their DNP degree" (p. 23). There was also no significant difference in the DNP degree's impact on nurse executive career fulfilment. This finding is not surprising given that most individuals with a DNP return to their same position, which equated to no substantial change in their responsibilities or compensation. As a result, this can often be perceived as low impact. This needs to be an ongoing area of research to measure the impact of the DNP-prepared executive. Due to the lack of employer knowledge about DNP-prepared executives, roles are not often designed to require a doctoral level of preparation, which also reduces options for DNP-prepared executives (Beeber et al., 2019).

In this chapter, the following areas are discussed: an operational definition of the clinical executive, an introduction to the AACN's *New Essentials of Doctoral Education for Advanced Nursing Practice*, and the position of the American Organization of Nurse Executives (AONE) regarding the DNP degree requirement for nurse executives. The objectives of this chapter are to give readers the opportunity to have a more in-depth view of the need for a DNP as a requirement for nurse executives and their influence by examining DNP program preparation.

▪ DEFINITION OF A CLINICAL EXECUTIVE

Nurse executives are responsible for aligning the mission, vision, values, philosophy, and culture of their organizations with nursing interventions, as well as communicating the corporate perspective to other nurses and clinicians (Clark, 2012). They are responsible for managing resources, organizing nursing care, planning and evaluating the services provided, and contributing to the achievement of optimal results for their organizations, patients, and staff (AONE, 2015). One cannot fully respect the role of the clinical executive without acknowledging the context in which it occurs. The clinical executive must oversee all aspects of clinical practice in healthcare organizations. The nursing practice within any organization has "24/7" accountability for processes, structures, and outcomes of care delivery (Fasoli, 2010). The responsibility of the clinical executive is ever changing, and the expectations of those in the role are greater. For the purposes of this chapter, the authors agree that senior-level nursing leadership (chief nursing officer [CNO], chief nursing executive, and vice president [VP] of nursing) and non-nursing chief executive roles in a healthcare setting is a form of advanced nursing practice. This would include nurses in executive roles in healthcare settings that are still practicing advanced nursing practice just not solely in nursing but more so clinical operations and at system-level platforms.

There has been emerging evidence of the connection between organizational performance and leadership (Frearson, 2002; Hallinger & Heck, 1996; Muijs et al., 2006). Health systems are complex and highly matrixed, requiring defined accountability structures and processes to ensure high-quality nursing practice. Moreover, these matrix relationships can expand from traditional dyad (nurse-physician) to triad (nurse-physician-administrator) to promote synergies and leverage systems. The need for focused executive academic preparation and ongoing development of leadership skills to work in highly complex, matrixed structures is clear (Gruebling et al., 2021). Now is the time to ensure that the well-prepared nurse executives are in key leadership positions, and that those individuals are ready to face the dynamic environment and associated challenges of the healthcare setting. Organizational performance during this unprecedented time in healthcare will be contingent on the effectiveness of the leadership team.

THE NEW AACN ESSENTIALS OF DOCTORAL EDUCATION FOR ADVANCED NURSING PRACTICE

The AACN (2006) identified seven core competencies for the DNP along with two additional differentiated competencies for nurses who choose to focus more on an advanced practice administrative role (i.e., clinical executive role) or an advanced practice–focused role (nurse anesthetist, nurse practitioner, midwife, clinical nurse specialist). The seven core essentials are (1) scientific underpinnings for practice; (2) organizational and systems leadership for quality improvement and systems thinking; (3) clinical scholarship and analytical methods for evidence-based practice; (4) information systems/technology and patient care technology for the improvement and transformation of healthcare; (5) healthcare policy for advocacy in healthcare; (6) interprofessional collaboration for improving patient and population health outcomes; (7) clinical prevention and population health for improving the nation's health; (8a—practice-focused) individual, family, and population-focused advanced nursing practice competencies for improving patient care processes and outcomes; and (8b—executive/administrative) systems or organization-focused advanced nursing practice competencies for improving patient care processes and outcomes.

Academic nursing has an obligation to transform nursing education in alignment with the current and future needs for healthcare. Nursing graduates, armed with a wide range of skills and competencies, are needed now and for the coming years (AACN, 2019). To meet this objective, in April 2021, member deans of the AACN approved new standards for nursing education, with competency-based education as its foundation. The revised Essentials framework includes competencies organized within 10 domains at two levels of nursing education: entry level and advanced level. An advantage of this approach is greater clarity and confirmation regarding the knowledge and skills of nursing school graduates (Giddens et al., 2022).

The Essentials: Core Competencies for Professional Nursing Education provides a framework for preparing individuals as members of the nursing discipline, reflecting expectations across the trajectory of nursing education and applied experience. *Competency-based education* is a process whereby students are held accountable for the mastery of competencies deemed critical for an area of study (AACN, 2021). *The Domains* constitute a descriptive framework for the practice of nursing. These Essentials include

10 domains that were tailored to reflect the discipline of nursing. The domains used in the Essentials are:

- Domain 1: Knowledge for Nursing Practice
- Domain 2: Person-Centered Care
- Domain 3: Population Health
- Domain 4: Scholarship for Nursing Discipline
- Domain 5: Quality and Safety
- Domain 6: Interprofessional Partnerships
- Domain 7: Systems-Based Practice
- Domain 8: Informatics and Healthcare Technologies
- Domain 9: Professionalism
- Domain 10: Personal, Professional, and Leadership Development

In addition to domains, there are featured *concepts* associated with professional nursing practice that are integrated within the Essentials. A concept is an organizing idea that represents important areas of knowledge. The concepts are Clinical Judgment; Communication; Compassionate Care; Diversity, Equity, and Inclusion; Ethics; Evidence-Based Practice; Health Policy; and Social Determinants of Health.

Competencies are organized within the domains, which are applicable across all areas of healthcare and across diverse patient populations. Concepts core to professional nursing practice are evident across the domains and competencies, reflecting broad application. Another key feature within the revised Essentials is a model that places all programs into one of two categories: entry-level and advanced-level nursing education. Level-1 entry-level programs will focus on preparing students for entry into professional nursing practice. Level-2 advanced-level programs will focus on the preparation of nurses for nursing practice in advanced nursing roles or advanced nursing specialties and thus includes requirements and competencies specific to the given specialty. These advanced-level subcompetencies complement and provide a foundation for the additional competencies required for achieving advanced role or advanced specialty practice. All DNP programs (post-baccalaureate and post-master's) demonstrate that graduates attain and integrate Level 2 subcompetencies and competencies for at least one advanced nursing practice specialty or advanced nursing practice role.

The new essentials are comprehensive to reflect the complex health needs of individuals and communities and the role of the nurse in meeting these healthcare challenges. One would expect substantial changes to nursing curricula as schools and universities implement these changes.

AMERICAN ORGANIZATION OF NURSE LEADERS (FORMERLY EXECUTIVES): NEWLY UPDATED (2019) – NURSE EXECUTIVE COMPETENCIES INCLUDING SYSTEM CNE

The American Organization of Nurse Executives/Leaders has positioned itself as the organization with expertise to excel in nurse executive practice (Waxman et al., 2017). At this time, the AONE/AONL has not endorsed the proposal that the DNP should be a requirement for either the clinical nurse executive or practice-focused nurse in advanced nursing practice roles. In their position statement, AONE (2007) supports the DNP as a terminal degree option for practice-focused nursing. They believe, however, that master's nursing degree programs in both generalist and specialty courses of study should remain intact. The Professional Practice Policy Committee of the AONE/AONL concludes that questions and concerns that have been voiced regarding patient outcomes, salary compensation, and financial impact on organizations have not been fully identified, investigated, or addressed as they relate to the DNP requirement.

Recognizing the significant challenges and unprecedented change in healthcare, the AONL (2022) has updated and published revised nursing leadership core competencies shared in a succinct and impactful expanded set of six. Overall, they are described as high impact, while acknowledging nursing leadership as a specialty that spans many healthcare organizations with a variety of roles that continue to evolve. The revised leadership competencies include elevating *Leader Within* to the core list (Hughes, 2022). As described by Hughes, this new competency recognizes the importance of personal experience, understanding, and intrinsic motivation as essential to successful performance as a leader (Hughes, 2022). The core competencies align well and are easily interpreted across a number of leadership roles, including manager, leader, executive, while spanning the acute and postacute setting, including population health. This is a meaningful change that nurse leaders should incorporate into their practice. The AONL Core Competencies are foundational to all nurse leaders from novice to expert which represent the six competencies described above with enhanced detail and specificity to encompass the breath of the expansive role. The competencies are particularly meaningful and helpful both to the new and experienced nurse leaders and organizations by providing clarity, specificity, and expansive areas of expertise that are attributed to and expected from individuals in this role. Leaders who embrace, engage, and embed these competencies personally and professionally should benefit.

The AONE/AONL considers nurse leadership as a subspecialty within nursing practice that requires competence and proficiency unique to the executive role. They believe that there are now six core competencies that are common to nurses in executive practice regardless of their educational level or title (AONE/AONL Nurse Executive Competencies, 2022). These six competencies are (a) communication and relationship building, (b) knowledge of the healthcare environment, (c) leadership, (d) professionalism, (e) business skills, and (f) leader within. These core leadership competencies align with specific core essentials of the AACN's *Essentials of Doctoral Education for Advanced Nursing Practice*, such as interprofessional collaboration, organizational and systems leadership, and clinical scholarship. The AONE/AONL recognizes that their competencies are core competencies and are not exhaustive of all areas of expertise for the nurse executive. They believe that the core competencies establish the standard for all levels of leadership and executive practice and can be used as a guideline for educational preparation of nurses seeking knowledge in executive practice.

The authors agree with the position of the AONE/AONL in that there needs to be more evidence to support making the DNP a requirement for those nurses functioning in clinical leadership advanced nursing practice roles. The authors, DNP graduates themselves, aver that this degree is scholarly, uniquely different from a graduate-level preparation for leadership, and is an educational process that prepares the nurse executive to think and function at an advanced level as evidenced by the positions held by these individuals and their accomplishments in these roles. Having said this, it is necessary to address some key questions before concluding that the DNP must be a requirement for any nursing leadership roles. In addition to the questions posed by the AONE/AONL, other questions need to be addressed as well. First, one must determine for what level of nurse leadership should the doctorate be required. It is the belief of the authors that it would be illogical to require all nurses in all levels of leadership to be doctorally prepared. As stated by Jones (2010), this becomes a scope of practice, connecting the level of preparation offered by the DNP as producing graduates functioning at a macroscopic level. The nurse executive at the most senior level in the organization needs to see the big picture that often transcends traditional organizational boundaries. Second, what impact, would such a requirement have on MSN programs? This issue is also raised by the AONE/AONL in their position statement. Some colleges have or are moving in the direction to eliminate MSN tracks as they create DNP degree options as part of their academic offerings. Second, what impact would the potential elimination of MSN programs have on the supply of nurse leaders? The AONE/AONL recognizes that nurses may choose other disciplines in which to acquire a master's degree, which may result in outward migration from the nursing profession. Overall, the reduction of the number of MSN programs or their elimination may result in some unintended consequences that may have long-term effects on the nursing profession and particularly on providing a steady pool of highly educated clinical nurse executives at a variety of levels. Does the MSN in nursing administration or health systems leadership benefit a mid-level manager/executive? We believe such preparation is highly beneficial for new directors. MSN education is well understood. When pursuing a doctoral program, it is important to understand the types of DNP, DNP/PhD programs offered and as a nurse leader understanding the value of an executive or health systems leadership focused DNP would be beneficial. Individuals should assess the programs available and make informed choices based on their career aspirations and goals. Seeking guidance from alumni is an excellent source of valuable information in addition to fully appreciating the curriculum, timeline, and project scope.

NURSE EXECUTIVE DNP PROGRAM PREPARATION: SIGNIFICANCE

The DNP program outcomes and curriculum prepare nurses at the DNP level to practice from a strong evidence-based foundation, effectively assessing healthcare policy, organizational effectiveness, population health, and economic trends in healthcare to provide interdisciplinary patient care in the communities in which they serve. The recent AACN report, *The State of Doctor of Nursing Practice Education in 2022*, reported that employers made the following curricular recommendations that are relevant to the DNP executive nursing role. Among these recommendations are to increase the focus on business education, including finance and statistics; increase the emphasis on policy and legislation; and include social media training.

One example is Duquesne University, where the DNP in Executive Leadership and Health Care Management was developed to address the needed knowledge and skills of the contemporary executive nursing leader and includes a partnership with the School of Business. Students take courses within the School of Business in addition to courses within the School of Nursing. These courses are designed to allow students to apply their current leadership experiences in a curriculum that advances their business acumen. Students collaborate with senior executives and leaders across various healthcare disciplines to identify problems, propose solutions, and implement change for healthcare systems as a whole. Students also gain the requisite knowledge of how finance, budgeting, human resources, and other aspects of business fit together to improve patient outcomes.

Several DNP courses, such as Health Care Policy and Finance; Ethical Leadership in Complex Organizations; Transcultural and Global Health Perspectives; Social Justice and Vulnerable Populations; and GPNS DNP Practice Practicum I and II expose students to individuals with diverse life experiences, perspectives, and backgrounds and increase students' knowledge of the local, state, national, and international communities that they serve. In Transcultural and Global Health Perspectives, students participate in a study-abroad trip to Rome. During their time in Rome, students witness a different health system and can compare it to the American healthcare system or to the system of their county. Students who do not participate in the study-abroad experience are required to seek out alternative cultures in their areas to enable them to participate in a comparative analysis. Residency preceptors at the sites where DNP students complete their projects provide feedback at the end of the residency. Evidence-Based Practice I and Evidence-Based Practice II were designed to develop the DNP student's ability to evaluate and use evidence to solve practice-based problems and improve overall quality of care. The DNP Practice Project provides an opportunity for the student to integrate their new skills into practice and to demonstrate many of the principles of nursing scholarship and the competencies delineated in the AACN Essentials (2021). The integration of these new or refined skills improves outcomes through organizational/systems leadership, quality improvement processes, and the translation of evidence into practice. The project focuses on program evaluation, quality improvement, and/or evidenced-based practice.

Duquesne's DNP Nurse Executive curriculum is described below.

THE DNP CLINICAL EXECUTIVE PRACTICA: ONE CLINICAL EXECUTIVE'S EXPERIENCE

Although all aspects of the DNP educational experience are important, additional focus will be spent on the practicum experience and the capstone scholarly project. The practicum experiences for each student are designed around the student's choice for specialization (administrative/executive or practice focused). The second author's (TT) practicum took place at Dartmouth Hitchcock Medical Center in Lebanon, New Hampshire, with the VP of nursing. During the experience, the VP of nursing along with other members of the senior leadership team undertook a restructuring of the organizational chart. The change, as you can imagine, was enormous. It not only was going to impact the hospital, but also had implications for change for other hospitals that were part of an alliance with Dartmouth. The VP of nursing was able to articulate the communication plan at every level of the facility and to those hospitals outside the physical boundaries of Dartmouth. The ability to participate in this monumental event at that hospital was vastly different from any of the clinical experiences in the MSN program experienced by this author 10 years before the DNP program.

During the practicum at Dartmouth, as a doctoral student, the second author functioned as a consultant and generated questions that might be posed by stakeholders and various team members within and outside the organization. During the residency, students are expected to exhibit critical thinking and participate in scholarly discussions. The key objective during the residency hours (practicum) is that the students drive the learning experience by being active participants who are not simply in an organization solely to shadow their mentors. Each course has objectives that provide guidelines for students' practicum experiences; however, the students also create unique objectives for each practicum experience, which results in ownership of the process and outcome of the residency. Although there were other practicum experiences (see Figure 7.1), the Dartmouth experience demonstrated the practice of an effective leader dealing with a very toxic change in a major healthcare organization. The overall focus of this practicum therefore was on the process of leadership and leadership style, and its effect on organizational culture.

A second practicum occurred at the University of Texas MD Anderson Cancer Center in Houston, Texas, one of the top oncology healthcare facilities in the nation. The

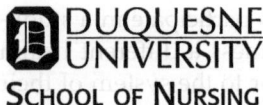

DNP-Executive Nurse Leadership Fall 2022 Start

Student: _____ Advisor: _____

Master's Degree Approved Hours: _____

Academic Year One								
FALL COURSES			**SPRING COURSES**			**SUMMER COURSES**		
YEAR	COURSE	CR	YEAR	COURSE	CR	YEAR	COURSE	CR
	GPNS 957 Evidence Based Practice I (50 Hours)	3		GPNS 959 Change Management and Project Analysis (50 Hours)	3		GPNS 955 Organizational Leadership in nursing and Health Care (50 Hours)	3
	GPNS 954: Analytical Methods for Evidence Based Practice and Practice Improvement (50 Hours)	3		MGMT 601 The Entrepreneurial Manager	3		GPNS 933 The Legal Environment in Nursing and Health Care	3
	TOTAL Credits	**6**		**TOTAL Credits**	**6**		**TOTAL Credits**	**6**
Academic Year Two								
FALL COURSES			**SPRING COURSES**			**SUMMER COURSES**		
YEAR	COURSE	CR	YEAR	COURSE	CR	YEAR	COURSE	CR
	GPNS 958 Evidence Based Practice II (50 Hours)	3		GPNS 960 Doctor of Nursing Practice Practicum I (Up to 350 Hours)	4		GPNS 961 Doctor of Nursing Practice Practicum II (Up to 350 Hours)	4
	MGMT 619: Budgeting and Finance for Managers	3		MGMT 620 Business Strategy	3			

FIGURE 7.1 Duquesne University DNP Nurse Executive Curriculum

focus of this residency revolved around my (TT) capstone project, which actually was a quasi-experimental pre- and post-test design study that investigated psychological distress among patients undergoing hematopoietic stem cell transplants. During this time, this second author was able to examine protocols and isolation practices used by experts in hematopoietic stem cell transplants. This practicum provided insight on current versus traditional practices for isolation and outcomes associated with various isolation interventions. The overall focus of this practicum was to evaluate the impact of leadership on the development of practice policies, standards, processes, and patient outcomes.

Throughout the DNP program, each student works with a patient population for which they must identify an evidence-based healthcare intervention to implement. Other critical components associated with the intervention and/or practice change includes cost-effective analyses, program evaluation, literature review in search of best practices, and identification of stakeholders that may influence the practice change and/or be affected by the change.

Another key focus of the DNP program is program evaluation. Several options for evaluation are introduced to students, which include utilization-focused evaluation, and formative and summative evaluations. In comparison to the master of science in nursing (MSN) administrative track, the detail with evaluation, research, evidence-based interventions, cost-effectiveness analysis, and policy development associated with healthcare

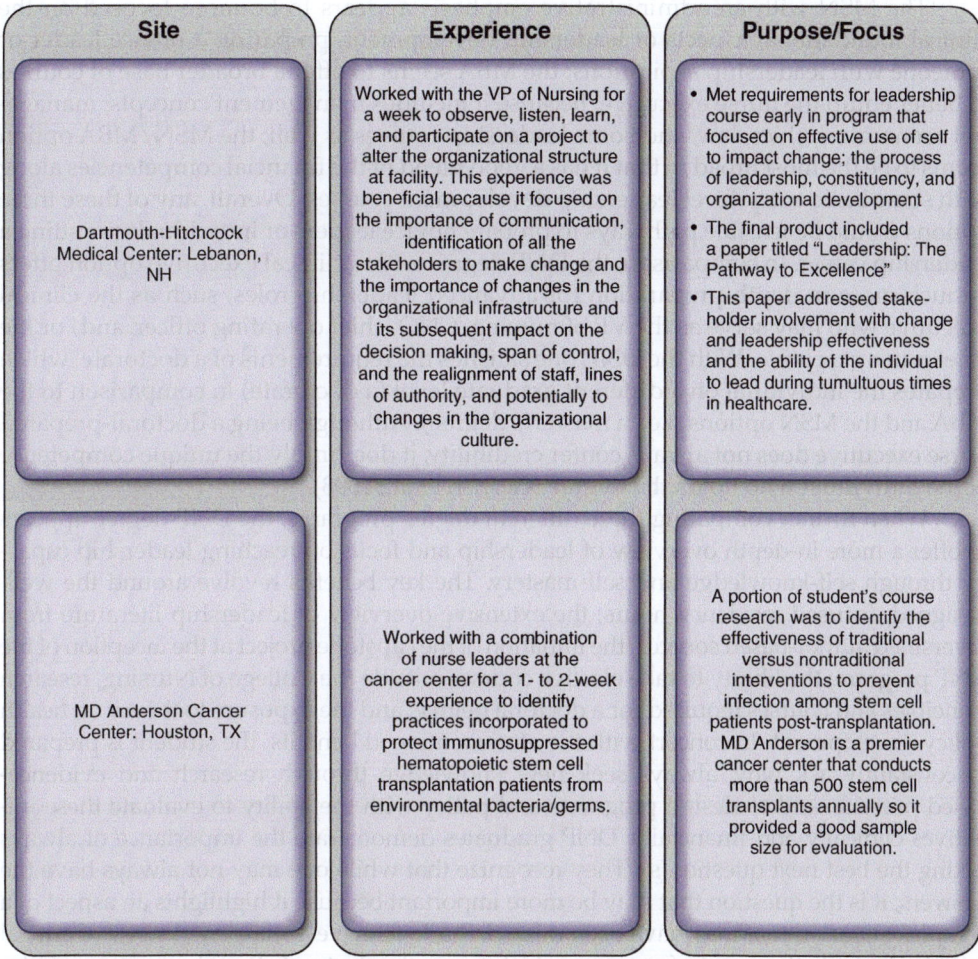

FIGURE 7.2 Student's Practica Experiences

initiatives, interventions, and outcomes was significantly different. Each of the authors believes that with the completion of the DNP program, we acquired a new level of thinking about program development and evaluation; identification and placement of best practices into practice settings; advanced practice in healthcare; interpretation of patterns from large data sets; and, most importantly, leadership in healthcare. Overall, the DNP practicum (residency) experiences greatly enhance the learning experience of students and enable them to view advanced practice from a macroscopic perspective, which is vastly different from the more microscopic approach experienced in the MSN administrative track. Figure 7.2 illustrates one author's experience as a DNP student.

■ NURSE EXECUTIVE PREPARATION: THE DNP VERSUS OTHER DEGREE OPTIONS

In terms of reviewing options to prepare the contemporary nurse executive, the options include an MSN degree with an administrative focus and a master of business administration (MBA); some colleges offer a combination of the MSN/MBA as a concurrent option.

The MSN with an administrative emphasis appears to be more focused on the clinical foundational aspects of leadership development, preparing a novice leader or someone with leadership aspirations; the MBA seems to offer a broader base of courses to better equip the nurse executive, because it includes management concepts, managerial economics, ethics, law, and some leadership courses as well; the MSN/MBA option seems to be the most broad in that it has a good blend of the financial competencies along with some basic entry-level leadership development courses. Overall, any of these three options would be feasible pathways to prepare novice leaders or individuals pursuing a leadership career. In comparison, the DNP degree with a clinical executive option offers a much more in-depth preparation for advanced leadership roles, such as the clinical executive who may serve as the VP of nursing, CNO, chief operating officer, and/or the chief nurse executive. With the DNP, one satisfies the requirements of a doctorate, which prepares the individual on a different graduate level (a doctorate) in comparison to the MBA and the MSN options (i.e., a master's degree). Although being a doctoral-prepared nurse executive does not always confer credibility, it does imply the unique competence of the individual who holds the degree (Gerrish et al., 2003).

When further comparing these different degree programs, the DNP degree appears to offer a more in-depth overview of leadership and focus on reaching leadership capacity through self-knowledge and self-mastery. The key benefits revolve around the well-designed, focused residency hours; the extensive overview of leadership literature from diversified author-based sources; the initiation of the capstone project at the inception of the DNP program; the liberty to take elective courses outside the College of Nursing, research principles and courses required for a doctoral degree; and the exposure to theory on health policy development. In concert with the aforementioned benefits, the student is prepared to constantly ask why, always seek new knowledge through research and evidence-based practice, and to design programs and policy with the ability to evaluate these initiatives clinically and financially. DNP graduates demonstrate the importance of always asking the best next question(s). They recognize that while one may not always have the answers, it is the question that may be more important because it highlights an aspect of a complex situation that may have been missed. Students have a sharpened sense of critical thinking outside the scope of nursing, which forces the doctoral clinical executive scholar to examine how healthcare is truly integrated both horizontally and vertically.

Very few nurse executives need to be convinced about the value of evidence-based practice (EBP) and its impact on safety, quality, cost, and elevation of the nursing profession. There is also evidence to suggest that hospitals have EBP models and activities, but there are still significant barriers to comprehensive implementation (Speroni et al., 2020). Nurse leaders with a deep understanding of EBP will be more effective in implementing EBP in their organizations as a standard of practice.

The DNP degree is an option that prepares nurse executives to perform at a higher level. We are not suggesting that the other degree options reviewed are inferior, because they are not. The authors believe that they offer a very sound preparation for one interested in leadership, while the DNP offers an advanced level of preparation for someone who desires more knowledge and preparation. The DNP is not more of the same, but a newer version or model of preparation for the nurse executive who functions as the senior nurse leader in organizations with other members of the executive team. The primary difference in the DNP is best described by Hader who states, "The curriculum and expectations of academic performance in the clinical doctorate programs are far more extensive than those in a traditional graduate program" (2010, p. 6). The focus of the DNP program is uniquely different and, in theory, does create a different type of graduate with the ability to think outside traditional boundaries and develop collaborative partnerships to move organizations forward successfully.

The AONL recognizes the MSN degree as critical for unit-level leadership and the DNP as appropriate for systems or executive-level leadership. Currently, AACN is forecasting the elimination of the MSN degree, moving to an all-DNP education option. Given the number of valuable work roles that benefit from having a master's degree but do not require the advanced competencies and expenses associated with obtaining a DNP degree, reaching consensus on this important point is needed (Morse & Warshawsky, 2021). It is important to note that in the 2014 AACN/RAND study on the DNP, three milestones were identified to achieve successful transformation to BSN-DNP track, which are: accreditation and certification requirements, student demand, and market demand. To date, none of these milestones has been achieved (Auerbach et al., 2015).

PREPARING THE CLINICAL NURSE EXECUTIVE OF THE FUTURE: WHY IT IS IMPORTANT

The U.S. Bureau of Labor Statistics estimates that the healthcare sector has lost nearly half a million workers since February 2020 (Yong, 2020). Statistics recently reported from a 2021 McKinsey & Company survey indicated that 22% of the remaining nurse workforce may leave their positions within the upcoming year (Hagland, 2022). A similar survey report from the AONL cited 17% of nurse leaders reporting that they were considering leaving the profession. Ninety percent of nurse leaders reported anticipating a staffing shortage beyond the pandemic (AONL, 2021). Many graduate nursing students did not enter or return to school for an advanced degree due to exhaustion or work demands related to the COVID-19 health emergency (Smith Glasgow, 2021). "The Role of the Doctoral Prepared Nurse Leader During the COVID-19 Pandemic: Lessons Learned" is discussed by Drs. Kingston and Zangerle, two seasoned chief nurse executives, in Chapter 19. Leaders and organizations that have best weathered various crises, most recently the COVID-19 pandemic, are those where leaders are in the trenches with the front lines. Institutions that have had the most challenging time have leaders who do not understand the real pain points people experience. Leaders who have excellent reputations stand behind their teams, and uphold nurses and other staff concerns and well-being as critical to high-quality patient care experiences. They are not focused solely on the bottom line. Nurse executives who are realistic, genuine servant leaders gain the respect of their staff (Gamble, 2022).

There is no doubt that the educational preparation and administrative-leadership acumen of the nurse executive are crucial to addressing these complex issues. In addition to the pressing nurse supply and morale challenges requiring creative solutions, broad long-term strategies and authentic leadership, nurse executives must remain committed to academic-clinical partnerships, diversity, equity, and inclusion evidence-based practice, quality nursing education for the workforce, and investment and elevation of the role of the nurse, particularly the bedside professional nurse. It is important for nurse executives to engage in reflective practice about the current crisis and the underlying factors resulting in the current state of the nursing workforce. Certainly, COVID-19 and its impact are major influences but what other considerations have contributed to the great resignation? The skill and advocacy level of the nurse executive are critical pieces of the puzzle if we are to stem the tide in nursing resignations and work toward a new and improved future of nursing that includes an inclusive work environment and representation at the bedside.

Since the inception of the DNP degree, there is growing evidence of its impact as demonstrated by successful graduates of the program functioning as effective clinical executives. Key indicators, as highlighted by the AONE, that need to be further investigated include the financial impact of increasing salary expectations of doctoral-prepared executives and the corresponding financial impact on organizations, patient satisfaction with holders of this degree, and specific degree-related patient outcomes as evidenced by organizations' performance with core measures established by the Centers for Medicare and Medicaid (CMS) and Hospital Consumer Assessment of Healthcare Providers and Systems (HCAHPS) scores. The majority of DNP graduates have reported that the DNP improved their competencies in quality improvement, evidence-based practice, and leadership (Kesten et al., 2021; Minnick et al., 2019). Jones (2010) indicates that executives at the top level of nursing administration are accountable for the executive level of patient services. She further states that executives will be expected to function at a macro level with decision making and actions that impact patients and others within the organization. Mid-level managers have a narrower focus and span of control within organizations and are more likely to function at a micro level by virtue of the organizational chart and structure of organizations. The nurse executive will work across both microsystem and macrosystem levels that include groups both internal and external to the organization. As stated earlier, one of the unique qualities of the DNP degree is its preparation of the nurse executive to think and function on a macrosystem level. Investigators must continue to monitor the market and demand for DNP graduates. In closing, the demand continues to create a need for clinical executives who are prepared beyond a master's level to address healthcare's enormous challenges. Since 2006, the racial and ethnic diversity in DNP programs has demonstrated steady growth (AACN, 2022). This finding is critical as it will hopefully increase the representation of BIPOC executive leaders who will assist with establishing the tone at the top for representation at the bedside and addressing health disparities among marginalized patient populations.

VOICES OF DNP EXECUTIVES: HOW A DNP INFORMED THEIR LEADERSHIP PRACTICE

Barbara Wadsworth, Chief Operating Officer

As a system CNE for the past 10 years, having completed my DNP in Health Systems Leadership from Vanderbilt University early in my tenure, I am incredibly grateful for the level of preparation, relevant learning, development, and understanding of the expectations of my executive role. Whether self-imposed, challenged by others, or advanced as a result of leading through a pandemic, the outcome is significant. The nurse executive steps up, leans in, and advocates for the community, patients, families, and workforce to assure sustainability, compassionate care, and well-being for all. My entire DNP learning experience was based on a foundational conceptual model that transformed my thinking and advanced my initiative, capability, and willingness to innovate, create, and make decisions. The level of collaboration needed throughout the pandemic was unprecedented and challenged by the speed to action required to assure a safe, responsive care environment. Having been promoted to chief operating officer while retaining the position of chief nursing officer from October 2020, the growth positionally, professionally, and personally continues. I find myself using the ANCC DNP competencies in my daily work and sharing them with the teams with which I work, constantly seeking understanding from others outside of our organization, including in non-healthcare fields, as that can be an excellent source of creativity and innovation for problem solving. It is imperative that as leaders, we challenge, support, and assure those we lead that failures will happen. We must model how to handle failure and how to support those to not fear failure. My role is to say yes, build people up by giving them opportunity, and reassuring them when they have failed, recognizing that without failure there is no growth and organizations flounder in mediocrity without innovation. As leaders we must carry the mission, vision, and values forward in the face of all adversity and communicate confidently that as a team our organization will rise to the occasion and meet the challenges ahead. Together we are stronger and it is our obligation to build resilience in our team.

As I reflect on the additional social challenges beyond the pandemic, a level of authenticity and compassion for the impact of societal issues on our workforce and the community cannot go unnoticed. Although far outside our walls and control, we can influence, control, and communicate expectations and standards that must be upheld day to day to support each other and to create a safe, welcoming, inclusive environment. I am proud to say that our organization has a level of authenticity that translates and is shared with all regularly as a way to acknowledge that we understand there is pain, anguish, and personal sacrifice, as well as challenges. Again, our ability to control those issues is limited; however, our heartfelt kindness, compassion, and ability to walk the talk benefits each of our team members and thus our patients and the community we serve.

Prior to my DNP education, I served in mid-level management. I would consider myself to have been successful in that role but with limited capacity and scope of practice based on the role and expectations. Following my DNP completion, I considered myself ready to take on increased levels of responsibility and a broader scope of advanced practice through leadership. Approximately 3 years following my DNP degree completion, I became the chief nursing officer of a community hospital where I worked along side other corporate officers to build and aid in the design of a new, replacement hospital. My responsibilities in this monumental event included working with architects on patient room design and headwall layouts, location of nursing stations, identification and placement of equipment. The replacement hospital culminated with the development of a plan to transport patients from the old hospital to the new location. This required an interdisciplinary team that involved nurses, physicians, local fire and police departments, and numerous others. This entire project required system-level thinking and planning. The scope was beyond the traditional boundaries of a mid-level manager. My confidence and capacity for understanding systems change on a broader scale was largely due to my DNP educational and residency experience.

Tukea Talbert, Chief Diversity Officer

Today, I serve as the chief diversity officer (CDO) for a major academic medical center (AMC). This role by far has been one of the most rewarding and challenging roles thus far. As the CDO, my work is all performed at a system-wide level. I work across many boundaries and with numerous interdisciplinary teams. The work expands beyond the hospital to the campus community and the community at large and includes all disciplines, not solely nursing. The scope of my work is expansive and requires that I build relational capital with people from all backgrounds in a myriad of settings ranging from front-line staff, patients, learners, senior executive peers, community leaders and advocates, campus/university colleagues, and city officials/leaders. Daily I build the business, clinical, and social justice case for diversity, equity, and inclusion (DEI). This work is possible because my DNP education and residency experience have taught me to think outside traditional boundaries and boxes to help create context for others to be a part of the DEI strategic plan and to create a system of accountability for the health system and our affiliates. Strategic objectives in the DEI space are predicated on my ability to view DEI literature and trends, network with industry colleagues, build power relationships in the community and across all settings. Ultimately, through communication/relationship management, leadership, professionalism, business skills/acumen, and my knowledge of the healthcare environment, I have been able successfully to build an inclusive, value-based culture, invest in our workforce impacting people from all backgrounds, provide more value-based care through stratification of quality outcomes based on race and ethnicity, and strategically advance care by influencing the presence of health programs in the community among populations made vulnerable through under-resourcing and power building relationships in the community.

My effectiveness in this role is linked to my skill sets that have been honed through my DNP educational experience. I have been able to create a DEI system of accountability and infrastructure that will be sustainable to ensure that all patients and people (workforce) have a fair opportunity to reach their highest potential in health and life success. As a leader, I have the privilege and responsibility to set the tone at the top. As a leader, I recognize the power and importance of people from all backgrounds not only having a seat at the table, but a voice at the table. As a leader, I must hold myself accountable to take bold actions to ensure representation at the bedside to eradicate health inequities. As a leader, I must demonstrate the use of people-centered language and bold actions to maintain an inclusive environment so that everyone can be their best selves and live their truth free of judgment.

Amanda Green, Director of Quality Monitoring and Reporting

The DNP program is where I first found my passion for leadership, as well as the power of my voice in improving patient outcomes through my nursing practice and skill set. My DNP program experiences allowed me to see first-hand the key role of nursing leaders. Many of these leaders have become my mentors and colleagues through my career and have taught me so much about nursing practice. The DNP program guided me in developing a leadership style and prepared me to take on the role of a nurse leader. It promoted my growth both professionally and personally and shaped me into the nurse and leader that I am today.

Kim Blanton, Associate Chief Nurse Executive

My doctoral degree assisted my leadership journey through further development of strategies and skills that have helped me navigate a complex healthcare system, while balancing the organizational and policy implications that arise in my new executive-level role. This degree increased my knowledge base of standardized practices that promote quality outcomes and healthcare system redesign. The doctoral program offered course work that focused on the changing healthcare reimbursement incentives, population health drivers, and promotion of innovative process improvement tactics, which help me address daily operational challenges at my facility.

Patty Hughes, Associate Chief Nurse Executive

The DNP provided me with opportunities for advancement and a set of skills that now allows me to more effectively navigate within the healthcare system. It also opened up access to a huge network of nurses across the country who face the same issues and concerns as me. With this network of DNP-prepared leaders, we can all work from our unique geographical perspectives and from our DNP knowledge base to offer resolution or best practices for our patients.

Lisa Thornsberry, DNP, Enterprise Nursing Director

The DNP program prepared me to be at the top of my educational background and competencies. The DNP program allowed me to focus on my development as a leader and to incorporate knowledge and use of transformation leadership in my daily role. I am better able to understand and manage all leadership styles and collaborate at the table with my peers and superiors. I am now better prepared on both local and state levels, as well as a national level, to focus on evidence-based practice and share my work with others at a higher level. Having my DNP has not only given me the tools to do so, but the confidence I need to pursue my goals within the healthcare field. It has allowed me to broaden my horizons outside of my healthcare institution.

Cecilia Page, Chief Information Officer

There are all the innate advantages of a DNP degree: the learning paradigms of critical thinking, research integration into practice, and courage to pursue innovations beyond your vision, which have all proven true in my growth as a leader who post-DNP was able to bridge clinical practice and information technology. Having achieved a DNP after more than 20 years of practice, it provided me a career differentiator not only to be awarded the role of chief information officer but also operate on a higher level, resulting in organizational impact. The toolkit gained in the educational process provided the foundation for success in addition to credibility around the executive table.

SUMMARY

Nurses in the clinical executive role are no longer invited to the table solely based on their clinical insight but more so for their ability and capacity to lead organizations based on their leadership competencies. The DNP is the optimal degree option for nurses seeking to expand their leadership skill set and knowledge to be better prepared to function in the increasingly complex healthcare environment.

In summary, because there are other strategies necessary to prepare nurses for clinical executive roles, the nursing profession cannot solely depend on an academic degree. Nurse leaders must be proactive in developing a framework that ensures ongoing development of leaders in executive roles that can be incorporated in the context in which they practice. These frameworks must include organizational charts that are aligned with the corporate strategic plan and that create the propensity for nurse leaders to have the capacity to lead and be involved in decision making at every level. The frameworks must provide ongoing opportunities for professional development, mentoring opportunities, and, last but not least, succession planning. Leadership development should not be by default or a second thought, but by design. It must be part of the culture established and supported by the nurse executive in collaboration with the other executive team members. We must regularly reexamine the process in which nurse executives are prepared for their leadership roles. Because leadership development is a process, it cannot be learned in a day or by completing another degree. The DNP degree offers an innovative educational experience that effectively prepares the nurse executive, but it is only the beginning of the process of leadership development. Nurse executives must be proactive and create organizational cultures that cultivate empowerment, ongoing professional development, and succession planning. The importance of ethical leaders who advocate vigorously for their constituencies cannot be underscored.

DNP-prepared nurses are focused on changing practice through the translation of evidence (Rodriguez, 2016). Nurse executives are far more focused on operational change and implementing change through leading practices that result in higher clinical quality, improved outcomes, and are patient focused. A DNP provides the needed academic advancement to meet the demands of the executive role and fully prepares the nurse leader to contribute in a meaningful way. DNP graduates add unique value in areas such as evidence-based practice, organizational change, quality improvement, and leadership. Many employers noted that DNP graduates have an enhanced ability to "look at the big picture" and bring about change at the organization or system level. This ability is being recognized increasingly by DNP employers such as hospitals and hospital systems, and there is some evidence that the number of leadership and executive positions that require or prefer a DNP is growing (AACN, 2022).

Swanson and Stanton (2013) report that current chief nursing officers believe that the DNP is relevant and is necessary to their practice. As we continue to focus on the DNP degree and its associated competencies, it will be important to continue to evaluate the impact of the DNP degree and hear what employers value among individual graduates and academic programs. As the largest profession within the healthcare workforce, nurses have an exciting opportunity to lead healthcare and make powerful positive changes and innovations. It will require well-prepared, courageous nurse executives at the helm willing to exhibit bold leadership even during the most tumultuous times in society and the industry.

LEADERSHIP CASE STUDY

The Nursing Shortage: Is International Nurse Recruitment the Solution?

In 2000, the number of full-time registered nurses (RNs) was estimated as 1.89 million, with an anticipated demand of 2 million (Bureau of Health Profession, 2004). The latter represents a 6% shortage (110,000) of full-time employed RNs nationally (Lee & Miller, 2005). Much of the increased demand is related to the projected number of nurses retiring, exceeding the number of new RNs entering the profession. Other drivers include the exodus of nurses related to burnout and stress especially at the height of the COVID-19 pandemic. Over an 11-year period, the number of nurses that have left the profession due to burnout has almost doubled from 17% to 31.5% (Wheeler et al., 2019). Understaffing is another driver for dissatisfaction and burnout during a time of high patient volumes and higher acuity patients that has resulted in burnout (Lasater et al., 2021). As vacancy and turnover rates increased, healthcare organizations focused on recruiting foreign-trained RNs or international recruitment.

Background

A major academic medical center (AMC) in the southeast was experiencing issues with RN supply to meet the demands of staffing units due to the pandemic challenges, nursing turnover, and challenges with recruiting domestic RNs. In the midst of the pandemic, a new 30-bed acute/progressive unit had been launched to meet demands and required RN staff. The unit was staffed predominantly with international and domestic agency RNs. In total, international RNs made up 50% of the staff used to care for the patients. The vacancy rate of this AMC ranged from 22% to 35% during the fiscal years 2021 and 2022.

The recruitment model used for this AMC was essentially an independent agency model in which an agency identifies and recruits international nurses for placement at healthcare facilities (Lee & Mills, 2005). Leaders were engaged in the interview process and were able to make final hiring decisions. The recruitment agency handled all of the contact and infrastructure assistance that included visa applications, experience and skill acquisition required by the hiring facility, and educational credentialing. Nurses were recruited from the Philippines, India, Kenya, and Nepal.

Challenges

Several of the international nurses ended their contracts early. Key drivers associated with the early exit of the RNs included (a) challenges with patient/RN assignments, (b) inability to adjust to practice differences between the AMC and their countries of origin, and (c) a lack of a sense of belonging and community (e.g., lack of trust in leadership, strained relationship with agencies, feeling of isolation).

The chief diversity officer (CDO) and the associate chief nurse executive (both DNP-prepared RNs) partnered to review and implement strategies to aid in the successful adjustment and recruitment of the international RNs. The CDO noted that the contract length of 3 years was actually longer or at least equal to the tenure of domestically recruited RNs. The CDO suggested that the AMC reimagine how the international nurses were from a lens of longevity versus temporary employment. Along with the associate chief nurse executive, they focused on onboarding, accessibility to community resources, especially those related to cultural enrichment and validation of the nurses, and measurement of impact (nurse-sensitive outcomes and employee engagement/satisfaction).

International Nurse Recruitment Questions to Consider

- What method is used to recruit international nurses?
- Are HCOs identifying ways to ensure that international nurses are connected to the community in which they will work?
  - Should there be a more intentional pathway to ensure that housing is a reasonably priced location that is proximal to the HCO?
  - Should efforts be made to ensure that international nurses are connected in their community by giving them housing locations in proximity to each other?
  - Should there be more intentionality to create an organized support group for international nurses so that issues can more easily be identified?
- Are HCOs conducting a formalized handoff with the recruitment agency that includes a thorough review of resources shared with the international RN such as:
  - Housing
  - Transportation (e.g., U.S. driver's license, vehicle, etc.)
  - Cultural supports/resources
  - Family absence/presence with RN

- Vacation allowances for travel to connect with family (locally or abroad)
- English as a second language accomodations
- Skill acquisition/competency assessment
- How are HCOs helping the RNs transition to practicing in the US?
- Are HCOs viewing the international RNs as temporary versus long-term (permanent staff)?
  - International nurses who are typically on 3-year contracts need to have comparable benefits for recognition and integration in nursing departments of HCOs
  - HCOs need to use the 3-year period as a time to recruit these individuals and ensure that they are fully acclimated into the healthcare system as their tenure is comparable to some domestically recruited RNs
- How are HCOs measuring the impact of the international RNs as it relates to nurse-sensitive outcomes (patient care) and the RNs, satisfaction, engagement, and sense of connection?

Strategies for Consideration

- Development of extended onboarding and recruitment plans customized for the international nurses that include:
  - Additional shadowing opportunities
  - Use of nurse clinical specialist to help with practice development at the elbow support
  - Use of staff development/educators to provide additional class instruction
- Creation of an international nurse navigator that would serve as a transition coordinator to the HCO and community (e.g., connect to cultural events, housing in close proximity to the HCO, connection to modes of public transportation, driver's license aids, vehicle rentals, car pools, etc.)
- Measurement of impact related to patient care/nurse-sensitive outcomes such as:
  - Catheter associated urinary tract infections (CAUTI)
  - Central line associated bloodstream infections (CLABSI)
  - Patient falls
  - Hypoglycemia management
  - Hospital acquired pressure injuries (HAPI)
  - Home grown questionnaire about transition (checklist) via a written or even focused interview with individuals
  - Utilization of curated questions related to sense of belonging/connection
- Ensure a handoff occurs between the HCO and recruitment agency for each nurse(s)

Case Summary Highlights

- Orientation and onboarding of international nurses must be structured in a way to ensure professional, personal, social acclimation, and clinical skill development
- HCO's must re-envision how the international nurse is viewed in that they are a permanent member of the team versus a temporary staffing solution
- Lessons learned include:
  o Leadership must take an active role in the recruitment, transition, and measurement of the impact of international nurses
  o Leadership must build relational capital with each nurse to ensure that they experience a sense of belonging and connection to the HCO, team, and leadership
  o Leaders must understand that foreign-trained RNs must adjust to new, more advanced technology, independent decision making/practice, new culture, new local vernacular, and different patient assignments
- Mentorships and sponsorships are essential for the foreign-trained RN
- Collaboration is critical to build a strong support system for international RNs; for example, this AMC used several experts within the system to build an infrastructure of support:
  o Chief diversity officer (created and identified system resources, for example, campus international affairs, general medical education coordinator, etc.)
  o Staff development specialist (focused on educational refresher for fundamentals in practice)
  o Clinical nurse specialist (served as a clinical practice development expert/resource)
- Frequent scheduled touchpoints with international nurses to facilitate timely feedback on their quality of life and transition
- Validation of services proved by the recruitment agency with the RN and its alignment with what is perceived by the international nurse

Case Summary

The supply and demand challenges with nursing will continue. The executive leadership teams in nursing and hospital leadership must reimagine the approach to recruit, retain, and promote nurses and the nursing profession. The DNP-prepared leaders are in a very unique position to play a critical role in the success of HCOs. They have been prepared to understand the practice challenges associated with nurses as well as to view the return on investment of having international RN colleagues at the bedside in the United States. This challenge in the profession is a time for DNP-prepared leaders to demonstrate their capacity to lead and use their education to know what questions need to be addressed along with who to invite to the table for a comprehensive approach that will lead to a sustainable solution.

It is also important to note that while nursing uses foreign-trained RNs, there are other disciplines that use individuals that are trained from other countries. This includes physicians and other disciplines. Solutions to address the recruitment, retention, and transition of foreign-trained individuals should be structured in a way to impact system-wide challenges and not singular departments. DNP-prepared leaders are often positioned to do boundary spanning and view matters from a system-level perspective that will aid in the development of a global solution that will benefit the HCO overall.

As trained DNP leaders, it is clear in the literature that foreign-trained RNs and domestically hired newer RNs will not inherit the wisdom, knowledge, or expertise of some of the more long-term RNs due to the massive exodus of RNs from the bedside (Yong, 2021). This fact must be a driving factor in how healthcare delivery, training, and recruitment are designed and performed. Part of the DNP education is looking at the translation of research to practice; the current plight of the profession makes this ability to translate research to practice even more critical.

CRITICAL THINKING QUESTIONS

1. Because leadership can be developed through learning and practice, what do you believe would be the essential content and experiences in a DNP program for a nurse either in or desiring to be in a clinical executive position?
2. Do you believe that having a doctoral degree would positively affect a clinical executive's authority and influence with other stakeholders?
3. Considering the differences in coursework and focus between PhD and DNP programs, which do you believe would be the most appropriate in development of the required skill set of a clinical executive?
4. What do you see as advantages of the DNP-prepared nurse executive taking both nursing and business courses as part of their educational preparation?
5. What would be the appropriate criteria to evaluate the effect of a DNP for clinical executives?
6. In your opinion, should the nursing profession address the issue of doctoral preparation for nurse executives and possibly establish a precedent and/or standard of preparation for other executives in top leadership roles? Why or why not?
7. What were your personal reasons for choosing a DNP program, and what track do you believe best meets your rationale for choosing a DNP program?
8. What do you believe are some of the current pitfalls with the preparation of nurse executives and how do you believe the DNP clinical track could address these issues/concerns?
9. What are the major issues facing the clinical nurse executive today? How will DNP preparation assist with addressing these issues?
10. What organizational steps must the clinical nurse executive take to rebuild the nursing workforce and improve morale in their organization?

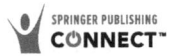

A robust set of instructor resources designed to supplement this text is located at http://connect.springerpub.com/content/book/978-0-8261-8137-4. Qualifying instructors may request access by emailing textbook@springerpub.com.

REFERENCES

American Association of Colleges of Nursing. (2004). *AACN position statement on the practice doctorate in nursing October 2004*. http://www.aacn.nche.edu/publications/position/DNPEssentials.pdf

American Association of Colleges of Nursing. (2006). *The essentials of doctoral education for advanced nursing practice.* http://www.aacn.nche.edu/DNP/pdf/Essentials.pdf

American Association of Colleges of Nursing. (2019). *AACN's vision for academic nursing.* https://www.aacnnursing.org/Portals/42/News/White-Papers/Vision-Academic-Nursing.pdf

American Association of Colleges of Nursing. (2021). *The Essentials: Core Competencies for Professional Nursing Education.* https://www.aacnnursing.org/Portals/42/AcademicNursing/pdfEssentials-2021.pdf

American Association of Colleges of Nursing. (2022). *The State of Doctor of Nursing Practice Education in 2022.* https://www.aacnnursing.org/Portals/42/News/Surveys-Data/State-of-the-DNP-Summary-Report-June-2022.pdf

American Organization of Nurse Executives. (2007). *Consideration of the doctorate of nursing practice.* http://www.aone.org/resources/doctorate-nursing-practice

American Organization of Nurse Leaders. (2021). *Nurse leadership COVID-19 study.* https://www.aonl.org/resources/nursing-leadership-covid-19-survey

Auerbach, D. I., Martsolf, G. R., Pearson, M. L., Taylor, E. A., Zaydman, M., Muchow, A. N., Spetz J., & Lee, Y. (2015). The DNP by 2015: A study of the institutional, political, and professional issues that facilitate or impede establishing a post-baccalaureate doctor of nursing practice program. *Rand Health Quality, 5*(1), 3. PMID: 28083356

Beeber, A. S., Palmer, C., Waldrop, J., Lynn, M. R., & Jones, C. B. (2019). The role of doctor of nursing practice-prepared nurses in practice settings. *Nursing Outlook, 67,* 354–364, https://doi.org/10.0116/j.outlook.2019.02.006

Boston-Fleischhauer, C. (2020). Chief nurse executive readiness for the here and now. *The Journal of Nursing Administration, 50*(6), 307–309. https://doi.org/10.1097/NNA.0000000000000889

Clark, J. S. (2012). The system chief nurse executive role: Sign of the changing times? *Nursing Administration Quarterly, 36*(4), 299–305. https://doi.org/10.1097/NAQ.0b013e3182669440.

Fasoli, D. R. (2010). The culture of nursing engagement: A historical perspective. *Nursing Administration Quarterly, 34*(1), 18–29. https://doi.org/10.1097/NAQ.0b013e3181c95e7a

Frearson, M. (2002). *Tomorrow's learning leaders: Developing leadership and management for post-compulsory learning: 2002 survey report.* http://lsda-acting.com

Gamble, M. (2022) *Hospitals' Ivory Tower Problem.* https://www.beckershospitalreview.com/hospital-management-administration/hospitals-ivory-tower-problem.html.

Gerrish, K., McManus, M., & Ashworth, P. (2003). Creating what sort of professional? Master's level nurse education as a professionalising strategy. *Nursing Inquiry, 10*(2), 103–112. https://doi.org/10.1046/j.1440-1800.2003.00168.x

Giddens, J., Douglas, J. P., & Conroy, S. (2022). The revised ASCN Essentials: Implications for Nursing Regulation. *Journal of Nursing Regulation, 12*(4), 16–22. https://doi.org/10.1016/S2155-8256(22)00009-6

Gruebling, N. Beckman, B. P., & Reeves, S. A. (2021). Wisdom shared: Health system nurse executives share success strategies for building high-performing nursing organizations. *The Journal of Nursing Administration, 51*(6), 307–309. https://doi.org/10.1097/NNA.0000000000001018

Hader, R. (2010). Who's the doctor, anyway? *Nursing Management, 41*(5), 6. https://doi.org/10.1097/01.NUMA.0000372024.76369.e8

Hagland, M. (2022). McKinsey Report: Nursing shortage will become dire by 2025. *Healthcare Innovation.* May 17, 2022, https://www.hcinnovationgroup.com/policy-value-based-care/staffing-professional-development/news/21268125/mckinsey-report-nursing-shortage-will-become-dire-by-2025

Hallinger, P., & Heck, R. H. (1996). Reassessing the principal's role in school effectiveness: A review of the empirical research, 1980-1995. *Educational Administration Quarterly, 32*(1), 5–44. https://doi.org/10.1177/0013161x96032001002

Jones, R. A. (2010). Preparing tomorrow's leaders: A review of the issues. *The Journal of Nursing Administration, 40*(4), 154–157. https://doi.org/10.1097/NNA.0b013e3181d40e14

Kesten, K. S., Moran, K., Beebe, S. L., Conrad, D., Burson, R., Corrigan, C., Manderscheid, A., & Pohl, E. (2021). Drivers for seeking the doctor of nursing practice degree and competencies acquired as reported by nurses in practice. *Journal of the American Association of Nurse Practitioners, 34*(1), 70–78. https://doi.org/10.1097/JXX.0000000000000593

Lasater, K. B., Aiken, L. H, Sloane, D. M., French, R., Martin, B., Reneau, K., Alexander, M., & McHugh, M. D. (2021). Chronic hospital nurse understaffing meets COVID-19: An observational study. *BMJ Quality & Safety, 30*(8), 639–647. https://doi.org/10.1136/bmjqs-2020-011512

Lee, R. J., & Mills, M. E. (2005). International nursing recruitment experience. *Journal of Nursing Administration, 35*(11), 478–481. https://doi.org/10.1097/00005110-200511000-00003

Minnick, A. F., Kleinpell, R., & Allison, T. L. (2019). DNP graduates' labor participation, activities, and reports of degree contributions. *Nursing Outlook, 67*(1), 89–100. https://doi.org/10.1016/j.outlook.2018.10.008

Morse, V., & Warshawsky, N. E.(2021). Nurse leader competencies today and tomorrow. *Nursing Administration Quarterly, 45*(1), 65–70. https://doi.org/10.1097/NAQ.0000000000000453

Muijs, D., Harris, A., Lumby, J., Morrison, M., & Sood, K. (2006). Leadership and leadership development in highly effective further education providers: Is there a relationship? *Journal of Further and Higher Education, 30*(1), 87–106. https://doi.org/10.1080/03098770500432096

Rodriguez, E. S. (2016). Considerations for the doctor of nursing practice degree. *Oncology Nursing Forum, 43*(1), 26–29. https://doi.org/10.1188/16.onf.26-29

Smith Glasgow, M. E. (2021). It is Time to Invest in Nurses [Letter to the Editor]. *Pittsburgh Post-Gazette.* December 2, 2021. https://www.post-gazette.com/opinion/Op-Ed/2021/12/02/Mary-Ellen-Smith-Glasgow-It-is-time-to-invest-in-nurses/stories/202112020012

Speroni K. G., McLaughlin M. K., & Friesen M. A. (2020). Use of evidence-based practice models and research findings in Magnet-Designated hospitals across the United States: national survey results. *Worldviews Evidence Based Nursing, 17*(2), 98–107. https://doi.org/10.1111/wvn.12428

Swanson, M. L., & Stanton, M. P. (2013). Chief nursing officers' perceptions of the doctorate of nursing practice degree. *Nursing Forum, 48*(1), 35–44. https://doi.org/10.1111/nuf.12003

Waxman, K. T., Roussel, L., Herrin-Griffith, D., & D'Alfonso, J. (2017). The AONE Nurse Executive Competencies" 12 years later. *Nurse Leader, 15*(2), 120–126. https://doi.org/10.1016/j.mnl.2016.11.012

Wheeler, M., de Bourmont, S., Paul-Emile, K., Pfeffinger, A., McMullen, A., Critchfield, J., & Fernandez, A. (2019). Physician and trainee experiences with patient bias. *JAMA Internal Medicine, 179*(12), 1678–1685. 10.1001/jamainternmed.2019.4122

Yong, E. (November 16, 2021). Why healthcare workers are quitting in droves. *The Atlantic.* https://www.theatlantic.com/health/archive/2021/11/the-mass-exodus-of-americas-health-care-workers/620713

CHAPTER SEVEN — Reflective Response

DIANE S. HUPP AND MARY CATHERINE LOUGHRAN

▪ EVOLVING ROLE OF THE CLINICAL EXECUTIVE

The role of the clinical nurse executive is as significant as it has ever been given the growing challenges in healthcare today. Nurse executives played instrumental roles during the 3 years of the COVID-19 pandemic. Managing the uncertainty, keeping our patients and staff safe, delivering quality care, and ensuring financial stability are a few of the key priorities placed upon nurse executives. There was no clear preparation or education to prepare for leading us through a pandemic. However, strong leadership including excellent communication skills and presence led most to success in holding their organizations together during the unprecedented and turbulent time.

Wadsworth, Talbert, and Glasgow define the clinical executive's primary responsibilities well, including aligning mission, vision, values, and philosophy which will ultimately build culture in one's organization. They include 24/7 accountability for nursing practice and patient outcomes. Outcomes are the driver of an individual's performance and an organization's performance. Successful clinical executives must be outcome driven with a focus on people, service, quality, growth, and finances.

Organizations today are challenged with recruiting and retaining top talent and opening access to manage demand, during a workforce shortage. The clinical executive is key to developing strategies to grow pipelines, retain staff, create new models of care, and deliver excellent patient and family experiences in the most cost-effective manner. These challenging times call for strong and educated nurse leaders.

▪ IMPORTANCE OF NURSE EXECUTIVE DNP PROGRAM PREPARATION

As a DNP graduate, I value the education that provided a more global view of healthcare that has helped me to prepare for progressing leadership roles, including the role of president of a large pediatric academic medical center hospital. I support the American Association of Colleges of Nursing's (AACN's) recommendation in *The State of Doctor of Nursing Practice Education in 2022* to increase the focus on business and finances as well as policy and legislation. Nurse executives must see beyond the walls of nursing and see the entire healthcare system as a whole. Improvement of patient and staff outcomes relies on all disciplines working together in an organization. New models of care that reduce the cost of care, while continuing to deliver on quality and service, are essential. Nurse executives partnering with chief financial officers is imperative.

One of the most meaningful experiences during my DNP program was the practicum. As chief nursing officer (CNO) at the time, I was offered the opportunity to step outside the hospital and provider space and into the payor side. Spending time at a health plan and learning the importance of value-based care was pivotal in my growth. The opportunity provided me knowledge and skills I would not have gained otherwise that have helped my understanding of both payor and provider strategies in the delivery of healthcare.

NURSE EXECUTIVE EDUCATION

The nurse executive practices in a business environment, which necessitates a skill set that is not traditionally taught in a graduate nursing curriculum. By utilizing their skills in organizational leadership, systems thinking, interprofessional collaboration, health policy, and direct patient care they contribute to the transformation of healthcare delivery to patient populations across the continuum of care. Therefore, a DNP nursing student needs to be adequately prepared to practice at the highest level of nursing practice to improve healthcare outcomes.

According to Giardinoa and Hickey (2020) students change personally and professionally as a result of course content, professional experiences, and collegial and faculty interactions. Students in our DNP program consistently comment on how they have changed both personally and professionally as a result of obtaining the DNP degree. They state that they can see the "big picture" when looking at issues in their organizations as well as identifying solutions from a systems perspective versus a departmental perspective. The students' educational journey helps them to redefine their professional roles of a DNP-prepared nurse leader.

We agree with Wadsworth, Talbert, and Glasgow, that the AACN is instrumental in shaping nurse executive education. The DNP Essentials (AACN, 2006) have provided the structure for the DNP executive nurse leadership curriculum along with the core competencies identified by the American Organization of Nurse Executives (AONE)/American Organization of Nurse Leaders (AONL). The DNP Essentials focus on advanced nursing practice but at the same time can support executive-level competency (Swanson & Stanton, 2013). In the past year, the AACN has introduced new Graduate Essentials (AACN, 2021) that we are reviewing and mapping to our current DNP courses. These new Graduate Essentials place a greater emphasis on population health, interprofessional partnerships, systems-based practice, professionalism, and personal, professional and leadership development. Additionally, the new Graduate Essentials include concepts that are integrated throughout the Graduate Essentials' competencies and subcompetencies. These include clinical judgment, communication, compassionate care, diversity, equity, and inclusion, ethics, evidence-based practice, health policy, and social determinants of health (AACN, 2021). Mapping these new essentials to our current courses provides us and other DNP programs with the opportunity to expand and/or include new content that will only support DNP students in their roles as nurse leaders and nurse executives. Faculty teaching in DNP programs need to continually assess their DNP curricula to make sure it is responding to the ever-changing healthcare environment and meeting the needs of nurse leaders and executives.

CHIEF NURSE EXECUTIVE PERSPECTIVES

Current chief nursing executives support increased emphasis on leadership, implementation science, and translation of evidence into practice along with business, information and technology management, and healthcare law (Embree et al., 2018). One way that we have supported the development of the business acumen of our DNP students in the Executive Nurse Leadership program was to collaborate with our School of Business to have our DNP students take courses in their MBA program (the terminal degree for finance majors). Their courses include entrepreneurial management, leading strategic change, budgeting and financial business operations, business strategy, human capital, diversity, and negotiation. The responses that we have received from students taking these courses have been positive and their interactions with the MBA students have provided them with different perspectives. We also hear from the School of Business that this collaboration has been positive for them as well and has exposed them to the world of nursing and healthcare. It serves as a model of interdisciplinary education and how schools within the same university can expose their students to diverse ways of examining issues from multiple perspectives.

According to Embree et al. (2018), CNO do perceive the DNP degree as appropriate for nurse executive roles. Application of the leadership skills that are enhanced and/or acquired as a result of their DNP education contributes to effective dialogue and decision making. It also ensures that nursing has a voice in decisions that affect patient care and the future of nursing practice.

As a former CNO of a large pediatric medical center hospital, I can appreciate firsthand what having a DNP degree brought to my tenure in that role. It allowed me to be more cognizant of working in both micro and macro systems, nursing research, and the importance of publishing nurse-led evidence-based practices and research in nursing and healthcare leadership journals.

CLINICAL NURSE EXECUTIVE OF THE FUTURE

The DNP nurse executive is uniquely qualified to influence the future of nursing and exemplify the standards of the profession. Wadsworth, Talbert, and Glasgow have noted the importance of ongoing research and information demonstrating the success of the DNP nurse executive or nurse leader in their roles in transforming healthcare delivery that supports improved patient care. Pursing the DNP degree also provides nurse executives with the opportunity to be role models for other nurses who are contemplating leadership roles in their professional career paths and provide for the next generation of nurse leaders.

As healthcare continues to evolve, we believe DNP programs will remain valuable in supporting nurse executives' professional growth and ability to see the broader picture in healthcare. It is both a challenging and exciting time in healthcare. As the AONE/AONL ponder the decision on whether a DNP should be required for the clinical nurse executive, let us continue to communicate the value of DNP programs and continue to ensure DNP programs evolve to meet the demands of the successful nurse executive.

REFERENCES

American Association of Colleges of Nursing. (2006). *The essentials of doctoral education for advanced nursing practice*. http://www.aacn.nche.edu/DNP/pdf/Essentials.pdf

American Association of Colleges of Nursing. (2021). The essentials: Core competencies for professional nursing education. *Journal of Professional Nursing Education*. https://www.aacnnursing.org/Portals/42/AcademicNursing/pdf/Essentials-2021.pdf

Embree, J. L., Meek, J., & Ebright, P. (2018). Voices of chief nursing executives informing a Doctor of Nursing practice program. *Journal of Professional Nursing*, 34(1), 12–15. https://doi.org/10.1016/j.profnurs.2017.07.008

Giardino, E. R., & Hickey, J. V. (2020). Doctor of nursing practice students' perceptions of professional change through the DNP program. *Journal of Professional Nursing, 36*(6), 595–603. https://doi.org/10.1016/j.profnurs.2020.08.012

Swanson, M. L., & Stanton, M. P. (2013). CNO perceptions of DNP degree. *Nursing Forum, 48*(1), 35–44. https://doi.org/10.1111/nuf.12003

CHAPTER EIGHT

The Nurse Educator Role

RUTH A. WITTMANN-PRICE AND DANA PERLMAN

■ NURSING FACULTY SHORTAGE

It has been more than 10 years since the first publication of this chapter describing the nurse educator shortage; unfortunately, the shortage has worsened. Even though the nurse educator shortage has become increasingly dire, nursing education continues to evolve, change, and become more regulated. Nursing regulatory agencies such as the National Organization of Nurse Practitioner Faculties (NONPF), the American Association of Colleges of Nursing (AACN), the National League for Nursing (NLN), and the National Council of State Boards of Nursing (NCSBN), have published recent information or regulations for nursing education yet expert nursing faculty needed to implement the changes are already overworked and underpaid when compared to academic faculty in other practice disciplines (Jarosinski et al., 2022). Besides heavy academic and clinical teaching workloads, as well as salaries that are less than those of clinically practicing advanced practice RNs, other factors also contribute to the nursing faculty shortage. Factors such as unsupportive leadership and stressful work environments have had devastating impacts and deter nursing faculty from staying in academic positions (Boamah et al., 2021).

The AACN has well-publicized the nurse educator shortage and rightly identifies it as a *national nursing crisis* due to the following data:

- The *Enrollment and Graduations in Baccalaureate and Graduate Programs in Nursing* (AACN, 2022) publication states that nursing schools and colleges in the United States turned away 91,938 qualified applications from baccalaureate and graduate nursing programs in 2021. Several reasons qualified students were turned away included an insufficient number of faculty, clinical sites, classroom space, clinical preceptors, and budget constraints. The number one reason for turning away candidates was the lack of nursing faculty.

- The AACN put out a *Special Survey on Vacant Faculty Positions* which revealed a total of 2,166 faculty vacancies in the United States that affected 909 nursing schools. Additionally, the survey, which had an 84% return rate, revealed that another 128 nursing faculty positions were needed to keep up with student demand (AACN, 2022).

A local example of the nurse faculty shortage is the numerous baccalaureate colleges/universities in the immediate Philadelphia, Pennsylvania, area (University of

Pennsylvania, Rutgers-Camden, Villanova, Drexel, Holy Family, Gwynedd Mercy, LaSalle, Widener, Easton, and Temple, to name a few), which are all reporting faculty needs. An internet search for nursing faculty positions in April 2023 revealed 76 positions in the Philadelphia area (within 25 miles of Center City, Philadelphia) on the Indeed website (2023).

A confounding factor in the nurse educator shortage is the need for diverse qualified nursing faculty as known by the demographics of the Philadelphia area and the country. The current nursing faculty in the United States does not mirror the demographics of the student or patient populations. There is an urgent need to diversify nurses and the nursing faculty workforce. Traditional hiring and nursing program admission techniques and implicit bias have deterred the progress of diversifying, providing equity, and being inclusive in nursing education (Bradford et al., 2022).

Some nursing regulatory agencies, the NONPF, AACN, NLN, and NCSBN, just to name a few, oversee much of the nursing education standards for undergraduate and graduate learners. Each agency updates its mission and regulations in response to the healthcare environment needs and provides nursing education with frameworks, standards, and competencies. Although there are other regulatory agencies, the four listed above are often cited; therefore, the influence that each of these organizations has on nursing education is discussed.

National Organization of Nurse Practitioner Faculties (NONPF)

The mission of the NONPF (2023) states; "The National Organization of Nurse Practitioner Faculties (NONPF) is the only organization specifically devoted to promoting high quality nurse practitioner (NP) education" (p. 1). The *2022 Standards for Quality Nurse Practitioner Education (6th ed)* provides guidance from a National Task Force (NTF) identifying the objectives of NP education (NONPF, 2022b). The NTF is comprised of representatives from the 18 nursing organizations listed in Figure 8.1. The NTF (2022) published four standards for nurse educators teaching in NP programs and within those four standards each standard has 7 to 15 criteria that need to be addressed.

1. Accreditation Commission for Education in Nursing
2. American Academy of Nurse Practitioners Certification Board
3. American Association of Colleges of Nursing
4. American Association of Critical-Care Nurses, Certification Corporation
5. American Association of Nurse Practitioners
6. American Nurses Credentialing Center
7. American Psychiatric Nurses Association
8. Association of Faculties of Pediatric Nurse Practitioners
9. Commission on Collegiate Nursing Education
10. Gerontological Advanced Practice Nurses Association
11. International Society of Psychiatric-Mental Health Nurses
12. National Association of Neonatal Nurse Practitioners
13. National Association of Nurse Practitioners in Women's Health
14. National Association of Pediatric Nurse Practitioners
15. National Certification Corporation
16. National Organization of Nurse Practitioner Faculties
17. National League for Nursing Commission for Nursing Education Accreditation
18. Pediatric Nursing Certification Board

FIGURE 8.1 Nursing Organizations Represented in the National Task Force

TABLE 8.1 AACN Domains and NONPF Corresponding Domains

AACN Essential Domains (AACN, 2021)	NP Domains (NONPF, 2022a)
Knowledge for Nursing Practice	Knowledge of Practice
Person-Centered Care	Person-Centered Care
Population Health	Population Health
Scholarship for the Nursing Discipline	Practice Scholarship and Translational Science
Quality and Safety	Quality and Safety
Interprofessional Partnerships	Interprofessional Collaboration in Practice
System-Based Practice	Health Systems
Informatics and Healthcare Technology	Technology and Information Literacy
Professionalism	Professional Acumen
Personal, Professional and Leadership Development	Personal and Professional Leadership

Additionally, the NONPF lays out competencies (NONPF, 2022a) that mirror the competencies published in 2019 by the AACN (Table 8.1). All 10 domains identified by the AACN Essentials are aligned with specific NONPF domains as well as an extensive list of subcompetencies that need to be met by learners in NP programs. Table 8.1 demonstrates the overarching domains of the AACN Essentials and the NONPF.

The NONPF, as a regulatory agency, does not address non-NP master's or non-NP doctor of nursing practice (DNP) degrees. Non-NP programs are accredited by the Commission on Collegiate Nursing Education CCNE (CCNE, 2023b), the accreditation arm of the AACN, one of the organizations prominent in developing the NTF standards and competencies.

Nurse educators who teach learners to become NPs are required to maintain the NONFP standards and competencies, as well as practice hours for continuing board certifications in their NP specialty. Board certifying organizations have their own set of topics that must be mastered, which are actualized in the certification test plan. Additionally, different board certifying organizations define "clinical practice" differently for NPs and NP faculty. For example, the American Nurses Credentialing Center (ANCC) provides a list of activities that can be used to satisfy the practice hours, including professional development (ANCC, 2022).

The American Association of Colleges of Nursing (AACN)

As stated before, the AACN recognizes the faculty shortage as published in the *Vison for Academic Nursing White Paper* (AACN, 2019). The AACN white paper states that nursing faculty should have a terminal degree and have current competencies for the subjects they are teaching. Additionally, the AACN proposes that nursing faculty have competency and knowledge about the AACN Essentials. The AACN indicates that additional educational courses and preparation are needed for nurse educators above and beyond holding a terminal degree, unless, of course, the terminal degree contains nurse educator courses. Specifically, those practitioners transitioning into an academic or clinical nursing education role should complete elective coursework in nursing education principles and be mentored into the educator role (AACN, 2019).

The AACN further encourages teaching teams to have diverse degrees, as well as curriculum design and instructional technology knowledge. Teaching should include didactic, simulation, and direct patient care. Nursing faculty should not only teach but engage in research related to clinical practice and educational issues (AACN, 2019).

1. Facilitate Learning
2. Facilitate Learner Development and Socialization
3. Use Assessment and Evaluation Strategies
4. Participate in Curriculum Design and Evaluation of Program Outcomes
5. Function as a Change Agent and Leader
6. Pursue Continuous Quality Improvement in the Nurse Educator Role
7. Engage in Scholarship
8. Function within the Educational Environment

FIGURE 8.2 Academic Nurse Educator Competencies

Source: National League for Nursing (NLN). (2022a). *CNE Handbook (2022).* https://www.nln.org/awards-recognition/cne/Certification-for-Nurse-Educatorscne/cne-handbook

The National League of Nursing (NLN)

The mission of the NLN is to "promote excellence in nursing education to build a strong and diverse nursing workforce to advance the health of our nation and the global community" (NLN, 2022d, p. 1). The NLN purports to be the voice of nurse educators and includes educators from all nursing education levels (diploma, associate, baccalaureate, master's, and doctorate). The NLN publishes four clear objectives as a strategic plan: (1) inclusiveness and (2) excellence in a diverse nurse educator workforce, as well as (3) integrity in education and (4) the building of a global nursing community (NLN, 2022d).

The NLN sponsors three certifications for nurse educators. The nurse educator certifications are the certified nurse educator (CNE), the academic novice educator (CNEn), and the certification academic clinical nurse educator (CNEcl). The NLN defines competencies for nurse educators in different roles (NLN, 2022a, b, c).

The NLN's eight competencies for academic nurse educators were introduced in 2005. The competencies have not changed and make up the CNE test plan. The competencies encompass the role of an academic nurse educator complete with teaching-learning and scholarship expectations. Figure 8.2 displays the eight NLN academic nurse educator competencies.

In 2018 the NLN defined competencies for the academic clinical nurse educator for faculty who teach in clinical settings. The academic clinical nurse competencies comprise the test plan for the CNEcl certification and are listed in Figure 8.3.

More recently (2020), the NLN defined competencies for novice academic nurse educators or faculty who are teaching for 3 years or less. The NLN novice academic

1. Function within the Education and Healthcare Environments
   1. Function in the Clinical Educator Role
   2. Operationalize the Curriculum
   3. Abide by Legal Requirements, Ethical Guidelines, Agency Policies, and Guiding Framework
2. Facilitate Learning in the Healthcare Environment
3. Demonstrate Effective Interpersonal Communication and Collaborative Interprofessional Relationships
4. Apply Clinical Expertise in the Healthcare Environment
5. Facilitate Learner Development and Socialization
6. Implement Effective Clinical and Assessment Evaluation Strategies

FIGURE 8.3 Academic Clinical Nurse Competencies

Source: National League for Nursing (NLN). (2022b). *CNEcl Handbook (2022).* https://www.nln.org/awards-recognition/certification-for-nurse-educators-overview/cne-cl/Certification-for-Nurse-Educatorscnecl/cne-cl-handbook

1. Facilitate Learning
2. Facilitate Learner Development and Socialization
3. Use Assessment and Evaluation Strategies
4. Participate in Curriculum Design and Evaluation of Program Outcomes
5. Function as a Change Agent and Leader
6. Pursue Continuous Quality Improvement in the Role of Nurse Educator
7. Engage in Scholarship
8. Function within the Educational Environment

FIGURE 8.4 Novice Academic Nurse Educator Competencies
Source: National League for Nursing (NLN). (2022c). *CNEn Handbook (2022).* https://www.nln.org/docs/default-source/default-document-library/cnen-handbook-2022_08.04.2022.pdf?sfvrsn=d53af4b9_3

nurse educator competencies comprise the test plan for the CNEn certification and are displayed in Figure 8.4.

All three lists of competencies and corresponding certifications for nurse educators have eligibility criteria and none of the criteria states that a person must have a terminal degree. The CNE and CNEcl criteria include at least 2 years of academic teaching as an alternative criterion for nursing educational courses. The CNEn criteria (which is the newest of the three certifications) requires nurse educator courses.

The National Council State Board of Nursing (NCSBN)

The NCSBN, being the watchdogs of the licensure and certification examinations for RNs and advanced practice RNs (APRNs), affects nursing education and the role of nurse educators. The goal of nursing education is to develop competent entry-level RNs and APRNs. The mission of the NCSBN is public health, safety, and welfare. The mission is accomplished through licensure and certifications. The licensure and certification examinations are an evaluative mechanism to ensure entry-level competencies. Therefore, the NCSBN regulates the most important outcome of nursing education and that is accomplished through practice analysis every 3 years (NCSBN, 2023b).

The NCSBN is enacting a new model in 2023 called the Next Generation NCLEX (NGN) which is predicated on a clinical judgment model. The clinical judgment model was developed because of the increased complexity of decisions that entry-level nurses have to make in clinical practice (NCSBN, 2023a).

The changes made by the NCSBN affect the current pedagogy used in nursing educational units and nurse educators must be able to apply new teaching/learning methodologies and assessment competencies in order to actualize RN candidate success. The clinical judgment model highlights how the changes in nursing practice affect the role of the nurse educator. Clinical practice updates are assumed into the licensure and certification assessments and become ongoing professional development opportunities for nurse educators.

Nurse Educator Qualifications

What qualifies a nurse to be a nurse educator is still not clear throughout the nursing discipline. Many nursing educational units will only hire a faculty member with a "terminal" degree, but since there is a shortage, many educational organizations are hiring faculty who are "in progress for their terminal degree". Master's degrees are usually the degree needed for associate and diploma nursing programs. Depending on the Carnegie classification of the college or university educational unit the terminal degree may be a DNP, EdD, or PhD. Other than the EdD there is no guarantee that a faculty member who has attained a DNP or PhD has nurse educator courses.

Most postgraduate nurse educator certification programs include at least three courses as essential knowledge for nurse educators. The three courses considered essentials address teaching-learning, curriculum development, and assessment and evaluation (NLN, 2022a). Many nurse educator certifications have additional courses, and many have practicum hours. The nurse educator course practicum hours usually consist of a preceptorship with a seasoned nurse educator.

The NONPF does not regulate nurse educators other than that they must maintain their APRN certification to teach in their specialty. Maintaining certification can be done in the form of current practice or professional development. The professional development required by the NONPF is not nursing education specific.

The AACN proposes that nurse educators have a terminal degree plus clinical competency above the level they are teaching, knowledge of the *"AACN Essentials"* and course work in nursing education. Nursing education is not considered an advanced practice by the AACN. Advanced practice designation is specific to the roles of certified registered nurse anesthetist (CRNA), certified nurse-midwife (CNM), clinical nurse specialist (CNS), and certified nurse practitioner (CNP; AACN, 2023).

The CCNE, the accreditation arm of the AACN, reviews academic units offering patient care–focused baccalaureate, master's, and practice doctorate degrees in nursing, as well as postgraduate (post-master's or postdoctoral) patient care–focused certificate programs, such as nurse practitioner or clinical nurse specialist. The CCNE recognizes that nurse anesthesia and nurse-midwifery have specific programmatic accrediting. The CCNE is not authorized to provide an accreditation process for nonclinical postgraduate certification programs, which includes the nurse educator track. Other nonclinical programs ineligible for CCNE accreditation are the nursing informatics and leadership tracks (CCNE, 2023a).

The NLN also has an accreditation arm, the Commission for Nursing Education Accreditation (CNEA), which accredits all levels and all programs (vocational, diploma, associates, baccalaureate, master, postgraduate, and DNP, 2023). Accreditation of nursing education programs is in alignment with the mission of the NLN. The NLN's oldest two certifications for nurse educators (CNE and CNEcl) provide an eligibility mechanism for nurse educators with experience teaching, yet the CNEn, the newest certification requires nurse educator courses.

The NCSBN does not regulate the educational process for nurse educators but determines the outcomes of the teaching process and is noted in this chapter to emphasize the changes that nurse educators need to adopt to foster successful educational outcomes for students. The new clinical judgment model must be understood and taught by nurse educators, many of whom have no formal education courses.

SUMMARY

The nursing profession's view, stance, and opinion of how to educate nursing faculty remains in disarray. Nursing education is not considered one of the advanced practice roles because it does not provide direct patient care, yet it affects direct patient care every day. The NONPF and CCNE do not recognize nursing education tracks or postgraduate certifications. The NLN does recognize nurse education tracks and postgraduate certifications but faculty without formal nursing education courses can be eligible for two out of three of the NLN certifications. Years of experience can be substituted for formal course work in the CNE and CNEcl certification, which is likened to the older apprentice-type model of learning.

Not having a direct path into nursing education, with the correct nurse educator courses, is a detrimental factor in the current nurse faculty shortage. Mentoring has been proposed as a positive step to faculty retention by the AACN and others (Hauck et al., 2022; Vanderzwan et al., 2023), but mentoring alone into an academic role, either at an MS(N), DNP, or PhD level is also denying academic nursing unit faculty with the formal knowledge needed in teaching-learning, curriculum development, and assessment and evaluation methods. Building confidence in nursing faculty may be imperative to retention strategies. Having the education needed for a role builds confidence (Gill & Newsome, 2023).

CRITICAL THINKING QUESTIONS

1. In 2004 the AACN made the decision to include the DNP Leadership Role but not Nursing Education. Why do you think they did that?
2. There is less debate about a new DNP FNP undertaking a full-time faculty role teaching other master's and DNP FNP students. How about the new DNP FNP teaching undergraduate students?
3. In your undergraduate program, what were the most effective teaching skills/methods that impacted you the most?
4. You are in your first full-time job as a DNP-prepared adult/gerontology primary care nurse practitioner. You decide you want to make some extra money as a part-time clinical instructor. How will you prepare yourself?
5. Why do you think there is a nursing faculty shortage?
6. BRAIN STORMING ACTIVITY: Spend 15 minutes and solve the nursing faculty shortage. Make two lists: 1) possible strategies and 2) fantasy strategies.
7. Discuss the link: fewer nursing faculty, fewer nurses trained (professional and advanced practice), fewer healthcare providers, less nurse-driven healthcare, equivalent to poorer national health outcomes?
8. What does the NLN mean by requiring teaching competencies?
9. Do you think nurses who get a PhD have these teaching competencies when they graduate?
10. Describe what you would consider the "Ethical Nursing Professor."

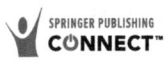

A robust set of instructor resources designed to supplement this text is located at http://connect.springerpub.com/content/book/978-0-8261-8137-4. Qualifying instructors may request access by emailing textbook@springerpub.com.

REFERENCES

American Association of Colleges of Nursing (AACN). (2019). *AACN's vision for academic nursing.* https://www.aacnnursing.org/News-Information/Position-Statements-White-Papers/Vision-for-Nursing-Education

American Association of Colleges of Nursing (AACN). (2021). *The essentials: Core competencies for professional nursing education.* https://www.aacnnursing.org/Portals/42/AcademicNursing/pdf/Essentials-2021.pdf

American Association of Colleges of Nursing (AACN). (2022). *Nursing faculty shortage.* https://www.aacnnursing.org/News-Information/Fact-Sheets/Nursing-Faculty-Shortage

American Nurses Credentialing Center (ANCC). (2022). *Certification renewal requirements.* https://www.nursingworld.org/~48fbb4/globalassets/certification/renewals/ancc-certrenewalrequirements.pdf

Boamah, S. A., Callen, M., & Cruz, E. (2021). Nursing faculty shortage in Canada: A scoping review of contributing factors. *Nursing Outlook, 69*(4), 574–588. https://doi.org/10.1016/j.outlook.2021.01.018

Bradford, H. M., Grady, K., Kennedy, M. B., & Johnson, R. L. (2022). Advancing faculty diversity in nursing education: Strategies for success. *Journal of Professional Nursing, 42,* 239–249. https://doi.org/10.1016/j.profnurs.2022.07.006

Commission on Collegiate Nursing Education (CCNE). (2023a). *Post-graduate APRN certificate programs & CCNE accreditation FAQ.* https://www.aacnnursing.org/CCNE-Accreditation/Resources/FAQs/Post-Graduate-APRN

Commission on Collegiate Nursing Education (CCNE). (2023b). *The CCNE accreditation process.* https://www.aacnnursing.org/CCNE-Accreditation/What-We-Do/CCNE-Accreditation-Process

Gill, M. E., & Newsome, W. M. (2023). A call to action for preparing nursing faculty to teach nursing theory. *Journal of Nursing Education, 62*(4), 191–192. https://doi.org/10.3928/01484834-20230323-01

Hauck, B., Seldomridge, L., Hall, N., Reid, T., Payne, B., & Jarosinski, J. (2022). Faculty academy and mentorship initiative partners with the Cohen Scholars Program to address the nurse faculty shortage. *Maryland Nurse, 24*(2), 17–17

Indeed. (2023). *Job search.* https://www.indeed.com/jobs?q=nurse+educator&l=Philadelphia%2C+PA&vjk=100d8bb397c054d9

Jarosinski, J. M., Seldomridge, L., Reid, T. P., & Willey, J. (2022). Nurse faculty shortage: Voices of nursing program administrators. *Nurse Educator, 47*(3), 151–155. https://doi.org/10.1097/NNE.0000000000001139

National Council State Board of Nursing (NCSBN). (2023a). *NCSBN launches next generation NCLEX exam.* https://www.ncsbn.org/news/ncsbn-launches-next-generation-nclex-exam

National Council State Board of Nursing (NCSBN). (2023b). *About NCSBN.* https://www.ncsbn.org/about.page

National League for Nursing (NLN). (2022a). *CNE Handbook (2022).* https://www.nln.org/awards-recognition/cne/Certification-for-Nurse-Educatorscne/cne-handbook

National League for Nursing (NLN). (2022b). *CNEcl Handbook (2022).* https://www.nln.org/awards-recognition/certification-for-nurse-educators-overview/cne-cl/Certification-for-Nurse-Educatorscnecl/cne-cl-handbook

National League for Nursing (NLN). (2022c). *CNEn Handbook (2022).* https://www.nln.org/docs/default-source/default-document-library/cnen-handbook-2022_08.04.2022.pdf?sfvrsn=d53af4b9_3

National League for Nursing (NLN). (2022d). *Mission and strategic plan.* https://www.nln.org/about/about/mission-and-strategic-plan

The National Organization of Nurse Practitioner Faculties (NONPF). (2022a). *NP role core competencies.* https://www.nonpf.org/page/NP_Role_Core_Competencies

The National Organization of Nurse Practitioner Faculties (NONPF). (2022b). *Standards for quality nurse practitioner education* (6th ed.). https://www.nonpf.org/store/viewproduct.aspx?id=20761806

The National Organization of Nurse Practitioner Faculties (NONPF). (2023). https://www.nonpf.org

Vanderzwan, K. J., Hiller, A., Carlucci, M., Amusina, O., Ryan, C., Krassa, T., McPherson, S., Tozer, C., Quinn, L., & Kent, D. (2023). A mentoring workgroup for academic role transition among clinical-track nursing faculty. *Journal of Nursing Education, 62*(3), 183–186. https://doi.org/10.3928/01484834-20230109-10

CHAPTER EIGHT
Reflective Response 1

BRITTANY GASPAR NETTLES

I graduated with my DNP in April of 2020, right as the world was effectively "shutting down." The global COVID-19 pandemic transitioned education to remote modes in what seemed like an instant, and both students and educators were grappling with the loss of in-person learning and clinical opportunities, as well as the sudden reliance on technology to ensure education in caring professions did not cease. Having worked as an adjunct clinical instructor for undergraduate nursing clinical while completing my DNP, I had already been planning a direct transition into teaching after graduation, but I now found myself facing the reality of transitioning into teaching at a time of extreme uncertainty. Undergraduate nurse educators were scrambling to figure out how to meet the unique needs of nursing students through the lens of a webcam while upholding academic integrity and rigor. Entering into education at this time provided both a unique challenge and an excellent opportunity for growth as I made my transition from an expert bedside registered nurse to an advanced beginner nurse practitioner and educator.

I think it is important to understand the context in which I transitioned into education post-DNP before reflecting on my experiences over the last 3 years. All things considered, my transition into education after obtaining my DNP was not as rocky or challenging as I had anticipated. I attribute some of my success in transitioning to the fact that I entered into education with a terminal degree. Completing my DNP project provided me with extensive experience in searching for, appraising, aggregating, and translating evidence into practice. These skills were essential in educating students throughout an ever-evolving pandemic, and they allowed me to be proactive in addressing student needs and in the utilization of technology to facilitate nursing education. I used research, student feedback, and my own personal experiences to develop more engaging remote educational sessions, quickly abandoning the traditional lecture format so many in education have relied on for so long because I was exhausted talking into the "void" to small, pictureless boxes on the Zoom screen. Attendance in my sessions improved. I did not shy away from discussions about the struggles of sudden shifts to remote learning and the physical and social barriers to accessing virtual education, as I had experienced education within the same setting. I made sure to check-in on the students whenever I had them "live," and made it a habit to email to check-in if I perceived there were any problems. I held virtual office hours with an "open door," meaning any student could pop-in on my Zoom link and discuss any issues, barriers, concerns, or questions they had. I felt as though I had the leadership and translation skills to help both students and faculty navigate these challenges.

I found myself acting as a mentor and leader for new faculty entering into my second year post-DNP. I am certain I would not have been in that position had it not been for the foundation of my DNP education and the ways in which I utilized my learned skills during that first unpredictable year. The resumption of in-person learning proved to be particularly challenging, as we were moving undergraduate nursing students who did skill checkoffs via Zoom into clinical courses that demanded solid skill and knowledge foundations on the first day of class. As faculty, we quickly identified fundamental knowledge deficits that we attributed to lack of engagement and breeches in academic integrity during remote learning. When we came back to in-person learning, we found that students were not prioritizing school, since their remote schedules had allowed them to work full-time while "attending" classes. Undergraduate students felt that we should be available and working on their schedules, when previously the schedule had always been set by the university. Given that this was many students' first experiences in college, they simply didn't know any different. Faculty resistance to returning to in-person learning was also a considerable barrier, with students receiving inconsistent guidance and communication. These challenges were overwhelming, and I found myself drowning between my desire to be student-focused but firm on my expectations of professionalism and rigor. In losing touch with our students, even just for a few semesters, we had lost our ability to infuse the principles of autonomy, accountability, integrity, excellence, and responsibility throughout all interactions—not just those that occur in a classroom.

To be frank, the past year (my third as a post-DNP educator) has been a struggle—not in the arena of facilitating course-specific nursing content, but in the arena of helping students understand the return to prepandemic expectations. Most students welcomed the return to in-person learning but addressing the few of those who are resistant to working within the new (old) program methodologies diverts time and energy away from working toward program and course-specific goals. As a faculty, we meet resistance to things like testing in person, attending clinicals on days that the hospital assigns, assignment deadlines, having to come to campus more than one day a week for classes and labs, and to meeting in-person to discuss course progression and challenges. The singular focus on National Council Licensure Examination (NCLEX) pass rates from local, state, and national interests have placed many points of emphasis on passing a test, rather than equipping our students with both the academic and professional skills necessary to navigate the complex world of nursing. As educators, we are challenged to consider the need for nurses due to the nursing "shortage," as well as the needs of this postpandemic generation of nursing students, all while balancing the unchanged expectations of the nursing profession. My DNP education has been, and will continue to be, essential in helping shape the "new normal" for undergraduate nursing students in the face of mounting barriers and demands.

CHAPTER EIGHT | Reflective Response 2

TIFFANY PRESSLEY

This chapter sheds light on many of the wonderful aspects of the nurse educator role. As nurse educators, we hold the future of nursing and advanced practice nursing in our hands. This is a tall task that requires preparation and well-rounded support to be successful. The chapter also creates a space for us to reflect on the challenges we face as nurse educators. In an effort to maintain a solution-focused reflection, I will expand on a few of the challenges mentioned within the chapter by sharing my experience with these hardships and offering words of wisdom for transforming these tribulations into triumphs.

ADDRESSING THE ELEPHANT IN THE ROOM

Let's first address the elephant in the room: the nursing shortage. According to a recent study, retirement and stress/burnout magnified by the COVID-19 pandemic contributed to approximately 100,000 registered nurses (RNs) leaving the workforce (Russell, 2023). By 2027, it is estimated that approximately 800,000 RNs and 184,000 licensed practical nurses/licensed vocational nurses (LPNs/LVNs) will have left the workforce since the beginning of the COVID-19 health emergency (Martin et al., 2023). Those numbers account for approximately 20% of nurses in the workforce today. All the while, many nursing schools across the country are seeing lower enrollment rates and an increase in the number of students struggling academically to meet the rigorous standards needed to enter and complete a nursing program. As nurse educators, we are vital to the future of nursing in the workforce. We are the foundation on which community trust in nursing and medicine is built. However, as nurse educators work toward this task of educating the next generation, we face our own shortages in the number of nursing and clinical faculty able to adequately perform the job at hand. This can leave one with the continual burden of needing to do more with less.

My first job as an advanced practice nurse was in the Air Force. Through the U.S. Air Force Health Professions Scholarship Program, the Air Force was generous enough to pay my way through my BSN to DNP program in exchange for years of military service. As a new provider, I quickly took on the weight of co-managing the psychiatric needs of the entire base with one other provider while also managing the roles and responsibilities of being an officer in the military. One day, I shared some of my frustrations with my mentor at the time. My mentor was higher-ranking than me and, fortunately for me, a licensed clinical social worker by trade. I remember expressing my frustration that I was struggling to do "more with less." After all, I had always prided myself on finding a way to make things work regardless of the resources given. That day, my mentor took a different approach and instructed me very clearly:

My mentor: "Captain Pressley, you will often hear that you are supposed to do more with less. Do you know what we *actually* do with less?"

Me: "No, sir. More?"

My mentor: "Less. We do less with less."

This conversation has stuck with me for years, as I carry and apply it daily to my career as a nurse educator as well as my ongoing part-time career as a psychiatric mental health nurse practitioner and U.S. Air Force traditional reservist. *We do less with less.* Sit with that for a minute. If we continue to push ourselves to do more with less, we fail to draw proper attention to the areas where more is needed. Simultaneously, we burn the candle at both ends, likely decreasing our overall effectiveness and self-care.

Words of wisdom: When discovering a situation where there is a need or push to do more with less, do less and professionally make the need(s) known. Instead of continuing to burn the candle at both ends, press pause and temporarily blow out the flame. Devote your energy instead to the appropriate way to advocate, search for, request, or procure "more." In nursing education, we come from various types of preparation and specialties that make a nursing program complete: DNP, PhD, EdD, MSN, MSN-Ed, CNE, etc. Regardless of our preparation, we are all taught the concepts of the nursing process, evidence-based practice, quality improvement, research, etc., which all require thorough assessment, careful planning, methodical intervention, and abundant advocation. To aptly educate the next generation of nurses, we must likewise apply these concepts to our daily challenges as nurse educators, using data and evidence to advocate for our needs and the needs of students.

GROWING FROM WITHIN AND MENTORSHIP

The chapter provokes reflection on the current faculty shortage as well as the weight of the expectations of nursing faculty. As nursing faculty, depending on the college/university, we are typically expected to be well-rounded in teaching, service, and scholarship in order to progress in our careers (and make tenure). How those three areas are defined and how well nursing faculty are supported in their quest to exemplify all three areas also depends on the college/university and the resources available. Let's take, for example, a nursing faculty member who is required to practice to maintain the licensure/certification needed to teach and clinically supervise nursing students. However, this faculty member is not given reduced teaching credits or compensated for any type of practice hours by their university. Let's also say this faculty member is at a university where the department of nursing is two full-time faculty members short, leading to an increase in teaching load. Where is the time for scholarship? Where is the time for service? Where is the time for self-care and the prioritization of personal needs? Is this faculty member being set up to fail the career progression/tenure expectations they are expected to meet? Let's add one more layer to the example: this nurse educator has no prior teaching experience or education around the pedagogy of nursing education. How are they expected to write curriculum, write test questions and assignments, etc., without adequate training and mentorship? What is adequate training and mentorship? How do we better empower our faculty members—especially those required to practice—to succeed?

Transitioning from full-time practice to full-time academia came with perks and challenges. Having a schedule that caters well (most days) to my personal life and responsibilities as a mother, wife, and community member is by far the biggest perk for me personally. I was fortunate enough to have training in my first undergraduate degree (prior to my nursing career) as a K–12 Spanish teacher as well as the opportunity to complete a nurse educator certificate during my BSN–DNP program. When I decided to switch from public secondary education to nursing, I suspected that teaching would find its way back into my career eventually. I am forever grateful for the nurse educator courses and practicum experience I had during my certification courses. These courses taught me pedagogy in nursing education and how to apply data, research, and evidence-based practice to my role as a nurse educator.

However, even with a respectable amount of preparation, training, and experience to take on a nursing faculty position, the weight of writing a new program, curriculum, and corresponding courses has been heavy at times. Seeking out other faculty members from my university and outside universities with education, training, and experience in nursing education (DNP in educational leadership, master's in nursing education, nurse educator certificate, etc.) has been monumental in my success as a faculty member and program coordinator. I have greatly benefited and am forever appreciative of the time and investment from my mentors and colleagues.

Words of wisdom: Universities and nursing departments must prioritize the mentorship model to support their faculty members, especially those without formal education or experience in nursing education. The mentorship model should include a pathway (financed by the university as professional development) for all nursing faculty to take courses to earn an additional degree/certification(s) in nursing education. The mentorship model should also include a peer mentor designated for new nursing faculty (regardless of experience). What is our most prized possession as humans? Time and money. (And arguably food for my fellow foodies out there!) These mentors should be paid for their mentorship, either with financial compensation or a reduction in course load.

Please remember to be kind to new faculty members coming in, even if it seems like they have everything they need according to their credentials and CV. Be kind and check in, even if they have worked at another university for years. For example, the solo act of moving from Blackboard to Canvas or vice versa can be overwhelming. If you are a new faculty member and you have not received a mentor, ask your leadership for one. Seek out support and wisdom from those who have education, training, and experience in nursing education.

DIVERSIFY AND SHOW ME THE MONEY

As nurse educators, we have recently been tasked with updating our curriculum from the 2006 version of *The Essentials* to the 2021 version, *The Essentials: Core Competencies for Professional Nursing Education* (American Association of Colleges on Nursing (AACN, 2021). What I appreciate most about the updated version is the increased emphasis on diversity, cultural competence, humility, and self-care. The Brookings Institution published a report with an analysis of the 2020 U.S. Census Bureau data that indicated that 40% of the U.S. population now identify as people of color: Latino or Hispanic, Black, Asian American, Native Hawaiian or Pacific Islander, and as two or more races (Frey, 2021). The report projected that by 2045, the majority of the U.S. population would be comprised of minority populations. We must teach and model the concepts of cultural awareness, cultural and linguistic competence, cultural sensitivity, cultural humility, and the impact of social determinants of health. We must work diligently to ensure our nursing workforce reflects the communities it serves. But how?

We established earlier that nursing education is the foundation of the future of nursing. Likewise, the future of diversity in nursing and nursing students is linked to increasing minority representation in our nursing faculty. As a nursing department, how are we exemplifying the need for minority representation in nursing and nursing education when many of our departments have one or fewer nursing faculty from minority backgrounds? For example, "according to 2021 data from AACN's annual survey, only

19.2% of full-time nursing school faculty come from minority backgrounds, and only 7.4% are male" (AACN, 2023). Successful recruitment of general nursing faculty as well as nursing faculty from minority backgrounds is dependent upon the equitable compensation of nursing faculty to nurses and advanced practice nurses in the workforce.

Words of wisdom: We must know and advocate for our worth as nurse educators. Negotiate your salary with comparative data from the workforce. Take advantage of tax breaks (in some states) for precepting, loan repayment for nurses and nursing faculty, scholarships/grants to continue your education, etc. As nursing faculty, we must advocate for and be active recruiters for a more diverse department.

RESILIENCY AND SELF-CARE

The nature of our roles as nurses and nurse educators often leaves us with superhero vibes. Frankly, we are superhuman in the ways we multitask, prioritize care, and save lives. However, we must be mindful of the danger of taking on the "superhero syndrome" by beginning to think we are the only ones who can "fix" a situation (Manning, 2021). This mindset promotes reactivity and prevents strategic planning and support. Most current research indicates that it is our younger RNs who are not surviving the stress and burnout of the nursing career. RNs ages 35 and younger are currently at the highest risk of burnout and leaving the workforce (Auerback et al., 2022). As nurse educators, we must set the example of what it means to care for ourselves to properly care for others.

Let me first say for any family, friend, or colleague that might also read this: I am "preaching to the choir" on this one. There are weeks throughout the semester when the candle is burning at both ends. Late nights and early mornings seem to be the only time to squeeze in those remaining six charts from patient care yesterday, grade those reflective journal assignments, write an exam, or create my daughter's costume for Sally from *The Cat in the Hat* for Dr. Seuss Day. I am a mother of three, a wife of one, a provider of the psychiatric needs of a panel of patients, a program coordinator and professor to graduate PMHNP students finding their way to the next step in their career, and a professor to undergraduate nursing students learning how to provide trauma-informed care to their patients while still sorting out their own identity and mental health challenges. When my cup runs empty, other people in my life with needs are still there, sucking with a straw to find any remnants of what is left.

Words of wisdom: The work is never done. Take caution not to allow your cup to run empty. The adage "never stop learning" takes on a whole new meaning and weight as a nurse educator. Our commitment to never stop learning is imperative for the future of nursing. Schedule time for yourself. Schedule time for your hobbies, your children, your partner, your friends/family, etc. Build a self-care routine by making one small change at a time and sticking to it. Find ways to destress that work for you and plan for them. Practice mindfulness-based interventions and strategies that have been linked with decreased stress among nurses and nursing faculty (Green & Kinchen, 2021). Find the appropriate time and professional manner to say "no." These acts are not selfish, but rather self-protective and empower us to model self-care and resilience to the next generation of nurses.

CONCLUSION

I admire the authors of this chapter for their willingness to highlight the importance of the nurse educator's role. I hope this reflection, my experiences, and my words of wisdom inspire advocacy for nursing faculty and nursing students, mentorship of junior faculty, recruitment of a diverse nursing faculty, and increased self-care and resiliency.

REFERENCES

American Association of Colleges of Nursing (AACN). (2023). *Fact sheet: Enhancing diversity in the nursing workforce.*

American Association of Colleges of Nursing (AACN). (2021). *The essentials: Core competencies for professional nursing education.*

Auerbach, D. I., Buerhaus, P. I., Donelan, K., & Staiger, D. O. (13 April 2022). *A worrisome drop in the number of young nurses.* Health Affairs Forefront. https://doi.org/10.1377/forefront.20220412.311784

Frey, W. (2021). New 2020 census results show increased diversity countering decade-long declines in America's white and youth populations. *Brookings Institute.* https://www.brookings.edu/research/new-2020-census-results-show-increased-diversity-countering-decade-long-declines-in-americas-white-and-youth-populations

Green, A., & Kinchen, E. (2021). The effect of mindfulness meditation on stress and burnout in nurses. *Journal of Holistic Nurses, 39*(4), 356–368. https://doi.org/10.1177/08980101211015818

Manning, M. (2021). *The step-up mindset for senior managers.* Panoma Press.

Martin, B., Kaminski-Ozturk, N., O'Hara, C., & Smiley, R. (2023). Examining the impact of the COVID-19 pandemic on burnout and stress among U.S. nurses. *Journal of Nursing Regulation, 14*(1), 4–12. https://doi.org/10.1016/S2155-8256(23)00063-7

Russell, K. (2023, April 14). About 100,000 nurses left the workforce due to pandemic-related burnout and stress, survey finds. *CNN.COM,* https://www.cnn.com/2023/04/13/health/nurse-burnout-post-pandemic/index.html#:~:text=Audio%20Live%20TV-,About%20100%2C000%20nurses%20left%20the%20workforce%20due%20to%20pandemic,burnout%20and%20stress%2C%20survey%20finds&text=About%20100%2C000%20registered%20nurses%20in,of%20State%20Boards%20of%20Nursing

CHAPTER EIGHT Reflective Response 3

JENNIFER LACY

Like many venturing into healthcare, my goal was to help people, although I initially wasn't sure nursing was the profession for me. A few courses and inspiring professors later, my love of nursing and dedication to further learning were sparked, eventually leading to a DNP degree. I enjoy the daily challenge of melding art and science to provide the best care. The humbling experience of helping people through their joys and sorrows each day continues to amaze me. I wanted to share this passion with the next generation of nurses who will care for others.

My desire to teach was partially satisfied in my nurse practitioner role. I loved seeing the students I precepted grow in confidence and skill during their individual time with me. The wish to share my knowledge and enthusiasm more widely, along with the education courses in my DNP program, motivated my shift from a clinical world to a faculty role. The shift to this new career proved to be seismic, as my skills and knowledge were stretched.

It is easy to slip into my clinical role for several hours a week. My confidence as an educator is still growing. This makes me appreciate my student's novice perspective more easily. Academic culture, language, and administrative structure are vastly different from the clinical world. It is more challenging to unpack my knowledge and provide it to novice nurses than I imagined, particularly through the use of innovative technology in a large classroom setting. But I enjoy this new challenge of combining the art and science of education, the humbling experience of teaching new learners, and my unique position to bridge the clinical and classroom worlds. And just as when starting any new role, having good mentorship and role modeling is essential.

I still love seeing the students' knowledge progression, albeit on a much larger scale now. Watching students become animated when talking about recent lectures or clinical experiences is immensely satisfying. And even a small word of thanks directly from a student is more gratifying than they will ever know. Seeing these sparks of passion from students makes me happy knowing that the next generation of excellent nurses will be carrying the torch, and I was able to have a role in that.

CHAPTER NINE

The Clinical Scholar Role in Doctoral Advanced Nursing Practice

BRIGIT VANGRAAFEILAND AND DEBORAH BUSCH

The emerging complexity and acuity of today's healthcare patient as well as the current consumer-driven environment that we live in makes clinical scholarship more important than ever before. The professional roles of nurses today require that nursing practice be consistent with emerging knowledge and translate the best evidence into practice. The COVID-19 pandemic has taught us that the roles and responsibilities of nurses will continue to expand, as they are key healthcare providers. Nurse leaders provide direction and management to ensure the best outcomes for the patient, system, and organization. To improve outcomes, clinical decisions must be grounded in clinical inquiry and evidence where nurses who practice in a scholarly manner work directly and collegially with other healthcare providers in other settings, in the discovery, application, and evaluation of new knowledge. Translation of evidence to the healthcare organization to improve health outcomes are ways other than through research that knowledge is generated in nursing practice (DePalma & McGuire, 2005; Melnyk & Fineout Overholt, 2021; Rolfe & Davies, 2009; Sigma Theta Tau International [STTI], 1999). This chapter defines clinical scholarship and the way it is continuing to evolve as advanced practice nurses (APNs) with practice-focused doctorates generate evidence/knowledge to translate evidence into practice and outcomes of care.

HOW IS CLINICAL SCHOLARSHIP DEFINED?

For several decades, nursing leaders have discussed the scholarship of practice (Benner et al., 1996; Carter et al., 2021; Dickoff & James, 1968; Diers, 1995). The PhD is rooted in the discovery of new knowledge, while the doctor of nursing practice (DNP) degree translates and connects discovery with application, which is a critical element for practice disciplines (Carter et al., 2021; Riley et al., 2002). This connection demonstrates the strength of clinical scholarship and addresses the historical bias that scholarship only comes from original research.

Clinical scholarship has been a theme in nursing and academicians have embraced that nursing practice should have a contextualization in clinical scholarship (Wilkes et al., 2013). However, operationalizing clinical scholarship has been fraught with various definitions and meanings. Most of the evidence suggests that clinical scholarship has elements of research. Clinical scholarship should be rigorous, creative, sustainable, assimilate theoretical and experiential knowledge, disseminated and replicative to advance the nursing profession and improve patient care outcomes and systems (AACN, 2018; Palmer, 1986). In Wilkes, Mannix, and Jackson's (2013) study on the definition of clinical scholarship they demonstrated that there are four elements of clinical scholarship: discovery, application, integration, and teaching. This concept aligns with Boyer's theory of clinical scholarship. Additionally, Limoges and Acorn (2016) recommend aligning clinical scholarship with Boyer's framework. Clinical scholarship has been rooted in nursing academics, but with a wide breadth of definitions. Similar concepts can be found in most definitions. Manley, McCormack, and Wilson (2009) defined clinical scholarship as evidence being made public, peer reviewed, and critiqued, and able to be reproduced and sustained. Similarly, O'Neil (2009) surmises that clinical scholarship is the translation of research into practice.

Scholars and researchers themselves have difficulty defining clinical scholarship (Wilkes et al., 2013). They argue that clinical scholars are those who build and disseminate nursing knowledge, participate in and lead practice-based research, share knowledge through translation, and link research and practice. When you examine the initial DNP white paper (AACN, 2015) those elements comprised the DNP education and role. The American Association of Colleges of Nursing (AACN) defines clinical scholarship as "those activities that systematically advance the teaching, research, and practice of nursing through rigorous inquiry that 1) is significant to the profession, 2) is creative, 3) can be documented, 4) can be replicated or elaborated, and 5) can be peer-reviewed through various methods."

The DNP degree and the AACN DNP Essentials (2005, 2021), have demonstrated a prime opportunity to grow clinical scholars. Melnyk and Fineout Overholt (2021) conceptualized clinical scholarship as evidenced-based practice (EBP). One of the foundational elements of the DNP degree and role is steeped in the competencies of *cultivate, ask, search, appraise, integrate, evaluate, and disseminate* (Melnyk & Fineout Overholt, 2021). Increased clarity on clinical scholarship has been at the forefront of DNP programs. The terminal degree has recognized that for advanced practice nurses, clinical scholarship is most valued when it is shared and disseminated with peers and organizations (Carter et al., 2019).

Clinical scholarship should not just be housed in the literature, it is a continuous process for the future development of nursing and the quest for continuous quality improvement to healthcare (Wilkes et al., 2013). Clinical scholarship includes application and dissemination—all of which result in a new understanding of practice and patient outcomes, system processes, and with nursing at the forefront of making change. Knowledge of different theoretical frameworks with various assumptions and theoretical propositions is critical for clinical scholars when choosing different types of evidence and in translating evidence into clinical practice. The DNP-prepared nurse can discover new ways of refining or transforming practice by using or adapting constructs and concepts in existing theoretical frameworks to solve everyday problems.

According to the AACN (2015), clinical scholarship is focused on generating new knowledge through innovation of practice change, the translation of evidence, and the implementation of quality improvement processes in specific practice settings, systems, or with specific populations to improve health or health outcomes. New knowledge generated by the DNP graduate can be transferred to other populations or systems but is not considered generalizable (AACN, 2015).

The main components of clinical scholarship include developing and disseminating nursing knowledge, participating in practice and evidence-based research, translation of knowledge and evidence, and joining research and practice. EBP, as described by Melnyk and Fineout Overhold (2021), has been widely adopted by DNP programs. Advanced practice to DNP and post-master's DNP programs include the use of Melnyk and Fineout Overholt's EBP as an integral part not only of program outcomes, but also as the cornerstone for DNP scholarly projects. The clinical scholar with a practice-focused doctorate will provide leadership for EBP with skills in translational research and sustainability. They are the conduit for bridging research and practice to optimize care and improved healthcare delivery models. This is accomplished by the discovery of clinical gaps, integration of the best evidence into practice, application of evidence into clinical arenas, and teaching others through dissemination of their work. This requires collaboration and leadership skills to ensure evidence-based research is translated to populations and organizations. Despite variations in the definition of what clinical scholarship means, the following are common themes that describe a scholar. Clinical scholars are characterized by a prominent level of vision and passion, critical thinking, continuous learning, reflection, and the ability to seek and use a variety of resources and evidence to improve the effectiveness of clinical interventions.

HOW IS CLINICAL SCHOLARSHIP DEMONSTRATED IN DNP GRADUATES?

In an era of unprecedented accountability for the delivery of quality, cost-managed healthcare, nurses are being challenged to demonstrate effective and efficient care. Well-informed consumers are demanding greater access to quality healthcare and have a greater awareness due to online sources of information. Clinical scholarship brings EBP to the forefront of healthcare delivery by meeting the quadruple aims in healthcare. According to Melnyk and Fineout-Overholt, EBP improves the patient experience through providing quality care, enhances patient outcomes, reduces costs, and empowers clinicians (nurses), which leads to higher job satisfaction for healthcare professionals (2019). Rising patient acuity, escalating complexity in healthcare needs, and the increasing infusion of technology in healthcare systems are creating daunting challenges for nurses. Additionally, nurses are practicing in environments with limited financial resources. As these challenges increase, nurses can no longer rely on traditional nursing practices or base their clinical decisions on intuition and years of clinical experience to plan and implement the care required by today's patients. Responding to this challenge requires collective and adaptive knowledge, clinical expertise, and commitment to provide EBP patient-care decisions on evidence and involvement of patients, cultivating a spirit of inquiry. Clinical scholarship is particularly important for APNs with practice-focused doctorates to provide leadership in establishing clinical excellence and informed healthcare policy.

The master of science in nursing (MSN) degree historically has been the degree for specialized advanced nursing practice. With the development of DNP programs, a clinical practice-focused doctorate, the DNP degree will become the preferred preparation for specialty nursing practice. The National Organization of Nurse Practitioner Faculties (NONPF) Standards for Quality Nurse Practitioner Education Report from the National Task Force (NTF, 2022), which has been endorsed by many of the major stakeholder nursing organizations, delineates the national standards for the development and assessment of nurse practitioner (NP) programs. The 2022 NONPF NTF guidelines include four standards of mission and governance, resources, curriculum, and evaluation to provide a framework for the development, maintenance, and assessment of NP educational programs and set the standards for NP education at the graduate level. The American Association of Colleges of Nursing (AACN) Essentials: Core Competencies for

Professional Nursing Education provides a framework and emphasizes the 10 Domains/Essentials, which have associated competencies and subcompetencies for both entry-level and advanced-level nursing education reflecting the discipline of nursing (2021). As noted by the AACN, these domains and competencies are meant to exemplify the uniqueness of nursing as a profession and reflect the diversity of practice settings yet share common language that is understandable across healthcare professions and by employers, learners, faculty, and the public (AACN, 2021, p. 1). The new era of nursing education is interweaving competency-based education with the foundational approach of EBP scholarship and practice.

Implementing EBP as a core competency within nursing represents a significant and critical skill for nurses, because they have a considerable amount of influence on healthcare decisions and in improving the quality, delivery, and safety of care (Dang et al., 2021). Clinical scholarship that incorporates EBP for the practice-focused doctorate should then build on what has been started by clinical scholars with the MSN degree to provide leadership for evidence-based practice. It has been noted that the knowledge of best care practices negatively correlates with years postgraduation, meaning that best practice knowledge declined exponentially as the number of years since graduation increased (Dang et al., 2021). Leveraging EBP into scholarly practice is one of the best strategies to enable and inform healthcare professionals of new practices, treatments, and technologies.

Evidence-based practice should result in better outcomes leading to a better quality of life for all citizens.

DNP graduates engage in advanced nursing practice and provide leadership for evidence-based practice. This requires competence in searching the literature and in knowledge application activities: the translation of research into practice, the evaluation of practice, improvement of the reliability of healthcare practice and outcomes, and participation in collaborative research (DePalma & McGuire, 2005).

The DNP Essentials (AACN, 2021) introduce 10 domains that represent the essence of professional nursing practice and the expected competencies for each of the 10 domains, which also interweave with the four spheres of care: 1) disease prevention/health promotion; 2) chronic disease care; 3) regenerative or respirate care; and 4) hospice/palliative/supportive care. To provide best practices that adhere to the DNP Essentials and four spheres of care, nurses must be taught and continue to apply the EBP process to their nursing practice. Graduates of nursing programs should be trained to use analytic methods to determine and implement the best evidence for practice; to design and implement processes to evaluate outcomes of practice, practice patterns, and systems of care against national benchmarks to determine variances in practice outcomes and population trends. In addition, nurses must have the skill sets and competencies to design, direct, and evaluate quality improvement methodologies and apply relevant findings to develop practice guidelines and improve practice and the practice environment. They need to be trained in the use of information technology and research methods to accomplish these. The DNP clinical scholar functions as a practice specialist/consultant in collaborative knowledge-generating research and disseminates findings from evidence-based practice and research to improve healthcare outcomes (AACN, 2021).

HOW IS EXPERTISE IN THE USE OF EVIDENCE-BASED PRACTICE ACHIEVED?

In practice, the utilization of research evidence does not occur in a vacuum, it must be incorporated into nursing education and supported in the professional environment.

A recent literature review identified that nurses may not be well prepared to apply EBP, and examined strategies for teaching EBP in nursing education and identified the need to integrate teaching strategies of EBP within all levels of nursing to further enhance students' knowledge and skills (Horntvedt et al., 2018). Continually building the foundational knowledge and competency of EBP to then be mastered by the DNP-prepared nurse is critical to prepare nurses for our ever-changing healthcare environment. A scoping review of nurse practitioners' (NPs') implementation of EBP into care demonstrated that NPs highly valued EBP yet encountered numerous obstacles such as lack of time, lack of EBP competence, lack of support from colleagues and managers, and inadequate resources (Clark et al., 2021).

The DNP's role in facilitating EBP needs to be conceived as that of a leader in best practices by examining, planning, implementing, analyzing, and disseminating outcomes of the EBP process. The Johns Hopkins EBP model identifies this as the PET process: Practice Question, Evidence, and Translation (Dang et al., 2021). Because DNP competencies are formulated at a higher level with more emphasis on leadership, quality improvement, healthcare delivery systems, and healthcare policy, the DNP-prepared nurse will be expected to provide leadership in creating working environments for evidence-based practice, with the expectation necessitating a certain level of skills and competency in translating science into practice. Clarke (2021) identified that NPs experienced barriers to implementing EBP in the professional setting, such as collaborative practice issues that affected EBP implementation, indicating that there is a need for the DNP-prepared nurse to be an instrument to build interprofessional collaborations and improve communication within the healthcare team for shared decision and goal making.

In terms of nurses' research values and skills, the DNP nurse can become a role model for change and transformation not only for the workplace environment, but also for the individual nurses working in that environment. This can occur at two levels by (a) increasing the nurse's confidence in evaluating the quality of the research evidence and (b) changing perceptions regarding the benefits of changing practice with the use of research evidence. The nurse leader who is prepared at the doctoral level can actively participate in formal or informal discussions on evaluating interventions reported in the research literature using the opportunity to increase nurses' knowledge and ability to evaluate research findings more wisely and logically. By taking on the role of an innovator, as an early adopter, the DNP nurse can create the climate for changing perceptions to one of increased respect for all individuals in the healthcare team and value for the scientific process and its outcomes.

As a leader in clinical practice, the DNP nurse can overcome limitations within the setting for practice. By allowing implementation of innovations through active support and provision of the needed structure and processes, the DNP administrator brings authority and accountability in facilitating the workplace environment for these innovations. This includes focusing on overcoming the limitations in how research is communicated. By providing the resources needed for the nurses and healthcare team to develop skills in reading, understanding, and evaluating research reports accurately and efficiently, the DNP administrator can promote, sustain, and maintain the implementation of evidence-based practice. In terms of barriers related to the quality of the research evidence, the DNP nurse can lead the effort to contribute further to the knowledge base by replicating investigations that evaluate the effectiveness of interventions. This requires a step beyond simply implementing and measuring the outcomes of interventions, to formally testing hypotheses regarding the impact of such interventions on nursing and healthcare. In effect, it requires the DNP-prepared nurse to be skilled in the conduct, use, and dissemination of translational research. In various leadership roles, the DNP-prepared nurse is uniquely positioned to innovate and experiment with various models for increasing the utilization of research in practice settings. With administrative authority that comes with these leadership roles, the DNP-prepared nurse should have multiple options available for integrating research into the workplace environment. Whether it is increased and more effective use of existing resources, building bridges of communication and collaboration, or the deployment of external support and expertise, the DNP nurse can raise the organization to higher levels of application of translational science into EBP practice. Particularly in promoting the translation of science into practice, the DNP nurse can engage in action research, which leads to the solution of everyday practical, as well as clinical, problems.

IS ACTION RESEARCH ORIENTED FOR DNP CLINICAL SCHOLARSHIP?

Methods to increase the quality and rate of research translation are increasingly becoming the focus of clinical practice. Leadership in clinical practice requires recognition that evidence-based practice is central to the achievement of effective and efficient healthcare delivery and to obtaining positive client outcomes (Mohide & Coker, 2005). Traditional approaches to building the evidence predominate in the current research enterprise. Nevertheless, there is increasing pressure upon the scientific community to look at alternative paradigms to increase the uptake of research evidence into community- and population-wide practice. Action research, one such alternative paradigm, is science designed to obtain practical results to solve a specific challenge. Engagement in action research is one area in which the DNP nurse is optimally positioned, with the strong leadership skills in community-based initiatives that of the education and preparation for DNP practice. In addition to the basic steps in traditional research of design, data collection, analysis, and communication, this alternative paradigm requires action, which is developmental in nature and has a wide range of applications in healthcare. This showcases the strengths and talents of the DNP nurse; it highlights the natural skills of the practitioner for practical solutions to real and actual problems in the clinical setting as they occur. In addition to skills and competencies in the application of multidimensional and multifaceted designs of participatory action research, the DNP nurse is prepared to lead communities to form collaborative partnerships with the academic scientists in community-based initiatives that aim to solve problems facing vulnerable populations (Stringer, 2007).

WHAT IS THE ROLE OF THE DNP CLINICAL SCHOLAR IN DISSEMINATION?

The role of the DNP nurse as clinical scholar has within it an inherent obligation and responsibility to disseminate knowledge and expertise gained from practice to various audiences. There are many reasons for engaging in the dissemination process. These include the sharing of ideas and new knowledge for the improvement of healthcare delivery and influencing healthcare outcomes. In addition, for practical purposes, dissemination activities are essential job requirements, including requirements for promotion and tenure in any work setting. The Fuld Institute has suggested clear guidelines that will assist nurses with the dissemination process (Dean et al., 2021). The guidelines provide a framework and outline for both submission and reviewing EBP scholarly work among nursing students and professional nurses alike (Table 9.1). As the numbers of DNP-prepared nurses increase, providing well-described, organized, and properly

TABLE 9.1 EBP Dissemination Guide

Title and Abstract	
Title	• Population/Problem & focus of project/initiative • Indicate this is an EBP project/initiative
Abstract	• Background and/or rationale • Aim or purpose of initiative • Implementation plan • Outcomes • Implications for practice
Keywords	Consider: • Population/Problem • Focus of the project/initiative • Outcomes
The Seven Steps of EBP*	
Step 0: Clinical Inquiry	*Tell the story of what problem/issue you were concerned about and wanted to address.* • Provide a brief narrative that describes the events that helped to identify the problem/issue that led to the clinical inquiry.

Background and Significance	*Why did the organization care about the problem/issue?*
	• Background of the problem/issue of interest
	• Significance of the problem/issue of interest
	  ○ Internal/external evidence and/or literature that identified/substantiated the problem/issue of interest
	• Strategic alignment
	  ○ How did solving the problem/issue of interest align with strategic goals and priorities of the organization?

Organizational Assessment	*How ready and prepared was the organization for EBP?* Organizational mission, vision, and values • Organizational culture, context for EBP • Organization's readiness for EBP (resources, preparedness, leadership commitment)

Framework	*What EBP framework or model guided the EBP work?*
	EBP framework examples include:
	• Organizational models:
	  ○ ARCC model
	  ○ PARIHS
	• Project models:
	  ○ ACE Star Model of Knowledge Transformation
	  ○ Clinical Scholar Model
	  ○ Iowa Model
	  ○ JHNEBP Model

Step 1: Formulation of a Searchable Question	*What searchable question did you formulate to guide your literature search?*
	Searchable question
	• Format:
	  ○ PICO
	  ○ PICOT
	  ○ Other

(continued)

TABLE 9.1 Evidence-Based Practice (EBP) Dissemination Guide (*continued*)

Step 2: Search for the Best Evidence	*How did you search for studies/articles to answer your question?*
	Results of literature search in a concise narrative or table/chart/diagram
	• Include:
	   ◦ Databases
	   ◦ Search strategies
	   ◦ Search terms/keywords
	   ◦ Filters
	   ◦ Number of studies/articles found

Step 3a: Critical Appraisal of Individual Articles	*How strong was the body of evidence?* • Evidence hierarchy or grading scale used to determine level of evidence of each study/article • Appraisal tool(s) utilized to assess quality of each study/article • Number of studies/articles retained ("keepers") • Number of studies/articles discarded and why

Step 3b: Synthesis of the Body of Evidence	*What recommendations did the body of evidence lead to?*
	• Synthesis of the body of evidence
	   ◦ Narrative and/or table format
	   ◦ Consider including narratives and/or tables for the following:
	      ▪ Levels of evidence
	      ▪ Effective interventions/best practices
	      ▪ Outcomes
	      ▪ Any other themes that emerged
	• Recommendation(s) made based on the synthesis of body of evidence

Step 4a: Integration of the Evidence: Implementation of the Evidence-Based Practice Change	*What did you implement or de-implement?*
	Evidence-based recommendation(s) integrated
	• Include:
	   ◦ Setting and context
	   ◦ Stakeholders
	   ◦ Implementation team assembled
	   ◦ Measurement plan
	      • Resources used to retrieve or collect data across the initiative
	         ▪ Instrument (survey, scale, or tool) used and the reported validity and reliability
	         ▪ Organization's internal database or dashboard
	   ◦ Approvals secured before implementation
	   ◦ Implementation strategies used
	   ◦ Facilitators and how they were leveraged
	   ◦ Barriers and how they were addressed
	   ◦ Resources used to implement the change
	   ◦ Evaluation plan
	   ◦ Sustainability plan

Step 4b: Integration with Clinical Expertise and Patient/Family Preferences	How were these other important aspects integrated in the practice change? • Clinical expertise • Patient preferences/values

(*continued*)

TABLE 9.1 Evidence-Based Practice (EBP) Dissemination Guide (*continued*)

Step 5a: Evaluation of Outcomes	*What did you measure and how did you know your practice change made a difference?*
	• Outcomes measured
	• Data collected and when (i.e., pre, post, specific interval)
	• Statistical analysis of data
	   ◦ Statistical significance
	   ◦ Clinical meaningfulness
	• Return on Investment (ROI)/Value of Investment (VOI)

Step 5b: Implications for Practice	*How was your experience useful in your setting and how could it help others?*
	• Lessons learned
	• Consider implications for the following (not all may apply):
	   ◦ Unit based
	   ◦ Organization wide
	   ◦ Other organizations/systems
	   ◦ Other settings (i.e., community, globally)

Step 6: Dissemination	*How will/did you tell your story?* • Internal and external dissemination completed and/or planned • Publications, presentations, posters ◦ Local, national, and/or international • Include approvals obtained for dissemination (if applicable).
Conclusion	*Summarize how using an evidence-based approach to address a problem/issue of interest enhanced solving the problem/fixing the issue.*

ARCC, Advancing Research through Close Collaboration; EBP, evidence-based practice; JHNEBP, Johns Hopkins Nursing Evidence-based Practice; PARIHS, promoting action on research implementation in health services framework; ROI, return on investment; VOI, value of investment

Source: © 8-17-2020 Dean, J., Gallagher-Ford, L., & Connor, L. Columbus, Ohio: The Helene Fuld Health Trust National Institute for Evidence-Based Practice in Nursing and Healthcare.

*Melnyk, B. M., & Fineout-Overholt, E., eds. (2019). *Evidence-based practice in nursing & healthcare: A guide to best practice*, 4th ed. Lippincott Williams & Wilkins.

prepared dissemination demonstrates to the scientific community and public that nurses are dually qualified to be leaders and participants in the EBP process, including dissemination of findings and knowledge.

Thus, DNP preparation includes experiences aimed at developing and increasing skills in manuscript writing as well as in oral presentations in the dissemination of ideas. In leadership roles, DNP nurses can create the climate for scholarship for those with whom they work. Increasingly, the endeavor to produce manuscripts for publication is carried on by writing teams that are engaged in common activities in healthcare delivery. Likewise, the tasks of preparing and delivering oral as well as poster presentations become less daunting and onerous if undertaken by teams of colleagues engaged in similar activities of dissemination. The DNP nurse provides the needed leadership to get the initiative started, to provide the resources for people to engage in these activities, and to encourage the work of continued and active scholarship. This also provides opportunities for mentoring and mentorship among nurses and other healthcare professionals who work together to achieve healthcare goals for groups of patients.

SUMMARY: THE FUTURE OF THE DNP CLINICAL SCHOLAR

Whether the creation of this degree enhances the progress of clinical scholarship for the profession of nursing and furthers the quality of patient care depends entirely on the nursing profession's willingness to address the critical issues related to educational quality, outcomes, and standards. Focusing on the issue of the preparation of the DNP as a clinical scholar is of particular importance. At the current time, when standards of DNP education are continuing to evolve, it is critically important that the skills and competencies that have been articulated to prepare the DNP for this role be coupled with specific parameters for identifying the outcomes of this preparation relative to this role. Albeit the transition and acceptance of the doctorally prepared DNP nurse has not been a smooth journey, there remains inconsistency and variation of beliefs among nursing schools, nursing leaders, and the marketplace (McCauley et al., 2020). Learning experiences in the educational and training curricula must emphasize increasing skills in the application of EBP and translational research, while at the same time the development of higher levels of competencies in the conduct of evaluation research and dissemination of critical findings must be facilitated and monitored before the DNP is granted the degree. The DNP graduate should be educated and trained for the increasingly interprofessional nature of practice within a transformed healthcare system. To prepare the DNP for the increased and enhanced roles in leadership, communication, and team practice, there must be opportunities for inter- and intraprofessional collaboration, both between DNP and PhD nursing students and between DNP students and students in other health professions. Increasingly, many DNP students have found opportunities to work with students in other fields, such as engineering, public health, healthcare administration, and business. Aligning with the AACN's DNP Essentials and Domains, along with the four spheres of nursing care, provides the foundation of purpose for the DNP nurse, and guides them to be a leader in improving healthcare outcomes and reducing disparities seen due to the inequities associated with population social determinates of health (AACN, 2021).

Nursing leaders and state and national organizations have spent considerable time and finances assuring the public, legislators, and other members of the healthcare community that the educational level that nurses currently possess results in high quality care. Although it is intuitively appealing that educational requirements and standards will address concerns of the National Academy of Medicine, formerly the Institute of Medicine (IOM), regarding patient safety and healthcare quality (IOM, 2000, 2001, 2003), there are inconsistencies in the educational preparation of DNP nurses that may not fulfill the promise on the quality of patient care and progress in the nursing profession (McCauley et al., 2020). Studies investigating the educational EBP content in nursing programs indicate the need to provide more EBP content in nursing programs and to integrate clinically interactive teaching strategies within nursing curricula to better prepare future nurses (Horntvedt et al., 2018). There are formative challenges being experienced by nurses attempting to incorporate the EBP process into clinical practice, and yet the findings indicate that nurses deeply value EBP and seek to incorporate EBP into their work to improve patient care outcomes (Clarke et al., 2021). The DNP-prepared nurse can be an instrument to promote collegial bridges within the interdisciplinary team, so that EBP can proliferate within the healthcare setting. These challenges must also encourage continuous dialogue about the best educational preparation for doctorally prepared APNs who will assume the role of clinical scholars (McCauley et al., 2020). This is critical as changes in technology, healthcare delivery systems, science, and changing and evolving roles for nurses all require that the nurses of tomorrow be prepared to participate in the healthcare system as it evolves. Additionally, employers and professional organizations should provide mechanisms for exercising leadership that support activities for clinical scholarship for DNPs, whose expertise in transformative EBP healthcare has the potential for significant improvements in healthcare outcomes and reduction of the ever-increasing disparities being experienced by vulnerable and marginalized populations. It is imperative that professional nursing groups and organizations endorse a call for more prolific clinical scholarship in this new cadre of DNPs as central to their mission and philosophy and as a rationale for a practice-focused doctorate.

CRITICAL THINKING QUESTIONS

1. Explain the differences in clinical scholarship between a practice-focused doctorate and a research-focused doctorate.
2. Describe the kind of clinical scholarship you believe is most appropriate for the practice-focused doctorate.
3. Explain why knowledge in theoretical frameworks is critical for clinical scholars with a practice-focused doctorate.
4. Why is clinical scholarship for APNs with practice-focused doctorates important?
5. How does a DNP APN achieve expertise in the use of evidence-based practice?
6. Explain how dissemination activities could be achieved by the DNP clinical scholar.
7. Discuss issues/barriers in the development of a DNP clinical scholar.
8. Explain the role of administrators in supporting DNP clinical scholars.

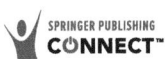

A robust set of instructor resources designed to supplement this text is located at http://connect.springerpub.com/content/book/978-0-8261-8137-4. Qualifying instructors may request access by emailing textbook@springerpub.com.

REFERENCES

American Association of Colleges of Nursing. (2015). *The doctor of nursing practice: Current issues and clarifying recommendations. Report from the task force on the implementation of the DNP.* https://www.aacnnursing.org/Portals/42/News/White-Papers/DNP-Implementation-TF-Report-8-15.pdf

American Association of Colleges of Nursing. (2021). *The essentials: Core competencies for professional nursing education.* Accessible online at https://www.aacnnursing.org/Portals/42/AcademicNursing/pdf/Essentials-2021.pdf

American Association of Colleges of Nursing. (2018). *Defining scholarship for the discipline of nursing.* https://www.aacnnursing.org/news-data/position-statements-white-papers/defining-scholarship-for-academic-nursing. Accessed 10/28/22.

Benner, P., Tanner, C., & Chesla, C. (1996). *Expertise in nursing practice: Caring, clinical judgment and ethics.* Springer Publishing Company.

Clarke, V., Lehane, E., Mulcahy, H., & Cotter, P. (2021). Nurse practitioners' implementation of evidence-based practice into routine care: A scoping review. *Worldviews on Evidence-Based Nursing, 18*(3), 180–189. https://doi.org/10.1111/wvn.12510

Dang, D., Dearholt, S. L., Bissett, K., Ascenzi, J., & Whalen, M. (2021). *Johns Hopkins evidence-based practice for nurses and healthcare professionals: Model & guidelines* (4th ed.). Sigma Theta Tau International.

Dean, J., Gallagher-Ford, L., & Connor, L. (2021). Evidence-based practice: A new dissemination guide. *Worldviews on Evidence-Based Nursing, 18*(1), 4–7. https://doi.org/10.1111/wvn.12489

DePalma, J., & McGuire, D. (2005). Research. In A. B. Hamric, A. Spross, & C. Hanson (Eds.), *Advanced practice nursing: An integrative approach* (3rd ed., pp. 257–300). Elsevier Saunders.

Dickoff, J., & James, P. (1968). Symposium on theory development in nursing. A theory of theories: A position paper. *Nursing Research, 17*(3), 197–203.

Diers, D. (1995). Clinical scholarship. *Journal of Professional Nursing, 11*(1), 24–30. https://doi.org/10.1016/s8755-7223(95)80069-7

Horntvedt, M. T., Nordsteien, A., Fermann, T., & Severinsson, E. (2018). Strategies for teaching evidence-based practice in nursing education: A thematic literature review. *BMC Medical Education, 18*(1), 172. https://doi.org/10.1186/s12909-018-1278-z

Institute of Medicine. (2000). *To err is human: Building a safer health system.* National Academies Press.

Institute of Medicine. (2001). *Crossing the quality chasm.* National Academies Press.

Institute of Medicine. (2003). *Health professions education: A bridge to quality.* National Academies Press.

Limoges, J., & Acorn, S. (2016). Transforming practice into clinical scholarship. *Journal of Advanced Nursing, 72*(4), 747–753.

Manley, K., McCormack, B., & Wilson, V. (2008). Introduction. In K. Manley, B. McCormack, & V. Wilson (Eds.), *Practice development in nursing: International perspectives* (pp. 1–16). Blackwell Publishing.

McCauley, L. A., Broome, M. E., Frazier, L., Hayes, R., Kurth, A., Musil, C. M., Norman, L. D., Rideout, K. H., & Villarruel, A. M. (2020). Doctor of Nursing Practice (DNP) degree in the United States: Reflecting, readjusting, and getting back on track. *Nursing Outlook, 68*(4), 494–503. https://doi.org/10.1016/j.outlook.2020.03.008

Melnyk, B., & Fineout-Overholt, E. (2021). *Evidence-based practice in nursing and healthcare: A guide to best practice* (4th ed.). Lippincott Williams & Wilkins.

Palmer, I. S. (1986). The emergence of clinical scholarship as a professional imperative. *Journal of Professional Nursing, 2*(5), 318–325.

Riley, J. M., Beal, J., Levi, P., & McCausland, M. P. (2002). Revisioning nursing scholarship. *Journal of Nursing Scholarship, 34*(4), 383–389.

Stringer, E. T. (2007). *Action research.* Sage Publications.

Wilkes, L., Mannix, J., & Jackson, D. (2013). Practicing nurses perspectives of clinical scholarship: A qualitative study. *BMC Nurse, 12*(1), 21.

CHAPTER NINE: Reflective Response 1

BRENDA DOUGLASS

Fittingly, Chapter 9 brings to the forefront the very essence of evidence-based practice (EBP) in improving outcomes of care corresponding to the advanced nursing practice clinical scholar role. In reflecting on the chapter authors' perspectives, it brings to light how in my own extensive nursing trajectory I have utilized EBP as a professional clinical nurse and nurse educator. One of the most powerful examples to share as a clinical scholar aligns to the "nurse as an educator" in preparing doctor of nursing practice (DNP) graduates. Educators have an obligation and responsibility to ensure that student learners are well equipped with the requisite EBP knowledge and skill set for the complex, contemporary healthcare landscape. Convergence of the nurse educator role with the practicing clinician role, application transpires where "practice what you teach" and role modeling occurs. In the clinical realm as a family nurse practitioner, practice contributes to the advancement of knowledge, application, and translation of evidence for clinical decision making (AACN, 2021). In this clinical scholar role and the context of caring, merging the science (research evidence) with clinical expertise along with patient preferences and values informs clinical decision making and thus, best practices for optimization of patient outcomes (Melnyk & Fineout Overholt 2021). Promoting a clinical environment of EBP and harnessing quality improvement opportunities lend to additional ways yielding to the clinical scholar role. Moreover, integration of the newly revised Essentials (AACN, 2021) with a competency-based education approach is integral to the clinical scholar role as a practice-focused DNP clinician and nurse educator informed by EBP. Over time, I have witnessed and experienced the evolution of the DNP role as a pioneer doctoral-prepared practice-focused nurse leader and remain passionate about being a nurse. While affected by some impediments, which were illuminated by the chapter authors, the DNP role has made gainful strides and exemplifies a clinical scholar. In closing, I bring forth a unique perspective from nursing career and firmly believe it is imperative that we prioritize EBP and embrace the benefit of DNP-prepared leaders guiding us into the future.

REFERENCES

American Association of Colleges of Nursing. (2021). *The essentials: Core competencies for professional nursing education.* https://www.aacnnursing.org/Portals/42/AcademicNursing/pdf/Essentials-2021.pdf

Melnyk, B., & Fineout-Overholt, E. (2021). *Evidence-based practice in nursing and healthcare: A guide to best practice* (4th ed.). Lippincott Williams & Wilkins.

CHAPTER NINE Reflective Response 2

JESSICA L. PECK

The chapter by VanGraafeilend and Busch presents an excellent framework for the clinical scholar role of the doctor of nursing practice (DNP)-prepared nurse. This is a much-needed intellectual dialogue that carefully considers both the merits and challenges inherent in the creation of a conceptual framework for the rapidly growing influence and contributions of DNP scholars as experts in translational science inherent in evidence-based practice (EBP). Since the inception of the DNP program of study in 2005, nurses have eagerly adopted this new clinical pathway to a terminal degree. As of 2022, there are 384 active DNP programs in institutions of higher learning (American Association of Colleges of Nursing [AACN], 2022a) with estimates of more than 60,500 DNP graduates entering the profession as DNP-prepared clinical scholars (AACN, 2022b). Most DNP graduates report their motivation in seeking a terminal degree as acquisition of specialized knowledge and not career advancement or employer recognition (AACN, 2022a). Early adopters have embraced the DNP role as clinical scholar. Contemporaneously, there has been a steady decline in the number of nurses seeking PhD preparation as nurse scientists over the last decade, currently accounting for less than 1% of the current nursing workforce. This is occurring despite high demand for PhD-prepared research scholars and a 14% increase in the number of PhD nursing programs with a program available in almost every U.S. state (AACN, 2022c).

Concern for the stability and future trajectory of the PhD-prepared nurse research scholar is justified and barriers, including role misperception, lack of education accessibility, and self-perceptions of inadequacy. These must be addressed as PhD-prepared nurse scientists are essential to the generation of new nursing knowledge through rigorous, original scientific research (Redeker, 2021). However, VanGraafeilend and Busch make an excellent observation about the need for DNP-prepared clinical scholars to shape nursing response grounded in clinical inquiry and EBP to the growing acuity and complexity of the healthcare environment, rapidly translating the best evidence to practice. As EBP experts, DNP-prepared clinical scholars can serve as an invaluable asset on PhD-led research teams both in academic and health systems settings, contributing clinical knowledge and expertise to clarify research questions and serving as expert liaisons for scholarship conducted in real-world practice settings with practical, sustainable clinical relevance and applicability.

Interprofessional tension emerged as PhD-prepared nurse academicians taught the first cohorts of DNP students in doctoral programs of study, grappling with the logistics of adopting and integrating the role of clinical scholar within the hierarchy of the profession. PhD-prepared nurse faculty are long accustomed to the privileges of academic rank and tenure structures inherent in academia. With growing numbers of PhD-prepared academicians and scholars nearing retirement and rapidly swelling ranks of DNP-prepared clinical scholars, critical skepticism festers over perceived lack of academic rigor of DNP preparation and value of the professional contributions of DNP clinical scholars, especially in academic teaching and scholarship (Groer & Clochesy, 2020). DNP-prepared faculty report feelings of marginalization and undervaluation by their PhD-prepared peers, organizational leaders, and academic structures in institutions of higher education. Self-reported professional growth barriers included lack of respect, inequity in hierarchal infrastructure, and discriminatory allocation of resources necessary for expected scholarship accomplishments (England & Lancaster, 2021). As every emerging DNP scholar is educated in the shadow of this academic paradigm conflict, it is essential for all doctorally prepared faculty to carefully consider their role in shaping attitudes and perceptions of the distinct but equally valuable contributions of both research and clinical scholars. The rigors of academic doctoral preparation for a career with an almost exclusive focus on research should not be held superior to the rigors of academic preparation required to prepare doctoral-level advanced practice clinicians with a comprehensive skill set as systems leaders and clinical scholars. Confusion still exists among graduate nursing faculty and students in differentiating the core constructs defining research versus clinical scholarship contributions (Jenkins et al., 2021). DNP and PhD scholars possess distinct yet complementary skill sets. Interprofessional respect for unique contributions to nursing scholarship with a collaborative approach best serves nursing as a profession to improve patient outcomes (Cygan & Reed, 2019).

Inequity can be seen in the myriad of academic hierarchal structures as universities designate clinical academic tracks for clinical DNP-prepared scholars and tenure tracks for PhD-prepared research scholars. For those universities in which DNP-prepared faculty are ineligible for tenure, there is often an assumption of inferiority as clinical track faculty feel their scholarship is less valuable, particularly in a research-intensive university pursuing or holding elite R1 status according to Carnegie Classifications of Higher Education Institutions. A recent survey found clinical-track public health faculty were more likely to hold a lower academic rank and report short contract duration with unclear expectations (August et al., 2021). A paucity of research exists to consider similar impacts in nursing academics. In consideration of the current faculty shortage that is projected to worsen (AACN, 2022d), academic nursing programs would be wise to consider a scientific, systematic framework (such as presented so articulately in this chapter by VanGraafeiland and Busch) standardizing definitions and expectations of clinical scholarship to prevent DNP-prepared faculty from leaving academia to pursue more lucrative clinical positions where the pay is better and respect is higher (Boamah, 2022).

Nursing has always been a profession that challenges traditional orthodoxy. It rapidly adapts and innovates to meet emerging health challenges, which brought the profession to the point of creating the role of DNP-prepared clinical scholar. Nursing has always been its own fiercest professional critic, with internal debate fueling forward-thinking, robust discussion that ultimately forges courageous new paths while safeguarding the public trust. It is time for the profession of nursing itself to clearly understand, articulate, and appreciate the contributions of a DNP-prepared clinical scholar.

REFERENCES

American Association of Colleges of Nursing [AACN]. (2022a). *The state of doctor of nursing practice education in 2022*. https://www.aacnnursing.org/Portals/42/News/Surveys-Data/State-of-the-DNP-Summary-Report-June-2022.pdf

American Association of Colleges of Nursing [AACN]. (2022b). *DNP fact sheet*. https://www.aacnnursing.org/News-Information/Fact-Sheets/DNP-Fact-Sheet#:~:text=In%20the%20years%20since,have%20graduated%20with%20a%20DNP.&text=Doctor%20of%20Nursing%20Practice%20(DNP,and%20translate%20research%20into%20practice

American Association of Colleges of Nursing [AACN]. (2022c). *Data spotlight: Trends in nursing PhD programs.* https://www.aacnnursing.org/News-Information/News/View/ArticleId/25233/Data-Spotlight-Trends-in-Nursing-PhD-Programs

American Association of Colleges of Nursing [AACN]. (2022d). *Nursing faculty shortage.* https://www.aacnnursing.org/news-information/fact-sheets/nursing-faculty-shortage

August, E., Power, L., & Anderson, O. S. (2021). What does it mean to be a clinical track faculty member in public health? A survey of clinical track faculty across the United States. *Public Health Reports, 137*(6), 1234–1241. https://doi.org/10.1177/00333549211048787

Boamah, S. (2022). Investigating the work-life experiences of nursing faculty in Canadian academic settings and the factors at influence their retention: Protocol for a mixed-method study. *BMJ Open, 12*(1), e056655. https://doi.org/10.1136/bmj-open-2021-056655

England, H. M., & Lancaster, R. J. (2021). Differences in perceived marginalization in doctorally prepared nurse faculty. *Journal of Professional Nursing, 37*(3), 626–631. https://doi.org/10.1016/j.profnnurs.2021.03.003

Cygan, H., & Reed, M. (2019). DNP and PhD scholarship: Making the case for collaboration. *Journal of Professional Nursing, 35*(5), 353–357. https://doi.org/10.1016/j.profnurs.2019.03.002

Groer, M. E., & Clochesy, J. M. (2020). Conflicts within the discipline of nursing: Is there a looming paradigm war? *Journal of Professional Nursing, 36*(1), 53–55. https://doi.org/10.1016/j.profnurs.2019.06.014

Jenkins, P., Meek, P., Amura, C., & Robertson, G. (2021). Inconsistency in faculty and student perceptions of DNP and PhD leader scholarship activity. *Journal of Nursing Administration, 51*(1), 49–54. https://doi.org/10.1097/NNA.0000000000000966

Redeker, N. S. (2021). Fortifying the pipeline of nurse scientists to assure the nation's health: A "career-span" approach. *Nursing Outlook, 69*(2), 246–248. https://doi.org/10.1016/j.outlook.021.02.005

CHAPTER NINE | Reflective Response 3
===

REGENA SPRATLING

In Chapter 9, clinical scholarship is clearly depicted as a critical component in the role of the doctor of nursing practice (DNP)-prepared nurse. Moreover, this scholarship has many forms that translate research into practice. It is this translational practice knowledge that needs to be shared with others in the profession, healthcare systems, and the public, and disseminated to diverse audiences using a variety of approaches (AACN, 2021). Dissemination includes written or oral reports presented to stakeholders, poster and podium presentations, manuscript submissions to journals, and even podcasts or news reports (Ayala et al., 2022). When clinical scholarship is peer reviewed, other viewpoints and perspectives are obtained and the scholarly work is evaluated for quality and rigor in its methods, and the clinical significance of its outcomes. Clinical significance is the clinical and practical importance of the project results for improving healthcare outcomes (Hayat, 2010). This peer feedback should be welcomed and, in my opinion, always improves the work of the scholar. Once disseminated, clinical scholarship is then critiqued and evaluated widely by colleagues for usefulness in their practice or practice setting. This peer review and wider critique is essential for the work to be reproduced and sustained, and ultimately used and adapted in the scholarly work of others. Dissemination is an essential part of clinical scholarship, and most importantly, advances clinical scholarship. Furthermore, I feel strongly that dissemination of clinical scholarship also improves satisfaction with the work and the role of the DNP scholar.

Additionally, the inclusion of writing teams and mentorship in this chapter is of great importance as they both are key components of successful clinical scholarship. In writing teams, there are strengths in a number of writers and in the expertise in members. Scholarship does not occur in isolation, and writing teams create a safe space for development of scholarly work, clinical writing, and addressing any obstacles or blocks in writing and completion of the work. Writing teams also build scholar confidence, accountability, and writing skills (Lavinghouze et al., 2022). Other viewpoints and perspectives, previously mentioned above as part of peer review, are encompassed in team writing as the team members are your peers. Writing team members may also be mentors, especially when a scholar is early in the DNP role. Mentorship is a dynamic relationship that begins in DNP education with the faculty mentor and student mentee. Upon graduation, the mentee often quickly becomes a mentor in the DNP role to other nursing and healthcare professionals. The pleasure in mentorship is the realization that the mentee has become a scholar who continually addresses healthcare outcomes in their clinical scholarship (Gonzalez & Finnell, 2020). Thus, it is essential to the DNP role to learn the writing process and the mentorship process, and then mentor others to become DNP scholars. Through writing and mentoring, I know that together we will continue to advance clinical scholarship and the clinical scholar role.

REFERENCES

American Association of Colleges of Nursing. (2021). *The essentials: Core competencies for professional nursing education.* https://www.aacnnursing.org/Portals/42/AcademicNursing/pdf/Essentials-2021.pdf

Ayala, F. J., DeBoard, E., Waldrop, J., Pereira, K., Oermann, M. H., & Silva, S. G. (2022). Dissemination of doctor of nursing practice project findings: Benefits and challenges associated with publishing in healthcare journals. *Nursing Outlook, 70*(6), 846–855. https://doi.org/10.1016/j.outlook.2022.07.011

Gonzalez, Y., & Finnell, D. S. (2020). Promoting and supporting a Doctor of Nursing Practice program of scholarship. *Journal of Nursing Education, 59*(9), 526–530. https://doi.org/10.3928/01484834-20200817-10

Hayat, M. J. (2010). Understanding statistical significance. *Nursing Research, 59*(3), 219–223. https://doi.org/10.1097/NNR.0b013e3181dbb2cc

Lavinghouze, S. R., Kettel Khan, L., Auld, M. E., Sammons Hackett, D., Brittain, D. R., Brown, D. R., Greaney, E., Harris, D. M., Maynard, L. M., Onufrak, S., Robillard, A. G., Schwartz, R., Siddique, S., Youngner, C. G., Wright, L. S., & O'Toole, T. P. (2022). From practice to publication: The promise of writing workshops. *Health Promotion Practice, 23*(1_suppl), 21S–33S. https://doi.org/10.1177/15248399221117477

SECTION THREE

Operationalizing Role Functions of Doctoral Advanced Nursing Practice

CHAPTER TEN

Law and Ethics in Decision Making in the Doctoral Advanced Nursing Practice Role

MICHAEL DAHNKE

Advanced roles in nursing bring greater responsibility and accountability for practitioners. Thus, greater attention and deliberation must be employed in decision making. A responsible practitioner will attempt to maintain personal, social, and professional standards of ethics. But a responsible practitioner will also understand the necessity of meeting legal standards, of following the law. There are important reasons for giving serious consideration to both and important reasons why the demands of each imperative increase with the expanding and elevating of professional roles. But in choosing how to act, should one focus primarily on being moral or on following the law? And is there a difference? Regarding the first question, one can answer in a principled or theoretical manner or a more practical manner. In principle, one should of course attempt to both follow the law and be a moral person and practitioner. Practically speaking, one may usually be able to achieve both; however, there may also be exceptional instances that make achieving both difficult, even impossible. Regarding the second question, in principle there are differences between law and ethics, between legal and moral obligations. In practice, often there is not. For example, the choice to report elder abuse is both legally and morally warranted. But sometimes there is a difference. Consider the case of a patient with a sexually transmitted infection who refuses to inform their spouse. The law would require maintaining confidentiality, but an ethical argument could point to a warranted breach of confidentiality. This type of case is why the conflicts related to the first question arise. To make clear and warranted decisions, these distinctions must be clarified and attention must be paid to both their respective importance their and demands.

What law and morality most fundamentally have in common is that they are normative systems, which means that they provide rules and values meant to direct human action. In the general course of life, they often coincide. Many acts are both moral and legal. Maintaining patient confidentiality under most circumstances is. Some acts are both immoral and illegal, like most cases of breaking confidentiality. But some acts are moral while illegal and others immoral while legal. Rushing someone in emergent medical need to the hospital, while breaking the speed limit, for example, is illegal but might be judged moral. There exists a complex and nuanced relationship between these two normative systems. And given their weight and the potential for conflict, it becomes important to understand each of them, especially in the context of increasing responsibility and accountability in expanded and advanced professional nursing roles.

LAW VERSUS MORALITY

Begin with a simple distinction. Laws are primarily aimed at regulating external actions or actions in the public realm, to protect the interests of individuals and promote the public good. In contrast, morality focuses on actions within one's private life and even one's private thoughts. The public sphere, in which we commingle with our fellow citizens in politics, commerce, and other areas of public life, is far more regulated by law. This is because one of the primary functions of law is to maintain civil order. Thus, those acts that could cause harm (physical harm, harm to property, violation of legal rights) are those primarily regulated by law. This is also why the legal and the moral are particularly commingled in the professional realm. Respect of the private sphere (i.e., noninterference) by law and government translates to respect for persons as individuals able to choose their own good, make their own personal decisions, build their own lives, and follow their own conceptions of morality. This view of legal regulation is sometimes conceptualized in terms of moral and political philosopher John Stuart Mill's (1910) harm principle: "the only purpose for which power can be rightfully exercised over any member of a civilized community, against his will, is to prevent harm to others" (p. 73). The implication is that the law should only interfere in individuals' actions when they pose a risk of harm to others but not a risk of harm to oneself. The assumption is that a rational, competent person who is performing an action with the potential for self-harm (heavy alcohol use, use of illicit drugs, cigarette smoking) has the ability to understand the consequences of their actions and choose to perform those actions nonetheless. It is not the state's place to protect someone against their self.

As attractive as this principle might sound, a couple of caveats must be noted. First, although most liberal democratic states likely operate under some explicit or implicit version of this principle, it is unlikely that any political state follows it with absolute stringency. Second, due to the uncertain nature of some underlying concepts, it may not even be possible for any state to follow this principle with absolute stringency in a clear and uniform sense. As to the first caveat, in our own society we arguably violate the harm principle with laws against recreational drug use, prostitution, and limitations on the selling of alcohol. As to the second caveat, there is uncertainty regarding what might count as harm and regarding the division between the private and public spheres. Mill (1910) conceptualized harm in terms of limitation or violation of individual interests or rights. This conceptualization is rather broad and not limited to physical harm but likely does not include emotional harm. But more importantly, if one follows the effects of a presumably self-regarding act far enough, one is likely to find some harm done to another. For example, rock-climbing might on its face seem like a choice that only places oneself at potential risk. However, if a rock-climber finds themselves in need of rescue, now rescuers may be at risk, and, if injured, payment for care may place a burden upon others. However, there comes a point at which following this line of causation becomes ridiculous. For this reason, Mill (1910) attempted to limit far-flung, fanciful claims of harm. The understanding of harm to others (in terms of which acts should be regulated or prohibited by the government) should be those harms caused "directly, and in the first instance," by one's actions (Mill, 1910, p. 75). In other words, "indirect" harms or harms caused indirectly by one's actions should not be reasons to legally prohibit or regulate an act or practice. This restriction does not fully resolve the problem, however, as the line between direct effect and indirect effect is not always clear. For this reason, debates arise in our society regarding laws concerning tobacco smoking in public spaces, wearing seatbelts in motor vehicles, and motorcyclists wearing helmets (CDC, 2011; GHSA, 2019; IIHS, 2019). In the practical realm of the clinic, one can think of public health laws, such as those regarding vaccination. Most states require students to receive certain vaccinations to attend public school. This can be seen as an imposition on one's private life and decisions regarding child-rearing. The fact that the vaccination is not directly mandated but only indirectly mandated through a requirement for public education can be seen as an attempt to compromise public welfare and personal rights. In addition, most states also allow for exceptions based upon religious or sometimes "philosophical" commitments as well, as a further compromise for personal rights.

Relatedly, the line between the private sphere and the public sphere is also not always clear enough to function as a distinct criterion for applying the law. Though theoretically distinct areas of life, according to German philosopher Jürgen Habermas (2000), they are equiprimordial, meaning that they are equally fundamental and also rely on one another's realization to be fully realized. Having a fully realized private life depends upon the proper and full realization of the public sphere and vice versa. Due to this codependence, the line between the public and private may not always be clear. The interpretation of the public and the private in relation to spheres of experience is by no means wholly objective or absolute. It was not long ago that domestic violence was considered by many as merely a private matter between a married couple, a private matter with which the government should not interfere (Solic, 2015). Also, currently, one of the primary points of contention regarding the moral/legal issue of abortion is whether the act is one of the private or public sphere. The discourse from the common pro-choice perspective is that abortion is a private act between a woman and her physician and thus should be free of government interference. According to the typical pro-life perspective, abortion is not merely a self-regarding act but one that harms others (fetuses) who should be viewed as having legal rights worthy of protection by the government. This does not mean that the public/private division in determining where the law applies is a useless standard, but it can't operate as a specific, purely objective, and absolute standard. It is one that is continuously undergoing negotiation and adjustment.

While the common distinction is that law addresses external or public activities and morality private ones, morality does still address public life. The areas of social ethics and professional ethics address our actions in the public sphere. Common social issues like abortion, the death penalty, and genetic engineering, while legal issues, are also issues of public ethical discourse. And of course, professional ethics—the ethics of physicians, nurses, lawyers, educators, etc.—address and regulate the actions of professionals as they practice and provide services among the public. Practitioners who work in areas related to genetics, reproductive health, and these other areas will need to understand the legal obligations involved as well as the deep ethical questions that arise. Potential conflicts between the two, as well as potential conflicts between personal and professional ethics, will have to be resolved for the virtuous and competent practitioner.

The idea that morality addresses the private sphere may even include the realm of thought. Beliefs and opinions are often judged moral or immoral. Racist, sexist, or homophobic beliefs may be considered morally improper. It is not just the acts that these beliefs inspire that are immoral, some may say, but the thoughts themselves. One of the most famous philosophical investigations into the morality of thought and belief is W. K. Clifford's (1999) essay "The Ethics of Belief." In this essay, originally published in 1877, Clifford argues that one has not only an intellectual obligation but indeed a *moral* obligation not to believe a claim until sufficient evidence is presented. Being credulous, that is, believing before sufficient evidence is presented (i.e., being gullible), is not only intellectually dishonest and possibly imprudent, but also morally dishonest and even socially and personally harmful, according to Clifford. Although the normativity of internal moral states are primarily regulated through ethics, there are even times when the law takes internal mental states into account. *Mens rea* is a legal concept that from Latin literally means "guilty mind." The principle of *mens rea* is that for one to be legally liable for a criminal act one must have a "guilty mind" and be aware of their actions; that is, one must have criminal intent. Certain external acts can be used to infer a guilty intent or *mens rea*. Similarly, federal law and state laws include different degrees of murder, some of which are identified by mental states like premeditation and malice aforethought. Authorities also cannot directly perceive these in the accused but can similarly infer them from actions.

Another distinction between law and morality relates to enforcement. Law has the force of the government behind it to enforce laws through the coercion of punishment. The enforcement of morality is comprised primarily of public disapprobation or tainted reputation. Social and professional ethics are the areas in which overlap with the law occurs the most. Our moral views on issues like abortion and the death penalty feed into the laws that governments pass regarding them. And the laws we have on these issues likely also have an influence on individuals' moral views regarding them (Mentovich & Zeev-wolf, 2018). Similarly, professional ethics often overlap with legal issues. Such overlap occurs every semester of a healthcare ethics or nursing ethics course when a student responds to a case involving questions of confidentiality with a simple invocation of HIPAA. Yes, the Health Insurance Portability and Accountability Act (HIPAA) of 1996 provides legal protections for patient confidentiality and outlines punishments for breaches of confidentiality. However, it is a mistake to assume that outside of or prior to HIPAA, there is no acknowledgment of the importance of confidentiality in patient care. Confidentiality was one of the moral principles emphasized in the original Hippocratic Oath, while respect for autonomy (considered by many currently as the most important of moral principles in healthcare ethics) was completely ignored. In 1996, the U.S. Congress sent the message that confidentiality in healthcare is so important that it should have the force of law and coercion of potential punishment behind it in order to provide even greater protection than mere moral disapprobation. Along these lines, it is also worth noting that in the formal study and education of social ethics and professional ethics, the analysis and evaluation of landmark legal cases is often central. To teach about abortion, cases like *Roe v. Wade* (1973), *Planned Parenthood v. Casey* (1992), and *Dobbs v. Jackson Women's Health Organization* are indispensable. To teach end-of-life ethics, the Quinlan case (*In re Quinlan*, 1976) and Cruzan case (*Cruzan v. Director, Missouri Department of Health*, 1990), along with *In re Helga Wanglie* (1991) and *Washington v. Glucksberg* (1997) cases provide rich context for discussion and exploration of central ethical issues. Whereas ethics in general only has the enforcement of reputation and social disapprobation behind it, professional ethics often include mechanisms of coercive enforcement such as loss or suspension of license to practice.

One simple distinction between law and morality is that laws are created and modified by legislative bodies. This imputes intentional and procedural qualities of laws. They can be merely created, modified, and annulled by a recognized body of authority. Ethical rules and principles do not work this way but develop or evolve organically within a community of valuers. They do undergo change, but an authoritative body cannot merely change moral rules with the wave of a hand. Ethics, in general, is not procedural in this manner. For example, in our society, various forms of gender and racial oppression have been viewed as morally acceptable, or even obligatory, in the past. These are changes influenced but not instantiated by legal change; changes that arose organically and continue to evolve. However, professional ethics can often take on a procedural quality as a means of more strictly and uniformly regulating conduct among members of the profession. Also, due to the procedural nature of law, the law only requires that one meet the specific inscribed requirements. Ethics often demands more than simply refraining from breaking rules but going beyond that to good and benevolent action. This is particularly true from a perspective of virtue ethics in which moral education and self-improvement and an ideal of moral excellence (not mere rule-following) is to be pursued. There are no laws prescribing actions related to bedside manner or actual *care* for a patient's position, difficulties, or challenges. However, an ethical practitioner will acknowledge and endeavor to meet these needs.

Finally, for the purpose of clear and just enforcement, law needs a degree of certainty, while morals have a greater degree of flexibility and variability. The law depends upon clear and distinct definitions, which may not always hold up outside the law. A simple example is the age of majority. In this society we recognize the age of majority in most contexts as 18. This means that there are certain rights, privileges, and responsibilities afforded 18-year-olds but not 17-year-olds, such as the right to vote and make one's own medical decisions. However, there is nothing magical that happens to one's mental or emotional maturity upon one's 18th birthday. And it is very possible to find 17-year-olds with greater maturity and decision-making abilities than some persons much older. Yet for the purpose of applying legal rights and responsibilities, a legal expediency is necessary. There are some exceptions regarding minors' rights built into the law like the mature minor doctrine in the context of medical decisions, the process of emancipation, and legal exceptions in relation to reproductive choices. But these are procedural exceptions that cannot of course locate and empower every minor capable of making mature decisions. This mechanism toward expediency does have its downsides, however. The cliché, "the law is an ass," appeals to one of these. Because of these dictated legal standards and rules applying universally but perhaps ill-fitting certain specific situations, the law receives a reputation for being stubborn and incompatible with common sense.

Because moral rules (outside of procedural professional ethics) are not distinctly delineated and dictated, some degree of flexibility and variability is inevitable and perhaps necessary. Moral principles often conflict and thus are in need of deliberation through the application of practical judgment in order to resolve conflicts. There is also the problem that moral judgments and systems vary even within a society and even more so among different societies. To reach consensus or have any fruitful moral discourse, some degree of flexibility will be needed.

OTHER INTERSECTIONS OF LAW AND MORALITY: IS IT MORALLY WRONG TO BREAK THE LAW?

Laws include coercive penalties to help ensure obedience and civil order. People of course try to avoid unpleasant repercussions, and so it is expected that they will generally follow laws. However, even absent penalties, is there a moral reason for following the law? Of course, in the case of some laws a legal violation qualifies as a moral violation as well. Acts like theft, murder, and rape are typically judged immoral as well as illegal. However, there are many laws the violation of which would not be patently immoral. Would there also be a moral imperative to respect and follow these laws?

There are two major theories regarding the foundation of law. The first, natural law theory,[1] maintains, according to the overlap thesis, that laws are founded in a preexisting understanding of morality (Bix, 2002, 2010; Weinreb, 2004). That is, a law (or a proper law) needs to be derived from a moral principle or value, which implies that a law that is not moral in itself is either not a law at all (Augustine, 1973; Blackstone, 2016), or does not meet the ideal of what a law *should be* (Finnis, 2011). This latter view is more famously expressed in Martin Luther King, Jr.'s (2018) "Letter from a Birmingham Jail": "there are *just* and there are *unjust* laws … A just law is a man-made code that squares with the moral law or the law of God" (p. 503). Because King (2018) affirmed this second interpretation of natural law, he maintained that one should accept the punishment for breaking even an unjust law. For, even though an unjust law is unjust, it is still a law: "One who breaks an unjust law must do it *openly, lovingly* … and with a willingness to accept the penalty" (King, 2018, p. 504).

Those who subscribe to the second theory, positivism, conceive laws as an expression of conventionalism and created by an authoritative body possibly out of whole cloth (Coleman & Leiter, 2010). According to this way of thinking, for a law to be a legitimate law it need not meet some test for morality. The authority and legitimacy of the law rests wholly in the authority and power of the lawmakers, not in some assumed moral foundation. Although there is no moral basis for law according to positivism, it may not be the case that laws are created in a purely arbitrary or self-serving manner. Law, even absent an essential relation to morality, can have the objective of maintaining social order or protecting and promoting the well-being of the populace.

Even absent an essential connection between law and morality, we can still explore the possibility of a moral obligation to follow the law. Most persons, it seems, are generally law-abiding. This is not to say that most persons have not broken some minor or trivial laws, even with impunity: speeding infractions, rolling stops, jaywalking. However, consider a person who intentionally violates what many would consider more serious laws: theft, armed robbery, murder, rape. Your typical (generally) law-abiding citizen will have negative feelings regarding such a person. These negative feelings are likely inspired by the moral quality of the lawbreaker's actions. These more serious infractions are often (as in the examples provided) perceived as both illegal and immoral. However, these negative feelings may be associated with something more than the purely moral nature of the actions. There may be a concern with the actual legal violations involved. But why? What is the source of this scorn for lawbreakers qua *lawbreakers*, not just as moral transgressors?

One possible answer to this question is that when one breaks a law, one disrespects the state and political apparatus that creates the law. Under this interpretation we, as citizens (or residents) have not only a legal but a moral obligation to the state in which we live. However, while it seems natural to understand a moral duty to an individual, a moral duty to a political state is a different type of thing and far more dubious. A state is a conceptual fiction, not a moral agent. There are other arguments for moral obligations toward the state, but these are similarly contentious and uncertain (Luban, 1988). If one does not clearly have a moral obligation to the state to obey laws, there may instead be actual persons (moral agents) to whom we could say that we morally owe a duty to obey the law. A common argument in support of this view is known as the "fair play argument," which is a species of social contract thinking (Hart, 1958; Luban, 1988; Rawls, 2001). Returning to the lawbreaker and the average citizen's scorn for the lawbreaker, one means of conceiving the lawbreaker and his actions is in terms of being a "free rider." A free rider is one who reaps the benefits of a system without contributing to that system. The lawbreaker places himself above others, as someone not beholden to the rules (laws) of society but benefiting from the goods of society nonetheless, one who rides for free. Such actions also suggest further moral failings such as arrogance, disregard for the needs of others, and selfishness. Without assuming an inherent morality in the law, the fair play argument identifies a moral duty owed to one's fellow citizens to follow the law nonetheless.

But is it always morally wrong to break the law? There are possible cases in which a free rider might be excused when their free riding is not born of moral failings like selfishness but of extenuating circumstances that make it difficult or impossible to contribute the same as the rest of the community. By analogy, could there be circumstances that might justify a failure to comply with a law, or even a blatant defiance of a law? If there are extenuating circumstances that make an individual unable to follow a law, then it seems reasonable to excuse that individual from that law. However, there may also be conditions regarding a law itself in which a violation could appear morally justified. The fair play argument holds that a law should be generally beneficial in order for an individual to be obligated to follow it (Luban, 1988). To say that a law is generally beneficial is to say that it secures, promotes, or encourages some good for society. Absent some beneficence, it would be difficult to assert that any individual should comply with any law. Only absolute coercion, thus injustice, could compel behavior in that manner. Further, to say that a law should be *generally* beneficial means that the law should not "confer benefits on one group at the expense of others" (Luban, 1988, p. 43). In other words, a law should not be discriminatory and unfair. This criterion is itself expressed in the 14th Amendment of the Constitution: "No state shall … deny any person within its jurisdiction the equal protection of the laws." To break a law for one's individual benefit and assumed exceptionalism speaks of moral failings, of "unilaterally exempting oneself from the shared conditions of the community" (Luban, 1988, p. 42). However, to break a law as an act of resistance against a law that does not meet basic standards of fairness can itself be seen as a courageous, moral act—an act aimed at seeking justice overall. Breaking laws for one's personal benefit reflects an arrogance and selfishness, a contempt for others that denies or neglects the personhood and equal interests of others in one's community. Breaking an unjust law, however, holds no such implications: "the fact that a law is wrong or is overwhelmingly stupid means that noncompliance with it exhibits no disrespect for one's fellows, and thus that there is no obligation to obey it in the first place" (Luban, 1988, p. 45).

■ PRIORITIES: LAW VERSUS MORALITY

As noted at the beginning of this chapter, law and morality comprise distinct normative systems and are more often than not congruent with one another. But sometimes law and morality may conflict. When we face such situations, which should we choose to follow if we cannot reconcile this conflict: the law or morality? The question here falls under the concept of normative dominance. When different types of normative systems conflict, which should be acknowledged as dominant? For example, fashion is another normative system. Fashion norms dictate or suggest the way people should dress. Consider the wearing of animal fur. There are people who find the cultivation, creation, and wearing of animal fur as highly immoral. Perhaps if we lived in a preindustrial society in which wearing animal fur was the only means of surviving very cold weather, the morality of the practice might be judged differently. But that is not the situation in which we find ourselves. We have many alternatives for warm clothing that do not pose the same level of harm to animals. And so, the cultivation and killing of animals to wear their fur or skins seems unnecessary, an unnecessary infliction of harm upon sentient creatures. Making such a sartorial choice in our milieu appears to have value only in terms of aesthetics and status. One wearing a fur who is confronted with the moral problems associated with the cultivation and wearing of fur might respond with a statement such as, "But it looks good." Many people, understandably, even those who do not consider themselves animal rights advocates, would find that response crass and insensitive; that is, morally bankrupt. For most people of any moral sensitivity, even those with refined fashion sense, morality is perceived as normatively dominant to fashion. But when addressing the question of normative dominance as it relates to law and morality, is the answer equally as clear?

We recognize the state as having power over us, even though in a representative democracy "we the people" are theoretically the government, or at least those who endorse and endow the formal government with power. The enforcement of law is part of that power. If we want to live prosperously and peacefully in society, then presumably it benefits us to obey the law. Living contrary to the law opens us up to civil litigation and criminal penalty. Of course, those consequences can befall even the most law-abiding citizens, but following legal strictures seems the best bet to avoid them. Thus, the motivation for obeying the law does not follow simply from a desire not to be punished. It also comes from a desire to live a good life within a particular social structure. Motivation for obeying the law may also be a matter of simple character. Some people merely may not have it in them to be a thief or to sell dangerous and illicit products to make money. Here, we begin to loop back to the theme of the previous section. If laws (or at least proper and legitimate laws) are founded in morality, then there are not merely prudential, self-serving reasons for obeying the law but moral ones as well. But even absent such a connection, there still may be independent, moral motivation to follow the law.

This progression also begins to point to an answer on normative dominance. Identifying the question of character in relation to law and the possible moral foundation of law suggests a greater normative dominance in morality. If morality indeed provides a foundation for law or a collective moral reason for obeying the law, as in the fair play argument, it does appear more fundamental and presumably more dominant. What this means is that in a conflict between law and morality, *ideally* one should choose to follow morality. It may not be prudent to establish that principle in any stricter or more absolutist sense than this. In any particular case one may have to consider the degree of moral and legal wrong involved and the moral and legal consequences involved. That is, it might be justifiable to commit a minor moral wrong in order to follow a more serious legal requirement, such as causing a nonemergent patient to wait in order to complete necessary bureaucratic duties. It may not be possible to foresee all such situations and thus not prudent to establish a stricter principle.

But what does it mean to say that a conflict may exist between law and morality? Laws *should* be moral, although they may not always be moral. Even if an immoral law merely does not meet the ideal of what a law should be, then we may, depending on the nature of the law, still have a moral duty to reform and repair the law, rather than simply disobey it. Even assuming legal positivism and the fair play argument, if there is a moral obligation under a sort of social contract to obey the law, that obligation breaks down when the law in question does not provide a general benefit to society or apply to people equally. In contemporary society, of course, the quintessential example of this type of situation is the American civil rights movement of the 20th century, particularly the activism and thought of Martin Luther King, Jr.

According to King (2018), what gave a law moral propriety and force was that it "squares with the moral law or the law of God" (King, 2018, p. 503). King was a man of faith, a Christian; thus, much of his thought and activism were inspired and driven by religious principle. More specifically, he had a moral interpretation of Christian doctrine which the discriminatory laws and social structures in the United States violated. King was a Baptist minister, so that of course makes sense. At the same time, he was open-minded and strategic enough to realize that he could not communicate to all merely within a narrow moral/religious point of view which not all who he may wish to contend with might share. So, in the quote above he disjunctively refers also to the "moral law." If an objective morality exists (in the form of moral law), then we can easily test law against it and know which laws we should have, which laws we should morally violate, which laws we should change. This question is of course a continuing and ongoing debate in philosophy. However, even if objective morality does exist, the situation is still not that simple.

Objective morality may exist, but our confidence in being able to access it and know what comprises it is not absolute. The employment of King as an example in this discussion is possibly a bit facile. From our current historical perspective, it is easy to look back upon King, his thoughts, and his activism and say he was right to challenge the law. He was right that the law was unjust and discriminatory. However, it is important to remember that many people at the time did not agree and saw him as a mere scofflaw or worse. Consider a similar activist today engaging in civil disobedience. Many could see that person as a troublemaker or mere provocateur. But in decades to come, they could become a great hero. Knowing whether a person is a troublemaker or a hero today is more of a challenge. Consider Timothy Quill. In 1991 palliative physician Dr. Timothy Quill (1991) "stunned the medical community" (Connolly, 1998, p. 201) when he announced in the pages of the *New England Journal of Medicine* that he had aided, at her request, a terminally ill patient in ending her life by prescribing barbiturates. In 1991, physician-assisted suicide was legal nowhere in the United States. Thus, in the act itself, and especially in the public nature of this announcement, he was placing himself at legal risk. He explains his moral view as inclusive of an advocacy for control and dignity in patients' deaths. Yet, previous to this event, ending of life was limited to legally sanctioned instances of withdrawal of life-sustaining treatment. But in crossing the line to *actively* contributing to the ending of a patient's life in this case, he refers to the value of his patient's independence, her fear of a lingering death, and *his* fear of the family dealing with a violent death. "I also felt strongly," wrote Quill (1991), "that I was setting her free to get the most out of the time she had left, and to maintain dignity and control on her own terms until her death" (p. 693). Yet, at the same time, he expressed some uncertainty when he writes of her request "stretching" him profoundly and of an uneasy feeling from exploring boundaries. This uncertainty or emotional disturbance is to be expected and is likely a sign of a thoughtful, conscientious person in the midst of a novel and difficult decision. Thus, in his mind at least, he was acting morally yet contravening widely accepted medical ethics at the time, as well as the law. Public opinion, the majority of the medical establishment, and the law would condemn his actions, yet he believed he was morally justified. As a result of this publication, he was investigated by authorities in Monroe County, New York. His case went before a grand jury, but the grand jury declined to indict. Today, physician-assisted suicide is legal in several states—though still not in the state of New York where Quill aided his patient. Quill (along with other physicians) was later involved in a suit against the state of New York claiming that the state's law prohibiting physician-assisted suicide violated the equal protection clause of the 14th Amendment (*Vacco v. Quill*, 1997). The U.S. Supreme Court ruled against Quill and his co-plaintiffs in a unanimous decision. A practitioner faced with a similar situation today may be placing himself at similar risk, depending on the specific location. If the practitioner agrees with their state's prohibition of such action, then personally they may face no conflict. Professionally, it may not be so simple. Is a practitioner who refuses a request such as this out of a sense of personal disagreement doing a disservice to their patient, not meeting requirement of fidelity? There is an argument to be made for that. However, for a practitioner to abandon sincere and well-considered personal moral values for the sake of perceived professional values, also raises problems of moral integrity. However, the central concern here is for the practitioner who disagrees with their state's legal prohibition of such actions in meeting patients' needs and desires. Even if their personal and professional morality cohere, such actions will be at odds with the law and legal obligations. To ignore those may seem heroic, but beyond what can be considered obligatory.

Given the state of our moral discourse on physician-assisted suicide, it may still be reasonable to be unsure whether Quill was responding morally to a law that may be immoral in itself. That is a matter we are still working through in terms of our social ethics. But is it enough that a moral dissenter of law thinks or believes that their act is moral? That, I believe, is not a question to which a general answer can be given. We have to consider the act in question and the thinking behind the act. What about when *you* face a situation like this? It is possible, though not likely, that the whole world is wrong while you are right. It is possible that you and a minority of others are right, while the majority is wrong. But it will ultimately come down to you, your reasoning, and your conscience. In class, I tell my students that I cannot, from the safety of a classroom, counsel them to break the law if they believe the law is immoral. That can only be their decision. You have to consider the values involved, the repercussions (legal and moral), and your own integrity and conscience. What is doing the (morally) right thing worth to you in this particular instance? Only you can answer that question.

CONCLUSION

As nursing roles advance, the decisions, responsibilities, and accountability that accompany these roles also advance and become more complex. The moral and legal demands then also become complicated. An understanding of these distinct obligations is needed. But these obligations are not merely distinct because the law and morality themselves are not wholly distinct. They wrap around each other, and the law is undergirded by moral obligations itself. This leads to inevitable conflicts between the two realms of normativity. Some such conflicts resist compromise, and a clear and distinct choice must be made. No general answer can be given as to which must always be given preeminence, despite the arguably more fundamental nature of ethics. Thus, the nature and weight of these differing imperatives must be understood to make specific judgments allowing for personal and professional values to be respected along with the precepts of the law.

CRITICAL THINKING QUESTIONS

1. How are law and morality (ethics) similar?
2. How do law and morality (ethics) differ?
3. What are the relative values of law and morality?
4. Of law and morality, which is more fundamental?
5. What is John Stuart Mill's harm principle?
6. How is Mill's harm principle manifested in social policy?
7. What are some limitations of Mill's harm principle?
8. What are the two major theories regarding the foundation of law? What are the strengths and weaknesses of each?
9. Is there a moral obligation to obey the law?
10. Is there ever a moral justification (or even obligation) to break the law?

NOTE

1 This theory of law should not be confused with the similar sounding natural law theory in the study of morality. While they share a name and some basic principles and intutions, one

addresses the essence of morality and the other the essence of law and the law's relationship to morality.

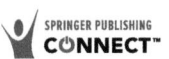

A robust set of instructor resources designed to supplement this text is located at http://connect.springerpub.com/content/book/978-0-8261-8137-4. Qualifying instructors may request access by emailing textbook@springerpub.com.

REFERENCES

Augustine. (1973). On free will. In A. Hyman & J. J. Walsh (Eds.), *Philosophy in the middle ages: The Christian, Islamic, and Jewish traditions* (pp. 33–64). Hackett Publishing Company.
Bix, B. (2002). Natural law theory: The modern tradition. In J. L. Coleman & S. Shapiro (Eds.), *Oxford Hand book of jurisprudence and philosophy of law* (pp. 61–103). Oxford University Press.
Bix, B. (2010). Natural law theory. In D. Patterson (Ed.), *A companion to philosophy of law and legal theory* (pp. 211–227). Blackwell Publishing Ltd.
Blackstone, W. (2016). *The Oxford edition of Blackstone's: Commentaries on the laws of England: Book I: Of the rights of persons*. Oxford University Press.
Centers for Disease Control and Prevention (CDC). (2011, April 22). *State smoke-free laws for worksites, restaurant, and bars: United States, 2000–2010*. https://www.cdc.gov/mmwr/preview/mmwrhtml/mm6015a2.htm
Clifford, W. K. (1999). The ethics of belief. In T. Madigan (Ed.), *The ethics of belief and other essays* (pp. 70–96). Prometheus.
Coleman, J. L., & Leiter, B. (2010). Legal positivism. In D. Patterson (Ed.), *A companion to philosophy of law and legal theory* (pp. 228–248). Blackwell Publishing Ltd.
Connelly, R. J. (1998). Death with dignity: Fifty years of soul-searching. *Journal of Religion and Health*, 37(3), 195–213.
Cruzan v. Director, MDH, 497 U.S. 261 (1990).
Finnis, J. (2011). *Natural law and natural rights*. Oxford University Press.
Government Highway Safety Association (GHSA). (2019). *Seat belts*. https://www.ghsa.org/state-laws/issues/Seat-Belts
Habermas, J. (2000). *The inclusion of the other: Studies in political theory*. MIT Press.
Hart, H. L. A. (1958). Legal and moral obligation. In A. I. Melden (Ed.), *Essays in moral philosophy* (pp. 82–107). University of Washington Press.
In re Quinlan. (1976). 355 A. 2d 647 – NJ: Supreme Court.
In Re the conservatorship of Helga M. Wanglie. No. PX-91-283. District Probate Division, 4th Judicial District of the County of Hennepin, State of Minnesota, 1991.
Insurance Institute for Highway Safety (IIHS). (May, 2019). *Motorcycles*. https://www.iihs.org/topics/motorcycles#helmet-laws?topicName=Motorcycles
King, Jr., M. L. K. (2018). Letter from a Birmingham jail. In S. M. Cahn (Ed.), *Exploring philosophy: An introductory anthology* (pp. 499–511). Oxford University Press.
Luban, D. (1988). *Lawyers and justice: An ethical study*. Princeton University Press.
Mentovich, A., & Zeev-wolf, M. (2018). Law and moral order: The influence of legal out comes on moral judgment. *Psychology, Public Policy, and Law*, 24(4), 489–502. https://doi.org/10.1037/law0000175
Mill, J. S. (1910). *Utilitarianism, Liberty, and Representative Government*. E. P .Dutton & Co. Inc.
Planned Parenthood v. Casey, 505 U.S. 833 (1992).
Quill, T. (1991). Death and dignity: A case of individualized decision making. *New England Journal of Medicine*, 324, 691–694. https://doi.org/10.1056/NEJM199103073241010
Rawls, J. (2001). Legal obligation and the duty of fair play. In S. Freeman (Ed.), *John Rawls: Collected papers* (pp. 117–129). Harvard University Press.
Roe v. Wade, 410 U.S. 113 (1973).
Solic, P. (2015). Private matter or public crisis? Defining and responding to domestic violence. *Origins: Current Events in Historical Perspective*, 8(10). http://origins.osu.edu/article/private-matter-or-public-crisis-defining-and-responding-domestic-violence
Vacco v. Quill, 521 U.S. 793 (1997).
Washington v. Glucksberg, 521 U.S. 702 (1997).
Weinreb, L. L. (2004). A secular theory of natural law. *Fordham Law Review*, 72(6), 2287–2300.

CHAPTER TEN Reflective Response

SHARON RADZYMINSKI

I commend Dr. Dahnke for tackling such a complicated and controversial subject. He provides a strong overview, supplemented with explicit examples, of moral and legal concepts involved in healthcare decision making. It is imperative that advanced practice nurses be aware of the implications these concepts have on their decision-making processes.

Law and ethics are two distinct concepts that govern human behavior, but they are often interrelated in many ways. Law refers to a set of rules and regulations that are enforced by a government or other authority, while ethics refers to a set of moral principles or values that guide an individual's behavior. Law is created by governments or other authorities through legislation, regulations, and court decisions, while ethics are shaped by social norms, cultural traditions, religious beliefs, and personal values. Law is enforced by the government or other authorities through the legal system, while ethics are enforced by social pressure, personal conscience, and professional codes of conduct. Violating the law can result in legal penalties such as fines, imprisonment, or other legal sanctions, while violating ethical principles can result in social or professional consequences such as loss of reputation, loss of trust, or loss of professional license. Law is generally universal and applies to everyone within a given jurisdiction, while ethics are more subjective and can vary across cultures, professions, and individuals.

In summary, law is a set of rules that are enforced by authorities, while ethics are moral principles that guide individual behavior. While law and ethics are related, they are distinct concepts that operate in different ways and have different consequences for violating them. Law and ethics are both important factors that influence decision making in nursing. Nursing practice is governed by legal and ethical principles that guide the nurse's behavior and ensure that patient care is delivered in a safe, effective, and ethical manner. Law provides the legal framework for nursing practice, establishing standards of care, defining the scope of practice, and outlining the legal obligations of nurses. Nurses are responsible for understanding and complying with the legal requirements governing their practice, including state and federal laws, regulations, and licensing standards. Ethics, on the other hand, provides a framework for making moral decisions in nursing practice. Ethical principles such as beneficence, nonmaleficence, autonomy, and justice provide guidance for nurses when they are faced with difficult ethical dilemmas in their practice. Nurses are expected to make ethical decisions that prioritize the patient's well-being and respect their autonomy and rights.

Dr. Dahnke makes a strong argument that laws must be moral and just. He cites the natural law theory, which claims a law needs to be derived from a moral principle or value, but also provides an alternative theory, positivism, which states that for a law to be legitimate it need not meet a test for morality. This certainly seems counterintuitive. However, upon closer inspection it raises significant questions. Who determines what is moral and what is not? Dr. Martin Luther King, Jr. is quoted as saying "a just law is a man-made code that squares with the moral law or the law of God" (King, 2018, p. 503).

What is missing is who determines that man-made code. What happens if each individual lives by a different code? What if the individual does not believe in God? For example, in some societies and in the minds of some individuals today, a spouse or child is considered as belonging to another through marriage or parenthood. There is a moral obligation to provide, care for, or act in their best interest. What happens if acting in their best interest means harsh discipline, bodily or mental harm, or confining them to a specified place? Who decides whether this behavior is moral or ethical? That is why we have laws.

Law is prevalent in healthcare because ethics is prevalent in healthcare, and in the United States we use the law to resolve ethical dilemmas (Scott, 2000). Law deals with ethics and in some circumstances determines ethics. Take for example, the situation I presented above. Although it was commonplace for husbands and fathers to proclaim ownership of their wives and children, and declared their right to treat them how they saw fit, at the turn of the 20th century, laws were enacted to protect women and children against abuse. The laws changed the moral code. During the second half of the 20th century, most difficult issues in healthcare that have raised profound ethical dilemmas (i.e., informed consent, confidentiality, right to die, professional negligence) have been addressed by law. Laws have reflected our society's evolving views on ethics. Laws also serve to enforce the socially agreed-upon views of right and wrong. Paradoxically when law becomes the primary enforcer of ethical views, its power can create problems for continued ethical reflection on the very issues that it was called upon to address in the first place (Scott, 2000). The process becomes a continuous circle. Individuals develop a moral code. When an individual's moral code conflicts with another's moral code then the collective opinion of society is called upon to settle the conflict. If conflict resolution is not attainable, then society looks to the law. Laws are created to represent the collective good, not a particular individual, so they are somewhat restrictive. Who determines the collective good are the lawmakers who are typically elected officials representing the society that elected them. If a law is considered unjust or unethical it is attributed to the lawmakers. How many lawmakers are elected and given power by members of society who know nothing about the person they are electing? What is the moral or ethical implications of that behavior? What are the moral and ethical professional behaviors of advanced practice nurses in the law-making process?

The law still reflects society's idealism. Immanuel Kant believed that: "The greatest problem for the human species, the solution of which nature compels him to seek, is that of attaining a civil society which can administer justice universally" (Kant, 1991, p. 45). Justice is an ethical concept of universal fairness for and among individuals Law is the vehicle by which a society attempts to achieve this lofty ideal. Oliver Wendell Holmes observed that: "The law is the witness and external deposit of our moral life. Its history is the history of the moral development of the race" (Holmes, 1897, p. 459). Thus, at any given point in time, it is the views of society that determine acceptable ethically appropriate behavior. In healthcare, our society has used the law to ask and answer questions about what are ethically appropriate behaviors among those who provide or receive or pay for healthcare services.

The intersection of law and ethics is where nursing needs to base its decision making. Law only sets the minimum for ethical behavior. Nurses are the ones who can choose whether they want to go beyond the law's minimums and strive for the ethical maximums. They can choose to start and end conversations with their patients quickly while obtaining informed consent or they can choose to engage the patient in thinking about their health and the ways it would best promote it, respect their choices, or allay their fears. Nurses need to obey the laws but advanced practice dictates that they do so at the highest level of professional ethics, which includes advocating for changes in the legal system.

REFERENCES

Holmes, O. W. (1897). The path of the law. *10 Harvard Law Review, 10*, 457–458.
Kant, I. (1991). *Political writings*, H. Reiss (Ed.), H. B. Nisbet (Trans.). Cambridge University Press.
King, Jr., M. L. K. (2018). Letter from a Birmingham jail. In S. M. Cahn (Ed.), *Exploring philosophy: An introductory anthology* (pp. 499–511). Oxford University Press.
Scott, C. (2000). Why law pervades medicine: An essay on ethics in health care. *Notre Dame JL Ethics & Public Policy, 14*(1), 245–303.

CHAPTER ELEVEN

DNP as Applied Statistician

JAMES SCHREIBER

INTRODUCTION

This chapter discusses core topics related to being an applied statistician. As roles and expectations change over time, along with external pressures, such as a limited pool of applied statisticians to hire, DNPs will need to increase their statistical knowledge. In this chapter, I focus on the supply of statisticians, common topics/common problems, data analysis, and where the applied field is evolving, along with some of the expectations in the field that now exist. The choice of topics in the chapter developed from 25 years of teaching, reviewing manuscripts and grants, and conversations and arguments with colleagues. Finally, a case study is provided.

SUPPLY LINES

Roles, responsibilities, and expectations change over time for individuals within every profession. The roles of nurses and the expectations of nurses have changed over time and this has been documented for decades (Saunders, 1954). DNP-educated nurses do not typically receive many educational experiences in research; that has been central to the PhD education. But most PhD-educated nurses are going to work in schools of nursing that are not research intensive (Oermann & Kardon-Edgran, 2018). And research skills, like all skills, deteriorate over time when not used. Therefore, those trained for research are, potentially, not conducting much research, and those not trained for research need these skills. Included in this mix, the employment forces at play could lead to the possibility of a massive shortage.

The overall employment of mathematicians and statisticians was projected to grow 33% from 2021 to 2031. There is a large need for individuals with this set of knowledge and skills (Bureau of Labor Statistics, 2022). There will be around 4,100 openings a year for mathematicians and statisticians over this same time period, and a 31% increase in need. Many of these will be replacement positions. These individuals will move to different jobs or leave the labor force, for example, to retire (Bureau of Labor Statistics, 2022). For reference, registered nursing positions are only expected to grow 6%, though other nursing specialties will be more in demand. Thus, it appears there is not an excess of mathematicians and statisticians being created, and applied statisticians are a subgroup of this field. The competition for these individuals is so intense that even the federal government has a public relations page about working as a statistician for the federal government (at https://stattrak.amstat.org/2012/11/01/federalstatisticalsystem).

There are numerous fields that use mathematicians and statisticians that are not university based: operations research positions in business, large technology companies, and smaller technology start-ups, along with organizations such as NASA and the JPL (Jet Propulsion Lab) to name a few. Those with mathematics and statistical backgrounds along with database management and coding experience are hired quickly with excellent salaries and benefits.

Finally, examining the changes in mathematics/computer science/statistics curricula over the past few years, there is a shift away from basic inferential statistical analysis to large data and machine learning. Education programs that are being developed and advertised are not focused on applied statistical analysis, such as independent t-tests, but on data science.

COMMON TOPICS/COMMON PROBLEM AREAS

p-Values

The p-value focus over the past 90 years has been problematic because most people simply do not understand what a p-value is, how it comes about, or how to interpret it. It has slowed down scientific progress. I will not go into depth on this, but highlight a few interesting aspects, as I and many others have written about the p-value elsewhere (The American Statistician Volume 73 March 2019; Schreiber, 2020; Ziliak & McCloskey, 2008). The p-value has made it to the United States Supreme Court (*Matrixx Initiatives Inc. v. Siracusano*, 2011). This case focused on information provided to shareholders and was a suit brought by investors. The plaintiffs were arguing that Matrixx did not disclose the fact that one of its products, Zicam nasal spray, caused loss of smell in some users because the results were not "statistically significant." Yet, the *risk* was real. The case was initially dismissed, but the U.S. Court of Appeals 9th Circuit reversed the decision, stating that "statistically significant" was up to the trier of the fact, such as a jury or investor. This led the way for the case to be pled before the Supreme Court. In a unanimous decision, associate justice Sonia Sotomayor wrote,

> We conclude that the materiality of adverse event reports cannot be reduced to a bright-line rule. Although in many cases reasonable investors would not consider reports of adverse events to be material information, respondents have alleged facts plausibly suggesting that reasonable investors would have viewed these particular reports as material. Respondents have also alleged facts "giving rise to a strong inference" that Matrixx "acted with the required state of mind."
>
> A lack of statistically significant data does not mean that medical experts have no reliable basis for inferring a causal link between a drug and adverse events. As Matrixx itself concedes, medical experts rely on other evidence to establish an inference of causation. See Brief for Petitioners 44–45, n. 22. [Footnote 7] We note that courts frequently permit expert testimony on causation based on evidence other than statistical significance. See, *e.g.*, *Best* v. *Lowe's Home Centers, Inc.*, 563 F. 3d 171, 178 (CA6 2009); *Westberry* v. *Gislaved Gummi AB*, 178 F. 3d 257, 263–264 (CA4 1999) (citing cases); *Wells* v. *Ortho Pharmaceutical Corp.*, 788 F. 2d 741, 744–745 (CA11 1986). We need not consider whether the expert testimony was properly admitted in those cases,

and we do not attempt to define here what constitutes reliable evidence of causation. It suffices to note that, as these courts have recognized, "medical professionals and researchers do not limit the data they consider to the results of randomized clinical trials or to statistically significant evidence."

The FDA similarly does not limit the evidence it considers for purposes of assessing causation and taking regulatory action to statistically significant data. In assessing the safety risk posed by a product, the FDA considers factors such as "strength of the association," "temporal relationship of product use and the event," "consistency of findings across available data sources," "evidence of a dose-response for the effect," "biologic plausibility," "seriousness of the event relative to the disease being treated," "potential to mitigate the risk in the population," "feasibility of further study using observational or controlled clinical study designs," and "degree of benefit the product provides, including availability of other therapies."

Essentially, the *p*-value should not be used for decision making in the way that it has been. As Wasserstein et al. (2019) have stated, do not assume that those values less than .05 indicate something is occurring and those over .05 that nothing is occurring. The applied statistician is more focused on what is going on with the data and where the variance is being accounted than on a specific magical value.

Error—Sampling Versus Measurement

There are two types of errors that need to be understood. The first is sampling error; the error due to the sampling process. Discussion of all the types of sampling processes is not warranted here, but a general understanding is. Imagine, as shown in Figure 11.1, the population distribution of a variable you are interested in (e.g., caloric intake, or anxiety) is normally distributed in the population. But the sample, you, the researcher obtains is the darker shaded distribution shown in Figure 11.2. The error you have is based on

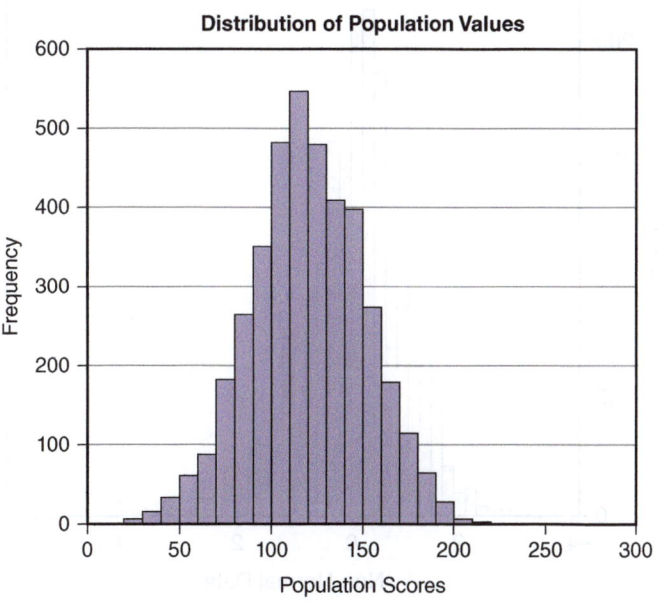

FIGURE 11.1　Normal Distribution for a Population

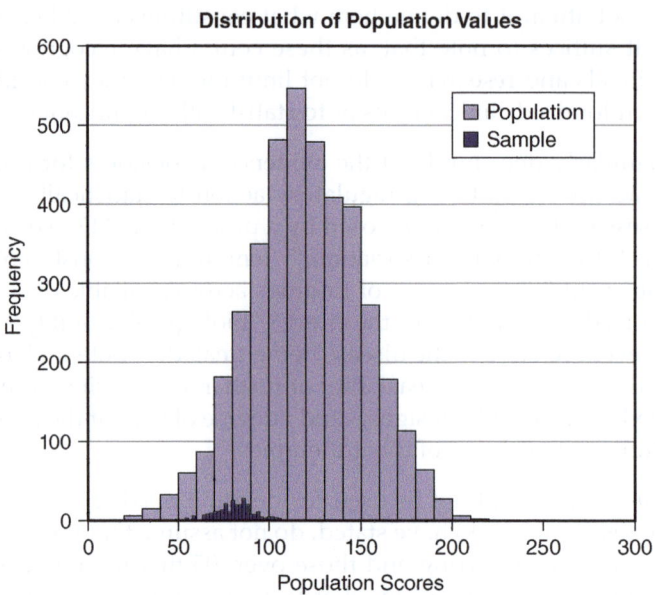

FIGURE 11.2 A Sample and the Population

the fact the that sample does not match the population—it is part of the lower end of the population. Thus, the mean, standard deviation, and other important information will be incorrect, that is, biased. This error can be exacerbated in data cleaning. Imagine, as shown in in Figure 11.3, that part of the sample is relatively far away—skewed to the right. Many researchers will immediately remove those participants because they are "outliers" on that variable and the researcher is trying to have a normal distribution shape. But those values are part of the population (personal communication, Gene V.

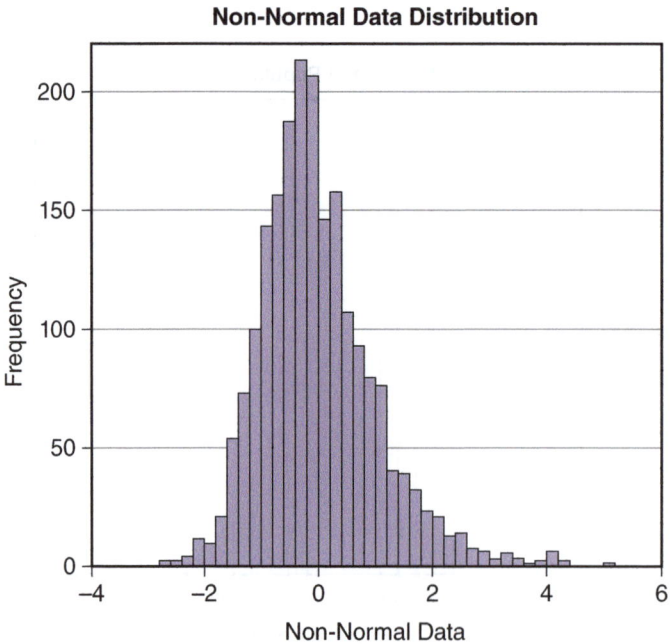

FIGURE 11.3 A Non-Normal Distribution

Glass). The results, after removal, potentially bias the parameters, such as the mean in this example; the adjusted mean value would be even lower than the population mean without those removed values. Even in Figure 11.2, the blue distribution is skewed and removal of data would bias the estimates. Note, again, that the mean of the sample is already lower than the population mean value.

Issues like these are why most of the time spent with the data should focus on data wrangling—getting to know your data and getting it into shape to analyze and documenting the changes you made to the data and why. This also allows you, as researcher, to understand the potential mistakes made from decisions based on the data at hand.

Measurement error, the second type of error, concerns the error in the data when using instruments (related to reliability, discussed later in the chapter). Instruments come in a variety of forms, such as psychological (e.g., generalized anxiety) or medical (e.g., thermometer), or physical (e.g., scale). Psychological instruments have a large amount of error. Researchers discuss this in the form of a model: $X = T + E$, where X is the observed score (e.g., anxiety score) and equals the true score, T (the participants' actual anxiety) plus error (E). We never really "know" a true score, we infer it based on the observed score and the amount of error we see. Data from an instrument with a reliability score of 0.80 has a 0.20 (20%) error. Thus, someone's true score with this much error could be much higher or much lower. Digital thermometers, an instrument that needs to measure accurately, can still have a an error of plus or minus 0.3 degrees (Sund-Levander et al., 2004). Blood pressure data is also error prone (Berg, 2019).

Sampling error has typically received the most attention because it is embedded in most statistics and research methods courses multiple times, but measurement error and measurement-related classes deserve a more central focus. The applied statistician is constantly worried about both because they negatively impact the inferences made from the data. Applied statisticians are constantly asking "how much do I have?" and "how far off might I be?"

Measurement

The types of data that are associated with different analyses continue to be a problematic area during manuscript reviews. Stevens (1946) argued for the four levels as nominal, ordinal, interval, and ratio (Table 11.1). Wright (1999) extended this group of four to more categories to include Peirce's (1931–1958) better system and argue for six steps to science. There are arguments that nominal and ordinal are not measurements (Bond & Fox, 2015; Wright, 1999). Nominal clearly has problems as a measurement because any value attached to a category is not a measure and does not have measurement qualities, for example, 1 = Male, 2 = Female. Even Stevens (1946) wrote that it is a "primitive form" and that as long as you do not assign the same numbers to different categories, "anything goes with the nominal scale" (p. 679).

Ordinal suffers from "distance" and "threshold" problems. Ordered categories (lowest to highest, or vice versa) assume that the distance between each category is the same. This expands to a larger problem when there are multiple categories, for example Likert-type scales (e.g., 1 = Agree, 2 = Somewhat Agree, 3 = Somewhat Disagree, 4 = Disagree). Also, there is an assumption that threshold (tipping point) moving from one category to the next is at the exact same position for each item and person. This is simply not true and has been demonstrated for decades.

Classical test theory (CTT) has been focused on the four levels of measurement working under the $X = T + E$ model. More generally within CTT, we also assume the error is random. Systematic error, such as bias, is not considered. Next, there is only one overall reliability typically based on a summed score, but this does not mean that

TABLE 11.1 Stevens' Categories of Data with Analysis and Research Questions

Scale Name	Stevens' (1946) Statement	Characteristic	Measures	Descriptive Statistics	Some Inferential Statistics	Generic RQ (How Much?)
Nominal (Categorical)	Determination of a quality	You can tell objects apart. Discrete units of categories. For example, gender, political affiliation	Measures in terms of names	Number of cases Mode Contingency Correlation	Contingency Correlation (also, Chi-Square)	Which is the most common?
Ordinal (Ordered Categorical)	Determination of greater or less	You can tell if one object is better or smaller, for example, school rankings	Measures in terms of more or less than	Median Percentiles	Rank correlation	Which is first? What is the middle?
Interval (Continuous)	Determination of equality of intervals or differences	You can tell how far apart objects are, for example, test scores, or temperature	Measure in terms of equal distances	Mean, median, standard deviation	Pearson product moment correlation, regression, t-tests, analysis of variance (ANOVA)	What is the average? How different are the means?
Ratio	Determination of equality of ratios	You can tell how big one object is in comparison to another, for example, velocity	Measures in terms of equal distances with an absolute zero point	Geometric mean, median, mode, standard deviation	Coefficient of variation, regression, correlation, t-tests, ANOVA	Same as above

reliability is permanently established. Reliability needs to be reestablished every time data are collected. For example, if you use a survey instrument that has been used before, you must calculate the reliability for *your* data. The fact that the data has had good or strong reliability scores previously is wonderful—we all want stable scores—but you have new data! That new data means you have to reestablish the reliability. Again, no data from any instrument are permanently reliable. There is also the issue that the reliability scores in many studies are not great. As stated earlier, if you have a reliability value of 0.80, remember, you have 20% error in that score.

For tests/examinations, CTT includes item difficulty (e.g., proportion correct) and/or item discrimination (e.g., people who scored high on this instrument also chose the answer for a specific item correctly). But the score is still just the summary of the items correct. This summary score is not very sophisticated. Item response theory (IRT) is fundamentally and, one could argue, philosophically different than CTT. IRT uses the person information and the item information to provide a probability model estimate-based score that is an actual measure at the interval level. The scoring system for the Next Generation NCLEX most likely will use an IRT-based probability model (Dickison et al., 2016). I use IRT-based scores in my undergraduate classes when I have traditional tests because it allows me to have more detailed information about the items and the respondents. Applied statisticians need to spend more time working on item response theory and less time in classical test theory.

Validity

No instrument is valid or has been validated, just like reliability. There is no other way to state this. Validity is about the quality of the inferences made from the *data*. Thus, validity is an inference making process based on the data and that process can go astray at any time. Additionally, one type of validity inference can be strong, such as content validity, and yet have poor construct or predictive validity evidence later.

Data Amount for Power Versus Accuracy

Power has been a consistent topic and concern to researchers, granting agencies, journal reviewers, and so on for decades. The reason for this focus has really only to do with trying to guarantee a *p*-value less than .05. Some readers might argue that the power is to make sure if there is a sample size large enough for a signal to be detected, that you observe it. But, in reality it has been about getting to .05 because 05 became "the" dominant signal for which to search. If you increase sample sizes enough, even extremely small relationships will be "statistically significant" at .05. The reason this occurs is because of the standard error, which is based on the sample size. For example, in a basic independent *t*-test the *t*-value is the difference of the two independent groups' mean values over the standard error; generically,

$$\frac{(observed\ values) - (expected\ value)}{standard\ error}$$

More technically, it is

$$t = \frac{(\bar{x}_1 - \bar{x}_2) - 0}{\sqrt{\frac{s_1^2(n_1 - 1) + s_2^2(n_2 - 1)}{n_1 + n_2 - 2}} * \sqrt{\frac{1}{n_1} + \frac{1}{n_2}}}.$$

Notice in the denominator the two sample sizes, n_1 and n_2. As those samples increase in size, the overall value in the denominator decreases. As the denominator value decreases, the ratio of the numerator to the dominator increases, thus creating a larger *t*-value. For example, five divided by four is smaller than five divided by three. This is why you hear many statisticians flippantly say increase your sample size and you will find what you want (i.e., $p < .05$). Even if you increase the sample sizes, where that sample is in relation to the population still matters (refer back to Figure 11.2). It would be better to focus on your measurement and sampling error. There is another way to think about sample size and accuracy, which is discussed later.

DATA ANALYSIS

Traditional data analysis, also called Fisher, Fisherian, or frequentist, includes independent *t*-tests, paired or dependent *t*-tests, analysis of variance (ANOVA), multivariate regression, exploratory factor analysis, principal component analysis, and the family of structural equation models (Schreiber, in press: Schreiber & Turk, 2022). These are all parametric analyses because the outcome variables are assumed to be continuous (interval or ratio) and normally distributed. There are nonparametric versions of these analyses when the outcome data are not normally distributed or are not continuous in nature, such as Kruskal-Wallace or logistic regression.

Common Data Analysis Errors

I have been a journal editor three times and an editorial board member or reviewer for dozens of journals. The topics discussed in this section do not encompass all of the errors, but are the most frequent ones in my experience. The first common error is that the research question, design, and analysis do not align. For example, the research questions discuss time-based mediation effects on an outcome: X comes before Y and M, where M also has to come before Y and changes (mediates) the size of the relationship between X and Y (Figure 11.4).

But the design is a survey where all the data are collected at the same time (thus negating the temporal argument). Or, there is a regression model with an interaction variable, when a mediation model or a separate path analytic model should have been implemented. Another similar example occurs when interactions are discussed in the theoretical framework and research questions, but are not tested in the analysis. These types of error occur more often than one might believe; I see them multiple times a year.

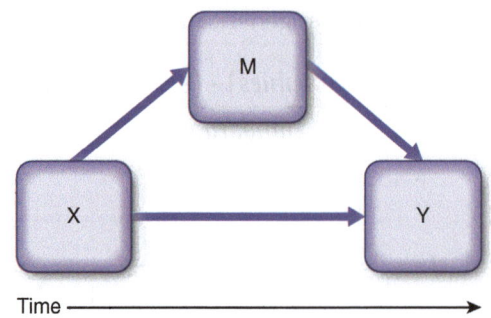

FIGURE 11.4. Mediation with Temporal Component

Next, the sample sizes do not add up from the stated sample size to the sizes in the tables or the analyses. If there are 450 participants in the descriptive statistics table, there should be 450 in the analysis, such as an ANOVA. Related, missing data or incomplete data are not thoroughly explained or dealt with properly. There are options for missing data and they do need to be justified, but ignoring or not discussing this issue continues to occur in manuscripts.

Another common error occurs when chi-square results are discussed as a measure of association when that is not what chi-square is; it is a measure of deviance of how different expected and observed values are. If you have data that are appropriate for chi-square analysis and want to discuss association, the value that needs to be calculated is phi, or possibly an odds-ratio in a case-control study. Related, Chi-square analyses constantly suffer from cell sizes (groups) that are small compared to the sample sizes in the rest of the cells. This happens a great deal in rare-event studies.

Correlations are commonly incorrect based on the data that were gathered. There are specific correlations for different types of data (Schreiber & Asner-Self, 2010). If the data of both variables are continuous and normally distributed, the traditional Pearson correlation is appropriate. As the data types change, such as skewed or more ordinal in nature (Likert-type), different correlations are needed (Schreiber & Asner-Self, 2010; Schreiber & Turk, 2022).

Mean values on frequency data still occur. The most common mean value on frequency data occurs with the binary gender classification. It should not be happening but still does. I think it happens because the author(s) are trying to make just one table. The descriptive tables should be created appropriately and separated by data type. With some more complex analyses, though, the author(s) should publish a covariance matrix that includes gender because of the analysis completed (e.g., structural equation model).

Effect sizes are still missing from studies (e.g., Cohen's *d*, Glass's delta, partial eta-squared, R-squared, Cox & Snell). If effect sizes are provided, very rarely will they be incorrect. If the error does occur, it is typically with Cohen, Glass, and Hedges. Cohen's *d* is appropriate if the standard deviations are about the same size and the sample sizes are the same or close. Hedges' *g* is used when group sizes are unequal, and Glass's delta (Δ) is calculated when there is a control group in an experiment.

Homogeneity of variance should be examined and discussed. Almost all software packages provide it automatically or it can be added with a click of a button. Homogeneity problems occur when the variances of data for the groups (e.g., independent *t*-tests and ANOVA) are meaningfully different. In Figure 11.5, the two distributions have the same variance; the same standard deviation.

In Figure 11.6 the control group has half the standard deviation shown in Figure 11.5. This smaller standard deviation reduces the value in the standard error for inferential tests. Note that in Figure 11.6, both of those distributions are normally distributed simulated data.

Extreme convenience samples generalized to population, and specifically populations far outside of the sample, is a continual issue. Many studies use convenience samples, and for some I would term extreme convenience samples. They violate the assumption of randomly selected participants, but convenience samples are common if not the norm. The fact is, many of these convenience samples are probably not representative of the population as a whole at all. First year students at Cal Tech are different than first year students at Duquesne. Quantitative analysis is about generalizing from sample to population, but it has become a bit ridiculous in some circumstances to make the claims being made given the sample, the measurement error, and the sample sizes involved.

Though difficult to tell in a manuscript, regression analyses, and correlations generally, suffer from transparency related to linearity. A correlation of any size can be

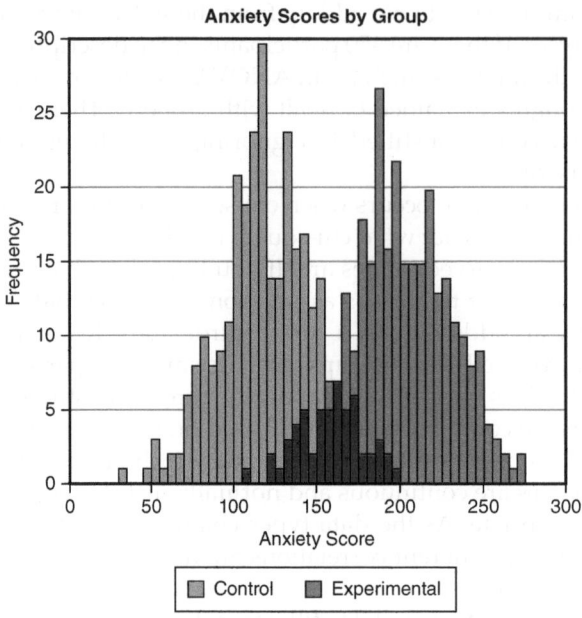

FIGURE 11.5 Overlapping Distributions—Equal Variances

represented by a variety of relations between two variables. This is commonly discussed as Ascombe's quartet (Figure 11.7). I have recreated the common visual most professors of statistics use to discuss this issue. Each of these scatter plots between two variables have one thing in common, their correlation is the same. The problem is the scatterplots are not, and some are nonlinear relations, which is an assumption of the traditional

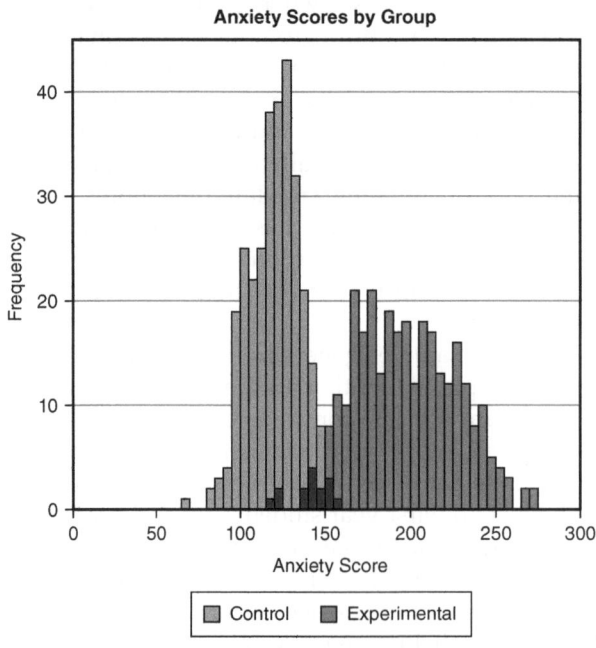

FIGURE 11.6 Overlapping Distributions—Unequal Variances

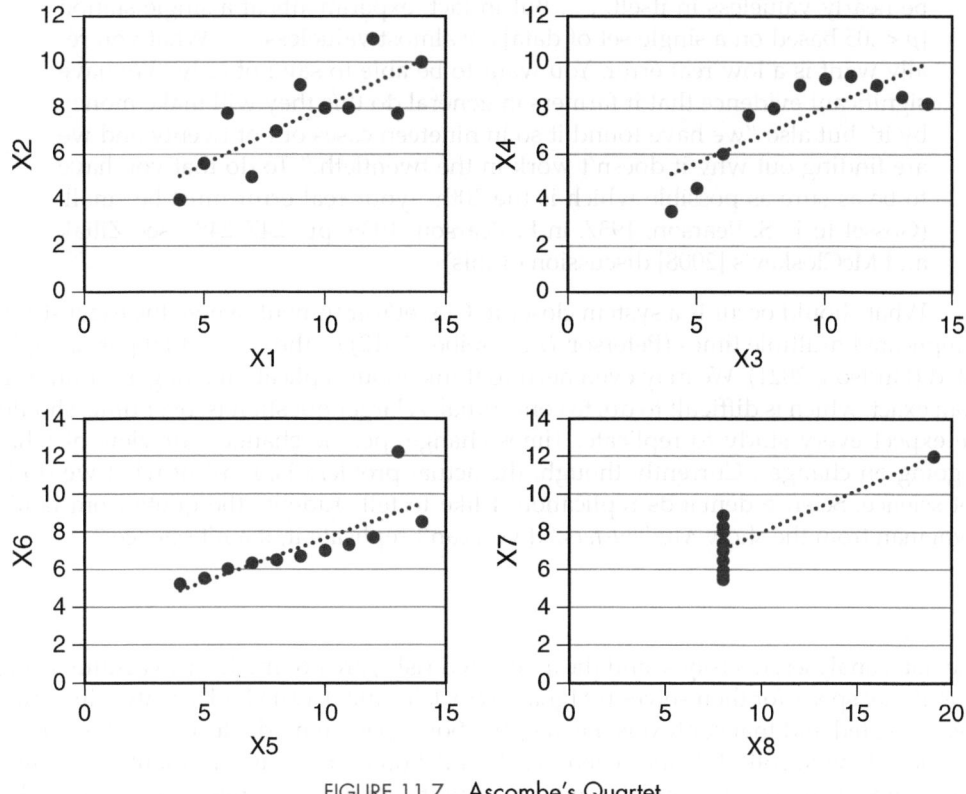

FIGURE 11.7 Ascombe's Quartet

Pearson correlation coefficient. This issue is also an argument for always visualizing data and their interrelations before analyses are undertaken.

Finally, there is a lack of discussion of residuals and error of the model. There are a variety of residuals that can be created, but most articles really bypass most of the residual discussion. At the most basic level, an in-depth understanding of the predicted outcome and the original outcome is critical. Residual analyses provide a pretty clear window into how well the model is working, but most researchers skim over this part of the analysis and just make sure the residuals are normally distributed.

EVOLVING AREAS AND THOSE WITH MORE VISIBILITY

The replication crisis has received a great deal of time in academic discussions. To me, there is no crisis of replication because the system is not designed for replication. Those who focus on the Type 1, Type 2, and p-value trifecta are using a system that is designed to run the study once with a large enough sample to reach .05. This trifecta is set up to *assume* replication or repeated studies over time, *not* actually do them. And the academic publishing system rewards that behavior—Skinner was not all wrong; people behave in relation to what is reinforced. What is interesting, especially related to p-values, is what William Gosset wrote to Egon Pearson about p-values and how Fisher had the logic reversed trying to get that 1 in 20 observation (0.05) instead of the reverse. He wrote,

> ...obviously the important thing in such is to have a low real error, not to have a "significant" result at a particular station. The latter seems to me to

be nearly valueless in itself. . . . But in fact, experiments at a single station [$p < .05$ based on a single set of data] *are* almost valueless. . . . What you really want is a low real error. You want to be able to say not only "We have significant evidence that if farmers in general do this they will make money by it" but also "we have found it so in nineteen cases out of twenty and we are finding out why it doesn't work in the twentieth." To do that you have to be as sure as possible which is the 20th—your real error must be small. (Gosset to E. S. Pearson, 1937, in E. Pearson, 1939, pp. 247–248—see Ziliak and McCloskey's [2008] discussion of this).

What should occur is a system closer to Gosset's argument, where the exact study is replicated multiple times (Peterson & Schreiber, 2012) or the conceptual part is replicated (Hudson, 2021). We may even need to think about replication along a continuum from exact, which is difficult to do, to conceptual. A larger question is, over time, should we expect every study to replicate. Times change, people change, our view of what is going on changes. Currently though, the actual problem is, most of what we do is not science. Science demands replication. I like to tell students the quote from Jamie Hyneman from the show *Mythbusters*. "If you can't replicate it, it ain't science."

Context

The data, analyses, decisions, and the associated risks, are not made in a vacuum. Data, thus, *do not* speak for themselves (D'Ignazio & Klein, 2020). Data had a context in which it was created and that context is meaningful. Some person made decisions about what to collect, how to collect it, and when to collect it. Sometimes it is important to examine what is not in a data set to understand it in order to conduct accurate and ethical analyses. There is also the context of the decisions made during analyses, which are rarely transparent. When you give different researchers the same data and same hypotheses, you can get very different results (Kha Breznau et al., 2021). The context matters.

Quality of Data and Data Bias

Understanding the type of data from a the viewpoint of measurement and basic reliability of the data and the ability to make valid claims from the data is the quality of the data. I am not discussing a reliability issue here, but the foundation, the core, of the data collected. Data can be stable or reliable and of extremely poor quality. A quote from Stamp (1929) relates the following anecdote:

> *Harold Cox tells a story of his life as a young man in India. He quoted some statistics to a judge, an Englishman, and a very good fellow. His friend said, "Cox, when you are a bit older, you will not quote Indian statistics with that assurance. The Government are very keen on amassing statistics—they collect them, add them, raise them to the nth power, take the cube root and prepare wonderful diagrams. But what you should never forget is that every one of those figures comes in the first instance from a chowty dar (village watchman), who just puts down what he damn pleases"* (pp. 258–259).

As with the context, quality examination requires the researcher to ask, How was the data collected? Who had the power to collect the data in that manner? For example, the way race and ethnicity have been collected over time is just one problematic area (Zuberi & Bonilla-Silva, 2008). In each U.S. Census you see the changes as the census takers try to get a better "measure" of race and ethnicity. Here they are trying to be more accurate with how individuals self-identify, but the original categories are not based on self-identification, but on constructs created by those in power. The existence of the data from the category does not mean that valid inferences can be made from the data based on the categories. Interrogating how and why the data were collected in a specific way leads one to interesting questions, such as with race and ethnicity: "Is this data acting as a proxy for something else?" This then leads to the question, "what was actually measured?"

One cannot talk about data quality, currently, without talking about the assumption of big data (also artificial intelligence [AI], algorithms, etc.); massive amounts of data solve all these problems. A massive amount of data does not equate to quality data. Even armed with the best intentions, a developer cannot account for all potential sources of bias, including implicit or unconscious bias (Project Implicit, 2020). Meredith Whittaker, executive director of the AI Now Institute, poses important related questions, "[w]hat assumptions about worth, ability and potential do these systems reflect and reproduce? Who was at the table when these assumptions were encoded?" (Rosenbaum, 2018). O'Neil's (2016) work on AI systems has demonstrated that mathematical models are not unbiased, and that the unregulated use of big data reinforces discrimination. O'Neil (2016) argues that the modelers of algorithms should take responsibility for the use of black box algorithms and charges policy makers to regulate their use (O'Neil, 2016). Power differentials focus on who is making the decision, how many people were involved in that decision, who is accountable for that decision, what counts as success, and who holds the decision makers accountable. What counts as success radically changes what is important (Muller, 2019). Decision points are human opinions embedded in a mathematical model (Alexander, 2018).

Research Versus Administrative Data

The original purpose of the data is becoming an area of concern, which has led to an increase in discussions concerning that purpose. Research data are collected for the purpose of conducting a research study, typically with specific research questions and specific variables of interest. Administrative data are collected for administrating an organization, and for purposes such as billing. The purpose and goals are very different, but increasingly, administrative data are being used for research purposes (Mazzali & Duca, 2015).

Administrative data have the advantages of size and up-to-date information, along with being able to link different sources of information. But these data can lack the exact clinical information a researcher needs, and the quality of the data is affected by its primary use, such as reimbursement. Then there are misclassifications of outcomes or exposure. Finally, there is the problem with the large datasets where "statistical significance" is easily achieved when in actuality there is little clinical relevance such as effect size or meaningful odds ratios (Mazzali & Duca, 2015).

Accuracy

The focus on power has driven researchers away from focusing on the accuracy of their estimates and how much confidence the researcher wants to have (Trafimow & McDonald, 2017). Reliability is different; reliability is about the stability of your scores—a researcher can have stable scores and have those scores be inaccurate. If there are real risks with making an incorrect inference from the results of a study, then the researcher should desire to have the highest accuracy possible with the highest level of confidence possible. For example, if the focus is examining the difference between two groups and the researchers want to be confident that their sample means are close to the population means, there are two important issues they must determine, how close and how confident (Trafimow & McDonald, 2017). Close can be defined with the distance in standard deviations away from the mean values and confidence can be a corresponding probability (Trafimow & McDonald, 2017). For example, if the researchers want the closeness to be within 0.1 standard deviation of the population means and feel very confident in those values (95%), then a sample size of about 500 is needed for a two-group analysis with the assumptions met. Again, this is not about statistical significance, this is about accuracy and confidence—a different way of viewing sampling. Historically, people have focused on getting to 0.05 for sample size, and have not focused on accuracy and confidence. A traditional power analysis of two groups would indicate a sample size of 128 is satisfactory.

Risk

Related to accuracy and confidence is risk. Risk is not a common topic in data analysis, but the risk or risks related to the decisions made from data analysis are important. As the decision risk increases, the importance of every part of the data analysis increases, and every part of the study, for that matter. Lately, this topic is growing among statisticians and researchers because of the problems with predictive analysis and artificial intelligence algorithms (Angwin et al., 2016; Broussard, 2019, 2023; Buolamwini & Gebru, 2018; Dastin, 2018; King et al., 2013; O'Neil, 2016). There are risks within a research study being conducted or a new mathematical model being developed. But there are postresearch risks that deserve to be openly discussed in more detail than has historically occurred.

Bayes

Bayes, or Bayesian, analysis is philosophically and mathematically different than traditional data analyses (t-tests, ANOVA, etc.). One critical difference is the addition of prior information into the analysis. Fisher-based analyses only deal with the data from the study, that is, the data at hand. Bayesian analysis considers prior information, such as the type of distribution of the data or previous research results. A second critical difference is the concept of probability. Fisher-based statistics views a single test of significance based on a single null hypothesis and if the probability of the data given the hypothesis is true ($P(D|H)$) is small enough ($p < .05$), then the hypothesis is rejected. You can also discuss this as the probability the hypothesis is true given the evidence. But that is not what most researchers want to know. What most researchers actually want to know is what is the probability of this evidence given the null hypotheses is true and only a Bayesian statistical analysis can do that (Carver, 1978). As computational power has increased and software has been developed, Bayes analyses are integrated into more and more software programs. As a result, there are easily implementable Bayesian versions of the traditional analyses.

Data Wrangling

Data wrangling has become an increasingly important topic due to the pervasiveness of large databases, but the foundation of this topic is traditional data cleaning. Researchers need to spend most of their time just looking at the data they have and any interrelations of interest. I spend the largest amount of time in a data analysis situation just seeing what is there, and sometimes how much is not there. This wrangling is related to the outlier data example from the sampling discussion. I might look at the data from a specific variable and notice there are data that appear to be outliers on that single variable. Then, when I look at that specific variable with another variable, the scatterplot does not look like there are outliers. This now looks like evidence for multivariate normality. Therefore, these multivariate normal data may not cause a residual problem later. This typically means I will run the analysis with and without the outliers to see what changes. Data wrangling takes time and many want to rush to the analysis. It is imperative that a significant amount of time is spent examining the data.

NURSES AND STATISTICS

I realize DNP-educated nurses are not trained for applied statistics. Traditionally, in an undergraduate nursing program there is a biostatistics/foundation of statistics course and one statistics course in MSN programs. Then the DNP program typically has no applied statistics courses and a quality improvement project as the capstone. This capstone may or may not include statistical analyses. In the 2006 Essentials, research and practice focus programs are separate research/PhD programs, specifically,

> Practice-focused doctoral programs are designed to prepare experts in specialized advanced nursing practice. They focus heavily on practice that is innovative and evidence-based, reflecting the application of credible research findings.

Yet, in the document it also states in Essential III (American Association of Colleges of Nursing, 2006) on page 12,
The DNP program prepares the graduate to:

1. Use analytic methods to critically appraise existing literature and other evidence to determine and implement the best evidence for practice.
   …
5. Use information technology and research methods appropriately to:
   collect appropriate and accurate data to generate evidence for nursing practice
   inform and guide the design of databases that generate meaningful evidence for nursing practice
   analyze data from practice
   design evidence-based interventions
   predict and analyze outcomes
   examine patterns of behavior and outcomes
   identify gaps in evidence for practice

These assume more than a basic experience with statistical analysis.

In the 2021 Essentials (American Association of Colleges of Nursing, 2021), this is completely gone. Yet, there are bits and pieces that imply this type of knowledge and skill sets are still expected. Domain 4: Scholarship for the Nursing Discipline descriptor states,

> The generation, synthesis, translation, application, and dissemination, of nursing knowledge to improve health care. Generation implies research and research implies analyses.

Further in the domain discussion, the document states,

> Scholarship is inclusive of discovery, application, integration, and teaching. While not all inclusive, the scholarship of discovery includes primary empirical research, analysis of large data sets, theory development, and methodological studies. The scholarship of practice interprets, draws together, applies, and brings new insight to original research.

Domain 8 also discusses nursing informatics and gathering data for making decisions. The data, whether large data sets or not, have to be analyzed. To fully implement these domains, DNP-educated nurses need to be exposed to more statistical analyses. I am not requesting everyone do this, but as a group who needs to know this, some will need to move into this role just to sustain the amount of designs, data collection, and analyses that are required. Many of the doctor of nursing practice programs in the country do not have enough courses or experiences that can create applied statisticians within the field. I have this same concern with PhD programs also—but that is not the focus here.

The idea of just "hiring a statistician" was never a viable business model and the scarcity of applied statisticians is going to get worse. Those who have data experience, computer programming experience, database knowledge, and any experience with large data sets are not going to rush into academe given the salaries and benefits (e.g., work from home—or anywhere in the world) that are available in other employment areas. Additionally, as a DNP you have the content area expertise that always makes understanding the data more efficient.

At some point, you have to create your own.

CONCLUDING THOUGHTS

Every field changes and the roles and responsibilities in that field change. At this juncture, the great attrition or great resignation has been affecting higher education (Hawes & Reynolds, 2022). Inside Higher Education's 2022 Survey of College and University Chief Academic Officers, 19% of provosts stated that faculty members are leaving at significantly higher rates than in the past. Sixty percent indicated that they are leaving at somewhat higher rates (Flaherty, 2022). In my own peer group of researchers who I am in contact with a great deal, 80% have looked for a job outside academe or have left within the past 2 years. A common phrase is, "I am done with the constant pressure and poor environment." The comments about pay aren't even a topic because the pay is so poor that it no longer warrants discussion. Specifically, for nursing, those with more training in applied statistics, that is, those with a PhD, are not a large group; there is already a current shortage of PhD-educated nurses, and again most of those do not end up in a research-focused institution.

I have tried to outline a few key areas that applied statisticians need to understand. Anyone can learn this information, but a dedicated focus to learning is necessary. There are so many free online resources; it is astounding. There are free statistical software programs such as JAMOVI (which has a free online book) or JASP—which also has a free online book. There are videos and tutorials also. There is the Khan Academy where the core aspects of data analysis can be learned. Even used statistics books at used book stores or online are an inexpensive way to get started. At the end of the references, I have left a few links for those who want to get started.

CASE STUDY

The director of professional practice, a DNP-prepared nurse, working within a large hospital system was approached by the chief nursing officer concerning the increase in turn-over rate during the past year. Recently, the director of professional practice was also approached by unit leaders concerning the number of medical errors, staff shortages, and behaviors that look like burnout.

Some beginning questions to get you thinking?

- What data may be available within the hospital system?
- Is it all administrative? Is it all in one database or many?
- How old is the data? How far back can you go?
- How are the error reports and shortages kept? Are they daily, weekly, monthly, quarterly?
- What type of data is it (e.g., nominal)?
- What are potential issues or concerns with the data that is available?
- What data may need to be collected?
- What are potential concerns or issues with data that will need to be collected?
- Are there related data that are accessible, such as a monthly wellness check in?
- If so, do you think people are answering honestly, or do you think the data is biased?
- Who will be in charge of this study? Will they get cooperation if there are multiple gatekeepers on the data?

CRITICAL THINKING QUESTIONS

1. Why should researchers focus on error instead of p-values?
2. Why should researchers design for accuracy and not power?
3. When should a researcher consider hiring a statistician versus learning how to run the analysis themself?
4. Why are repeated studies more important than p-values? How is this related to the concepts of reliability and validity?
5. Why are instruments never valid or reliable?
6. What is the critical reason correlations between continuous variables must be graphically displayed in addition to the calculation of the value?
7. Why is the replication crisis not really a crisis?
8. How does the context of the data collection matter for analysis? How is this related to the difference between research and administrative data?
9. How is data quality (e.g., accuracy, bias) related to the concept of validity?
10. How are replication and accuracy related to the level of risk of the results of a study?

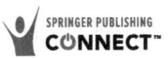

A robust set of instructor resources designed to supplement this text is located at http://connect.springerpub.com/content/book/978-0-8261-8137-4. Qualifying instructors may request access by emailing textbook@springerpub.com.

REFERENCES

Alexander, M. (2018, November 8). *The newest Jim Crow*, N.Y. TIMES, https://www.nytimes.com/2018/11/08/opinion/Sunday/criminal-justice-reforms-race-technology.html

American Association of Colleges of Nursing. (2006, October). *The essentials of Doctoral Education for Advanced Nursing Practice essentials*. https://www.aacnnursing.org/Portals/42/Publications/DNPEssentials.pdf

American Association of Colleges of Nursing. (2021, April 6). *The essentials: Core competencies for professional nursing education.* https://www.aacnnursing.org/Portals/42/AcademicNursingn/pdf/Essentials-2021.pdf

The American Statistician. (2019). Special Issue on *p*-values: Statistical inference in the 21st century: A world beyond $p < 0.05$. Volume 73, Sup1. https://www.tandfonline.com/toc/utas20/73/sup1

Angwin, J., Larson, J., Mattu, S., & Kirchner, L. (2016, May 23). *Machine bias*, PROPUBLICA, https://www.propublica.org/article/machine-bias-risk-assessments-in-criminal-sentencing.

Berg, S. (2019, June 13). *4 big ways BP measurement goes wrong, and how to tackle them.* https://www.ama-assn.org/delivering-care/hypertension/4-big-ways-bp-measurement-goes-wrong-and-how-tackle-them

Bond, T. G., & Fox, C. M. (2015). *Applying the Rasch Model: Fundamental measurement in the human sciences,* (3rd ed.). Routledge. https://doi.org/10.4324/9781315814698

Broussard, M. (2019). *Artificial unintelligence: How computers misunderstand the world.* MIT Press.

Broussard, M. (2023). *More than a glitch: Confronting race, gender, and ability bias in tech.* MIT Press.

Buolamwini, J., & Gebru, T. (2018). Gender shades: Intersectional accuracy disparities in commercial gender classification. *Conference on fairness, accountability and transparency* (pp. 77–91). PMLR.

Bureau of Labor Statistics. (2022, October 10). *Occupational outlook handbook: Mathematicians and statisticians.* https://www.bls.gov/ooh/math/mathematicians-and-statisticians.htm

Carver, R. (1978). The case against statistical significance testing. *Harvard Educational Review, 48*(3), 378–399. https://doi.org/10.17763/haer.48.3.t490261645281841

Dastin, J. (2018, October 10). Reuters, *Amazon scraps secret AI recruiting tool that didn't like women.* https://www.reuters.com/article/us-amazon-com-jobs-automation-insight/amazon-scraps-secret-ai-recruiting-tool-that-showed-bias-against-women-idUSKCN1MK08G

D'ignazio, C., & Klein, L. F. (2020). *Data feminism.* MIT press.

Dickison, P., Luo, X., Kim, D., Woo, A., Muntean, W., & Bergstrom, B. (2016). Assessing higher-order cognitive constructs by using an information-processing framework. *Journal of Applied Testing Technology, 17*(1), 1–19.

Flaherty, C. (2022, July 5). *Calling it quits.* https://www.insidehighered.com/news/2022/07/05/professors-are-leaving-academe-during-great-resignation

Hawes, C., & Reynolds, S. (2022, August 01). Radical retention: How higher education can rise to the challenges of the great resignation and beyond. *National Association of College and Employers.* https://www.naceweb.org/career-development/best-practices/radical-retention-how-higher-education-can-rise-to-the-challenges-of-the-great-resignation-and-beyond

Hudson, R. (2021). Explicating exact versus conceptual replication. *Erkenn, 88,* 2493–2514. https://doi.org/10.1007/s10670-021-00464-z

Kha Breznau, N., Rinke, E. M., Wuttke, A., Nguyen, H. H. V., Adem, M., Adriaans, J., Alvarez-Benjumea, A., Andersen, H. K., Auer, D., Azevedo, F., Bahnsen, O., Bazler, D., Bauer, G., Bauer, P. C., Baumann, M., Baute, S., Benoit, V., Bernauer, J., Berning, C., ... Żółtak, T. (2021, March 24). Observing many researchers using the same data and hypothesis reveals a hidden universe of uncertainty. *Proceedings of the National Academy of Sciences, 119*(44), e2203150119. https://doi.org/10.1073/pnas.2203150119

King, J. D., Buolamwini, J., Cromwell, E. A., Panfel, A., Teferi, T., Zerihun, M., Melak, B., Watson, J., Tadesse, Z., Vienneau, D., Ngondi, J., Utzinger, J., Odermatt, P., & Emerson, P. M. (2013). A novel electronic data collection system for large-scale surveys of neglected tropical diseases. *PloS one, 8*(9), e74570. https://doi.org/10.1371/journal.pone.0074570

Matrixx Initiatives, Inc. v. Siracusano, 563 U.S. (2011). https://www.supremecourt.gov/opinions/boundvolumes/563BV.pdf

Mazzali, C., & Duca, P. (2015). Use of administrative data in healthcare research. *Internal Emergency Medicne, 10,* 517–524. https://doi.org/10.1007/s11739-015-1213-9

Muller, J. Z. (2019). *The tyranny of metrics.* Princeton University Press.

Oermann, M. H., & Kardong-Edgren, S. (2018). Changing the conversation about doctoral education in nursing: Research in nursing education. *Nursing Outlook, 66*(6), 523–525. https://doi.org/10.1016/j.outlook.2018.10.001

O'Neil, C. (2016). *Weapons of math destruction.* PUBCCC

Pearson, E. S. (1939). "Student" as statistician. *Biometrika, 30*(3/4), 210–250.

Peirce, C. S. (1931–1958). *Collected papers of Charles Sanders Peirce.* C. Hartshorne & P. Weiss (Eds.), Harvard University Press.

Peterson, S. E., & Schreiber, J. B. (2012). Personal and interpersonal motivation for group projects: Replications of an attributional analysis. *Educational Psychology Review, 24*(2), 287–311.

Project Implicit. (2020, January 22). *About us*. https://implicit.harvard.edu/implicit/aboutus.html

Rosenbaum, E. (2018, May 30). *Silicon Valley is stumped: AI cannot always remove bias from hiring*. CNBC. https://www.cnbc.com/2018/05/30/silicon-valley-is-stumped-even-a-i-cannot-remove-bias-from-hiring.html (quoting Meredith Whittaker, co-founder of the AI Now Institute at New York University and founder of Google's Open Research group).

Saunders, L. (1954). The changing role of nurses. *The American Journal of Nursing*, 1094–1098.

Schreiber, J. B. (2020). New paradigms for considering statistical significance: A way forward for health services research journals, their authors, and their readership. *Research in Social and Administrative Pharmacy, 16*(4), 591–594. https://doi.org/10.1016/j.sapharm.2019.05.023

Schreiber, J. B. (in press). *Analyses for health and social sciences*. DEStech Publishing

Schreiber, J. B., & Asner-Self, K. (2010). *Educational research*. Wiley and Sons.

Schreiber, J. B., & Turk, M. (2022). *Statistics and data analysis for nurses*. Springer Publishing Company.

Stamp, J. (1929). *Some economic factors in modern life*. PS King and Sons.

Stevens, S. S. (1946). On the theory of scales of measurement. *Science, 103*(2684), 677–680.

Sund-Levander, M., Grodzinsky, E., Loyd, D., & Wahren, L. K. (2004). Errors in body temperature assessment related to individual variation, measuring technique and equipment. *International Journal of Nursing Practice, 10*(5), 216–23. http://doi.org/10.1111/j.1440-172X.2004.00483.x. PMID: 15461691

Trafimow, D., & MacDonald, J. A. (2017). Performing inferential statistics prior to data collection. *Educational and Psychological Measurement, 77*(2), 204–219.

Wasserstein, R. L., Schirm, A. L., & Lazar, N. A. (2019). Moving to a world beyond "$p < 0.05$". *The American Statistician, 73*(sup1), 1–19.

Wright, B. D. (1999). Fundamental measurement for psychology. In S. E. Embretson & S. L. Hershberger (Eds.), *The new rules of measurement: What every psychologist and educator should know* (pp. 65–104). Lawrence Erlbaum Associates Publishers.

Ziliak, S., & McCloskey, D. N. (2008). *The cult of statistical significance: How the standard error costs us jobs, justice, and lives*. University of Michigan Press.

Zuberi, T., & Bonilla-Silva, E. (Eds.). (2008). *White logic, white methods: Racism and methodology*. Rowman & Littlefield Publishers.

JAMOVI FREE WARE

https://www.jamovi.org
Jamovi Books
https://www.learnstatswithjamovi.com
https://vorpress.com/health/index.htm
Videos
Jamovi https://datalab.cc/jamovi/
SPSS
https://datalab.cc/spss/
JASP Freeware
https://jasp-stats.org
JASP books
https://vorpress.com/health/index.htm
https://jasp-stats.org/jasp-materials/

CHAPTER ELEVEN Reflective Response

MARIA GILSON DEVALPINE AND MATTHEW A. JONES

Chapter 11 gives a primer on statistical tools, issues, and recommendations for the DNP-prepared nurse. Schreiber also proffers an interesting argument for preparing DNP students to serve in roles as applied statisticians. However, as Schreiber also points out, DNP programs rarely have applied statistics courses, and many nurses' last exposure to statistics was in their undergraduate or remote master's education. This begs the question that if we think nurses should be acting in some capacity to use statistics, shouldn't they receive more formal, applied training in this area? Schreiber points to a myriad of open-source resources (the amount of free quality education *is* outstanding), but there are also many resources out there that are not high quality and, in some cases, give incorrect information. How does one with little to no training in basic statistics evaluate the quality of the resources they consume, evoking the old adage: *you don't know what you don't know*. Schreiber's review of the *p*-value and its misunderstanding is a prime example of how a little more formal training could go a long way.

The *p*-value is a subject we (authors) have specifically focused on in discussing the use of statistics with nursing students and educators. We regularly hear from DNP students that they just need a *p*-value in their capstone project, often to satisfy their committee. The presence of a *p*-value may incorrectly infer statistical rigor; in many cases sample sizes for DNP projects are so small that they are statistically underpowered. The interpretation of the *p*-value might not be the most appropriate approach in this situation (Jones & deValpine, 2018). There are many limitations and abuses regarding the *p*-value that are thoroughly covered elsewhere and as Schreiber notes, this value should not be used for decision making in the way it has been. Reinforcing Schreiber's point about basic statistical education, we still see definitions of the *p*-value in nursing articles that seem to be at odds with the American Statistical Association's clarification and definition. Moreover, with very small sample sizes, the use of *p*-values might not make sense.

Sample sizes for DNP projects are typically small (Kuerban, 2018) and as Schreiber points out, often focus on quality improvement projects. Thus, attention to effect sizes would be beneficial for DNP student projects. We do agree with Schreiber that missing effect sizes are a problem: they receive little to no attention in DNP literature, programs, and projects. And, in our consultations across the United States, we find DNP students are often surprised to hear about effect sizes at all. Fortunately, they are equally surprised to hear how easy they can be calculated, especially with the availability of free, online calculators.

We agree with Schreiber's premise that DNP students need more or better exposure to statistics, not only for their projects, but more important, in practice. The timeline of the degree is one of the biggest constraints for incorporating more exposure to statistics and we recognize that preparing DNP students to be "applied statisticians" is a tall order. Schreiber points out that the 2021 version of the DNP Essentials notes the generation of knowledge, which inherently implies research and analysis. We would even go one step further beyond implying, rather, suggesting that the generation of knowledge cannot take place without proper research, which of course means that analysis needs to take place, and that DNP students need to understand the results of this (their) analysis. When the DNP Essentials speak of *discovery*, therefore, research, analysis, and an understanding of analysis needs to take place. All of which means DNPs *are* necessarily applied statisticians, at least for the duration of their programs, and that more (or better) exposure to statistics in DNP programs is required. To translate and apply nursing knowledge, as the DNP Essentials expect, graduates need to be not only critical consumers of research, but *generators* and *discoverers* of knowledge. To evaluate research for application, nurses need to understand the strengths and weaknesses of research and statistical pitfalls AND be able to apply or avoid them in their own projects and eventual practice (Jones et al., 2021).

The market has been an increasingly utilized mechanism to address the statistical issues in DNP projects. Yet, as Schreiber suggests, "hiring a statistician" is not viable. Not only is there a limit in the marketplace, but there is a limit of those qualified to dispense advice. In a gig market economy, anyone can hang out a statistician for hire sign. For DNP students pressed for time completing projects, they might understandably gravitate toward the cheapest and quickest source advertising statistical consulting services. Additionally, it is not realistic to assume that if we want DNP graduates in practice to engage in *synthesis, translation, application, and dissemination* of nursing knowledge to improve healthcare (further requirements from the Essentials) they will continue to hire a statistician after graduation. Those working in larger systems might have some access to professional, dedicated research staff (i.e., research associates, biostatisticians, epidemiologist, etc.), but this would be a rare occurrence for DNPs working in smaller, less formal settings.

Given the credit and time limitations of these now well-established programs, we have advocated just-in-time statistics to ensure students' exposure, however limited (Jones et al., 2021). In reality, however, nursing faculty are not prepared to be statistical generalists, ready to teach any method that is needed for a particular DNP project. This leaves the student only able to use the methods that are available among the faculty's expertise, rather than those best suited to their question or population. Branching out into sister math and statistics departments has been limiting because of communication barriers between the professions and the time burden that these consultations impose. Our best approach to increasing exposure to statistics for students had been to use a paid consulting methodologist (author) who advised students, not only which statistics to best apply, but also fostered more robust and accurate conceptual formulation of projects in a cohesive approach. Unfortunately, this, our best solution, suffered budget reductions and our consulting methodologist was replaced with a statistical applications package, leaving the connection between conceptualization and methods abandoned. Students need to understand the whole knowledge generation process, not just the selection of statistical tools. With current credit, time, and budget limitations, the role of DNPs as applied statisticians is unlikely to develop from DNP education alone. If we want DNP-prepared nurses to utilize statistics more in their DNP projects and practice, then dedicated methodologists, whether part or full time, need to exist for these programs. Whatever the format of inquiry for the DNP project (there are many), if the statistical techniques and analyses used are improper or weak, their work product will be unpublishable.

REFERENCES

Kuerban, A. (2018). Statistic methods used in scholarly projects of doctor of nursing practice graduates. *International Journal Nursing and Clinical Practices.* 5(276), 2. https://doi.org/10.15344/2394-4978/2018/276.

Jones, M., & deValpine, M. (2018). A gentle reminder about *P*-values: What are we actually teaching? *Nurse Education Today*, 62, 134–136. https://doi.org/10.1016/j.nedt.2018.01.001

Jones, M., McDonald, M., Schubert, C., & deValpine, M. (2021). Use of statistical tests in doctor of nursing practice projects. *The Journal for Nurse Practitioners, 17*(9), 1118–1121. https://doi.org/10.1016/J.NURPRA.2021.06.006

CHAPTER TWELVE

The Role of the DNP in Addressing Health Equity

DENISE LUCAS, SR., MARY MEYERS, AND JANET BISCHOFF

INTRODUCTION

This chapter encompasses the role of the doctorallyprepared advance practice registered nurse (APRN) and the key responsibilities they have in addressing health equity in the United States. The education of these APRNs prepares them to be leaders at the highest level of nursing practice with the goal of improving patient outcomes and utilization of current research in all practice settings. This initiative is led by the American Association of Colleges of Nursing (AACN) and their 2021 *The Essentials: Core Competencies for Professional Nursing Education* (AACN, 2021b). The National Task Force (NTF) *Standards for Quality Nurse Practitioner* (NP) *Education* (NTF, 2022) plays an important part in the doctor of nursing practice (DNP) role by providing congruent standards for all NP programs, no matter the population foci. There are multiple definitions and components of health equity in the literature. The Centers for Disease Control and Prevention (CDC, 2022a) states health equity is achieved when individuals are afforded the opportunity to reach their full health potential. The AACN uses the thoughts from Kranich (2001) to broadly define health equity, meaning the ability to recognize differences in resources or education that allow an individual to fully participate in society and overcome obstacles, ensuring fairness (AACN, 2021b) The social determinants of health (SDOH) are clearly interrelated with health equity, and inequity exists when there is an uneven distribution of education, housing, transportation access, employment opportunities, healthcare, or public health systems (Community Guide, 2022). SDOH are "conditions in the places where people live, learn, work, and play that affect a wide range of health risks and outcomes" (CDC, 2021a, para 1). The determinants are grouped into five domains and include:

- Economic stability—employment, food insecurity, housing instability, poverty
- Education—early childhood development, enrollment in higher education, highschool graduation, language, and literacy
- Health and health care—access to health services, access to primary care, health literacy

- Neighborhood and built environments—access to food that supports health, crime and violence, environmental conditions, quality housing
- Social and community context—civic participation, discrimination, incarceration, social cohesion (CDC, 2021a)

When barriers are identified that create inequity, the system should develop practices that overcome them. Inequities are "reflected in differences in length of life, quality of life, rates of disease, disability, death, and access to treatment" (CDC, 2022a, para 2). To ensure equitable systems, all individuals should be treated fairly, unhampered by artificial barriers, stereotypes, or prejudices (Cooper, 2016). As the DNP role expands into practice settings and direct patient care, the benefits of the advanced practice knowledge and skills possessed by DNP-prepared NPs make them essential stakeholders in conversations concerning inequities. These practitioners are infused with knowledge and actions that design, integrate, role model, and evaluate how NP can further health equity in their practice and profession (AACN, 2021b).

The Future of Nursing 2030 report (National Academies of Sciences, Engineering, and Medicine, 2021) and the NTF (2022) state that nurses will play a critical role in the pathway to advancing and achieving health equity by addressing the SDOH. These standards exist to ensure ongoing DNP program quality and include an overarching framework addressing mission and governance, resources, curriculum, and evaluation. Established criteria such as these, with support from 17 key national nursing organizations, solidifies the quality and consistency of DNP education, leading to curricula that are based on known evidence and wellunderstood by others. The magnitude and consistency of this work supports addressing and lifting any barriers or restrictions that limit advanced practice nurses to practice at their highest level of education, which includes the DNP-educated nurse. The demand for doctorallyprepared nurses will only increase in the decades ahead, as will the multifaceted needs of patients with chronic health conditions. This clearly demands that the DNP must navigate complexities in all phases of the workforce, while also reducing inequities.

The United States outspends other wealthy nations in healthcare yet continues to have paltry and last-place rankings in several measures, such as access to care, overall health outcomes, and health equity (Kuehn, 2021). The Affordable Care Act remains controversial and while a start to address inequities it does not address all individuals who are vulnerable, and many Americans remain uninsured or underinsured. As a key player in promoting equity the DNP-prepared nurse has an important role in identifying and addressing deficiencies, especially surrounding the concept of health equity. The DNP nurse can be an integral part of designing and implementing policies and interventions that lead to both systems and individuals with improved outcomes. A well-established framework for this exists with the Healthy People 2030 SDOH (U.S. Department of Health and Human Services [U.S. DHHS], 2022a). As mentioned above, the SDOH are not concrete medical concepts, rather a constellation of factors recognizing other social factors that are key in a person's life and the contributions or detriments the factor provides in relation to that person's health (Braveman, 2022). Some determinants are specific to care, such as healthcare access and quality, and others more abstract, such as education, neighborhoods, community, and economic stability. The aim of these determinants is to promote an environment where social and physical factors may lead to better health (National Center for Health Statistics, 2016).

Since the beginning of the Healthy People initiative in 1980 the focus on health equity as an SDOH has advanced through the years. The 1990 decade was focused on reduction of deaths, and the iteration in 2000 began to mention a reduction in health disparities, and in 2010 moved from reduction of disparities to their elimination. The initiative in 2020 identified the need to achieve equity and in 2030 calls for health equity as the highest level of health for all people (U.S.DHHS, 2022b). This chapter focuses on the SDOH and the role the DNP APRN has in promoting health equity. A clear description of the determinant and how it may be embraced follows, along with a threaded case presentation depicting the role a DNP-prepared nurse implemented in a patient scenario.

SOCIAL DETERMINANTS OF HEALTH

SDOH are used to describe the nonclinical factors that do not include medical care yet have an impact on an individual's health. Although the United States spends more on medical care than other industrialized nations, it ranks near the bottom on key measures of health (infant mortality, life expectancy). This brings to the forefront how factors such as where individuals are born, grow, live, worship, and work intersect with health (World Health Organization [WHO], 2021). Medical care does influence health, but it is not the only influence. SDOH key issues such as poverty, housing, literacy, graduation rates, crime, environmental conditions, incarceration, and civic participation can have a profound effect on both the incidence and prevalence of morbidity and mortality, as well as quality of life (CDC, 2021a). During the last two decades, there has been much research on these social factors and their effect on health outcomes. It is reported that SDOH can have as much as a 50% effect on health outcomes and these conditions can become risk factors that affect an individual's wellness and longevity (Whitman et al., 2022).

An initial step toward identifying and addressing SDOH involves screening of individuals by health providers and health systems. There are various ways to screen for SDOH that could be included in health histories. Some of the screening tools available for utilization include the Protocol for Responding To and Assessing Patient Assets, Risks, and Experiences (PRAPARE), the Social Needs Screening Tool (American Academy of Family Physicians [AAFP], 2019), or the Accountable Health Communities Health Related Social Needs Screen Tool from the CDC (Lathrop, 2020). Each of the five domains of the SDOH are described and applied to the DNP APRN role in reducing health inequities.

Education

Health and educational outcomes for individuals can be closely linked to each other. People with less education live shorter and less healthy lives compared to people with higher education. Inequalities in health and education are linked as education can provide opportunities for individuals to earn higher incomes, which in turn give them social and psychological benefits, encourage healthier lifestyles, and provide them access to good healthcare. Individuals with higher levels of education tend to live longer and are heathier. On the other side, poor health can put educational attainment at risk—a process that affects people from early childhood throughout their lives (U.S.DHHS, 2021). Education is primarily funded at the local level in the United States, which is based on the community's tax base. This creates disparity as those communities with higher local property tax have better school funding and access to more fiscal resources for education (Ahluwalia, 2021). Both high school graduation and/or college education can improve health and well-being. The home environment, quality of schools, size of schools/classrooms, availability of student loans, and family support can impact the potential to improve population health. By promoting and supporting education from pre-kindergarten to post-high-school programs, education has a positive impact on employment options, job retention, and higher social status (U.S.DHHS, 2021).

In support of the above information, the Rural Health Information Hub (2020a) declares increased education as the SDOH that is most modifiable leading to healthier behaviors and better overall outcomes. Adults tend to have greater economic growth with more education. The Rural Health Information Hub describes five levels of education:

- Early childhood is foundational in building social and emotional skills.
- High school completion programs improve the likelihood students graduate or receive their general educational diploma.
- Out-of-school-time academic programs help improve focused academic achievement areas such as science and math.
- Community schools allow schools to serve as community hubs to support students and families with a variety of services.
- College access programs expand educational offerings for students who are low-income or from minority communities to prepare them to apply to and enter college (Rural Health Information Hub, 2020b).

Forward-thinking communities need to recognize and take measures to consider educational needs across the life span from very early childhood to adulthood. Programs such as Head Start, after-school programs, vocational and community colleges promote a healthier community, safer neighborhoods, and most likely a higher tax base that supports schools. Lastly, we are seeing from the global pandemic the impact of school closures, remote learning, and social isolation on students overall as they return to school with behavioral and learning barriers and poor performance metrics on standardized testing (Lancet Public Health, 2020), with many communities showing very concerning standardized test scores (Kuhfeld et al., 2022).

A gap exists with individuals that have limited English language skills and are more likely to show lower literacy rates. Literacy overall can include listening, speaking, writing, reading, and numeracy. Health literacy is the ability to use and understand health-related information. This inability to understand and use English creates a barrier to accessing healthcare, medications, preventative care, and understanding basic health information. This communication barrier extends to the ability of the provider to understand the patient, as well as of the patient to understand the provider (U.S.DHHS, 2021). Nurses have traditionally asked education questions on patient histories to determine the last level of school completed and whether the patient can read and write, but the issue of health literacy goes beyond a grade completed in school. The doctorally-prepared NP must incorporate this expansion of language in literacy in their interactions with patients and families. As cultural diversity increases in APRNs, addressing literacy in their communities becomes embraceable as the patient/provider cultural connection improves.

Economic Stability

Economic stability, or financial health, is a multifaceted concept. It encompasses the ability to manage expenses, handle unexpected financial stress, have minimal debt, and save for the future (Weida et al., 2020). The phenomenon of poverty having a deleterious effect on health outcomes has been documented as far back as 1817. Rene Villermé reported clear differences in health outcomes between the rich and poor neighborhoods of Paris (Boozary & Shojania, 2018), reflecting some of the earliest work on SDOH. As

Boozary and Shojania (2018) point out, 200 years later, despite many advances in healthcare, the economic inequity people experience still exerts significant influence on health outcomes.

For many Americans, particularly after the COVID-19 global pandemic, an already fragile economic environment has given way to increasing poverty. In every aspect of life poverty affects the experience of overall health and access to care. Persons who are poor suffer anxiety and distress leading to depression and may form harmful coping mechanisms such as substance abuse, smoking, and other risky behaviors (Price et al., 2018).

Economic instability is often a multigenerational problem for many people. Children born into poverty do not have access to nutritious food, high-performing schools, and safe housing (Green et al., 2021). According to the U.S. Census Bureau the official poverty rate in the United States was 13%, with 40 million people in poverty. Of the total number of people living in poverty, 5% of the total were children (Shrider et al., 2021). When children start their lives in poverty, there is a huge economic cost to the United States. Parenting styles are adversely affected by economic instability. In poverty there is less time to spend with children as parents struggle to survive, and their children are at a much higher risk for chronic conditions like asthma and obesity (Walker, 2021). The stress of poverty on mothers and children was examined in 2021 in a small study measuring cortisol levels in children living in poverty. Toddlers were found to have elevated cortisol levels because of the stress of their mothers, coping with holding together their daily lives in a patchwork approach, juggling costs of rent, food, childcare, clothing, and other daily obligations (Bates et al., 2021). Economic instability becomes a stumbling block right at the beginning of a child's life, affecting their health and their ability to thrive and experience a level playing field with other children who suffer fewer inequities.

In the United States, access to healthcare is usually determined by the ability to make a living, with employer-sponsored insurance being the largest source of coverage for individuals and families. For those between the ages of 18 and 65, insurance is attained by one's ability to find full-time employment with benefits as part of the employment package, and approximately 156 million people (Kaiser Family Foundation, 2019) receive health care in this fashion. However, there remains a large gap in coverage due to rising premiums and small businesses that are not mandated to offer work-related healthcare coverage. The loss of a job has a devastating effect on an individual and family and results in the loss of insurance covering provider visits, medications, and hospitalizations. While the COVID-19 pandemic has certainly stressed health insurance access, even in normal times any change in household structure or employment creates health insurance transitions, which can include transitioning to uninsured status, underinsured status, or from commercial insurance to no insurance or Medicaid, which can create health and financial security risks (Bivens & Zipperer, 2020).

The impact of SDOH is illustrated well with the story of Marge S., age 62, who came to a free health center in her community after 5 years without health insurance or healthcare. Marge and her husband married shortly after graduating from high school and purchased a two-bedroom home in a quiet neighborhood and were still living in that home. Marge's spouse was unexpectedly disabled and unable to work, which resulted in the loss of insurance benefits for his family. Marge had been employed full time early in her marriage but when her son was born 30 years earlier, she became a stay-at-home mom. Her son is married and works as an accountant at a small firm in a neighboring town, where he lives with his wife and young daughter. The loss of the sole source of income combined with loss of health insurance and financial stability placed severe economic stress on Marge's family. Marge's husband's disability enabled him to receive Social Security Disability Insurance; however, since Marge was only 62 years old she was not yet eligible for Medicare, and could no longer afford her medications or provider visits for her chronic hypertension and cardiac problems. Because Marge had been dealing with chronic problems, she was not well enough to hold a job. However, until the economic instability caused by her husband's disability, she was able to manage well and see the healthcare providers necessary for her conditions. Adequate health insurance had made the bills manageable. Now with the sudden financial stress, they were barely able to manage on their drastically reduced income. Once her medication refills expired, she could no longer afford any of the numerous prescription medications that she required, nor could she afford to pay out-of-pocket for provider visits.

Marge's story is illustrative of what happens when there is a sudden loss of income combined with dual health problems for individuals and families. The American Academy of Physicians has long advocated for universal healthcare as a right for all people (Butkus et al., 2020). In a position paper written in 2018, the World Health Organization (Kuehnert et al., 2022) defined health as a complete state of mental and social well-being and not just the absence of disease. In their *Call to Action*, Butkus et al. (2020) recommend a health system that ameliorates all social factors that contribute to poverty and inequitable health.

Extreme poverty has a profound impact on life expectancy. According to Price et al. (2018) there is a 15-year life expectancy difference for men and 10 years for women between the top and bottom 1% of income distribution in the United States Adding an exclamation point to this statistic this difference in life expectancy is equal to the damage done to a person who has been a lifetime smoker (Chokshi, 2018).

Providers are educated to prevent and treat illness. Patients are educated about "modifiable risk factors" as a way to help them take control of health behaviors. Doctorallyprepared APRNs are key drivers in examining both poverty and economic instability as modifiable risk factors (Chokshi, 2018). APRNs work with vulnerable populations and are key to changing the trajectory of health outcomes and have an opportunity to affect the patient's ability to achieve good health. Economic factors must become part of the initial assessment as much as vital signs, health behaviors, and past medical history. The components of an economic assessment are only a first step.

Further examining Marge's situation, as she moved further away from healthcare, her medical conditions deteriorated. Her blood pressure was out of control and her legs swelled to twice their size. Eventually she began to notice that the swelling in her legs was starting to weep a foul-smelling drainage. In the midst of all of this economic turmoil, COVID-19 occurred. The need for community lockdown mandates further isolated her and her family for almost 2 years, limiting her access to health and healthcare and widening the inequity gap for Marge. Poverty, a well-known detriment to health, was wreaking havoc on Marge's well-being.

Clinicians must consider poverty as a detriment to health and must pay attention to the cost of healthcare, which is bankrupting many people in the United States. Boozary and Shojania (2018) make an excellent point when they suggest that the adage of "first do no harm" be expanded to include the impact of exorbitant healthcare costs keeping people in poverty. There are some glimmers of hope in this battle. Congress reauthorized the Children's Health Insurance Program (CHIP), which addresses a root cause of lifelong health problems starting in childhood. The city of Philadelphia had a novel plan for this by instituting a tax on sugary beverages and used that money to fund children's programs, libraries, and parks (Boozary & Shojania, 2018). The American Academy of Nursing suggests that economic instability is central to most SDOH (Dunbar-Jacob et al., 2013). DNP-prepared nurses can use their skill set to address upstream social issues by working within coalitions to affect policy by lobbying, media campaigns, direct protest actions, and personal messaging to lawmakers (Kuehnert et al., 2022). DNP nurses have the ability to affect positive change in individual patients and in populations, all the while taking the lead in these changes. Healthcare in the United States has become more complex over the past decade, offering DNP-prepared nurses opportunities for leading various teams in any of these arenas.

Desperate to get help, Marge finally listened to a friend who told her about a free health center in her town and urged her to make an appointment. Finally, out of options and greatly concerned for her declining health, she called the health center. When she arrived, she was greeted by an NP who held a DNP. The DNP APRN did an initial assessment incorporating the SDOH. It quickly became apparent that the NP needed to assemble a multidisciplinary team, which included a dietician, pharmacist, licensed counselor, and patient navigator to address both her immediate and ongoing health issues. Multiple pressing health problems were addressed at her initial visit. She received dressings for her legs, lab work and an EKG, and all of her previous medications were provided. Because of the complexity of her needs and the length of time she had been without any healthcare, a one-time appointment was made for her to see the medical director of the health center, who happened to be a cardiologist. Marge was brought back to the clinic weekly for several months to monitor and address her ongoing health concerns. Every effort was made to provide Marge with the supplies she needed to address her bilateral weeping edema; supplies she would not have been able to afford at that time.

The strength of the DNP APRN lies in their commitment to safety, health promotion, and care within the community setting, all aimed at addressing inequity. Their impact is felt at the organizational, state, regional, and national levels as awareness of the DNP role advances. Through promotion of evidence-based practices via mentoring, precepting, publishing, and speaking in the community the DNP-prepared nurse achieves scholarship and advances the DNP role. APRNs who earn a DNP do not see themselves as "supplements" in the healthcare arena, but rather as leaders and innovators facilitating change. They contribute strong leadership to complex healthcare environments enabling DNPs to impact health outcomes using multiple levels of engagement (Boswell et al., 2021).

Health and Healthcare

There are many barriers to health and healthcare interfering with a person's access to needed services. These barriers can include, but are not limited to, health insurance coverage, access to primary or specialty care, diagnostic testing and evaluations, transportation limitations, and access to medications (Kullgren et al., 2012). The cumulative impact of these barriers have a significant effect on under-resourced communities. In turn, the overall detrimental effect is increased risk of poor health. This was clearly evident in Marge's story.

The DNP provider assessed Marge's physical, emotional, and social needs. She was enrolled in a study taking place at the health center that would track her progress over time and provide her with a food box once a month containing groceries appropriate for someone with hypertension. She was able to receive pill boxes to keep track of her medications and a blood pressure cuff for use at home. The DNP APRN arranged for a senior nursing student who was on a clinical rotation at the health center to teach Marge to check her blood pressure. She was offered free counseling services provided at the health center to help her cope emotionally with all that was occurring in her life. The NP noted that she had not been able to get a mammogram or gynecological exam in about four years, so Marge was referred to a local program specifically for women without insurance. The mammogram revealed that she had a suspicious lesion, leading to a diagnosis of breast cancer requiring surgery and radiation. These were medical bills that would have bankrupted Marge's family, but her NP was able to work with the insurance navigator at the health center to obtain Medicaid coverage. The addition of health insurance for Marge opened doors to other healthcare products and services, reducing many inequities that come with the barrier of no health insurance. Now she could get into the local wound clinic and receive additional supplies she needed. Once Medicaid was in place, Marge had her breast surgery and four weeks of radiation followed. She was given a clean bill of health, and for the first time in about 5 years, she felt healthy, productive, and hopeful for the future.

As shown in Marge's story, lack of insurance is one of the largest barriers to healthcare; inadequate insurance coverage can be even more common. This often leads to avoidance of care and increased out-of-pocket medical expenses, overwhelming medical debt, and unused preventative services. In 2020, following the enactment of the Affordable Care Act, the number of uninsured, nonelderly individuals declined by 20 million people and the uninsured rate fell 8%. In 2020 the uninsured rate among children remained at 6%, even with increased availability of Medicaid and CHIP. The uninsured are primarily nonelderly adults, Black, and working families with low incomes who live in the South or West. Most who are uninsured have been without insurance coverage for long periods of time (Tolbert et al., 2020).

Provider access for both primary care and specialty healthcare remains a challenge. Those individuals who do not have insurance or are underinsured are less likely to have an established primary care provider, and subsequent access to provider specialists when needed. Limited provider access due to fewer providers in nonurban or rural communities makes it harder for individuals to obtain primary care or preventative health services. Provider shortages exist at all levels of healthcare, which can include primary, dental, and mental health care providers (Health Resources and Service Administration [HRSA], 2022). And shortages are not just affecting medical providers. By 2025, the United States is estimated to have a shortage of approximately 446,000 home health aides, 95,000 nursing assistants, 99,000 medical and lab technologists and technicians, 275,000 registered nurses, and more than 29,000 NPs (Johnson, 2022). Telehealth has made improvements with both access and communication between patients and providers, but this requires technology that not all have and can afford (Healthy People 2030, 2020).

The availability of ancillary healthcare services creates even more healthcare access issues. About 50% of Americans do not have vision insurance nor can they enroll in a plan that is financially feasible. One of the biggest fears of many Americans is blindness, which is often preventable with screening and care (CDC, 2021b). Vision care, for example, primarily in the elderly, has not been adequately addressed and is often missing as part of the overall healthcare provided. Medicare does not include benefit coverage for items like routine eye exams or eyeglasses, although it does cover glaucoma testing and various eye surgeries. The elderly may also have trouble securing an eye appointment or getting transportation to the eye appointment (Spencer, 2020). Blindness and other visual impairments are included in the 10 most common causes of disability among those over the age of 65. And it's not only the elderly with vision issues: 25% of children under the age of 17 have been identified as having vision issues. Fewer than 15% of preschool children receive an eye assessment and fewer than 20% receive vision screening (American Public Health Association [APHA], 2020). Uninsured and underinsured individuals have poor access to vision services due to the high cost of out-of-pocket expenses, distance to providers, cultural barriers (language), or low levels of health literacy (Chheda et al., 2019). Addressing disparities could involve better understanding and communication of community resources, appointment times expanding to evening or weekend hours, providers accepting Medicare insurance, and better access to vision screening programs (Williams & Sahel, 2022).

Not all Americans have the same access to dental care. Many of the dental barriers are identical to other healthcare services: transportation, insurance, and cost. Poor oral health accumulates and becomes serious as individuals go through life, resulting in progressive, chronic conditions. This can affect academic performance, employment, earnings, and general overall health (Valachovic, 2018). Regular preventative dental care is essential for good oral health. The CDC (2021b) advocates for integrating oral health programs into existing chronic disease prevention care. Blacks, Hispanics, Alaskan natives, and American Indians statistically have the poorest oral health compared to other U.S. racial/ethnic groups.

Physical therapy (PT) and occupational therapy (OT) services are aimed at improving functional outcomes. SDOH can affect identification of functional issues, referral to postacute services, and access to PT/OT services. Arthritis and chronic back pain disproportionately affect individuals who are non-White, have less than a high school education, are unemployed, homeless, or those living in the inner city or rural areas (Conoc et al., 2021). There is an underrepresentation of PT/OT services in rural areas which limit appointments and treatment duration (Gkiouleka et al., 2022).

Transportation systems can play a huge role in access to healthcare, especially in the care of chronic disease, when addressing health disparities. This can involve planning that would benefit many vulnerable populations related to low-income communities, homeless populations, the disabled, the elderly, and racial/ethnic disadvantaged groups (Ingram et al., 2020). Healthcare access is more than just access to a provider or acute care services, but also includes outpatient clinic appointments and pharmacy access. Transportation interventions can include access to bus passes, taxi vouchers, transport reimbursement vouchers, and free shuttle services (Starbird et al., 2019).

One aspect of transportation that is often overlooked is simply roads and sidewalks—making sure that sidewalks are available and in good condition when the individual needs to walk to access healthcare, grocery shopping, or the pharmacy. Many areas have construction in progress and sidewalk access is limited, or the individual needs to go into the street to bypass the construction area, which can cause hazards for both the pedestrian and the motorist (Ingram et al., 2020).

Inconvenient or unreliable transportation is another barrier that is evident when considering SDOH. While access to public transportation is considered a given, many communities, especially less urban and rural communities, do not have bus, taxi, or ride-sharing options available. This lack of public transportation can impede an individual's access to healthcare due to distance and time burden (Starbird et al., 2019). Take into consideration the time spent waiting for the bus, the bus connection schedules, and available bus stop locations (seating access, awnings, structures for wind or snow breaks) that can lead to inaccessibility to the most vulnerable populations in low-income, inner-city residents, or the elderly.

For Marge, there was initially a lack of both health insurance as well as providers that would accept her as a patient. These barriers to access caused a gap in treatment of hypertension, also allowing the extreme swelling of her legs and early cellulitis to progress. Lack of insurance also limited her access to ongoing preventative care, such as mammography. The solution in this situation was her ability to access a free health center in her community that consisted of NP primary care services. The health center was also able to connect Marge with other community resources. Fortunately, Marge's home was on the public bus line and Marge has an annual bus pass provided by the health center and she is able to use this mode of transportation for most of her needs.

Access to pharmaceuticals can impede quality chronic care due to availability or pricing of medications. Healthy People 2030 advocates the need to integrate SDOH into all aspects of the pharmacy workflow, meaning comprehensive medication management. This management extends from the medications themselves to obtaining the medications, and to patient education regarding their actions and side effects (Pastakia et al., 2022). Many pharmaceutical companies do offer cost-effective subsidies to individuals that qualify according to income, which makes many medications accessible. This may favor medications that are less expensive rather than medications that deliver the greatest health gain based on medication efficacy (DiStefano & Levin, 2019). Pharmaceutical applications for patient assistance programs require one to have technology, be able to follow directions to manage the request, and to submit necessary documents, such as proof of income to be considered and qualify.

The DNP role expands the traditional nurse role in that it is not enough to identify and understand the patient's insurance status, but to encompass the concepts of caseload and reimbursement. The above discussion outlined common health disparities existing in today's healthcare arena. The DNP-educated nurse is a key member of the healthcare team that can make a difference in the care of all patients, especially those that are disadvantaged, in the same way nursing approaches care holistically. It is not enough to prescribe medications and interventions. The DNP-prepared nurse must also consider the resources the patient has access to and what treatment plan is feasible and design care within these parameters, all the while focusing on the reduction of any health inequities.

Neighborhood and Built Environment

The neighborhood one lives in can have a profound impact on health for individuals. Until recently, healthcare focused mainly on prevention and treatment of illness in individuals. However, it is coming into sharp focus that there must also be attention given to those things outside of "medical care" that impact health. Neighborhoods that are unsafe during the day are not places where children can play, or where adults can recreate (Rollston & Galea, 2020). This became intensely obvious during the recent COVID-19 pandemic. Rollston and Galea (2020) predicted there would be 60,000 deaths from COVID-19. The United States surpassed that number within years after the beginning of the pandemic. According to the latest CDC statistics, from February 2020 to October 2022, 1,061,364 people died as a direct result of COVID-19, with 90% of death certificates listing COVID-19 as the prime cause of death, and the remaining 10% listing it as a causative factor (Santiago et al., 2021). The reason for this lies in the disinvestment of the United States in the social drivers of health, such as education, early childhood intervention, housing, and public health itself (Rollston & Galea, 2020). Our focus on curative care rather than looking at conditions that cause disease cost the United States dearly during the pandemic. People in poorer neighborhoods tend to have jobs that did not allow for work from home. They had to show up or risk losing their already poverty-level income. This exposed them frequently to the COVID-19 virus during the early days of the pandemic, before there was any vaccine, medication, or adequate personal protective equipment. It became clear that the neighborhood you lived in played a huge role in whether you were infected with COVID-19 and the quality of care you received.

Nejad et al. (2021) examined the impact on health of those living in slums. Factors such as increased pollution, substandard housing, and overcrowding create an environment that is unsafe for mental, physical, and social health. Neighborhoods that lack green spaces, transportation, and accessible healthcare decrease the likelihood of living healthy lives. If there are no clinics to treat those without insurance, health problems remain unaddressed, as happened with our patient Marge. By the time she heard about the health center in her town offering free care, she had significant, immediate, and looming medical problems.

The effect of poor neighborhoods on children is well documented. It is proposed that three out of ten neurodevelopmental disorders can be linked to environmental conditions in the neighborhoods they live in, particularly for Latino and Black children (Santiago et al., 2021). In order to effect change it is important for primary care and pediatric practitioners to understand the structural and racist factors that have created inequities in housing (Green et al., 2021). Throughout the history of the United States, there have been efforts to keep people of color segregated in what is often substandard housing. Despite the civil rights movement of the 1960s, as well as the Fair Housing Act of 1968, which prohibited housing discrimination based on color, race, religion, or nationality, poor enforcement of housing laws continued due to the societal pressures of the time. In addition, there was a trend in the late 20th century by the federal government to disinvest in housing. There are four housing domains that impact child and family health: quality, stability, affordability, and the neighborhood. In regard to neighborhoods, concentrated areas of poverty lead to health disparities, as well as poor educational opportunities. Green et al. (2021) make a case for primary care and pediatric healthcare providers having a "neighborhood level lens" to begin to address this problem.

Older people are also adversely affected by unsafe and poor neighborhoods. As people age and become less mobile, it becomes more difficult to have access to healthy foods, particularly if the neighborhood does not have a grocery store, creating a food desert. Older adults begin to rely on processed foods, which are high in sodium and generally unhealthy. Often these poor neighborhoods have multiple fast-food establishments, contributing to unhealthy food choices. Unsafe neighborhoods where there is widespread crime pose another problem for vulnerable elders. Research has shown that outdoor activities in senior communities are beneficial to the mental and physical health of older individuals. Australia created models of outdoor gyms for older people. They have worked to secure spaces for seniors to use gym equipment safely with others who are exercising. This has created connections for elders they might not have had as it engages them in a healthy active lifestyle (Levinger et al., 2018).

Feeling unsafe in a neighborhood, whether one is young or old, is a constant source of tension that affects all aspects of physical and mental health. The inability to walk and exercise even during the day can lead to a sedentary lifestyle, which is proven to result in higher rates of obesity, type 2 diabetes, and metabolic syndrome. The lack of green space and blighted neighborhoods with high rates of crime caused primarily Black (91%) participants to report feelings of being unsafe, which led to higher stress, depression, and weight gain (Pearson et al., 2021).

Neighborhoods have a profound effect on the health of everyone, from prenatal life to elders. And these needs will vary from community to community. Practitioners must view this as something that should be assessed, and on a policy level DNP-prepared nurses must become activists to assist all in their care to find safety in the places they live. Using community engagement strategies, the entire healthcare team, NPs, providers, public health nurses, and community leaders must work together to achieve equitable solutions that meet the neighborhood needs.

Social and Community Context

Social barriers to healthcare, such as community violence, substandard housing, low or no monetary income can correlate with poorer health outcomes. All of these factors create stress, which has a direct effect on chronic disease and premature aging. The way social factors have a direct effect on the physical body is complex, as are physical and emotional stress, all of which the DNP-prepared nurse can address (Lathrop, 2020).

Healthy People 2030 aims to assist individuals in obtaining relevant social support in the places where they live, work, learn, and play. Building social capital by civic participation not only builds communities but produces secondary health benefits such as increased physical activity, decreased anxiety, and better nutrition. Expanding social networks through community engagement can be accomplished through working in community gardens, joining groups (book clubs, Scouts, the Red Hat Society), or simply by volunteering (food banks, hospitals, church activities, visiting shut-ins). Civic participation can also be accomplished by voting. This feeling of belonging, especially community belonging, promotes well-being and improves community life (U.S. DHHS, 2019b).

Social cohesion is another concept that includes social capital. High levels of social support positively affect health outcomes by reducing emotional stress, leading to improved cardiovascular, neuroendocrine, and immune systems. Social isolation caused by the recent pandemic has affected individuals of all ages in the past few years. With older adults, isolation can be prevalent as contact with friends and family decreases with age. Individuals that live in low-income, high-crime communities can often have lower levels of social cohesion due to the potential for harm (U.S.DHHS, 2019a).

Discrimination can negatively impact health and can occur at both the structural and individual level. Discrimination is action that is unfair or unjustified that harms individuals or groups. It can be based on race, gender, sexual identify, age, or the presence of disabilities. Structural discrimination can limit opportunities, resources, and even the well-being of those less privileged. This can be evident in housing choices, healthcare service choices, or access to educational opportunities. Individual discrimination can have both physical and emotional health costs. Individuals with lower income had subsequent decreased emergency room visits that were associated with discrimination in healthcare (Abramson et al., 2015).

Incarceration of individuals who are confined in a prison or jail for more than one year are more commonly seen among certain groups such as Black, Indigenous, and People of Color (BIPOC), creating additional disparities with health (Zucker et al., 2022). These individuals are more likely to exhibit a higher incidence of hepatitis C, HIV, and tuberculosis. Women who are incarcerated face a greater burden of disease with HIV/AIDS, HPV, and other sexually transmitted infections. Those released from incarceration have difficulties securing employment, transportation, and housing, which can pose threats to well-being, thus making healthcare a low priority. The individual's family is also affected by incarceration, especially children. They are more likely to live in poverty, witness domestic violence, witness substance abuse, or be homeless. These children also have a higher rate of learning disabilities, developmental delays, speech/language issues, attention disorders, and aggressive behaviors (Sugarman et al., 2020).

The result of adverse childhood experiences and a life growing up with identified disadvantages (poverty, malnutrition, crime, low education attainment, lack of medical care) is something the DNP APRN should be acutely aware of when evaluating the community where practice takes place. Collaboration with additional community partners such as police departments, correctional institutions, health departments and addiction services, other social services, and various child and adult protective services is key, and the DNP-prepared nurse should begin these conversations and connections. A truly unique opportunity exists in pulling these community players together in a proactive rather than punitive fashion. Communities with high incarceration rates typically have higher BIPOC living in them and pulling together to reduce disadvantages and disparities for individuals and families is a deeply caring and humbling opportunity.

DNP EDUCATION AND PREPARATION FOR THE DNP ROLE

The latest educational revisions in graduate nursing education have occurred in tandem. The AACN released *The Essentials: Core Competencies for Professional Nursing Education* in

2021 with the idea of transforming nursing education to meet future needs in healthcare (AACN, 2021a), while providing more consistency in graduate program outcomes. With this comes a competency-based education approach where "... students demonstrate that they have learned the knowledge, attitudes, motivations, self-perceptions, and skills expected of them as they progress through their education" (AACN, n.d., para 1). The *Essentials* (AACN, 2021a) driving nursing education now consist of 10 domains with competencies written at two levels to include those at the entry level of nursing education and for those seeking an advanced nursing degree. The competencies "mature" as the student advances their education. The National Organization of Nurse Practitioner Faculties (NONPF, 2018) has called for all APRNs to earn a DNP by the year 2025. The NONPF position of committing to have all entry-level NP education at the DNP level by 2025 promotes the inclusion of health equity concepts in all phases of the NP providing healthcare. One of the key roles of the DNP is to help ensure the fair distribution of available resources regardless of age, gender, race, ethnicity, or socioeconomic status.

In 2021 the fifth iteration of the NTF criteria was published and reviewed by stakeholders in NP education. In 2022 the final version was released for adoption after two years of exploration and development. The document presents four standards all NP programs must recognize, no matter the population focus of the program:

- Standard I: Institutional mission/philosophy/values and governance necessary to advance NP program excellence
- Standard II: Fiscal, human, student support, and physical resources required for a quality NP program
- Standard III: Curriculum necessary to prepare students for the nurse practitioner role, including meeting national standards and outlining the depth and breadth of requisite knowledge and skills for student success
- Standard IV: Systematic evaluation process for ongoing quality improvement through assessment of program outcomes, resources, curriculum, faculty, and students (NTF, 2022)

What does this mean for the education of doctorallyprepared NP students? First, the NTF, AACN, and NONPF language and aims align, specifically around formal program accreditation language. The NTF criteria closely aligns with the AACN's evaluative arm, the Commission on Collegiate Nursing Education, and the standards used for accreditation of nursing programs and health equity are specifically noted. Second, many NP programs across the country will now move to a competency-based format and planned experiences or simulation opportunities working with underserved individuals may be included. While competency-based education is a common occurrence in some healthcare disciplines, such as medicine, it is a change for many in nursing. Third, the number of clinical hours required for students has increased from a minimum of 500 hours to 750 hours, allowing planned experiences with direct patient care and with DNP scholarly projects that focus on health equity and how the DNP may take a leadership role in improving this for patients. Last, the opportunity for NP students educated at the doctoral level presents itself full center in many ways. In the new *Essentials* three domains support students as they begin their work addressing health equity issues.

- Domain 2: Person-Centered Care focuses on supporting an individual in multiple complex ways while providing holistic, individualized, and respectful care
- Domain 3: Population Health examines the delivery of care across the continuum and speaks specifically to equitable population health outcomes

- Domain 6: Interprofessional Partnerships teaches the DNP student about collaborative experiences that intentionally enhance healthcare and improve health equity (AACN, 2021a).

The current revisions in graduate nursing education provide educational underpinnings that put the DNP-prepared advanced-practice nurse in a position to take the lead in healthcare in both focused and larger settings. DNP programs prepare their graduates to expertly appraise research findings and the literature. They are able to identify, modify, and plan opportunities that will promote success while reducing inequity in their organization or community. Programs have the opportunity to address SDOH at the course level and follow this learning into direct patient care experiences where a DNP scholarly project could easily be identified. This will support the three key domains of providing person-centered care, examining population health issues with the underserved group chosen, and work with an interprofessional team to enact change, all the while learning to lead the interprofessional team. Both faculty and students have the opportunity to explore and establish themselves with community agencies that focus on underserved individuals and health disparities. Considering agencies that cross the lifespan is unique, such as health departments that fulfill many pediatric, contraceptive, and sexually transmitted infection needs, agencies that care for older adults, food pantries that reach individuals and families, and homeless shelters are all opportunities that exist outside of traditional settings such as free clinics and federally qualified health centers. This establishment with underserved community agencies may be a paradigm shift for faculty who hold individual or academic practices. This allows faculty and the university to be known and recognized in the community for their interest in underserved individuals while providing direct clinical and project experiences for students.

CONCLUSION AND SUMMARY

There has been great confusion over time as to what place the DNP has in the healthcare milieu, especially in nonacademic settings (Beeber et al., 2019). In fact, because the DNP is a practice doctorate, many DNPs practice in clinical settings and can fade into the background of being simply an APRN. This presents an opportunity for DNPs to begin to distinguish their role in addressing health equity, calling on the SDOH as an applicable framework and creating real change for patients (Beeber et al., 2019).

Evidence-based practice is widely recognized as essential to healthcare quality and safety (McNett et al., 2021). Until 2004, the only doctorallyprepared nurses held PhDs. Traditionally, PhDs are recognized as researchers. With the addition of the DNP degree, a new cadre of doctorallyprepared nurses were poised to translate the research findings of the PhDs into clinical practice. Despite the ambiguity of the role of the DNP, this moment in our history is an opportunity for DNPs to enact real change in a fractured healthcare environment. While PhDs embrace the research role, the DNP is best suited to implement research evidence for patients and populations (McNett et al., 2021).

Until recently DNPs have been primarily located either in academia or as leaders in hospital administration. The situation with healthcare in the United States presents a unique opportunity for an increased role for DNPs in clinical practice settings by enhancing quality and performance and concretely addressing the SDOH within their practice (Dobrowolska et al., 2021). DNPs find themselves serving as administrators of free clinics or federally qualified health centers, working in health departments, establishing independent practices, leading community focus groups, and occupying seats on community boards of directors.

This chapter aimed to present the significant role the DNP-prepared nurse has in reducing health inequities. The focus on health equity has strengthened with each iteration of the Healthy People directive. Nurse practitioners often find themselves practicing in arenas where they care for those who experience health inequity daily. This allows for a keen eye on the places where their patients live, learn, work, and play that affect their health just as much as chronic conditions such as diabetes or high blood pressure. Through their education and career path as nurses these providers are poised to become key players in supporting the Healthy People aims and helping those they care for achieve health equity. They are prepared to recognize deficiencies, organize, and lead community teams, and engage in larger health policy initiatives at the organization, community, state, and national levels. As healthcare providers caring for people of all ages the DNP-prepared nurse learns what community resources are available and helps their patients navigate these life-changing community resources. They also recognize gaps in these resources and put their strengths in quality improvement and abilities in navigating systems to move patients and communities in directions to level the health inequity playing field. Marge went without basic healthcare for a period of time. Her needs progressed, she had multiple comorbid problems, and once she was in the midst of receiving care more significant problems were discovered that involved a malignancy. Marge's problems, even taking each problem in isolation, were overwhelming to a person who had no idea where to turn for care. However, once she found her way to her DNP NP provider, doors were opened for her, and her conditions were addressed and improved. She was able to regain a sense of dignity and hope and feel respected. The DNP-prepared nurse plays a clear role in addressing the SDOH and health equity in this exemplar, which speaks to the essence of the role for which these individuals are prepared. This practice doctorate in nursing is key in moving the needle forward in addressing and mitigating SDOH in vulnerable populations.

Our patient Marge is an example of many who find themselves vulnerable financially, medically, and emotionally who can benefit greatly from the expertise of DNP-prepared healthcare providers. Marge experienced both a lack of health insurance and a lack of providers that would accept her as a patient. These barriers to access caused a gap in treatment of her hypertension, also allowing the extreme swelling of her legs and early cellulitis to progress. Lack of insurance also limited her access to ongoing preventative care. The solution in this situation was her ability to access a health center in her community that consisted of doctorallyprepared NP primary care providers who accepted those who were uninsured. The center was also able to link Marge with other community resources. Despite the fact that this center does not bill insurance and relies completely on donations, fundraisers, and grants to sustain services, Marge received comprehensive care that put her back on the road to health. The doctorallyprepared NPs were able to work together with the rest of the staff at the center to provide an interdisciplinary, holistic approach to her care—at absolutely no cost to her. Knowledge of resources in the community were crucial to assisting her with her breast cancer diagnosis and treatment, resources she was unaware of despite their close proximity to her home. This is a real but simple example of the ability of DNPs to provide top notch quality care to patients who are uninsured. This exemplar is the essence of the education of the DNP who is at the front lines of making a profound difference for people at risk.

CRITICAL THINKING QUESTIONS

1. What is the DNP's role in promoting health equity? How can health equity be strengthened from a curricular perspective?
2. How can DNPs impact health policy at a local and national level to achieve health equity?

3. How can DNPs become more visible in the media to bring attention to health equities in their respective communities?
4. How should our insurance structure change to promote health equity?
5. What individual and family resources need to be provided to low-income families to achieve health equity?

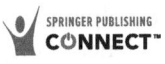 A robust set of instructor resources designed to supplement this text is located at http://connect.springerpub.com/content/book/978-0-8261-8137-4. Qualifying instructors may request access by emailing textbook@springerpub.com.

REFERENCES

AACN. (n.d.). *AACN's definition of competency-based education*. Definition of Competency-Based Education (aacnnursing.org)

AACN. (2021a). *Diversity, equity, and inclusion in academic nursing*. AACN_Position_Statement.pdf (utexas.edu)

AACN. (2021b). *The essentials: Core competencies for professional nursing education*. https://www.aacnnursing.org/AACN-Essentials

Abramson, C. M., Hashemi, M., & Sánchez-Jankowski, M. (2015). Perceived discrimination in US healthcare: Charting the effects of key social characteristics within and across racial groups. *Preventive Medicine Reports, 2*, 615–621. https://doi.org/10.1016/j.pmedr.2015.07.006

Ahluwalia, M. (2021). Addressing education and wages to close the gap in health disparities. *Voices in Bioethics, 7*. https://journals.library.columbia.edu/index.php/bioethics/article/view/7578/3941

American Public Health Association (APHA). (2020, October 24). *Increasing access and reducing barriers to children's vision care services*. https://www.apha.org/policies-and-advocacy/public-health-policy-statements/policy-database/2021/01/12/increasing-access-and-reducing-barriers-to-child-vision-care-services

Bates, R. A., Ford, J. L., Jiang, H., Pickler, R., Justice, L. M., Dynia, J. M., & Ssekayombya, P. (2021). Sociodemographics and chronic stress in mother-toddler dyads living in poverty. *Development Psychobiology, 63*(6), e22179. https://doi.org/10.1002/dev.22179

Beeber, A. S., Palmer, C., Waldrop, J., Lynn, M. R., & Jones, C. B. (2019). The role of doctor of nursing practice-prepared nurses in practice settings. *Nursing Outlook, 67*(4), 354–364. https://doi.org/10.1016/j.outlook.2019.02.006

Bivens, J., & Zipperer, B. (2020, August 26). Health insurance and the COVID-19 shock. *Economic Policy Institute*. https://www.epi.org/publication/health-insurance-and-the-covid-19-shock

Boozary, A. S., & Shojania, K. G. (2018). Pathology of poverty: The need for quality improvement efforts to address social determinants of health. *BMJ Quality Safety, 27*(6), 421–424. https://doi.org/10.1136/bmjqs-2017-007552

Boswell, C., Mintz-Binder, R., Batcheller, J., Allen P., & Baker, K. (2021). Capturing the impact of the doctor of nursing practice degree on west Texas health care. *The Journal of Continuing Education in Nursing, 52*(4), 192–197. https://journals.healio.com/doi/abs/10.3928/00220124-20210315-08

Braveman, P. (2022). *Maxcy-Roseman-Last public health and preventive medicine* (16th ed.). In M. L. Boulton & R. B. Wallance (Eds.). McGraw Hill.

Butkus, R., Rapp, K., Cooney, T. G., & Engel, L. S. (2020). Envisioning a better U.S. health care system for all: Reducing barriers to care and addressing social determinants of health. *Annals of Internal Medicine, 172*(2 Suppl), S50–S59. https://doi.org/10.7326/m19-2410

CDC. (2021a). *About social determinants of health (SDOH)*. https://www.cdc.gov/socialdeterminants/about.html

CDC. (2021b, April 23). *Our vision: Regular, affordable eye exams*. https://www.cdc.gov/diabetes/library/spotlights/eye-exams.html#print

CDC. (2022a, March 3). *Health equity*. https://www.cdc.gov/chronicdisease/healthequity/index.htm

CDC. (2022b, March 5). *Cost-effectiveness of oral diseases interventions*. https://www.cdc.gov/chronicdisease/programs-impact/pop/oral-disease.htm

Chheda, K., Wu, R., Zaback, T., & Brinks, M. V. (2019). Barriers to eye care among participants of a mobile eye clinic. *Cogent Medicine, 6*(1). https://doi.org/10.1080%2F2331205X.2019.1650693

Chokshi, D. A. (2018). Income, poverty, and health inequality. *Journal of the American Medical Association, 319*(13), 1312–1313. https://doi.org/10.1001/jama.2018.2521

Community guide. (2022). *Health equity.* https://thecommunityguide.org/topic.healthequity

Conoc, R. Z., Geis, C., & Vincent, H. K. (2021). Social determinants of health in physiatry: Challenges and opportunities for clinical decision making and improving treatment precision. *Frontiers in Public Health. 9,* 738253. https://doi.org/10.3389%2Ffpubh.2021.738253

Cooper, C. L. (2016). *The Blackwell encyclopedia of management.* Blackwell Publishing. http://www.blackwellreference.com/public/book.html?id=g9780631233176_9780631233 176

DiStefano, M. J., & Levin, J. S. (2019). Does incorporating cost-effectiveness analysis into prescribing decisions promote drug access equity? *American Medical Association Journal of Ethics, 21*(8), e679–685.

Dobrowolska, B., Chruściel, P., Markiewicz, R., & Palese, A. (2021). The role of doctoral-educated nurses in the clinical setting: Findings from a scoping review. *Journal of Clinical Nursing, 30*(19–20), 2808–2821. https://doi.org/10.1111/jocn.15810

Dunbar-Jacob, J., Nativio, D. G., & Khalil, H. (2013). Impact of doctor of nursing practice education in shaping health care systems for the future. *Journal of Nursing Education, 52*(8), 423–427. https://doi.org/10.3928/01484834-20130719-03

Gkiouleka, A., Aquino, M. R. J., Ojo-Aromokudu, O., van Daalen, K. R., Kuhn, I. L., Turner-Moss, E., Thomas , K., Barnard R., Strudwick, R., & Ford, J. (2022).Allied health professionals: A promising ally in the work against health inequalities- a rapid review. *Public Health in Practice, 3,* 100269. https://doi.org/10.1016/j.puhip.2022.100269

Green, K. A., Bovell-Ammon, A., & Sandel, M. (2021). Housing and neighborhoods as root causes of child poverty. *Academic Pediatrics, 21*(8Suppl.), S194–S199. https://doi.org/10.1016/j.acap.2021.08.018

Healthy People 2030. (2020). *Access to health services.* Access to Primary Care – Healthy People 2030 | health.gov

Health Resources and Service Administration (HRSA). (2022). *What is workforce shortage.* https://bhw.hrsa.gov/workforce-shortage-areas/shortage-designation

Ingram, M., Leih, R., Adkins, A., Sonmez, E., & Yetman, E. (2020). Health disparities, transportation equity and complete streets: A case study of a policy development process through the lens of critical race theory. *Journal of Urban Health, 97,* 876–886. https://doi.org/10.1007/s11524-020-00460-8

Johnson, S. R. (2022). Staff shortages choking U.S. health care system. *US News & World Report.* https://www.usnews.com/news/health-news/articles/2022-07-28/staff-shortages-choking-u-s-health-care-system#:~:text=By%202025%2C%20the%20U.S.%20is,industry%20market%20analytic%20firm%20Mercer.

Kaiser Family Foundation. (2019, Feburary 1). *Coverage at work: The share of nonelderly Americans with employer-based insurance rose modestly in recent years, but has declined markedly over the long term.* https://www.kff.org/health-reform/press-release/coverage-at-work-the-share-of-nonelderly-americans-with-employer-based-insurance-rose-modestly-in-recent-years-but-has-declined-markedly-over-the-long-term

Kranich, N. (2001). *Libraries and democracy,* American Library Association, pp.15–27.

Kuehn, B. (2021). US health system ranks last among high-income countries. *Journal of the American Medical Association, 326*(1), 999. https://doi.org/10.1001/jama.2021.15468

Kuehnert, P., Fawcett, J., DePriest, K., Chinn, P., Cousin, L., Ervin, N., Flanagan, J., Fry-Bowers, E., Killion, C., Maliski, S., Maughan, E. D., Meade, C., Murray, T., Schenk, B., & Waite, R. (2022). Defining the social determinants of health for nursing action to achieve health equity: A consensus paper from the American Academy of Nursing. *Nursing Outlook, 70*(1), 10–27. https://doi.org/10.1016/j.outlook.2021.08.003

Kullgren, J. T., McLaughlin, C. G., Mitra, N., & Armstrong, K. (2012). Nonfinancial barriers and access to care for U.S. adults. *Health Service Research, 45* (1 Pt. 2), 462–485. https://doi.org/10.1111/j.1475-6773.2011.01308.x

Kuhfeld, M., Soland, J., Lewis, K., & Morton, E. (2022, March 3). The pandemic has had devastating impacts on learning. What will it take to help students catch up? *Brookings Institute.* https://www.brookings.edu/blog/brown-center-chalkboard/2022/03/03/the-pandemic-has-had-devastating-impacts-on-learning-what-will-it-take-to-help-students-catch-up

The Lancet Public Health. (2020). Education: A neglected social determinant of health [Editorial]. *The Lancet Public Health, 5*(7). e361.https://doi.org/10.1016/S2468-2667(20)30144-4

Lathrop, B. (2020). Moving toward health equity by addressing social determinants of health. *Nursing for Women's Health, 24* (1), 36–44. https://doi.org/10.1016/j.nwh.2019.11.003

Levinger, P., Sales, M., Polman, R., Haines, T., Dow, B., Biddle, S. J. H., Duque, G., & Hill, K. D. (2018). Outdoor physical activity for older people-the senior exercise park: Current research, challenges and future directions. *Health Promotion Journal of Australia, 29*(3), 353–359. https://doi.org/10.1002/hpja.60

McNett, M., Masciola, R., Sievert, D., & Tucker, S. (2021). Advancing evidence-based practice through implementation science: Critical contributions of doctor of nursing practice- and doctor of philosophy-prepared nurses. *Worldviews on Evidence Based Nursing, 18*(2), 93–101. https://doi.org/10.1111/wvn.12496

National Academies of Sciences, Engineering, and Medicine. (2021). *The future of nursing 2020–2030: Charting a path to achieve health equity.* The National Academies Press.

National Center for Health Statistics. (2016). Social determinants of health. *Healthy People 2020 midcourse review.* https://www.cdc.gov/nchs/data/hpdata2020/hp2020mcr-c39-sdoh.pdf

National Organization of Nurse Practitioner Faculty. (2018). *The doctor of nursing practice degree: Entry to nurse practitioner practice by 2025.* Microsoft Word - NONPF DNP Statement May 2018 (3) (ymaws.com)

National Task Force (NTF) for Quality Nurse Practitioner Education. (2022). *Standards for quality nurse practitioner education* (6th ed). https://www.nonpf.org/page/NTFStandards

Nejad, F. N., Ghamari, M. R., Mohaqeqi Kamal, S. H., Tabatabaee, S. S., & Ganjali, R. (2021). The most important social determinants of slum dwellers' health: A scoping review. *Journal of Preventive Medicine and Public Health, 54*(4), 265–274. https://doi.org/10.3961/jpmph.21.073

Pastakia, S. D., Clark, A., Lewis, K., & Taugher, D. (2022, October 24). Expanding comprehensive medication management considers to include responses to the social determinants of health within the BD Helping Build Health Communities Program [Editorial]. *Journal of the American College of Clinical Pharmacy, 5,* 793–797. https://doi.org/10.1002/jac5.1679

Pearson, A. L., Clevenger, K. A., Horton, T. H., Gardiner, J. C., Asana, V., Dougherty, B. V., & Pfeiffer, K. A. (2021). Feelings of safety during daytime walking: Associations with mental health, physical activity and cardiometabolic health in high vacancy, low-income neighborhoods in Detroit, Michigan. *International Journal of Health Geographics, 20*(1), 19. https://doi.org/10.1186/s12942-021-00271-3

Price, J. H., Khubchandani, J., & Webb, F. J. (2018). Poverty and health disparities: What can public health professionals do? *Health Promotion Practice, 19*(2), 170–174. https://doi.org/10.1177/1524839918755143

Rollston, R., & Galea, S. (2020). COVID-19 and the social determinants of health. *American Journal of Health Promotion, 34*(6), 687–689. https://doi.org/10.1177/0890117120930536b

Rural Health Information Hub. (2020a, March 6). *Improving information to address social determinants of health.* Improving Education to Address Social Determinants of Health - RHIhub SDOH Toolkit (ruralhealthinfo.org)

Rural Health Information Hub. (2020b, March 6). *College access programs.* College Access Programs – RHIhub SDOH Toolkit (ruralhealthinfo.org)

Santiago, A. M., Berg, K. A., & Leroux, J. (2021). Assessing the impact of neighborhood conditions on neurodevelopmental disorders during childhood. *International Journal of Environmental Research and Public Health, 18*(17). https://doi.org/10.3390/ijerph18179041

Starbird, L. E., DiMaina, C., Sun, C., & Han, H. (2019). A systematic review of interventions to minimize transportation barriers among people with chronic diseases. *Journal of Community Health, 44,* 400–411. https://doi.org/10.1007/s10900-018-0572-3

Sugarman, O. K., Bachhuber, M. A., Wennerstrom, A., Bruno, T., & Springgate, B. F. (2020, January 21). Interventions for incarcerated adults with opiod use disorder in the United States: A systematic review with a focus on social determinants of health. *PLOS One. 15*(1), e0227968. https://doi.org/10.1371/journal.pone.0227968

Shrider, E. A., Kollar, M., Chen, F., & Semega, J. (2021). *Income and poverty in the United States: 2020.* United States Centus Bureau. Income and Poverty in the United States: 2020 (census.gov)

Tolbert, J., Orgera, K., & Damico, A. (2020, November 6). *Key facts about the uninsured population.* Kaiser Family Foundation. Key Facts about the Uninsured Population | KFF

U.S. Department of Health & Human Services (U.S.DHHS). (2019a). *Social cohesion.* Social Cohesion – Healthy People 2030 | health.gov

U.S.DHHS. (2019b). *Civic participation.* https://health.gov/healthypeople/priority-areas/social-determinants-health/literature-summaries/civic-participation

U.S.DHHS. (2021, August 2). *Education access and quality*. https://health.gov/healthypeople/objectives-and-data/browse-objectives/education-access-and-quality

U.S.DHHS. (2022a). *Health equity in healthy people 2030*. https://health.gov/healthypeople/priority-areas/health-equity-healthy-people-2030

U.S.DHHS. (2022b). *History of healthy people*. https://health.gov/our-work/national-health-initiatives/healthy-people/about-healthy-people/history-healthy-people

Valachovic, R. W. (2018 May 5). Implications for the dental care of vulnerable populations if medicaid is cut back. *Academic Medicine, 93*(5), 687–689. https://doi.org/10.1097/ACM.0000000000002161

Walker, D. K. (2021). Parenting and social determinants of health. *Archives of Psychiatric Nursing, 35*(1), 134–136. https://doi.org/10.1016/j.apnu.2020.10.016

Weida, E. B., Phojanakong, P., Patel, F., & Chilton, M. (2020). Financial health as a measurable social determinant of health. *PLoS One, 15*(5), e0233359. https://doi.org/10.1371/journal.pone.0233359

Whitman, A., DeLew, N., Chappel, A., Aysola, V., Zuckerman, R., & Sommers, B. D. (2022, April 1). Addressing social determinants of health: Examples of successful evidence-based strategies and current federal efforts. *Assistant Secretary for Planning and Evaluation (ASPE)*. https://aspe.hhs.gov/reports/sdoh-evidence-review

Williams, A. M., & Sahel, J. A. (2022). Addressing social determinants of vision health. *Opthalmology Therapy, 11*, 1371–1382. https://doi.org/10.1007/s40123-022-00531-w

World Health Organization (WHO). (2021). *Social determinants of health*. https://www.who.int/health-topics/social-determinants-of-health#tab=tab_1

Zucker, D. M., Reagan, L., Clifton, J., Abdulhamed, A., Roscoe, L., Wright, R. M., Penix, D., Shelton, D., & Loeb, S. (2022). NPs caring for people who are incarcerated and negatively impacted by social determinants of health. *The Nurse Practitioner Journal, 47*(6), 38–46.

CHAPTER TWELVE | Reflective Response

ROBERTA WAITE AND DEENA A. NARDI

ENSURING HEALTH EQUITY REQUIRES INTENTION, BOLD ACTION, EMPATHY, AND COMPASSION

Ensuring health equity for all is multifaceted, but importantly it requires nursing practice informed by research and a commitment to advocate for social justice across sectors and settings, including research, governance, practice, education, policy, and leadership. Social justice, "full participation in society and the balancing of benefits and burdens by all citizens, which in most cases involves social reconstruction" (Hosseinzadegan et al., 2021, p. 119), is a core tenet within nursing's code of ethics and must drive the work of DNPs, where they will have to be intentional and demonstrate bold and courageous action in executing this principle. DNPs can identify social determinants of health (SDOH), often focusing at the individual level. Micro-, meso-, and macro-level approaches by DNPs are fundamental, however, in creating habits of social justice, requiring their "learning and predominant way of thinking to shift from merely the individual client to collective society and from tertiary (reactive) care approaches to primary (preventive) care approaches" (Hosseinzadegan et al., 2021, p. 127). This would demonstrate a manifestation of social justice in the health system that surmounts the traditional biomedical lens.

Just as integral to health equity and social justice is the attention we give to our patients, awareness of their values and needs, as well as having an in-depth understanding of the social and structural processes that create inequities in health. Health equity is social justice in health because disparities in health can only be remedied by obstructing calculated or unconscious social and structural forms of discrimination that fortify social disadvantage (Fraser et al., 2019). For example, in the United States, one's perceived race is often a barrier to ensuring optimal health. DNPs must understand how race is intertwined with structural mechanisms from a social stance. Race is socially constructed; however, just saying this alone is no longer acceptable. To appreciate how race plays out in the lives of their patients (from birth to death), DNPs must be able to clearly discern what social construction means and the purpose that it serves, especially in settings that have been colonized. This has huge implications in policy development that DNPs can be engaged in, as well as ensuring that practice does not perpetuate harm toward patients (e.g., biological/race essentialism).

The pursuit of health equity and social justice requires that we use our empathy, coupled with compassion, which requires an intention to "be with" the patient at hand. Focusing solely on the facts, the data, best practices, or guidelines in place can reduce nursing practice to a healthcare app, which can be informed by the newest published research, as long as we keep updating it, but cannot respond to the primary human need of our patients—to be seen, heard, understood, respected, and valued. This use of empathy to "know" each patient provides a doorway, a portal, into our patient's experience of living with and working around health conditions, including SDOH challenges, that obstruct their being able to "reach their full health potential," another description of health equity (Austin, 2017, p. 76). Using empathy allows us to see the obstacles in their way, while compassion, which is the drive to alleviate suffering, creates the intention to harness resources and use them to sustain, support, or improve a patient's health, as the DNP-prepared nurse was able to do in a therapeutic alliance with Marge in the preceding chapter.

This chapter identified economic instability as affecting the other SDOH, playing a central role in her slide to unwellness and chronic disease states. Marge did not have health insurance, the lack of which is recognized as the biggest of many barriers to receiving basic healthcare, including necessary medications, in a nation that relies on private insurance from for-profit corporations to fund healthcare services. The DNP provider took a deep dive into the system, connecting Marge with medical specialists, including a nurse navigator, who would arrange for her oncology treatment. We note here, however, that it took the diagnosis of breast cancer for Marge to become eligible for Medicaid, which then "opened the doors" of funding for treatment that otherwise "would have bankrupted her," as it does many other cancer patients and their families in the United States. Social processes and values held in our society inform health policy and aligned resources, therefore DNPs, understanding of social structures enables them to identify ways in which economic, political, and institutional forces can inflict direct injury or harm to patients. While it is important for DNPs to integrate social context into healthcare delivery, merely focusing on a clinical context is too narrow to address systemic influences of the SDOH. Structural and legal interventions are requisite to effectively tackle root drivers of SDOH. Incorporating assistance from medical-legal partnerships (MLP) was an additional option that Marge could have benefited from. MLP is able to promote positive changes in the health and well-being of patients; make improvements in institutions, services, and practices; and finally, enact improvements in policies and laws that affect populations that are made vulnerable (Teitelbaum & Lawton, 2021). It is important for DNPs to recognize the role of law in forming health systems and environments that are premised on and can aid in constructing health equity, which is created by more than individual choice or simple randomness. Rather, health equity is a consequence of the historic and ongoing interplay of inequitable structures, policies, and norms that inform the lives of all in society. Ensuring health equity requires ameliorating long-term discriminatory structural systems and practices, and leading with actions aligned with social justice, empathy, and compassion to provide quality healthcare that is not contingent on race, gender, location, or socioeconomic status. Today, economic instability, with no healthcare insurance and no means of affording needed medications, equates to the end of the journey to ensure health equity in the United States.

REFERENCES

Austin, W. (2017). Global health ethics and mental health. In E. Yearwood & V. Hines-Martin (Eds.), *Routledge handbook of global mental health nursing* (p. 76). Routledge.

Fraser, K., Brady, J., & Lordly, D. (2019). Taking social justice to a different stage: How poetry promotes emancipatory health narratives. *Journal of Critical Dietetics*, 4(2), 18–27. https://doi.org/10.32920/cd.v4i2.1108

Hosseinzadegan, F., Jasemi, M., & Habibzadeh, H. (2021). Factors affecting nurses' impact on social justice in the health system. *Nursing Ethics*, 28(1) 118–130. https://doi.org/10.1177/0969733020948123

CHAPTER THIRTEEN

The DNP and Academic-Service Partnerships

SANDRA RADER, SANDRA ENGBERG, SHELLEY WATTERS, AND JACQUELINE DUNBAR-JACOB

Nursing has a long history of collaboration between service settings and academic settings in the education of nurses. From the initial educational model of apprenticeship to the placement of formal educational programs within hospitals to the education of nurses over the past half century in universities and community colleges, the relationship between the clinical setting and the educational setting has been central to the education of the next generation of nurses. This relationship is consistent with other disciplines with a strong practice focus. Medicine has long situated much of its education within the clinical practice setting as have numerous other health professions. Professions such as education and social work also include practice experiences in work settings. The nature of the partnerships established between academic and service settings has varied from shared ownership to affiliation agreements designed to provide opportunities for learning. The agreements have focused principally on student education, with the service personnel cooperating with academic instructors or serving as direct educators themselves.

In 2004 the American Association of Colleges of Nursing (AACN) determined that advanced practice education should move from the master of science to the doctor of nursing practice (DNP) level. This was followed by the 2007 decision of the nurse anesthesia Council on Accreditation (CoA) and the 2015 statements by the National Association of Clinical Nurse Specialists (NACNS) and the National Organization of Nurse Practitioner Faculties (NONPF) to move these advanced practice specialties to the DNP. These decisions have expanded the possibilities for academic-service partnerships. Additional education in leadership, policy, finance, quality improvement and evaluation methodologies, translation of research, as well as further advances in clinical or administrative education, have made the DNP a highly contributing professional for both the academic and practice sides of the partnership. These skills provide added value for the inclusion of the DNP in academic-service partnerships.

■ MOVING FROM AFFILIATION TO PARTNERSHIP

The presence of the DNP in both practice and academic settings provides opportunities for collaborations extending well beyond the traditional affiliation for student education.

Not the least of these is the opportunity to contribute to the quality and innovation of both practice and education. For example, as a component of the University of Pittsburgh Medical Center (UPMC)/UPitt (UPMC Health System and University of Pittsburgh School of Nursing) Partnership, doctorally prepared senior staff at UPMC serve on the school leadership team, as well as a variety of academic councils. Similarly, doctorally prepared faculty serve on the nursing leadership group, as well as on nursing and interdisciplinary committees. The benefit of this form of partnership is improvement of communication and broadening of the perspective in these critical working groups.

In this model, DNP-prepared senior staff serve on the undergraduate, master's, and DNP councils. The councils design curriculum, review specific learning activities, review student progress, and ensure that programs are addressing future healthcare workforce skills. In addition, the DNP staff serve as members of DNP student projects, deliver lectures to classes, and precept students. The addition of the DNP staff from the health system provides information on the vision for practice, confirmation of educational directions, opportunity for the service partners to learn about changes in educational initiatives, and input on the positive and negative experiences of students, faculty, and clinical staff in the education of students. The educational background of the DNP staff in quality improvement, mentorship/preceptorship, and an advanced level of practice enriches the conversation between the academic and service partners.

Reciprocally, the DNP (and PhD) faculty of the School of Nursing serve on a variety of practice councils. For example, faculty serve on the health system nursing informatics council and evidence-based practice council for Nursing. Faculty also serve on interdisciplinary committees, such as recruitment committees, ethics committee, scientific review committee, infection control and patient safety committee, as well as the quality committees/boards. In addition, faculty serve as consultants at selected hospitals and collaborate in selected quality initiatives. Faculty are able to bring the perspective of both education and advanced practice to the work of these councils enriched by the advanced clinical, translational, policy, and quality improvement DNP education they received. The shared participation means that clinical staff are aware of educational innovations and academic staff are aware of practice changes without accidental discovery. This makes interactions around students and educational processes more efficient and reinforces trust between the two groups.

The connections between the practice environment and the academic environment that are enriched by the education of the DNP faculty member or clinical setting staff promote a deeper level of engagement in both the academic and service environments. The emphasis on personal opinion driving educational and practice decisions is replaced with a commitment to and understanding of the translation of research findings to education and practice along with both an appreciation for and the competence to evaluate such innovations in real world (educational/practice) settings. Further the shared perspective of the DNP in both settings facilitates collaboration in advancing the profession.

One of the strongest areas of partnership is in the education of the next generation of DNP students. Two models of education currently exist. One of those models, supported by the AACN, NONPF, NACNS, and CoA, advocates for advanced practice education at the BSN to DNP level. In this model the student has 1,000 or more hours of supervised clinical practice, as well as education in systems, evidence-based practice and translation, policy, and leadership. Programs that follow this model may offer post-master's programs within the specialty track. The second model offers leadership, evidence-based practice translation, policy, and systems educational content as a general post-master's DNP program without a specialty focus. Thus, there may be some variation in the contribution to advanced practice innovations between the two groups.

Whichever the program, the education of the DNP is heavily dependent upon a clinical partnership that can support that level of education.

ACADEMIC-SERVICE PARTNERSHIPS IN THE EDUCATION OF THE DNP

The August, 2015, report from the AACN Task Force on the Implementation of the DNP, included a statement reaffirming the importance of academic-service partnerships in creating and sustaining progressive education and practice. The Task Force recommended that DNP programs follow the AACN-AONE Task Force on Academic-Service Partnership guiding principles when establishing partnerships (AACN Task Force on Implementation of the DNP, 2015). Partnerships should be formalized relationships based on "mutual goals, respect and knowledge" (p. 1). As educational programs establish academic-service partnerships, they should consider potential partners beyond traditional healthcare systems. A broad range of partnerships should be considered (AACN-AONE Task Force, 2012).

Academic-service partnerships have the potential to benefit students as well as the partnership sites. A broad range of partnerships will allow DNP students to engage in practice experiences that allow them to attain and demonstrate the DNP Essentials. Practice experiences for the DNP student should include more than direct patient care. They should also include indirect care opportunities that allow students to broaden their expertise in relation to the skill set defined in the DNP Essentials. Having a broad range of practice partners will facilitate DNP programs' ability to provide these experiences for students. They will also help to ensure adequate numbers of high quality direct patient care experiences for advanced practice DNP students. The 2015 AACN Report from the Task Force on the Implementation of the DNP states that all DNP programs are required to document and validate that graduates have met all of the DNP essential outcomes. This includes BSN to DNP and MSN to DNP students and students in programs focusing on leadership and health policy, as well as direct patient care roles. In addition, the report recommends practice immersion experiences where students have the opportunity to apply, integrate, and synthesize knowledge related to the DNP Essentials and to demonstrate achievement of outcomes in relation to advanced nursing practice (AACN Task Force on Implementation of the DNP, 2015). Meeting these requirements and recommendations requires access to a variety of practice settings. Academic-service partnerships can help ensure this access.

More recently, the AACN has adopted and published a new set of essentials, identifying the core competencies essential for practice (AACN, 2021). These competencies, marking a significant change from past essentials, were developed by an academic-service task force to ensure that both practice leadership and educational leadership generated and agreed upon the educational core of nursing. The DNP essentials are drawn from a general core with advanced levels of practice and knowledge expected of the advanced practitioner. These essentials are now expected to be combined with the specialty organization requirements for the education of the advanced practice registered nurse (APRN). Of particular note is that three of the five advanced practice roles have deadlines for DNP to become the entry-level education: nurse anesthesia, nurse practitioner, and clinical nurse specialist. DNP students will be evaluated on their level of performance of these competencies, reflecting a shift in the education of advanced practice nurses. This will require a developmental partnership between education and practice as both revise the teaching/learning processes for the APRN.

Academic-practice partnerships are also important beyond direct clinical learning and the implementation of the new essentials and their evaluation in that education. The partnership is also critical to the development of the DNP student in the identification, design, and conduct of their culminating project. In this respect the academic partner, with design expertise, and the practice partner, with opportunity for implementation, collaboratively can provide DNP students access to settings and persons where they can plan, implement, and evaluate their project with mentorship shared across the partners. According to the white paper, all DNP projects should:

- Be designed to effect healthcare outcomes through either direct or indirect care
- Have a micro-, meso-, or macro-level systems focus or a population/aggregate focus
- Be implemented in the appropriate practice setting
- Include a plan for sustainability
- Include evaluation of process and/or outcomes that guide practice or policy
- Provide the basis for future practice-related scholarship (AACN Task Force on Implementation of the DNP, 2015)

DNP projects should demonstrate the cumulative knowledge and skills students have gained during their program (Waldrop et al., 2014). Having an adequate number and range of academic-practice partnerships is important in providing DNP students with access to practice settings and their expertise, along with knowledgeable faculty, where they can develop, implement, and evaluate a project that meets the above criteria.

In addition to the benefits that these partnerships afford DNP programs and their students, there are potential benefits for the practice settings (Dunbar-Jacob et al., 2013). Two recent reviews of academic-practice partnerships have identified numerous beneficial foci (Markaki et al., 2021; Sadeghnezhad et al., 2018). Benefits to education included increasing educational capacity, supportive learning environments, joint curriculum improvements, opportunities for collaborative practice and interprofessional experiences, and the potential for financial support. Benefits to service included improved transition to practice, staff development opportunities, and improvement in patient outcomes. Benefits to both included access to the expertise across the education-service settings, strengthening capacity in the community, and enhanced satisfaction with the service learning component of education.

A focus on Magnet recognition and improvement in the quality of care, as well as the requirement for quality monitoring, are among the forces driving interest in academic-practice partnerships (Kleinpell, 2016). DNP programs are designed to prepare experts in specialized advanced practice as well as leadership. Students are educated for practice that is innovative and evidence-based, applying credible research findings to improve healthcare outcomes. Additionally, the DNP student is prepared to undertake quality improvement initiatives. When the DNP student has the opportunity to collaborate with practice partners in the design, implementation, and evaluation of their terminal project, the practice site as well as the student benefits from the knowledge gained. DNP program faculty with expertise in the various methodologies relevant to DNP practice, such as quality improvement, program evaluation, evidence implementation, and N=1 can partner with members of the clinical team and the student in the design, implementation, and evaluation of projects that improve quality and evidence-based care. Faculty can also collaborate with clinical partners on the development of APRN residency programs. Finally, academic-practice partnerships can enhance the ability of practice sites to recruit and retain DNP-prepared APRNs.

Although we did not identify any academic-practice partnership models that were specifically designed to provide clinical experiences for DNP students, several of the models in the literature involved graduate students and could serve as effective DNP program-practice models. Thabault et al. (2015) described an academic-practice partnership between Minute Clinics and Northeastern University School of Nursing. The goals of the partnership were to recruit and retain APRNs in Minute Clinic practice sites, support academic progression, and provide teaching expertise to develop the knowledge and skills needed to lead interprofessional teams in retail and other community settings. Service and faculty partners developed an APRN postgraduate residency within the Minute Clinics that included a two-credit online leadership course at the completion of the residency program. Tuition for the course was funded through the residency program. Preceptors as well as residents were invited to take the course.

Killeen and colleagues (2015) described a practitioner-teacher model in which APRNs in practice settings served as advanced practice nurses and preceptors. In 2012 Rush University Medical Center was selected as a graduate nursing education (GNE) site, administered by the Centers for Medicare and Medicaid Services. As a GNE site, Rush was able to trial new models of care. One of the models included one in which acute care NPs provided 24/7 patient coverage for the cardiac intensive care unit. Development of the practice model included a teacher-practitioner model for NP training.

Some educational programs are expanding the clinical opportunities for DNP students, and subsequently graduates, through the introduction of novel sites for partnerships. Shurson et al. (2021) also described an academic-service partnership designed to support workforce capacity and the education of DNP students in veterans' health. Here DNP students worked within the variety of Veterans Administration clinical sites. The school of nursing provided a dedicated faculty and preceptor development. Students had the opportunity to engage with leadership and to develop doctoral projects designed to stimulate practice innovation. Hooshmand et al. (2019) expanded the clinical practice and project development further through community partnerships. Expansion of the academic-practice partnership has gone beyond the multiplicity of types of clinical settings. Norman et al. (2021) describes a unique partnership with a state board of nursing to enrich the students' learning of policy. This included participation in state-wide meetings, and contribution to a subsequent report.

An increasing number of academic service partnerships are collaborating on the projects that students carry out, with the projects designed to benefit real world problems experienced by the service partner. For example, Wright and Cranmer (2018) describe a program in which DNP students study complex problems in the practice arena through their statistics and complex systems courses. Williams et al. (2022) describe incorporation of process improvement in DNP student projects to advance leadership initiatives.

Fairchild (2012) described an academic-practice partnership between a university and rural hospitals that focused on APRN students in a graduate online nursing informatics course. The partnership led to the development of an online nursing informatics service-learning course. Students worked with healthcare providers and nurse administrators in the partner rural healthcare settings to assist with various health information technologies (HIT) needs. During the semester, student teams (two to three students) were assigned to the rural health setting, where they worked with the personnel in the setting to identify HIT continuing education needs and then worked via telecommunications with their rural healthcare partners to design, conduct, and evaluate a project related to and/or supported by informatics or HIT. For DNP programs, projects such as this would allow students to develop and demonstrate skills related to DNP Essentials focusing on information systems and technology, as well as interprofessional collaboration and teamwork.

In addition to these examples of partnerships, there are opportunities in nurse-run clinics. Nurse-run clinics can benefit the academic setting by providing a practice setting for APRN DNP faculty and an opportunity for faculty to precept and evaluate students' skills. These clinics increase access to care, with many providing care to underserved populations (Sullivan-Marx et al., 2010; Xippolitos, 2011). Indeed, one such example was described by Humphreys et al. (2004) in which faculty serve as providers as well as preceptors for the students.

CREATING A STRONG INFRASTRUCTURE TO SUPPORT ACADEMIC SERVICE PARTNERSHIPS: A CASE STUDY

Collaboration is an essential skill for nurse leaders. As nurses, we often find ourselves in the middle of communication between multiple partners. Many times, these partners are physicians or other clinical disciplines. But it is also the case that, where multiple schools or multiple health systems exist, these partnerships might include one health system and multiple educational partners as well as one academic unit and multiple service partners. This chapter provides an exemplar of effective collaboration and communication through educational and service organizations serving Pittsburgh, Pennsylvania; UPMC and its surrounding academic partners. This work is in the form of an academic service partnership council (ASPC).

UPMC is characterized as a global health enterprise. It is made up of various entities, including an insurance arm, an international division, and an enterprise services arm known for its innovation and broad strategic thinking. The system is comprised of over 40 hospitals, including operations in Italy, Ireland, and soon China. There are over 400 doctors' offices, extended care facilities, and outpatient sites. This provides for expansive clinical opportunities for students at every level, particularly for the DNP student from varying specialties.

Partnering with schools of nursing has been a long-standing UPMC practice. The UPMC Health System is closely affiliated with the University of Pittsburgh, a major academic institution with a top-ranked nursing program. This structure represented a strong foundation from which an academic service partnership could be formed.

Beyond the University of Pittsburgh School of Nursing, there are many nursing academic institutions in the region. They represent programs with DNP, PhD, master's, baccalaureate, associate, and hospital-based diploma degrees. The Academic Service Partnership Council (ASPC) began with the UPMC Health System and its university affiliate and nine other nursing programs within the region. The first task was to create structure and work—a purpose to come together.

The ASPC was first somewhat formal. The invitation list included academic representation in the form of deans, program directors, and faculty. Service representation included chief nursing officers, directors of nursing education, program administrators, and practice nurse educators. Meetings were held monthly, and the journey began with the mission to create systems that support the finest clinical experiences, the most highly prepared nurses, and a focus on hiring and retaining the best nursing talent locally and nationally.

The goals were lofty and it was easy to see that relationships needed to be built to achieve these goals and for effective collaboration to occur. The first goal was to establish trust. Participants would only then feel comfortable discussing issues with those with whom they traditionally competed. The council began by identifying the challenges each faced. These included increasing patient complexity, faculty shortages, legislative changes, quality metrics and reimbursement implications, rapid technological changes, and preceptor development.

It was important to identify the first project that all would have a stake in. The cochairs included a DNP-prepared clinical education leader and a DNP-prepared chief nursing officer within the UPMC Health System. The DNP leadership role in bridging the service and academic settings made exceptional use of the advanced clinical, leadership, and education competencies developed through DNP education. It was clear that the UPMC Health System lacked standardization across each clinical setting. Each academic institution held an affiliation agreement with the UPMC Health System. Each clinical site managed affiliation agreements differently and held different standards for student placement. This meant that multiple and different affiliation agreements needed to be processed even though all hospitals were part of the same health system. Similarly, the educational partners held affiliation agreements with practice partners outside of this large system, both for acute and specialty care and for community practice, meaning they too were needing to process multiple affiliation agreements. Further, students cleared for clinical rotations at one site might not be cleared for clinical rotations within another site. Standardizing the affiliation agreements and creating a "universal agreement" and a process whereby one centralized committee reviewed and made decisions regarding student background checks and clinical rotations within this health system would be the first big project of the ASPC.

This standardization improved efficiencies for the clinical sites and the academic institutions. Overcoming the various nuances, such as how we processed the agreements and who held the clearance documents, required open dialogue on both sides. The work included a representative from the UPMC Health System corporate legal department who was involved and at the table. This helped to clear legal concerns in real time and with a great degree of credibility.

The success of this inaugural project opened the doors for the development of many projects to come. There are open discussions regarding recruitment needs of the hospitals and enrollment information from each of the participants is collected. Information is shared openly across schools of nursing. This is something that would not have happened without the trust and collaboration built within the ASPC. The council communicates and celebrates its academic partnership success while providing cutting edge industry information on an annual basis. This takes shape in the form of an annual ASPC retreat. This retreat brings together deans and faculty from each academic partner with practice and education leaders from the hospitals. Topics and presenters usually include some successful key partnership projects, as well as experts on national topics in healthcare. The event is sponsored by the UPMC Health System in thanks and appreciation for past and future engagement.

The issue of faculty shortages is very real among the education partners. Natural collaboration began to occur based on geographical location between various university partners and UPMC Health System hospitals. Soon, dedicated education units were born.

A dedicated education unit takes staff nurses on a hospital-based unit and pairs them with students serving as their clinical instructor as they collaboratively care for a group of patients. The nurses receive special training in providing nursing education and guidance as they work with students on their unit. This training focuses on education practices, ethical-legal aspects of clinical education, teaching-learning strategies, and clinical evaluation. This model mimics the physician clinical education model and has been successfully replicated across the UPMC Health System.

With the rapidly changing landscape of healthcare reform, the council provides a regular legislative update from the health system by government relations staff. Additionally, the council also works to tackle the rapid technological changes. Health system informatics nurses were invited to the table and developed a coordinated plan to provide electronic medical record access to faculty and students and one standardized class to educate academic partners. That has transformed into sharing electronic medical record weekly communication updates with education partners and involving them in documentation optimization work. This provides opportunity to explain the details of meaningful use and the healthcare system is working to standardize and build in electronic strategies to facilitate quality standards of care.

The health system traditionally participated in student feedback surveys. The methodology for distributing the surveys, however, was not consistent between schools. There was also not a clear mechanism to communicate results. This provided minimal opportunity to determine how well the health system was serving students and no ability to trend results. This was clearly another body of work for our council. The group developed and approved a standardized methodology. Surveys for faculty and students and preceptors are distributed at the end of every semester. Results are then shared openly and transparently across hospitals and education partners. It is particularly important for the hospital chief nursing officers to see this valuable information by unit. This gives the opportunity to assess unit culture and influence new nurse success rates. Equally important is the information to the school as it assesses the contribution of the practice partner to its student development.

The work of the ASPC continues. It has grown from a partnership with nine educational institutions to over 15 education partners. The council continues to address the shared challenges in healthcare. This partnership has promoted innovation and collaboration in striving for excellence. The partnership program was initiated based on mutual potential benefits. Today many of those benefits are realized. The council members have moved from competitors to collaborators on many levels. This has involved creating a stakeholder coalition, shared decision making, and a shared structure. The council now enjoys partnerships in clinical education and staff development. The outcomes have been beneficial to the health system and academic partners. This foundation serves as a strong springboard for clinical partnerships at all nursing education levels.

This culture of collaboration and partnership has created a fertile ground for the DNP student and graduate. The UPMC Health System has opened its doors to many DNP clinical experiences and quality projects. Many of those experiences help shape innovative leadership and care models. Further, the UPMC Health System enjoys the leadership and practice of many DNP nurses across its ranks. This model has served to strengthen the practice of nurses within the health system and the education of nurses and students within the academic settings. The academic-service partnership has benefit for all.

CRITICAL THINKING QUESTIONS

1. What added benefit does the DNP bring to the academic-service partnership?
2. What can the DNP in the service setting contribute to the academic setting?
3. What can the DNP in the academic setting contribute to the service setting?
4. Given the two models of preparation of the DNP, what are the unique contributions of each to the academic-service partnership?
5. Where in the setting(s) is the DNP best positioned to enrich the academic-service partnership?
6. What are the optimal expectations for the DNP in the service setting and the DNP in the academic setting?
7. How does the academic-service partnership collaborate best to prepare the strongest DNP graduate?

8. What areas of DNP practice within the academic-service partnership that are in need of evaluation?
9. What is the value of the DNP student project to the service and academic sides of the partnership?
10. How might an academic-service partnership be structured that maximizes the contributions of the DNP graduate?

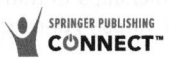 A robust set of instructor resources designed to supplement this text is located at http://connect.springerpub.com/content/book/978-0-8261-8137-4. Qualifying instructors may request access by emailing textbook@springerpub.com.

REFERENCES

AACN-AONE Task Force on Academic-Practice Partnerships. (2012). *Guiding principles*. http://www.aacn.nche.edu/leading-initiatives/academic-practice-partnerships/GuidingPrinciples.pdf

AACN Task Force on Implementation of the DNP. (2015). *The doctor of nursing practice: Current issues and clarifying recommendations*. http://www.aacn.nche.edu/aacn-publications/white-papers/DNP-Implementation-TF-Report-8-15.pdf

American Association of Colleges of Nurses. (2021). *The essentials: Core competencies for professional nursing education*. https://www.aacnnursing.org/Portals/42/AcademicNursing/pdf/Essentials-2021.pdf

Dunbar-Jacob, J., Nativio, D. G., & Khalil, H. (2013). Impact of doctor of nursing practice education in shaping health care systems for the future. *The Journal of Nursing Education*, 52(8), 423–427. https://doi.org/10.3928/01484834-20130719-03

Fairchild, R. M. (2012). Hold that TIGER! A collaborative service-learning academic-practice partnership with rural healthcare facilities. *Nurse Educator*, 37(3), 108–114. https://doi.org/10.1097/NNE.0b013e318250415b

Hooshmand, M., Foronda, C., Snowden, K., de Tantillo, L., & Williams, J. R. (2019). Transforming health care through meaningful doctor of nursing practice community partnerships. *Nurse Educator*, 44(3), 132–136. https://doi.org/10.1097/NNE.0000000000000577

Humphreys, J., Martin, H., Roberts, B., & Ferretti, C. (2004). Strengthening an academic nursing center through partnership. *Nursing Outlook*, 52(4), 197–202. https://doi.org/10.1016/j.outlook.2004.04.009

Kleinpell, R. M., Faut-Callahan, M., Carlson, E., Llewellyn, J., & Dreher, M. (2016). Evolving the practitioner-teacher role to enhance practice-academic partnerships: A literature review. *Journal of clinical nursing*, 25(5–6), 708–714. https://doi.org/10.1111/jocn.13017

Killeen, K. M., Rudy, D., Delaney, K. R., Kleinpell, R., Hinch, B., Barginere, C. (2015). Academic/service integration advances APRN practice. *Nurse Leader*, 13(2), 57–62, https://doi.org/10.1016/j.mnl.2015.01.009

Markaki, A., Prajankett, O. O., Shorten, A., Shirey, M. R., & Harper, D. C. (2021). Academic service-learning nursing partnerships in the Americas: a scoping review. *BMC Nursing*, 20(1), 179. https://doi.org/10.1186/s12912-021-00698-w

Norman, L., Wells, B., & Edwards, A. P. (2021). From policy to practice: A DNP student perspective. *Nursing Forum*, 56(3), 630–634. https://doi.org/10.1111/nuf.12582

Sadeghnezhad, M., Heshmati Nabavi, F., Najafi, F., Kareshki, H., & Esmaily, H. (2018). Mutual benefits in academic-service partnership: An integrative review. *Nurse Education Today*, 68, 78–85. https://doi.org/10.1016/j.nedt.2018.05.019

Shurson, L., Godfrey, T., Flamm, K., Bertsch, M., Broughton, E., & Prettyman, A. (2021). Utilizing academic–service partnerships to advance the care of veterans, *The Journal for Nurse Practitioners*, 17(5), 605–610. https://doi.org/10.1016/j.nurpra.2021.01.013

Sullivan-Marx, E. M., Bradway, C., & Barnsteiner, J. (2010). Innovative collaborations: A case study for academic owned nursing practice. *Journal of Nursing Scholarship: An Official Publication of Sigma Theta Tau International Honor Society of Nursing*, 42(1), 50–57. https://doi.org/10.1111/j.1547-5069.2009.01324.x

Thabault, P., Mylott, L., & Patterson, A. (2015). Describing a residency program developed for newly graduated nurse practitioners employed in retail health settings. *Journal of Professional Nursing:*

Official Journal of the American Association of Colleges of Nursing, 31(3), 226–232. https://doi.org/10.1016/j.profnurs.2014.09.004

Waldrop, J., Caruso, D., Fuchs, M. A., & Hypes, K. (2014). EC as PIE: Five criteria for executing a successful DNP final project. *Journal of Professional Nursing : Official Journal of the American Association of Colleges of Nursing, 30*(4), 300–306. https://doi.org/10.1016/j.profnurs.2014.01.003

Williams, T., Hande, K., & Kleinpell, R. (2022). Linking process improvement with DNP projects: Strategies to advance clinical leadership initiatives. *Nurse Leader, 20*(5), 444–450. https://doi.org/10.1016/j.mnl.2022.04.010

Wright, P. P., & Cranmer, J. N. (2018). Leveraging graduate academic-practice partnerships to transform health system outcomes. *Nursing Administration Quarterly, 42*(4), 324–330. https://doi.org/10.1097/NAQ.0000000000000311

Xippolitos, L. A., Marino, M. A., & Edelman, N. H. (2011). Leveraging academic-service partnerships: Implications for implementing the RWJ/IOM's recommendations to improve quality, access, and value in academic medical centers. *ISRN Nursing, 2011*, 731902. https://doi.org/10.5402/2011/731902

CHAPTER THIRTEEN Reflective Response

MARIE ANN MARINO AND KATE FITZPATRICK

We applaud Rader et al. in this chapter for amplifying the integral role nurses with a doctor of nursing practice (DNP) degree play in academic-service partnerships. Since the American Association of Colleges of Nursing (AACN) released its 2004 position statement calling for nurses with advanced degrees to provide higher levels of care and leadership to accelerate quality patient and population outcomes and mitigate the looming nurse faculty shortage, the number of schools/colleges of nursing offering DNP degrees has multiplied exponentially. With skills in the translation of evidence to practice, financial and strategic planning, information technologies, patient quality and safety, population health, advocacy and change theory, interprofessional collaborative practice, and systems-level leadership, among others, DNP graduates are expected to lead in healthcare delivery transformation, advance clinical practice, and serve as health policy advocates.

Since the inception of the DNP degree, nurses with DNPs have been filling pivotal roles in healthcare and academia. In addition to academic roles, DNPs serve at all levels, including traditional clinical roles (nurse practitioner, nurse anesthetist, clinical nurse specialist, or nurse midwife); nurse manager, supervisor, or practice administrator; and executive leaders in large healthcare settings and systems, including academic medical centers.

While much has been written about the role of DNPs in academic settings, the role of DNPs in practice settings, and in particular, academic-service partnerships, has not been widely explored. Academic-service partnerships serve as collaborative relationships between academic institutions and healthcare organizations whereby leveraging of resources, talents, and assets are optimized. The relationship between the practice setting and the academic setting is central to improving quality and patient outcomes, translating evidence into practice, developing innovative and nurse-led care models, addressing the nursing shortage and building a strong nursing workforce, and providing leadership, mentorship, and advocacy. In our opinion, the role of the DNP in academic, service partnerships and the strength of this relationship can be transformative.

Jefferson Health (JH) and Jefferson College of Nursing (JCN) have shared a long-standing academic-service affiliation, beginning with the creation of the Jefferson Medical College School of Nursing in 1891. Through a series of mergers and acquisitions, the clinical and academic divisions integrated, forming the foundation of the present integrated structure for the Jefferson enterprise. The emergence of COVID-19 created situations that were completely unprecedented, and it became evident that relying upon prior solutions and programming would not yield sufficient results. Using a formalized and strong academic-service partnership, JCN and JH collaborated to develop a shared vision. This vision leverages our relationship to develop innovative programming designed to strengthen nursing education, research, clinical practice and competency, to support nurse wellness, and to create a robust hiring pipeline. Led by Dr. Kate FitzPatrick (a DNP), jointly appointed as executive vice president and

Connelly Foundation chief nursing executive and professor and associate dean at JCN, and Dr. Marie Ann Marino, jointly appointed as dean and professor at JCN and vice president of nursing academic partnerships and innovation within JH, the partnership is committed to advancing nursing across the continuum. The partnership is under the day-to-day management of Dr. Beatrice Leyden (a DNP), senior vice president of nursing practice, learning and scholarship for JH and assistant professor, and Dr. Jennifer Bellot, JCN associate dean of academic practice integration. The unique contributions of DNPs as leaders, educators, mentors, change agents, practice innovators, and advocates are integral to the success of the partnership.

The presence of DNPs in the clinical setting greatly improves quality and patient outcomes and spurs practice changes to achieve them. DNPs are academically and experientially prepared to analyze data, identify areas for improvement, and develop strategies to enhance the quality of care. They are also acculturated to lead change initiatives and to influence policy at the organizational and system levels. These skills help to drive innovation and improve healthcare outcomes.

One of the primary roles of the DNP in academic-service partnerships is to bridge the gap between academia and clinical practice. DNPs are educated to translate research into practice and to implement evidence-based interventions that improve patient outcomes. This is a crucial skill as it ensures that the latest research findings and evidence are incorporated into clinical practice. DNPs are also highly skilled in mitigating barriers to evidence-based practice (EBP), such as inadequate knowledge and skills, staff resistance, and resistance in the organizational climate. In this role, DNPs serve as role models to new nurses entering the profession by highlighting the impact nurses can have on patient outcomes. As part of the JCN-JH partnership, five nurse scientist faculty have 0.2 of their time (full-time equivalent or FTE) dedicated to supporting research and EBP initiatives within JH, primarily working with DNP leaders on patient care units. Faculty effort costs are jointly supported by JCN and JH. The nurse scientist program has greatly enhanced the implementation of EBP and research at the bedside.

By virtue of their education and training, DNPs are skilled in the development and implementation of innovative and nurse-led care models that provide value and meet the needs of patients. With the transition from a volume- to value-based system of care, conventional assumptions about healthcare delivery must be challenged and a transformational shift in the way we think about healthcare delivery must be undertaken. It is precisely in this landscape that DNPs can drive system improvement, adaptive change, and increase stakeholder engagement. Skills in interprofessional collaboration position DNPs to work effectively across disciplines and to break down silos. Through improved communication among healthcare professions, team-based care models that position nurses as leaders, improve patient outcomes, and reduce workforce burden can be developed. These models can impact equitable care delivery by increasing access and improving patient outcomes for vulnerable populations. Further, through interdisciplinary teamwork, DNPs can help to address patient care concerns and organizational operational issues.

DNPs can play a pivotal role in addressing the nursing shortage. Through their work with universities and colleges, DNPs can expand nursing programs to ensure a robust pipeline of highly qualified, entry-level and advanced-practice nurses, nurse leaders, and nurse scientists. The JCN-JH partnership supports innovative, bidirectional programming to mutually benefit nurse retention and enrich student education. Service and academic leaders from JH and JCN regularly attend each other's shared governance and strategic planning meetings to discuss and facilitate workforce and strategic planning. This bidirectional participation has highlighted the role of the DNP in partnered initiatives such as RN early hiring, standardization of clinical ladders to include advanced degrees and preceptor service, and the nurse scientist program. This shared participation has been critical to the clinical staff's understanding and awareness of educational innovations and academic staff are more fully aware of practice changes in real time. Additionally, DNP-prepared JH nurses have been a critical source of clinical adjunct instructors within the JCN. The preference for JH-affiliated clinical adjunct faculty with a DNP has deepened JH's understanding of JCN's curriculum and standards. It has also increased JCN's understanding of JH and workforce needs and challenges.

Academic-service partnerships facilitate collaborative and informed development of curricula and programs. Specifically, JH and JCN have partnered to develop a DNP in executive leadership track, designed to ready master's-prepared nurses for roles in executive leadership across all care delivery sites and at the system level. The contributions of DNP-prepared nurse executives across JH ensured that the curriculum was cutting edge, relevant, and transformative. The JH-JCN partnership provides valuable opportunities for DNP students and graduates to hone their leadership skills and to advance their careers. The partnership also allows DNPs to work alongside other DNP-prepared nurse leaders, clinicians, and researchers, as well as other healthcare professionals, to develop, implement, and lead initiatives that drive change, improve quality of care, and innovate models of care.

DNPs are also a powerful agency for healthcare policy advocacy, activism, and change. With their advanced knowledge and expertise in these areas, DNPs are well positioned to influence healthcare policy at all levels. DNPs can advocate for policy changes at the local, state, and national levels that support the nursing profession, such as increased funding for nursing education and research and equitable reimbursement rates for nursing services. They can provide expert testimony and advise policymakers on key healthcare issues, such as access to care, patient safety, and healthcare equity.

Academic service partnerships bring numerous benefits to healthcare organizations and academic institutions and are an essential component of healthcare delivery. The role of the DNP in academic service partnerships is instrumental in driving healthcare delivery innovation, advancing nursing's evidence base, and critical to improving patient outcomes, enhancing the quality of care, and promoting evidence-based practice. The DNP's role as mentor, leader, and educator facilitates sharing of knowledge and expertise with other healthcare professionals ensuring that nursing practice is constantly evolving and transforming. DNP-prepared nurses within academic-service partnerships enhance the value and quality in health systems and play a vital role in the transformation of healthcare delivery.

REFERENCE

American Association of Colleges of Nursing. (2004). *AACN position statement on the practice doctorate in nursing.* http://www.aacn.nche.edu/DNP/pdf/DNP.pdf

CHAPTER FOURTEEN

Coaching in the DNP Executive Role: Linking Personal Development and Performance Enhances Leadership Athleticism

MICHAEL SMITH AND ROSALIE MAINOUS

The newly minted doctor of nursing practice (DNP) will face many challenges given the rapid state of change seen in the U.S. healthcare system, academia, and patient care. The public must be able to rely on the DNP to lead change in response to system fluctuations. Political pressures on policy generation, the need for quality and safety to be integrated into decision-making, and outcomes that affect the fiscal bottom line add a burden on the DNP graduate to perform at an elevated level consistently. One way to accomplish this goal is through an executive coach (EC).

Many of today's problems are amenable to the executive coaching relationship. Capitalizing on one's experience, moving out of a silo to add perspective, and receiving support to prevent personal burnout in the high-stress healthcare environment are all positive outcomes (Sagin, 2016). The EC can help with communication issues and conflict; having an independent, objective assessment and support has been found by most executives to be extremely valuable (McNally & Cunningham, 2010). Since 2020, critical professional nursing-related publications are driving professional practice and moving forward with an aggressive agenda, including identifying competencies for the DNP (both in practice and during the academic experience). Two publications are addressed below as they have implications for and demonstrate the value of an executive coaching relationship.

First, *The Essentials: Core Competencies for Professional Nursing Education* (AACN, 2021) states that advanced nursing roles or specialties must be founded on 10 domains, which are areas of competence. Domain 9, Professionalism, holds professional identity as core to the meeting of the competency. Professional identity allows for developing emotional intelligence, moral courage, and effective decision-making. It continually evolves from one's personal development through the development of others. Using a national think tank, four domains of professional identity for nursing were identified: values and ethics, leadership, discipline-specific knowledge gleaned from research and other disciplines, and comportment (Godfrey, 2022). While the Essentials guide nursing education, we posit that Domain 9 and professional identity are central to all elements of nursing, whether it be practice, education, policy development, entrepreneurship, or research. In a 2021 study, researchers found that two significant aspects of professional identity are linked to continuing a nursing career, which is critical in an acute and ever-expanding nursing shortage. Findings included belongingness (also a component of diversity, equity, and inclusion) and the ability to mentor future generations (Kristoffersen, 2021).

Professional identity is a component of leadership presence intrinsically. This area of investigation is booming and has been the focus of researchers across the health professions. The development of this identity and the adoption of professional precepts is part of what makes us nurses, physicians, physical therapists, or dentists. As we enter professional practice, it helps us know where our practice stops, and the subsequent profession's practice begins. It is also an area expanding as roles continue to evolve and parameters are defined. In the 1970s, registered nursing practice was much more restrictive than it is in the 2020s; the physician was most certainly the "captain of the ship." However, like nursing, the other health professions were still evolving. It was not unusual for nursing, as an example, to *dispense* medication, now the purview of the pharmacist. Regulatory practice boards, which exist to ensure the public's safety, have curtailed in some ways and expanded in others the professional practice arena for each health profession, while trying to define the overlap between the professions. We also now work as an interprofessional team for best practice. The COVID-19 pandemic elevated the sense of professional identity in nurses, especially for those not on the frontline versus those not on the frontline (Li et al., 2021).

A systematic review of the health professions' literature on professional identity measures was performed, and only two instruments had significant, psychometrically sound evidence (Matthew et al., 2019). Even those two only met some of the criteria. What was found was that most of the work has been qualitative, and what has been done has yet to be reported to have reliable and valid measures. Therefore, the interpretation of the literature to date must be cautionary. It is advised to take a fresh look at professional identity formation, which should start early in a student's educational process. A leader is often judged by their ethics, values, response to wrongdoing, professionalism, and code of conduct. Engendering public trust, focusing on strengths instead of weaknesses, and increasing socialization as a professional nurse are all fundamental to developing professional identity (Crigger & Godfrey, 2014) and contribute to leadership presence. Growth in these areas can be achieved through coaching.

The modern healthcare system must be flexible, agile, and innovative in a post-pandemic world. People's performance will drive success. Understanding the report, *The Future of Nursing 2020–2030: Charting a Path to Achieve Health Equity* (National Academies of Sciences, Engineering, and Medicine, 2021), recognizes the importance of the social determinants of health (SDOH), health equity, and health outcomes. This report outlines the role nurses must play, the outcomes that must be achieved, and the skill set necessary to accomplish these goals. For nurses to impact health equity, they must be prepared as leaders and action oriented. They must have organizational support and critical expertise to perform in a complex, continuously evolving system. Individuals can only perform at this level with the benefit of many resources over time, including mentors, coaches, experiential opportunity, and the development of a health equity lens.

Leadership competencies are promulgated by the American Association of Colleges of Nursing (AACN), Association of Nursing Leadership (AONL), Sigma Theta Tau International (STTI), and many other prominent professional associations, outlining outcomes a nursing leader must meet. Many leadership development programs exist that are noteworthy. But from a behavioral perspective, adding a coach to a leadership program, as the Society for Behavioral Medicine does, was highly rated by the participants as support for their role (Cheesbrough et al., 2020)

SPORTS AND BUSINESS LINK

"Coaching" has been part of sports for more than a century (Potrac et al., 2013). Sports serve as the first, if not the only, context for many people about the coach's role in leading a team. That image often includes a coach patrolling a sideline of a field or court, screaming at their players with a rolled-up paper, or writing on a chalkboard developing the perfect plan to win a game. However, sports coaches perform many more leadership functions than we see in the crowd or on television. In fact, sports provide many examples of leadership and performance that corporate America has adopted.

Former UCLA men's basketball coach John Wooden is one of the most successful coaches in collegiate sports history. UCLA, under Coach Wooden, won 10 national championships during the 1964–1975 seasons (Gallimore & Tharp, 2004). One would think at the surface that this sustained success was achieved through superior player talent or brilliant strategy. While players and strategy are essential, the success experienced by UCLA transcended multiple graduating classes, and there are many teams with talented players and coaches. How did Coach Wooden and UCLA build a dynasty for more than a decade? His behavioral framework was a catalyst and a role model for leaders in business and elsewhere.

Early in his life as a 24-year-old basketball coach, Wooden began to ponder what factors drove athletic success. Over the next 15 years, he compiled and revised his cornerstones and building blocks until he completed his "Pyramid of Success," shown in Figure 14.1 (*Pyramid of Success*, n.d.). The pyramid demonstrates values and traits that lead to "Competitive Greatness." The framework's innovation was the focus on the *journey* and not the *destination*. Wooden emphasized the importance of effort and preparation before the game and less on the outcome. To Coach Wooden, if a player did his best in the preparation, the results would be satisfactory regardless of whether it was a win or loss. This philosophy was unique in the sports landscape: "As long as you try your best, you are never a failure" (Wooden, 1997). The culture and accountability instilled with the pyramid proved to be enduring well past his UCLA tenure.

Coaching in business has existed since the 1950s (Ellinger & Kim, 2014). These early relationships took the form of apprenticeships as personal development. In the 1970s, coincidentally around the time of Wooden's retirement, executive coaching began to gain popularity as sporting concepts were integrated into the personal development work. Coaching in the business context focuses more on leadership behaviors, with many companies publishing organizational values and desired leadership competencies like the Pyramids of Success framework. It is standard now for organizations to subscribe to a tailored competency model integrated into their assessment and development processes. Coaches can play different roles depending upon the leader but all are in service of supporting leader behaviors to drive better personal and corporate performance. A significant focus in most coaching relationships involves ways to enhance the leader's team performance, such as improving communication, motivation, and quality. These discussions often have the coach guiding the leader to be a coach for their teams. Teams coached by their manager see improved relationships, engagement, and personal development (Jones et al., 2016), the hallmarks of a coaching relationship.

While coaching may have been used in some settings to work with an underperforming employee, it is a common and best practice to utilize a coaching resource for the highest-performing and most impactful leaders. Executive coaching is a vehicle for

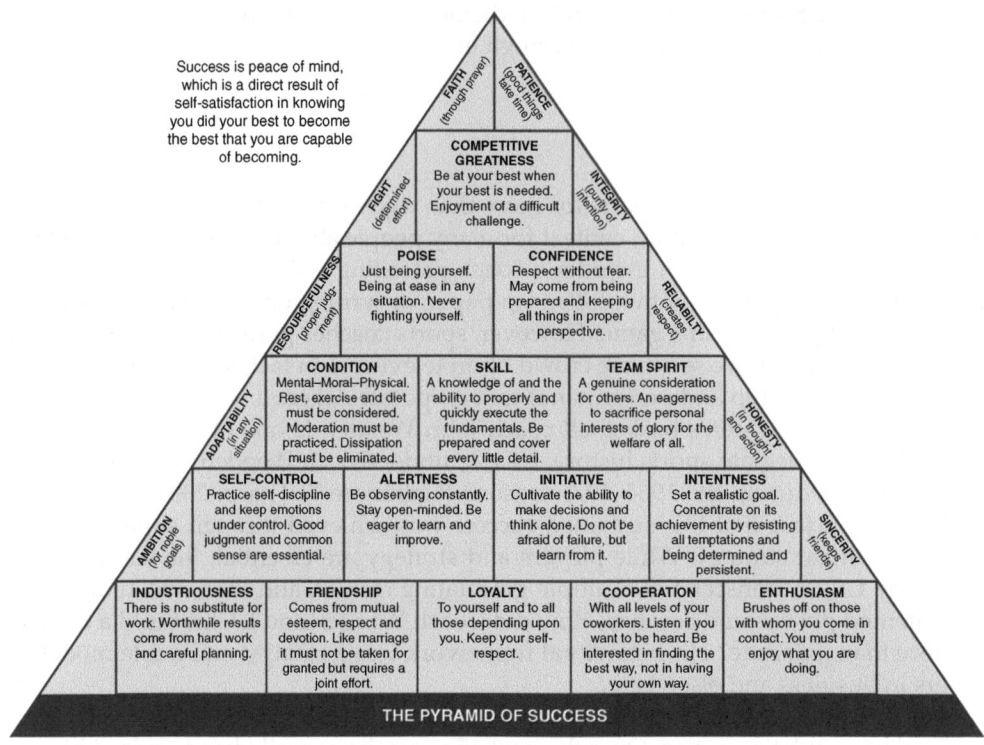

FIGURE 14.1   John Wooden's Pyramid of Success
Source: Pyramid of Success, n.d.

peak performance from a company's "leadership athletes." This integration of personal development and performance links to a sports context as the world's most successful athletes view their performance as determined by the quality of their training. Tennis player Serena Williams is perhaps the most accomplished tennis player of all time, winning 39 Grand Slam titles (*Tennis Grand Slam Titles*, n.d.). Serena says about her success: "Luck has nothing to do with it because I have spent many, many hours, countless hours, on the court working for my one moment in time, not knowing when it would come" (Devaney, 2020). Serena knows that her personal development is the predictor of her performance.

Executive coaching's impact on corporate performance is becoming increasingly apparent. Today, executive coaching is a $14 billion industry in the United States (IBIS World, n.d.). Many famous CEOs evangelize coaching as a critical contributor to their success. According to Bill Gates in his 2013 TED Talk:

> "Everyone needs a coach. It doesn't matter whether you're a basketball player, a tennis player, a gymnast, or a bridge player.... We all need people who will give us feedback. That's how we improve."

While coaching will always have a sports linkage, corporate America has embraced the practice as a critical performance driver. Why are the lessons learned from Coach Wooden and corporate America relevant to a healthcare or an academic environment? Like sports and business, healthcare and academia are results-based industries. The principal concern is the health and wellness of individuals, communities, and societies. Enhancing our ability to lead, communicate, and "coach" our teams is the best way to maximize patient outcomes.

WHAT IS EXECUTIVE COACHING?

Executive coaching, a somewhat misunderstood resource, often given to leaders to help them excel, has at its heart the development of one's strengths (Biswas-Diener, 2010). However, it sometimes elicits a negative response due to the lack of standardization, competencies, and operational definitions and the many who now label themselves "coaches" (D'Antonio, 2018).

There are four main support paradigms: consulting, mentoring, therapy, and coaching. Providing a consultation means helping the nurse leader reach a stated outcome. However, the difference between consulting and coaching is that the consultant provides information, assessments, and reports, and the consultant may become involved in the work of the business. "Consulting is defined as the practice of providing a third party with expertise on a matter in exchange for a fee" (https://www.consultancy.org/career/what-is-consulting, November 17, 2022). There is no reason to keep confidential what the employees share with them while doing business within the company. Mentorship, however, is a different kind of relationship, and some believe you cannot "assign" a mentor to someone. They would have you believe that a mentor-mentee relationships must develop organically; however, such relationships do involve trust and mutual respect, a meeting of the minds. While not all mentoring relationships work, our experience has been that many paired mentor-mentees have very productive, long-term relationships that are meaningful to both parties. Mentoring is the "transfer of role- or industry-specific knowledge from a more experienced mentor to a less experienced protégé" (McNally & Cunningham, 2010, p. 8). Therapy deals with long-term issues that require a look to the past to manage the present and the future. Coaching, specifically executive coaching, leads the nurse leader to the answers they hold within themself. Coaches help one reach a satisfactory conclusion through assessments, feedback, and reflection. The definition of coaching that is used by the Center for Creative Leadership (CCL) is "Partnering with someone else formally or informally, in thought-provoking and inquiry-based conversations intended to produce positive personal and professional changes" (CCL, 2018, p. 6). An EC keeps confidential all information garnered from the employee but may provide a summary written report based on outcomes to the employer. The relationship between the EC and the nurse leader is a safe one that allows for full disclosure without fear of retribution, and it should not matter if the employer is paying for the service contract or not, although this would typically be dealt with in the contracting process (ICF, 2021).

There are many broad coaching categories, including executive, academic, life, developmental, transitional, internal versus external, etc. In the world of coaches, anyone can hang out a shingle and charge what the market will bear. Hourly rates vary widely. With many types of coaches, there is no training, certification, compliance, regulatory mechanisms, policies, or credentialing. The school of hard knocks may be the foundation for a life coach practice, and they may excel as a result. Academic coaching has vital steps such as establishing a relationship, conducting an assessment, forming an action plan, evaluating, and revising based on the outcomes (Deiorio et al., 2016). Some coaches have been trained in a standard, approved curriculum, by master coaches, with experiential competence and a required number of sessions logged that meet the standard set by the International Coaching Federation, headquartered in Lexington, Kentucky. This nonprofit entity sets credentials, standards, and educational guidelines for coaches (www.coachingfederation.org). Another credentialing group, the National Consortium for Credentialing Health and Wellness Coaches, has developed standards for health and wellness coaching (Jordan et al., 2015). These credentials provide legitimacy but do not mean that those that are uncredentialed may not be stellar coaches and the right fit for you. Some of the best coaches have had training but have yet to see it necessary to pursue the credential. Their success in the field has been their validation.

The latest trend is team coaching, which requires a skilled practitioner that is more directive (ICF, 2020). Conflict resolution is integral to the model, and the interaction usually lasts months and leads to sustainability (ICF, 2020). D'Antonio (2018) lists some approaches used in coaching, including motivational interviewing, mindfulness, positive psychology tenets, neurolinguistic frameworks, and coaching based on science. Coaches can also be short-term focused with a direct coaching approach or more of a long-term focus that is developmental and challenges one's thinking (CCL, 2018).

Some may choose an internal or external coach, depending on the situation. Internal coaches work for the employer, have had some training, can have more impact across the organization, and may be the only fiscally viable option (usually a much less expensive approach). The external coach, however, can build trust in the process and should be used for senior team members (Schalk & Landeta, 2017). External coaches are generally viewed as instilling more trust in the process. Positive psychology coaching (PCC) has provided many instruments for use in the coaching relationship based on the science of positive psychology. Several were classified and tested for their use in PCC. Strength spotting is a handy tool, as is journaling, guided self reflection, and goal setting (Richter et al., 2021).

There are leadership interventions that have an element of coaching. Internal members of an organization can be identified for development as coaches; it has been suggested that it takes 6 months to be proficient with this new skill set (Grant, 2010). Utilizing a theory of coaching-based leadership, 41 executives were split into two groups. One group received feedback based on a baseline assessment, a workshop, and three executive coaching sessions. The intervention group was given a program based on strengths conducted by ECs. Both groups improved from baseline statistically but did not differ statistically between them, possibly due to the instrumentation relying on self-reports. When the study was complete, some in the control group received the strengths-based intervention due to its perceived value. The intervention group improved on coaching-based leadership skills, the development of psychological capital, work engagement, and performance (Zuberbuhler et al., 2020).

WHEN IS COACHING MOST USEFUL?

Transitions and change are a constant for the DNP. Transitioning to a new job, role, or project requires an assessment of one's strengths and weaknesses and how to be one's best. Within executive coaching, helping an individual through career transitions is a common theme. One qualitative study sought to determine which coaching techniques contribute most to "transformative individual learning" (Terblanche, 2021, p. 11) during a transition. Nurse leaders value new knowledge that allows for reflection and experimentation. Career transition insights are gained when the nurse leader can use what they have learned experientially and then immediately reflect to gain new insight (Terblanche, 2021). Providing actual knowledge to the nurse leader is not embraced by all but seems highly valued by the recipient.

Many situations arise when the need for an EC becomes readily apparent. Among those, one of the first encountered will be the ability to navigate conflict, which can be significantly enhanced through executive coaching. ECs are trained to ask the right questions and know how to probe, elicit, and provide feedback (Sherman, 2019). In what is often perceived as a muddy, tangled quagmire, an EC can tease out the pertinent points and assist the individual in developing a plan to defuse the situation. *Carefronting*,

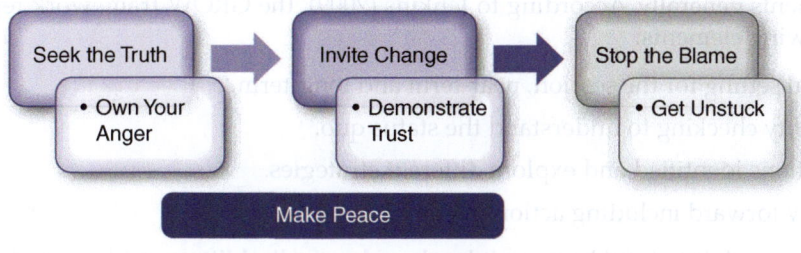

FIGURE 14.2 Carefronting

especially useful in healthcare settings, is a method to manage conflict that is used by some coaches and has the parameters shown in Figure 14.2.

One of the biggest challenges is the alignment of the DNP's background and experience with the needs of the practice partners. There is a critical need for DNP graduates to have a broader understanding of the larger institution, the healthcare environment, and system-level factors at play (Wright & Cranmer, 2018, digital version). Conversations within these environments can fall back on basic tenets practiced within a coaching relationship and part of the coach's repertoire that can be role modeled. For example, use words that have a positive impact or connotation on the organizational system.

Some DNPs will move into either academic leadership or practice leadership. An EC, mentors, and other resources are extremely valuable in that transition. A detailed case study of an MD who was moving into an institutional leadership position with a model of leadership coaching demonstrated critical transitions that occurred at timed intervals. In the first 6 months, communication was emphasized, as well as procedures, policies, and identifying strengths and weaknesses. Both coach and MD or nurse leader can see this as a co-created experience. During coaching in the second 6 months, professional identity solidifies, fragilities are exposed, and biases are examined. An examination of the importance of relational expertise and managing one's emotions become apparent (Rathmall et al., 2019). These experiences may easily translate to another practice doctorate, the DNP.

■ WHAT TO EXPECT?

While there are many different coaching approaches, they have similar process steps (Thach, 2002). Coaching engagements generally begin with a discussion between the coach and nurse leader regarding the catalyst for a coaching engagement and potential desired outcomes. The second phase would involve data collection to validate the initial discussions and inform the formal development plan. Data can be both qualitative and quantitative. Qualitative data would be detailed self-assessment questionnaires and interviews with the nurse leader stakeholders such as the manager, peers, direct reports, external partners, and even family and friends. Quantitative data could incorporate the use of psychological assessments. The last phase would involve coaching sessions discussing where there are opportunities for the nurse leader to experiment with new behaviors. The coach needs to display many competencies during these sessions. This chapter focuses on the most prevalent aspects of coaching engagements.

Many formalized models incorporate these process steps, with GROW being one of the most popular frameworks. Developed by Graham Alexander, Max Landsberg, and John Whitmore, GROW was initially intended to serve as a coaching conversation tool (Sir John Whitmore, 2009). Now that framework serves as the basis for coaching engagements generally. According to Jenkins (2009), the GROW framework represents the following elements:

- **G**: Goal setting for the session, near-term and long-term.
- **R**: Reality checking to understand the status quo.
- **O**: Options identified and explore different strategies.
- **W**: Way forward including action planning.

This framework is helpful because it has broader applicability outside a coaching relationship. The process of identifying a goal, the context in which the goal needs to be accomplished, identifying different paths available, and executing the plan, can be utilized in decision-making and other crucial conversations. It also serves as an available toolkit for managers when coaching their teams.

Data collection is essential in the coaching process due to the potential lack of self-awareness. Psychological studies have consistently shown that people frequently have inaccurate perceptions of themselves and how others see them. We tend to have a more optimistic perception of ourselves than others, making it more likely that we will disagree with constructive but critical feedback (Cannon & Witherspoon, 2005). Perhaps no form of data is more crucial than feedback from internal and external colleagues. Feedback from individuals we work with is one of the best ways to increase self-awareness of our strengths and development opportunities (Thach, 2002). This form of data collection, known as 360 feedback, can be facilitated differently.

A coach will work with the nurse leader to develop a list of people whose perspectives would be valuable. This list can range from a few individuals to 15 or more. It is important that the individuals selected are a realistic representation of their ecosystem and not just their "cheerleaders." Often, the best feedback comes from those with whom we have had past challenges. The EC either administers an online questionnaire or meets with individuals in person. The questions asked are usually tailored based on the nurse leader's coaching goals. The most important aspect of this work is the absolute confidentiality of the participant responses. The freedom to provide feedback as honestly as possible is dependent on anonymity. Sometimes, feedback is grouped by participant type, for example, peers or direct reports, to gather themes from different vantage points. 360 feedback does have disadvantages. It is not objective data. The participants offer subjective perspectives that rely on the coach to reconcile where biases may exist. A skilled coach relies on the power of inquiry and maintains professional skepticism to ensure that a critical perspective is not fully transparent or missed. This data gathering technique is most useful when the nursing leader has been an existing employee at the organization, not for new leaders who are unknown.

Another common source of data collection is psychometric assessments. One popular tool is the Myers-Briggs Type Indicator or MBTI. The MBTI measures personality dimensions to analyze preferences in behavior, decision-making, and communication (*MBTI Basics*, n.d.). While MBTI is a popular tool, a coach can be certified in many tools with different use cases. In addition to personality, tools attempt to describe and measure factors such as thinking style, communication preferences, conflict traits, behavioral tendencies, core competencies, and many more. These assessments range in scientific validity. Regardless of whether the tool is scientifically valid, they can be useful to spur conversation and self-reflection. A coach will incorporate these assessments with 360 feedback and self-assessment questionnaires to form a complete picture of a person's current reality. The coach and nurse leader then discuss the data obtained and reconcile this information with the nurse leader's initial self-assessment to incorporate into a development plan. See Table 14.1 for an illustrative development plan.

TABLE 14.1 Illustrative Development Plan

Development Goal	Action Plan	Outcome
Enhanced Decision-making	• Approach smart risk taking with a "fail forward" mindset; if we must fail, do it quickly and ensure the learning from it is communicated broadly. • Identify an important upcoming decision you must make where you feel you lack some clarity or needed information. Chart deliberate, small steps you will take to arrive at that decision; make connections to prior experiences that will assist you in feeling comfortable moving quickly. • Add a recurring weekly block to your calendar that is dedicated to working on the strategic components of your job. Make this time as prioritized as any meeting on your calendar.	Improve decision process, pace, and quality; manage time to grow strategic abilities
Political Acumen	• Understand and join the informal network and participate by keeping people informed; "pre-meetings" can help seeking to understand parties' positions and concerns. • Remember that you do not need to undertake opportunities alone. Make it a collaborative effort by asking valued coworkers to help you out. Seeking feedback and opinions of others will build trust, strengthen relationships, and help close any existing perception/reality gap; identify and execute a new formal routine of feedback gathering, • When listening to the ideas of others, try to find the merit of their ideas. Ask questions and work together to ensure that ideas include a practical implementation and result. Repeat someone else's message back to them in your own words to ensure understanding and demonstrate empathy.	More comprehensive understanding of potential obstacles to goal accomplishment (people, process, resource, or otherwise); increased partnership throughout organization; better perspective taking to arrive at mutually satisfactory outcomes.
Coaching and Developing the Team	• Work to build capacity in self and team by leading with questions not opinions; provide more detail on rationale and potential options when guiding team. • Focus on maintaining open lines of communication and work on "delegating to develop." Monitor and minimize tendency to "close the door" and do things yourself. • Restructure individual and team meetings to allow for maximum time allocation to strategic dialogue regarding coaching, problem solving.	Build skills & leadership capability in your team; free up your own time for more strategic leadership; improve personal coaching skillset.

The nurse leader and the coach partner to create development plans. While these plans address the original identified goals, it is not uncommon for new goals to emerge because of the data collection process. Development plans can be goal-oriented or process-oriented (Williams & Lowman, 2018). Goal-oriented plans focus on accomplishing specific outcomes, whereas process-oriented plans focus more on interpersonal skills. Either focus can lead to a successful coaching engagement (Williams & Lowman, 2018). Once a nurse leader has identified their development focus areas and specific tactics to employ, it is common for an alignment meeting with the nurse leader's supervisor to occur. Alignment with the supervisor allows the nurse leader to solicit support during the engagement. It also creates transparency in measuring the development plan's success.

Once the development plan is finalized, coaching moves forward with clarity. Coaches use questions as a vehicle to both challenge and support the nurse leader during their journey to maximize their potential. Coaches rely on the power of inquiry to accelerate learning and growth in the nurse leader. Questions can take many forms, including the following (Cox, 2013):

- Information seeking related to facts, actions, events, thoughts, feelings
- Exploratory to probe scenarios, options, convictions
- Clarification to check for understanding

As the goal is to increase the nurse leader's self-awareness and capacity to adopt new behaviors and skills, the coach rarely tells a nurse leader what to do. Using powerful questions enables the nurse leader to learn for themselves more substantively. Depending upon the experience level of the nursing leader, the coach may lean less on questions and more on conversation as a tool. Often, more senior nursing leader coaches play an advisory role, helping the leader think through options and approaches.

This phase of the coaching journey introduces the human side of change. People vary in terms of how quickly and significantly they are adaptable to change. A coach and nurse leader will usually discuss their prior history of change during the feedback process, but if the nurse leader is new to coaching, this will be a different experience. Langley et al. (2009) summarize critical areas from the fields of psychology and change management that are useful to consider in a coaching engagement:

1. People are different. Our learning styles and thinking preferences impact how to introduce change. Data collected during psychometric assessments and the 360 processes can clarify the best communication method.
2. Discovering motivation is paramount. Motivation drives behavior and linking leaders' and teams' work to motivation can have lasting benefits. There are two types of motivation: intrinsic and extrinsic. Intrinsic motivation refers to motivation from within us related to the task, like values alignment, while extrinsic motivation is from an outside influence, such as a reward (Carsrud & Brannback, 2011). Linking to intrinsic motivation tends to have more lasting benefits.
3. Attract people to change. Identifying all the technical and normative elements involved is essential to seeing the entire system and ensuring the nurse leader drives the change process. Change does not occur in a silo. As you go through your coaching journey, you need to engage others in your change process. The participants in your 360 processes are generally an excellent place to start.

Both the coach and the nurse leader considering the human side of change will result in the best probability that the development plan will result in its proper execution and sustainability.

COMMON FOCUS AREAS

While every coaching engagement and development plan is individually tailored, common focus areas emerge as leaders face similar challenges across settings. This section will highlight some of the more common focus areas for leaders working with an EC.

Emotional Intelligence

Intuitively, more than technical and operational acumen are necessary to be successful. So-called "soft skills" such as motivating and inspiring, building relationships, navigating conflict, or stress management are critical to a high-performing leadership athlete. These soft skills are sometimes called our emotional intelligence, or "EQ." The term has been used in various forums for decades. However, psychologists in the 1980s became open to forms of intelligence other than the Intelligence Quotient, or IQ, which represents our cognitive or rational ability (Chan & Mallett, 2011). Daniel Goleman propelled emotional intelligence (EQ) into the mainstream in the mid-1990s. Every successful leader has some EQ. Emotional leadership styles dictate success, and those unable to navigate this territory, self-regulate, and improve their self-awareness are destined to have a short-lived career (Goleman et al., 2001). Executive coaching, in general, is thought to facilitate the development of emotional intelligence (D'Antonio, 2018).

The first area a coach will focus on for EQ is emotional awareness. We must understand what we do and why we do it. Doing this requires being aware of your emotions at the moment. Emotions are neither positive nor negative, so understanding them without passing judgment can be challenging. Becoming more in tune with the physical reaction to certain emotions and identifying the people or situations that trigger you create a foundation for being more intentional about your reactions (Stein, 2011). Often a coach will suggest keeping a journal to write down your emotions so you can spot patterns and work on a plan to anticipate similar situations differently.

Once you are more self-aware, managing yourself becomes the focus. Self-management requires using your emotional awareness to be intentional about your behavior. Self-management enables you to tailor your communication to people and situations, regulate emotions when necessary, and dial back urges so near-term impulses do not hinder longer-term goals (Stein, 2011). Coaches may explore self-management techniques such as pausing before reacting, asking a question to allow time for composure, or taking slow, deep breaths. Gratitude can also be helpful. Thinking of a person or situation you are grateful for can help ease stressful moments.

Once your emotions are more under your control, a coach will then focus with you on others' emotions. Being able to assess the emotions of others represents an essential component of EQ (Stein, 2011). It requires being open to other viewpoints and being completely present to listen and observe. A coach may work with nurse leaders on techniques such as reading body language and nonverbal cues, being intentional about time and place when communicating, and asking clarifying questions to ensure alignment during a crucial conversation.

Last, these EQ skills then allow for enhanced relationships. Relationships are critical to personal and professional success, and a coach may focus on forming more robust networks, managing conflicts, and effective communication across different settings and personality types (Stein, 2011). A coach may have you practice relationship techniques such as identifying trust barriers, being vulnerable, giving and receiving feedback, and being transparent regarding your thought process.

Individual and Organizational Alignment

Enhancing self-awareness is critical to any coaching journey. Some engagements involve identifying your personal values system and leadership style. While understanding yourself first is crucial, you must also understand whether your organization has a culture aligned with your preferences. An organization's values are an essential driver of its culture. The values that count are what the organization lives, rewards, and promotes, not the inscription on lobby doors or paperweights (Bolman & Deal, 2017). Understanding the integration of self and organization is essential to unlocking the maximum organizational effectiveness and individual performance. One helpful framework to diagnose these factors is the competing values framework developed by the University of Michigan (Cameron, n.d.). This framework creates four dimensions based on the rate of change and autonomy compared with an internal or externally focused orientation. Based on the desired quadrant, culture, values, and leadership traits are shown that maximize effectiveness (see Figure 14.3). The optimal traits in each quadrant represent extremes, so understanding what you and your organization's current situation is vital to developing a game plan to maximize your performance and development. A coach would help you diagnose your organization's quadrant and areas of alignment and gaps with your values and preferred leadership approach. What is noteworthy is that culture and values systems are not static. A constant evaluation of yourself and the organization is required to ensure alignment. The role of a leader sometimes is to navigate the conflicts that emerge between value systems and emerging technical and institutional demands (Besharov & Khurana, 2015). The coach can be an effective sounding board to explore conflicts when they emerge.

The Coaching Journey Is a Learning Journey

Even when you are aligned with your organization's culture, it is essential to consider the broader organizational environment in which you operate. It is also essential to consider the coaching journey as a learning journey. As you experiment and practice with your coach, learning new behaviors and skills will not occur in a vacuum. According to Lave and Wenger (1991), learning is not a separate process. We do not turn learning on and off. Learning integrates into our everyday practices within our specific context. This perspective posits that thoughts and behaviors arise from cultures and social practices (Turner & Nolan, 2015). Recognizing the role of our environment in shaping our learning and actions is a critical insight that can accelerate progress. This everyday learning experience involves participation with people and information continually. Therefore, our learning and personal development do not have an "end." It becomes a trajectory we follow daily (Greeno & Gresalfi, 2008). Coaches frequently have nurse leaders construct a stakeholder map to understand environmental influences on performance or have the nurse leader document personal and department goals relative to broader strategic initiatives. This sheds light on broader organizational dynamics that may impact personal learning. Coaching sessions will often unpack events through a lens of the environment's role in what transpired, the corresponding learning, and the appropriate game plan for future similar events.

Political Acumen

Understanding that our performance is influenced by the organizational culture in which we participate, an essential skill for leaders is advocating and advancing agendas or policy changes. Having good ideas is not enough. A coach will work with their nurse

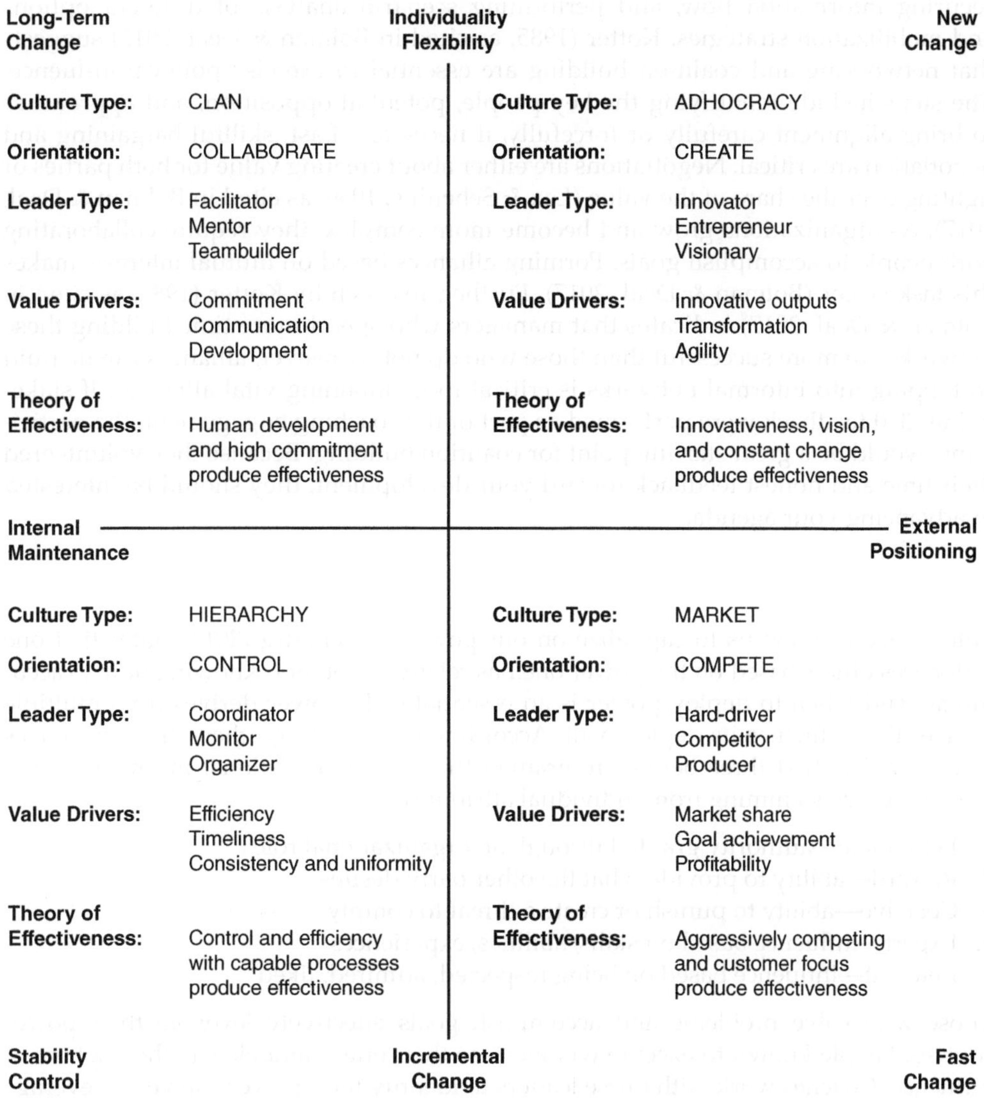

Long-Term Change	**Individuality Flexibility**		**New Change**
Culture Type:	CLAN	**Culture Type:**	ADHOCRACY
Orientation:	COLLABORATE	**Orientation:**	CREATE
Leader Type:	Facilitator Mentor Teambuilder	**Leader Type:**	Innovator Entrepreneur Visionary
Value Drivers:	Commitment Communication Development	**Value Drivers:**	Innovative outputs Transformation Agility
Theory of Effectiveness:	Human development and high commitment produce effectiveness	**Theory of Effectiveness:**	Innovativeness, vision, and constant change produce effectiveness
Internal Maintenance			**External Positioning**
Culture Type:	HIERARCHY	**Culture Type:**	MARKET
Orientation:	CONTROL	**Orientation:**	COMPETE
Leader Type:	Coordinator Monitor Organizer	**Leader Type:**	Hard-driver Competitor Producer
Value Drivers:	Efficiency Timeliness Consistency and uniformity	**Value Drivers:**	Market share Goal achievement Profitability
Theory of Effectiveness:	Control and efficiency with capable processes produce effectiveness	**Theory of Effectiveness:**	Aggressively competing and customer focus produce effectiveness
Stability Control	**Incremental Change**		**Fast Change**

FIGURE 14.3 The Competing Values Framework for Culture, Leadership, Effectiveness, and Value Drivers

Source: Cameron (n.d.). An introduction to competing values framework, *Haworth*.

leader on the best mechanism to take the idea to execution in the given environment. This work is done through understanding and embracing your organization's politics. Admittedly, the word "politics" often comes with negative connotations. However, politics are not negative. They are how organizations make decisions and allocate scarce resources when parties have competing interests. Often, managers are one of two extremes in organizational politics, either naïve or cynical (Kotter, 1985, as cited by Bolman & Deal, 2017). A coach will work with you to formulate a plan to increase your political acumen. The outcome of your plan will create a healthier political mindset between those extremes.

So, what do we mean when we say political acumen? According to Pichault (1993, as cited in Bolman & Deal, 2017), this skill includes identifying influence holders, securing information flow, and performing scenario analysis of different options and mobilization strategies. Kotter (1985, as cited in Bolman & Deal, 2017) suggests that networking and coalition building are essential to exercise political influence. The steps include identifying the key people, potential opposition, and approaches to bring alignment carefully or forcefully, if necessary. Last, skillful bargaining and negotiation are critical. Negotiations are either about creating value for both parties or fighting over the share of the value (Lax & Sebenius, 1986, as cited in Bolman & Deal, 2017). As organizations grow and become more complex, they require collaborating with people to accomplish goals. Forming alliances based on mutual interests makes this task easier (Bolman & Deal, 2017). Further, research by Kotter (1982, as cited in Bolman & Deal, 2017) indicates that managers who spend more time building these networks are more successful than those who do not. However, alliances can be fluid so tapping into informal networks is critical to maintaining vital alliances. If stakeholder 360 feedback were performed as part of the coaching engagement, the participants would be a great starting point for coalition building. Because they volunteered their time and honest feedback toward your development, they should be interested in advancing your agenda.

Power

Political skills allow us to capitalize on our power. Lunenburg (2012) states that one influences others based on the power one has relative to others. Knowing how to accumulate and when to deploy power is an essential skill. Power derives from multiple sources that influence its deployment. According to Lunenburg, there are five sources of power. The first three below are granted through organizational means, with the remaining two stemming from individual attributes:

1. Legitimate—authority granted through an organizational role
2. Reward—ability to provide what the other party desires
3. Coercive—ability to punish or create a threat to comply
4. Expert—influence based on skills, abilities, experiences
5. Referent—influence based on being respected, admired, liked

Those who solve problems and accomplish goals effectively leverage their power sources. People known to execute will increase their brand and elevate their sphere of influence. Coaches work with nurse leaders to identify their power sources to leverage them effectively. It is worth noting that expert and referent power tend to be more long-lasting and effective, but all can be effective in advancing one's agenda.

CONVERSATION PLANNING AND OVERCOMING BIAS

A common topic for a coaching session is planning or reviewing a critical conversation. Establishing relationships and using political acumen occur through discourse. Planning conversation strategies and even role-playing are common coaching topics during sessions. One good frame to analyze conversations is each party's position relative to the conversation. Harre and Van Langenhove (1991) probe language and power structures through positioning and conversations. Positioning often is a function of our power source in our environment, which influences the strategy we employ to achieve our desired outcome. According to them, conversations are the foundations of social activity, and all conversations involve positioning. Stone et al. (2010) discuss that each conversation has three distinct layers that we are not always aware of: (a) what took place, (b) people's feelings, and (c) people's identity or self-image. To plan and then deconstruct a conversation, they suggest we examine what is said and what went unsaid. During conversation strategy sessions, coaches probe each party's power source and positioning. These strategy sessions include scenario planning to anticipate where conversations may lead to build confidence ahead of the meeting. Afterwards, these techniques help nurse leaders unpack conversations that help the current situation and build skills for the next.

As we think about conversation planning, a coach will challenge nurse leaders' assumptions to ensure they use a sports expression, "seeing the field clearly." Everyone has cognitive biases that impact decision-making, communication, and relationships (Bazerman, 2001). While biases are powerful, we also know that mental models are fluid. We can intentionally create a new belief we do not currently hold (Senge et al., 1994). A tool for more effective communication is the ladder of inference (Argyris, 1990, as detailed in Senge et al., 1994). This tool recognizes that our heuristics form beliefs continuously reinforced from select data based on our experience. This heuristic influences how we see the field and engage with others. Senge et al. (1994) offer a sequence of events that occur in our conscious and subconscious when dealing with the external environment (see Figure 14.4):

1. Experience occurs—Objective data as you would record on video.
2. Individual selects—We select experiences based on preconceived notions, mindset, or present bias.
3. Meaning is made—Selected data filters through a lens of our beliefs, and we make sense of the experience.
4. Assumptions are made—The sense we make drives us toward assuming motives and facts.
5. Conclusion formed—We believe we have assessed the situation.
6. Beliefs adopted—Another data set is formed and added to our belief system, driving future behavior.
7. Action taken—We act and feel confident based on the perceived accurate processing of the events.

Awareness of this cycle of events is powerful when planning a conversation to influence others and advance your agenda. We need to see things as they are to act most productively. Senge et al. (1994) share a three-step process to aid this effort: *reflection, advocacy,* and *inquiry*. *Reflection* involves self-awareness of your mindset based on potential biases identified through the ladder of inference tool. *Advocacy* involves ensuring the other party is aware of your thinking and the substance of your position. When advocating your viewpoint, "I" statements are helpful to avoid the other party feeling defensive. For example, rather than saying, "You did that on purpose, which was so frustrating!" say, "when that situation happened, it left me feeling frustrated." This form of advocacy will encourage a more productive conversation. *Inquiry* involves probing for the substance of the other party's position. Typical questions could involve, "This is how I see this. What am I missing?" These practical conversation skills have utility across many leadership settings. See Case Study #2 for an example of where these tools could be implemented.

Harnessing Diversity, Equity, and Inclusion (DEI)

When we talk about diversity, we discuss *differences*. Diversity is the differences that impact our interactions with each other and our relationships. These differences can be actual or perceived and relate to both the visible and invisible (Nkomo et al., 2019). Diversity in teams and organizations creates the potential to harness complementary perspectives. It is a necessary raw material to achieve the highest performance potential.

336 ▪ III: OPERATIONALIZING ROLE FUNCTIONS

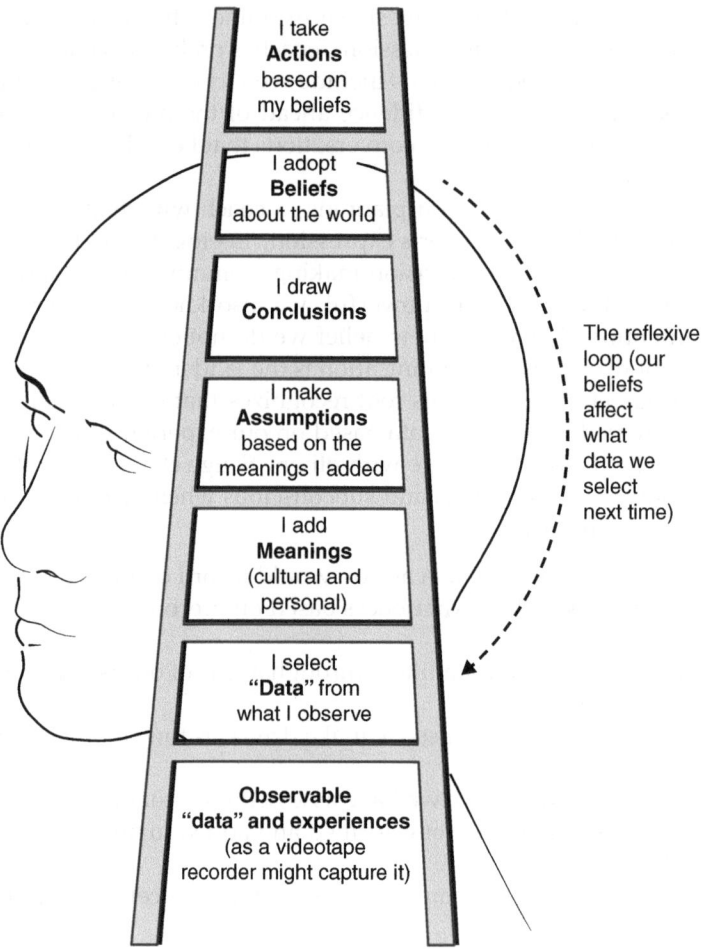

FIGURE 14.4 Ladder of Inference

Source: Senge, P., Kleiner, A., Roberts, C., Ross, R., Smith, B. (1994). *The Fifth discipline fieldbook: Strategies and tools for building a learning organization*. Currency, Doubleday.

Having a diverse team is just the start. It merely creates the foundation for success. To capitalize on that foundation, an environment must allow everyone to show up as the best version of themselves and utilize their strengths (Shore et al., 2018). A coach will work with the nurse leader on how to be an inclusive leader. Inclusive leaders ensure that people are comfortable being their most authentic selves and speaking their minds. A critical difference between diversity and inclusion is that inclusion can be more challenging. We know it when we see it *if we are looking*. The first step in leading inclusively is to be intentional. Pay attention to who is invited to meetings. Pay attention to who is speaking at meetings. Pay attention to whose ideas are celebrated and whose ideas are ignored. Nevertheless, inclusiveness can feel amorphous, also. Behavior that excludes some does not impact others the same way. At a minimum, leaders can be comfortable and supportive of differences (Shore et al., 2018). Finally, being equitable does not mean treating everyone equally. It means treating them fairly. Some people will need more or different things to be successful. A coach will work with the leader on tailoring approaches to individual team members.

A challenge for nursing leaders can be where DEI ranks as a priority in your organization. DEI is a stated focus for most organizations, but it is generally competing with other priorities that are more immediate and easier to measure. Organizations lack endurance because of leadership changes, short-term incentives, or business crises. We are asked to do too many things with too few resources to do it all. Lacking focus impacts initiatives with clear financial impact, let alone initiatives like DEI, where the financial impact is not always clear. The research on links between DEI and results is mixed (Kochan et al., 2003). This underperformance is due to poor execution of DEI initiatives. The good news is that leading inclusively can be improved organically, even if it is not the primary focus. A successful DEI strategy synergizes with other cultural initiatives, such as creating a psychologically safe environment (Guillaume et al., 2013).

Leadership Presence

When you present yourself to others, you are quickly "sized up." First impressions are essential. There are six categories of nonverbal communication that an EC can help you become more aware of and manage effectively (McNally & Cunningham, 2010). First, your *body movements* are significant and include such things as your facial expressions, which can often be interpreted differently in different cultures. Listening, openness to the other individual, and a relaxed stance indicate your interest in the other. *Touch* is perceived differently in different cultures, and some texts will help guide you in this haptic, for example, *Kiss, Bow, or Shake Hands* by Morrison and Conway (2006). *Voice* or speech can provide insight into emotion, attitude, or authority. *Use of Space* indicates the individual's boundaries and is part of the communication style. *Time* can be cultural or can be dictated by your professional environment. Are you on time, or are you early? Do you make people wait to see you? And finally, *appearance* is part of the nonverbal complex. How are you dressed? Are tattoos permissible in your environment? If not, how do you communicate with those external to your company? Grooming, attention to detail, and jewelry are all considered (McNally & Cunningham, 2010), and an EC can address all facets of the nonverbal complex. Diversity, equity, and inclusion have opened the door to more acceptance of different styles of dress and grooming. However, we are not where we need to be broadly, so it is essential to be mindful of industry or sector norms. Recognizing that we are not where we need to be, nursing leaders should advocate for the broadest possible inclusivity within these norms instead of narrowly interpreting them.

BRINGING EXECUTIVE COACHING TO THE LEADERSHIP TEAM

When building the leadership team, individuals with varying perspectives and skill sets are sought. Each will come to the team from a different starting point in their leadership journey. Each would benefit from an EC in the formative stages of a leadership trajectory and should be advocated for by the leader. Strategic outlays to support policies enhance the institutional climate and readiness for change (Guerrero & Kim, 2013). A baseline assessment of leadership gaps should be performed, and with the assistance of an EC, these gaps can be addressed for each, fleshing out their abilities for a fully functioning team. Every leadership team is different and has different strengths and weaknesses. A team climate inventory is an instrument often used in leadership team scenarios to identify areas that need improvement and those that are working well. The form is anonymous and can tease out comments that team members are unwilling to vocalize due to perceived negative consequences (Jones & Gorell, 2015). The best thing a leader can do is be surrounded by individuals who shore up their shortcomings and give honest feedback to the leader. The new leader who assumes an already established team will need to learn to make necessary changes diplomatically without demoralizing the remaining team members. Their EC can help them through this emotion-laden process. The willingness to support change, the ability to remain agile, maintaining a focus on goal setting, and the promotion of self-efficacy are all challenges that can be addressed in a successful coach-nurse leader relationship (Theeboom et al., 2017).

Readiness

When selecting a coach, there are certain traits that one should seek: the mutual feeling of trust, empathy, transparency, predictability, reliability, benevolence, and integrity (Terblanche et al., 2022).

In most case study scenarios, communication is an issue. Trusting your coach and allowing for an honest assessment is fundamental to the relationship and the only way to move forward. The coach must ask the right questions; you must provide illuminating answers. Both you and the coach need to be active listeners. This means being fully present, allowing for silence, and addressing open-ended questions (Sherman, 2019). Another common issue addressed within a coaching relationship is managing conflict or ethical issues that may arise, or sometimes both. Partnering with your coach is an essential technique and component of the ICF competencies (ICF, 2021).

You must be ready to be coached. This may be stating the obvious, but if you do not believe in the technique, lack trust, and are unwilling to co-create and define what needs to be accomplished, investing in an EC may not be the best use of resources. There are four signs that a nurse leader is not ready for coaching. According to Brubaker and Mitchell (2018), a lack of self-awareness and an unwillingness to own a problem may indicate a lack of receptivity. In addition, an unwillingness to book a session because you are trying to find just the right fit or you need help finding the time demonstrates a lack of buy-in. Finally, some fundamental, long-held beliefs may be challenged, which could be fear-producing and generate defensive behavior (Brubaker & Mitchell, 2018). Each nurse leader must embrace the value of EC and be willing to engage in receiving a benefit, especially given the time and money investment necessary.

To have a successful coaching relationship, there must be trust. You must trust the individual as well as the process. In a military setting where there were 74 coaching pairs, the ability to establish rapport, mutual trust, and commitment led to positive coaching outcomes (Boyce et al., 2010). The relationship between the coach and nurse leader is fundamental to the success of the coaching experience. This trust does not seem to be predicated on similarity in gender or otherwise perceived similarity. In an international study, there was insignificant effect on outcomes from similarity and perceived similarity did not impact career satisfaction (Bozer et al., 2015).

Does My Coach Need Nursing or Healthcare Experience?

Like most contextual questions, the answer to whether your coach needs nursing or healthcare experience is "it depends." Research has shown that while the coach-nurse leader match is essential, improved results are driven by rapport building and trust. Shared experiences and credibility were relevant only if they enhanced the coaching parties' relationship (Boyce et al., 2010). Further, gender and perceived similar styles or values have not significantly impacted outcomes. This is likely because the more structured the coaching process is, the less critically coach characteristics influence the results (Bozer et al., 2015). You may not necessarily need a highly experienced subject matter expert to guide you toward improved performance, depending upon your goals and expectations of the engagement. There are benefits and considerations to having a coach with subject matter or industry experience; there are advantages to having a coach who can objectively look beyond discipline-specific demands as an outsider and recognize the nuances of the problem.

A coach who is a former nursing leader or has significant knowledge of the role's demands can minimize the learning curve of culture, terminology, and stakeholder roles. Coaches with subject matter expertise may have experiences in similar situations the leader is confronting. The coach can anticipate scenarios and ask relevant questions based on their experiences. Often, a coach with a nursing leadership background can relate to the practical challenges in a way that makes the nurse leader more confident in the direction of the coaching journey. This firsthand knowledge of what worked or did not work in their career can help build rapport and trust and accelerate growth. The risk is that the coach leans on their background to offer solutions rather than focusing on building the nurse leader's capacity to solve problems themself.

Conversely, there are benefits to having a coach who is an outsider to nursing and healthcare. Being new to the role and industry forces the nurse leader to explain situations deliberately. The introductory phase may be frustrating with an outsider as a coach. However, slowing down to explain people and circumstances often leads to the coach testing assumptions that a subject matter expert may take for granted. It may also allow a coach to draw parallels to other industries where a new healthcare best practice can emerge. It is important to remember that the coach's purpose is to guide the leader to build their "leadership athlete muscles," not necessarily advise them on what to do. Because an outsider cannot advise from personal experience, this background guides the nurse leader to the answer from within the nurse leader's personal experience. This process can be an effective way to build leadership capacity.

The best answer is alignment between the nurse leader's needs and the coach's role at the specific moment in time. The coach needs to serve the nurse leader's agenda regardless of their background. This agenda involves understanding the nurse leader's context, aspiration, and the best path to get there. Often, this involves creating clarity to guide the nurse leader to the right questions before focusing on the solutions. As you build that leadership capacity, your enhanced assessment and problem-solving skills lead to better decision-making. Sometimes, the best coach is external to the field but fully understands the coaching process, the right questions to ask, and the nuances of interpersonal relationships.

Negotiating for a Coach in an Employment Contract

When applying for an executive leadership position, whether in the academic world, practice arena, governmental affairs, or some other venue, it is advantageous to one's personal development to negotiate for an EC as part of the employment package. Most C-suite executives today are offered an EC as part of their package. This has not trickled down to nursing as the standard, but it should be. There is much that can be learned in your academic program. There is much more that you will learn in your practice setting. Being forward-thinking instead of reactionary will instill confidence in your team.

Most employers will expect to go through some negotiation for high-level positions—a director position, nurse manager, chief nursing officer, program director, associate dean, or dean—to name just a few. Employers will present a package and ask you to respond. This is your opportunity to advocate for yourself and to request an EC. You may negotiate for a package, for example, 5 to 10 sessions, or for something more substantial, depending on the position, such as a 6-month contract with an experienced EC to get you through the onboarding and assessment of issues in your new environment. They can be instrumental in effective leadership communication. Some things that are out of your control will occur, and beginning with an awareness of how you speak, interact, and listen can be fundamental to your success (Ebner, 2018).

Depending on your new company and whether it is in the private or public sector will dictate how much they will be willing to offer as a benefit. Pricing in your package could vary from just enough for a few sessions ($1,000–$5,000) to a 6-month commitment or more for $50,000. Coaching fees vary widely depending on background, time in the field, and, frankly, how good they are. Do some research before requesting to ensure a good match between what will be reasonable for the employer to offer and what will get you what you need as you move into the new position.

There are leadership companies with a panel of ECs from which to choose and individuals that work independently. Look at each coach's biography—look at more than one. Compare and contrast. Some companies have a process where you are matched after you pick your top three choices. Other scenarios allow you to select your own. Once matched, and moving through the steps of executive coaching, ask yourself if there is value in the relationship. Has this been the right match? Much like therapy and mentoring, you might not find the perfect fit the first time. However, perseverance allows you to find the right coach for you and your scenario. You must also be motivated to do the work and to get results. Meeting with the EC to make your boss happy will likely not allow for the many benefits one can realize in a positive coaching relationship.

CASE STUDY #1   Influencing Without Authority

As the leader of the clinical nurse practitioner team, you have identified a quality improvement initiative that revolves around outcomes related to patients being overmedicated and suffering from multiple drug interactions. You work with three physicians in the practice; two of them are careful and follow the standard of care for various primary care diagnoses, while the third always prescribes multiple drugs with interactions that compound the adverse side effects seen. Two of your nurse practitioners also follow the practice model of the over-prescribing physician. You plan an in-service training on the standard of care for these diagnoses and then start collecting data to determine if the practice update changes prescriptive practice in your clinic. The three providers have changed nothing since the update based on the best evidence. You hire an EC to help you work this scenario satisfactorily and to learn how to lead the team better.

The EC introduces the topic of "influencing without authority." You form a development plan with the following steps: (a) analyze the stakeholders for an entry point, (b) focus on mutual benefit, (c) get buy-in, and (d) build coalitions. You meet with the provider you have known the longest and start with points of agreement. Since you know this provider is data-centric, you use facts and data to support your position and build slowly with your request. Finally, after incrementally agreeing on a position, you then work to build a coalition with the next provider who is more open to change, recognizing the other provider's change in position. You continue your coalition-building one by one.

- What do you think of the coach's recommendations?
- Which of these steps makes you the most uncomfortable?
- How would you modify the approach if you were in this situation?

> **CASE STUDY #2 Conversation Planning**
>
> You are a department head, and annual budget submissions are due. You have an important initiative you want to spearhead but learn that a fellow department head is attempting to launch a similar initiative. This initiative is clearly within your department's scope of responsibility, but you believe that your peer is ambitious and wants to use the initiative to elevate their stature. You and your peer are different stylistically. You have been told that you are supportive, collaborative, and people oriented. Your peer is more demanding, assertive, and task oriented. You are apprehensive about approaching your peer because you have seen them become defensive previously and use conflict to their advantage. Unfortunately, your supervisor has not been interested in resolving personnel issues in the past. They want people to sort it out themselves. You engage your coach to seek guidance on navigating the conversation.
>
> The coach uses the ladder of inference tool and the steps of (a) reflection, (b) advocacy, and (c) inquiry to guide planning. You recognize during reflection why you are apprehensive about the conversation. It is not because the peer can be assertive and defensive. It is because you do not think your peer is putting the organization first. During the advocacy phase, you script your talking points by focusing on the situation and how it impacts you, carefully using "I" statements and avoiding "you" statements. Finally, you plan several questions to understand your peer's perspective. You feel more confident in the conversation and set up a one-on-one meeting.
>
> - What do you think of the coach's recommendations?
> - How would you predict the situation evolves from here?
> - What would you have done differently?

SUMMARY

Executive coaching can be of value to the new graduate, the mid-career leader making a transition, and the senior leader faced with the complexities and challenges of today's healthcare environment. There are several key points to consider when evaluating the merits of an EC.

There are many challenges as a leader in a constantly evolving global healthcare platform. Leadership occurs at every level, not just at the system level. Key reports from both the American Association of Colleges of Nursing and the National Academy of Medicine identify challenges and offer strategies. The use of a coach is a well-accepted resource to address the many goals promulgated by national thought leaders. But there are scenarios when the use of an EC is particularly warranted. These include during transitions (movement within the institution, movement across institutions with similar missions, movement across sectors, such as from the practice to the academic environment), promotions, and reorganizations. Conflict and how to resolve it is a strategy often amenable to a coaching relationship as well as culture and how to *assimilate* if moving into an unfamiliar environment or to *change* a poor culture as part of a collaborative plan with an EC.

There is a process for engagement with a coach and the steps necessary to establish a relationship. Many models incorporate these steps, but the GROW process includes goal setting, reality checking, options, and way forward (Jenkins, 2009). Using this framework, the EC helps the nurse leader to identify those that might help to offer an external perspective. A development plan is offered as an illustrative guide to demonstrate the types of goals, action items, and outcomes one might have in an executive coaching relationship.

The development of leadership athleticism, often obtained through an EC, will help ensure the leader's longevity. There are key concepts that impact the development of this athleticism. Emotional intelligence, individual and organizational alignment, the complexity of competing values, and political acumen—all can be explored through the coaching relationship. There are many types of power that can also be leveraged to improve one's impact. Overcoming bias and a focus on inclusivity are part of critical conversations that the nurse leader and the EC will have. Challenging one's assumptions to move past bias and using the ladder of inference tool helps one reflect and sort through data and its cultural meanings.

The EC for the nurse leader with a DNP does not need to be a nurse. In some cases, an outside perspective is what is needed. However, others, when using trade jargon and scenarios that must drill down into a very specific way of being, may necessitate a nurse EC. Further, one must be ready to be coached and open to this type of relationship. Influential, honest, soul baring conversations about how the nurse leader comes to the table are critical. If in a transition from one job to another, strategies may be used to negotiate for access to an EC in the employment contract.

CRITICAL THINKING QUESTIONS

1. What is executive coaching? In what ways might executive coaching provide leadership development for you in your leadership position?
2. What professional transitions have you already experienced in your career development? What were the challenges you faced in making those transitions?
3. If you were promoted into a position of authority over those who are current peer colleagues, what challenges do you think you would face?
4. What are the likely transition challenges that the DNP will face in the near future?
5. What expectations or political naivetes about leadership may inhibit smooth transitions into positions of increased authority?
6. Discuss leadership athleticism and executive coaching strategies that promote success.
7. What do you consider your strengths and weaknesses as a leader?
8. Describe an experience of your professional "personal best." What have you accomplished professionally that you are most proud of? What leadership qualities of yours contributed to your success in this endeavor?
9. During times of crisis or stress, how do you lead? How could an executive coach assist you to be more effective?
10. Discuss a challenging personal leadership situation. How could an executive coach assist you in navigating this challenge.

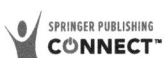 A robust set of instructor resources designed to supplement this text is located at http://connect.springerpub.com/content/book/978-0-8261-8137-4. Qualifying instructors may request access by emailing textbook@springerpub.com.

REFERENCES

AACN. (2021). *The essentials: Core competencies for professional nursing education*. AACN.
Bazerman, M. (2001). Common biases. *Judgement and managerial decision making* (pp. 13–41). Wiley.

Besharov, M. & Khurana, R. (2015). Leading amidst competing technical and institutional demands: Revisiting Selznick's conception of leadership. *Research in the Sociology of Organizations, 44*, 53–88. https://doi.org/10.1108/S0733-558X20150000044004

Biswas-Diener, R. (2010). *Practicing positive psychology coaching: Assessment, activities, and strategies for success*. Wiley.

Bolman, L., & Deal, T. (2017). *Reframing organizations: Artistry, choice, and leadership* (6th ed.). Jossey Bass.

Boyce, L. A., Jackson, J. R., & Neal, L. J. (2010). Building successful leadership coaching relationships [Article]. *The Journal of Management Development, 29*(10), 914–931. https://doi.org/10.1108/02621711011084231

Bozer, G., Joo, B.-K., & Santora, J. C. (2015). Executive coaching: Does coach-coachee matching based on similarity really matter? *Consulting Psychology Journal, 67*(3), 218–233. https://doi.org/10.1037/cpb0000044

Brubaker, M., & Mitchell, C. (2018). 4 signs an executive isn't ready for coaching. *Harvard Business Review*, The Daily Alert, July 09, 2018.

Cameron, K. (n.d.) An Introduction to the Competing Values Framework. *Haworth, 11*(11), 4. https://www.thercfgroup.com/files/resources/an_introduction_to_the_competing_values_framework_white_paper-pdf-28512.pdf

Cannon, M., & Witherspoon, R. (2005). Actionable feedback: Unlocking the power of learning and performance improvement. *Academy of Management Executive, 19*(2), 120–134. https://doi.org/10.5465/AME.2005.16965107

Carsrud, A. & Brannback, M. (2011). Entrepreneurial motivations: What do we still need to know? *Journal of Small Business Management, 49*(1), 9–26. https://dx.doi.org/10.1111/j.1540-627X.2010.00312.x

Center for Creative Leadership. (2018). *Better everyday conversations*. Center for Creative Leaderships.

CarolinaChan, J. T., & Mallett, C. J. (2011). The value of emotional intelligence for high performance coaching. *International Journal of Sports Science & Coaching, 6*(3), 315–328. https://doi.org/10.1260/1747-9541.6.3.315

Cheesbrough, K. R., Bronzert, J., & Frazier-De La Torre, E. (2020). Leadership, academia, and the role of career coaching. *Translational Behavioral Medicine, 10*(4), 870–872. https://doi.org/10.1093/tbm/ibaa057

Consultancy.Org. (n.d.). *What is consulting*. https://www.consultancy.org/career/what-is-consulting

Cox, E. (2013). *Coaching understood: A pragmatic inquiry into the coaching process* [Book]. SAGE Publications.

Crigger, N., & Godfrey, N. (2014). From the inside out: A new approach to teaching professional identify formation and professional ethics. *Journal of Professional Nursing, 30*(5), 376–382. https://doi.org/10.1016/j.profnurs.2014.03.004

D'Antonio, A. C. (2018). Coaching psychology and positive psychology in work and organizational psychology. *The Psychologist-Manager Journal, 21*(2), 130–150. https://doi.org/10.1037/mgr0000070

Deiorio, N. M., Carney, P. A., Kahl, L. E., Bonura, E. M., & Juve, A. M. (2016). Coaching: A new model for academic and career achievement. *Medical Education Online, 21*(1), 33480. https://doi.org/10.3402/meo.v21.33480

Ebner, K. (2018, December 5). *Making the most of coaching*. Success strategies for engaging and working with coaches. [Webinar]. Producer: Nebo. https://nebocompany.com/making-the-most-of-coaching-webinar

Ellinger, A. D., & Kim, S. (2014). Coaching and human resource development: Examining relevant theories, coaching genres, and scales to advance research and practice. *Advances in Developing Human Resources, 16*(2), 127–138. https://doi.org/10.1177/1523422313520472

Gallimore, R., & Tharp, R. (2004). What a coach can teach a teacher, 1975–2004: Reflections and reanalysis of John Wooden's teaching practices. *Sport Psychologist, 18*(2), 119–137. https://doi.org/10.1123/tsp.18.2.119

Godfrey, N. (2022). New language for the journey: Embracing a professional identity of nursing. *Journal of Radiology Nursing, 41*(1), 15–17. https://doi.org/10.1016/j.jradnu.2021.12.001

Goleman, D., Boyatzis, R., & McKee, A. (2001). Primal leadership: The hidden driver of great performance. *Harvard Business Review, 79*(11), 42–53.

Grant, A. M. (2010). It takes time: A stages of change perspective on the adoption of workplace coaching skills. *Journal of Change Management, 10*(1), 61–77. https://doi.org/10.1080/14697010903549440

Greeno, J., & Gresalfi, M. (2008). Opportunities to learn in practice and identity. In P. A. Moss, D. C. Pullin, J. P. Gee, E. H. Haertel, & L. J. Young (Eds.), *Assessment, equity, and opportunity to learn* (pp. 170–199). Cambridge University Press.

Guerrero, E. G., & Kim, A. (2013). Organizational structure, leadership and readiness for change and the implementation of organizational cultural competence in addiction health services. *Evaluation and Program Planning, 40*, 74–81. https://doi.org/10.1016/j.evalprogplan.2013.05.002

Guillaume, Y. R. F., Dawson, J. F., Woods, S. A., Sacramento, C. A., & West, M. A. (2013). Getting diversity at work to work: What we know and what we still don't know. *Journal of Occupational and Organizational Psychology, 86*(2), 123–141. https://doi.org/10.1111/joop.12009

Harré, R., & Van Langenhove, L. (1991). Varieties of positioning. *Journal for the theory of social behaviour, 21*(4), 393–407. https://doi.org/10.1111/j.1468-5914.1991.tb00203.x

IBIS World. Business coaching in the US - market size 2003–2028. (n.d.). IBIS World. Retrieved August 9, 2022, from https://www.ibisworld.com/industry-statistics/market-size/business-coaching-united-states/#:~:text=past%205%20years%3F,The%20market%20size%20of%20the%20Business%20Coaching%20industry%20in%20the,average%20between%202017%20and%202022.

ICF. (2020). *ICF team coaching competencies: Moving beyond one-to-one coaching*. V.13.11. International Coaching Federation. 1–21.

International Coaching Federation. (2021). *Updated ICF core competencies*. International Coaching Federation.

Jenkins, H. (2009). *Confronting the challenges of participatory culture: Media education for the 21st century*. MIT Press.

Jones, G., & Gorell, R. (2015). *50 top tools for coaching: A complete toolkit for developing and empowering people* (3rd ed.). Kogan Page.

Jones, R. J., Woods, S. A., & Guillaume, Y. R. F. (2016). The effectiveness of workplace coaching: A meta-analysis of learning and performance outcomes from coaching. *Journal of Occupational and Organizational Psychology, 89*(2), 249–277. https://doi.org/10.1111/joop.12119

Jordan, M., Wolever, R. Q., Lawson, K., & Moore, M. (2015). National training and education standards for health and wellness coaching: The path to national certification. *Global Advances In Health and Medicine, 4*(3), 46–56. https://doi.org/10.7453/gahmj.2015.039

Kochan, T., Bezrukova, K., Ely, R., Jackson, S., Joshi, A., Jehn, K., Leonard, J., Levine, D., & Thomas, D. (2003). The effects of diversity on business performance: Report of the diversity research network. *Human Resource Management, 42*(1), 3–21. https://doi.org/10.1002/hrm.10061

Kotter, J. P. (1995). Leading change: Why transformation efforts fail. *Harvard Business Review, 73*, 59–67.

Kristoffersen, M. (2021). Does professional identity play a critical role in the choice to remain in the nursing profession? *Nursing Open, 8*(4), 1928–1936. https://doi.org/10.1002/nop2.862

Langley, G. J., Moen, R., Nolan, K. M., Nolan, T. W., Norman, C. L., & Provost, L. P. (2009). *The improvement guide: A practical approach to enhancing organizational performance* (2nd ed.). Jossey-Bass Publishers.

Lave, J. & Wenger, E. (1991). *Situated learning: Legitimate peripheral participation*. Cambridge University Press.

Lax, D. A., & Sebenius, J. K. (1986). The measure of negotiation. *Negotiation Journal, 2*(1), 73–92. https://doi.org/10.1111/j.1571-9979.1986.tb00339.x

Li, Z., Zuo, Q., Cheng, J., Zhou, Y., Li, Y., Zhu, L., & Jiang, X. (2021). Coronavirus disease 2019 pandemic promotes the sense of professional identity among nurses. *Nursing Outlook, 69*(3), 389–398. https://doi.org/10.1016/j.outlook.2020.09.006

Lunenburg, F. C. (2012). Power and leadership: An influence process. *International Journal of Management, Business, and Administration, 15*(1), 1–9.

MBTI Basics. (n.d.). *Myersbriggs.Org*. https://www.myersbriggs.org/my-mbti-personality-type/mbti-basics

McNally, K., & Cunningham, L. (2010). *The Nurse Executive's Coaching Manual*. Sigma Theta Tau International.

Morrison, T., & Conway, W. A. (2006). *Kiss, bow, or shake hands: The bestselling guide to doing business in more than 60 countries* (2nd ed.). Adams Media.

National Academies of Sciences, Engineering, and Medicine. (2021). *The Future of Nursing 2020–2030: Charting a Path to Achieve Health Equity*. The National Academies Press. https://doi.org/10.17226/25982.

Nkomo, S. M., Bell, M. P., Roberts, L. M., Joshi, A., & Thatcher, S. M. B. (2019). Diversity at a critical juncture: New theories for a complex phenomenon. *Academy of Management Review, 44*(3), 498–517. https://doi.org/10.5465/amr.2019.0103

Potrac, P., Gilbert, W., & Denison, J. (2013). Routledge handbook of sports coaching. In *Routledge Handbook of Sports Coaching*. https://doi.org/10.4324/9780203132623

Pyramid of Success. (n.d.). *Uclabruins.com*. https://uclabruins.com/sports/2013/4/17/208274583.aspx

Rathmall, W. K., Brown, N. J., & Kilburg, R. R. (2019). Transformation to academic leadership: The role of mentorship and executive coaching. *Consulting Psychology Journal: Practice and Research, 71*(3), 141–160. https://doi.org/10.1037/cpb0000124

Richter, S., van Zyl, L. E., Roll, L. C., & Stander, M. W. (2021). Positive psychological coaching tools and techniques: A systematic review and classification. *Frontiers in Psychiatry, 12*, 1–19. https://doi.org/10.3389/fpsyt.2021.667200

Sagin, T. (2016). The case for executive coaching. *Healthcare Executive, 31*(4), 60–61.

Schalk, M., & Landeta, J. (2017). Internal versus external executive coaching. *Coaching: An International Journal of Theory, Research and Practice, 10*(2), 140–156. https://doi.org/10.1080/17521882.2017.1310120

Senge, P., Kleiner, A., Roberts, C., Ross, R., Smith, B., (1994). *The Fifth discipline fieldbook: Strategies and tools for building a learning organization*. Currency, Doubleday.

Sherman, R. O. (2011). Carefronting: A new approach to managing conflict. *Emerging RN Leaders*. https://emergingrnleader.com/carefronting/

Sherman, R. O. (2019). *The nurse leader coach: Become the boss no one wants to leave*. Sherman.

Shore, L. M., Cleveland, J. N., & Sanchez, D. (2018). Inclusive workplaces: A review and model. *Human Resource Management Review, 28*(2), 176–189. https://doi.org/10.1016/j.hrmr.2017.07.003

Stein, S. (Steven J.). (2011). *The EQ edge: Emotional intelligence and your success* (H. E. Book, Ed.; 3rd ed.) [Book]. Jossey-Bass.

Stone, D., Patton, B., & Heen, S. (2010). *Difficult conversations: How to discuss what matters most* (2nd ed.). Penguin Books.

Susan Devaney. (2020, October 5). 15 inspirational quotes from the formidable Serena Williams. *Vogue*. https://www.vogue.co.uk/arts-and-lifestyle/gallery/serena-williams-quotes

Tennis Grand Slam Titles. (n.d.). *Serenawilliams.Com*. https://www.serenawilliams.com/pages/tennis

Terblanche, N. (2021). Coaching techniques for sustained individual change during career transitions. *Human Resources Development Quarterly, 32*(1), 11–33. https://doi.org/10.1002/hrdq.21405

Terblanche, N., Molyn, J., deHaan, E., & Nilsson, V. O. (2022). Comparing artificial intelligence and human coaching goal attainment efficacy. *PLOS One, 17*(6), e0270255. https://10.1371/journal.pone.0270255

Theeboom, T., Van Vianen, A. E. M., & Beersma, B. (2017). A temporal map of coaching. *Frontiers in Psychology, 8*, 1–12. https://doi.org/10.3389/fpsyg.2017.01352

Thach, E. C. (2002). The impact of executive coaching and 360 feedback on leadership effectiveness. *Leadership & Organization Development Journal, 23*(4), 205–214. https://doi.org/10.1108/01437730210429070

Turner, J., & Nolan, S. B. (2015). Introduction: The relevance of the situative perspective in educational psychology. *Educational Psychologist, 50*(3), 167–172. https://psycnet.apa.org/doi/10.1080/00461520.2015.1075404

Whitmore, J. (2009). *Coaching for performance: Growing human potential and purpose—The principles and practice of coaching and leadership* (4th ed.). Nicholas Brealey Publishing.

Williams, J. S., & Lowman, R. L. (2018). The efficacy of executive coaching: an empirical investigation of two approaches using random assignment and a switching-replications design. *Consulting Psychology Journal, 70*(3), 227–249. https://doi.org/10.1037/cpb0000115

Wooden, J. (1997). *Wooden: A lifetime of observations and reflections on and off the court*. McGraw-Hill Professional.

Wright, P., & Cranmer, J. N. (2018). Leveraging graduate academic-partnerships to transform health system outcomes. *Nursing Administration Quarterly, 42*(4), 324–330. https://doi.org/10.1097/naq.0000000000000311

Zuberbuhler, M. J. P., Salanova, M., & Martinez, I. M. (2020). Coaching-based leadership intervention program: A controlled trial study. *Frontiers in Psychology, 10*, 1–21. https://doi.org/10.3389/fpsyg.2019.03066

CHAPTER FOURTEEN Reflective Response

KAREN KAUFMAN AND DAVID GRAD

This chapter, "Executive Coaching in the DNP Executive Role: Linking Personal Development and Performance Enhances Leadership Athleticism," by Michael Smith and Rosalie Mainous, is a deeply comprehensive exploration of the value that professional coaching can provide DNP graduates who are entering or have already established themselves in the fields of healthcare, patient care, and academia. Leadership athleticism provides a fitting and useful analog for personal leadership development and performance in an executive capacity outside of sports. For a DNP executive leader to effectively navigate complex organizational systems and relationships, healthcare mandates, political hierarchy, and the rigorous expectations of the patient experience, one must maintain a keen awareness of oneself, as well as one's position within a social system, and have the ability to build and manage relationships effectively. Effective leaders must be politically and socially astute and possess mental and physical stamina, along with the emotional intelligence to stay afloat in a relentlessly fast-paced environment.

In this reflective response, we draw parallels between the resilience of athletes and athletic leaders and the persistence required to succeed in an executive role. The two positions demand a similar drive toward sustained high performance against a backdrop of ever-increasing pressure and rapidly changing circumstances. Considering these transferable lessons and ideas also allows us to gain valuable insight by contrasting the expectations of each position. One key difference, for example, that we see between the athlete and the executive comes from how rest and relaxation is viewed as an important tool for productivity in the athletic world, but disregarded in the world of business, despite similar demands for performance and improvement. The discipline to retrain our brains away from natural, instinctual impulses, and toward trained, managed action is praised in both the business and sports worlds. But, as evidenced by the COVID-19 pandemic, the factors contributing to our brains' responses to stimuli are sometimes not under our control. This is where the diligence and discipline of rest and healing come into play; leadership becomes a delicate balance of knowing when to sharpen your tools and when to use them.

The authors begin the chapter by providing an overview of the core competencies in which nurse professionals must demonstrate proficiency, emphasizing the elevated stakes caused by the rapid state of change within the industry. They go on to outline the importance of developing skills related to leading oneself and others, specifically those pertaining to professional identity and performance. These skills and abilities, according to Smith and Mainous, are vital for high achievers in any industry looking for success in the mercurial, ever-changing world of the modern workplace. Acknowledging the effect that the COVID-19 pandemic had on elevating the sense of professional identity in nurses, the authors assert that "People's performance will drive success," defining performance to incorporate actions taken beyond the technical skills and abilities necessary for being a nurse. "For nurses to impact health equity," they continue, "they must be prepared as leaders and action-oriented. They must have organizational support and critical expertise to perform in a complex, continuously evolving system. Individuals can only perform at this level with the benefit of many resources over time, including mentors, coaches, experiential opportunity, and the development of a health equity lens." In fact, so important are leadership skills in determining success in the new and complex environment of modern nursing, the authors suggest that beyond simply providing leadership development programs, adding a coach to supplement such programs could provide new nurses with a profound advantage. Sharpening emotional intelligence, interpersonal and relationship skills, effective communication, proficiency in navigating change, leading through conflict, winning buy-in for necessary shifts in policy and procedures, and countless other skills not traditionally within the purview of nursing can make for more well-rounded nurses and leaders. Specifically, Smith and Mainous credit this growth to the additional long-term support participants would receive from a coaching relationship, much like how an athlete with great skills and abilities has the potential to perform to their full potential under proper coaching. Extending the comparison between sports and business deeper still, the chapter then explores the impact of coaching on team organization, focusing on the approach of one of the most successful coaches in college sports history, UCLA's John Wooden. The chapter explores Wooden's "Pyramid of Success," a model that demonstrates values and traits that lead to "competitive greatness" by focusing on the journey and not the destination. This makes for an effective entry point into the history of coaching, including some context for effective use cases of executive coaching, and provides an impressive array of models, frameworks, and approaches a coach might take with those with whom they work.

This chapter provides a comprehensive examination of, and a compelling testimonial for, the importance of coaching in the nursing profession, outlining the challenges involved in today's healthcare, academic, and patient support environments. It makes for a powerful resource for nurses and those who would prepare them for further professional success, detailing the benefits of coaching and best practices for its application. One area that the chapter does not explore, but which we feel is critical to peak performance and longevity as a leader, is the sustainability of learning. New connections are emerging between the field of learning science and instructional design, causing a reevaluation of leadership development programs and approaches to executive coaching.

CHAPTER FIFTEEN

Negotiation Skills in New Doctoral Advanced Nursing Practice Roles

H. MICHAEL DREHER

Doctoral advanced practice nurses are creating new frontiers in the field of nursing and, as practitioners, they are contributing significantly to the overall healthcare system. To fulfill this role, they will encounter many situations requiring negotiation skills. Successful negotiation skills are important in most professional careers, including nursing. Negotiation falls within the realm of both strategy and tactics. This chapter focuses primarily on the strategic role of the doctor of nursing practice (DNP) graduate and provides tactical examples that may be faced in actual practice.

This chapter begins with the context of organizational culture and systems theory as the setting in which negotiation takes place. Discussion includes the traits of successful negotiators and the crucial elements for successful negotiation, sources of power, and the five-step process for negotiation. Since not all individuals approach negotiation from a collaborative stance, skills are required for negotiating at an "uneven table," when rank and privilege affect the strategies. The new bachelor of science in nursing (BSN)-to-DNP graduate has had no opportunity to negotiate for a first professional position and (a) has a first graduate degree with no career experience, (b) has a still relatively new doctoral nursing degree known by many healthcare professionals but not all, (c) with limited knowledge by the public of the DNP degree itself, and (d) is particularly disadvantaged as a new DNP graduate as and a new nurse practitioner (compared with a post-master's advanced practice registered nurse [APRN] with years of experience). In a study of new residents and fellows entering academic medicine, Berman and Gottlieb (2019), write that negotiation skills are essential for women and underrepresented minorities to reduce disparities in compensation and resources that begin upon entry into the workforce. It is obvious that the new DNP graduate, with or without professional or advanced practice experience, needs to develop effective and—maybe as a goal—even sophisticated negotiation skills. It can be done. The chapter ends with strategies for overcoming barriers to successful negotiation, such as the "Four Horseman of the Apocalypse," (not the four horsemen in the chapter of Revelations in the Bible predicting the arrival of the Antichrist, war, famine, and death, of course).[1]

Negotiation is a crucial skill for successful relationships (Gates, 2022; Gottman, 2011; Shapiro, 2015). To have the necessary collaborative relations within and between disciplines, DNPs should aim to develop these skills and strategies, even those practiced by diplomats. For example, individuals who take a win-win approach to conflict resolution, even as this is sometimes a difficult undertaking, view conflicts as problems to be solved and seek solutions that achieve both their own goals and the goals of the other person. Individuals with this orientation see conflicts as opportunities for improving relationships by reducing the tension between two people (Chambers, 2023; Gottman, 2011; Katz & Patterini, 2008). Therefore, the purpose of negotiation is to resolve differences over, for example, information, values, or goals. Fisher et al. (2011) provide the following working definition of negotiation: "Two or more parties, with common and conflicting interests, come together to put forth and discuss explicit proposals for the purpose of reaching an agreement" (p. 10).

It is important in any negotiation to begin with common interests to create rapport. The purpose of negotiation is to reach an agreement that is based on a thorough discussion of each party's ideas and where an agreement is reached to meet the needs of both parties. The solution assures commitment to follow through to completion by each party. This differs from compromise, which is based on both parties' willingness to *settle* on an option. Compromise might best be described as "win-lose." And while compromise may be the antithesis to a good negotiation, new DNPs entering their first job may find negotiating for a position intimidating.

THE ROLE OF THE DNP IN NEGOTIATION—THE STRATEGIC VIEW

Before completing her DNP degree, Dr. Schmidt was a nurse practitioner (NP) in the stroke center of an academic medical center. Because of her years of experience in the acute care of stroke patients, she decided to do her DNP clinical practicum in a rehab unit. This rounding out of her experience with stroke patients and her career extensive knowledge base, focused her to conclude that stroke rehab needs to focus on all domains—social and functional—for patients to recover a sense of self and the roles in their lives and with their families. Unfortunately, she was met with resistance to this change. The first issue here is why was there resistance to what appears to be a positive advance in health in this circumstance. Is the DNP NP facing resistance more to the degree and role? What new ideas can we offer Dr. Schmidt in negotiation?

This section addresses a system context for using negotiation skills, the organizational culture as a context for change, and how gender and culture influence the role of the DNP. Helping Dr. Schmidt understand the organizational culture in which she finds herself and using the principles from CRR Global (formally known as the Center for Right Relationships, founded in 2007 and renamed in 2011), which is a systems approach described in the following paragraphs, could help her better negotiate the change. Perhaps, because of her gender, she is more focused on maintaining a relationship than in clearly and directly arguing for change for the patient's sake (Donaldson & Frohnmayer, 2007).

This compromising style was a gender difference that Holt and Devore (2005) found in a meta-analysis of 36 studies of self-reported data on conflict-resolution tendencies. Thomas et al. (2008), in a study of gender differences in conflict, found that men scored significantly higher in competing styles at low, medium, and high levels of responsibility in the workplace. Berdahl et al. (2018) describe a masculine style of organization that can be characterized by toxic leadership, bullying, and harassment associated with poor individual outcomes for men as well as women as the target of gender bias and hostility to any effective negotiation. Chang and Milkman (2020) describe contrary organizational dynamics such as blinding decision-making, substituting, and articulating new social norms, as strategies to create more equity in the workplace and these "soft tactics" **(rational persuasion, socializing, exchanging, personal appeals, consultation, and inspirational appeals)** should elevate the platform for less gender bias in negotiating.

Systems Theory as a Context for Negotiation

The DNP role in negotiation requires a high level of systems thinking and an ability to apply expertise in systems theory and functioning. The role includes being a participant in the larger system and being a catalyst for systemic change through negotiation. Therefore, there is a compelling leadership dimension to negotiation at this higher level.

Historically, negotiation took place within top-down, patriarchal organizational systems. The 21st century is unfolding a new (albeit imperfect) dimension in systems work. The dimensions are multifaceted and include a focus on the relationships within systems; organizational theory; emotional, social, and systems intelligence (Goleman, 2012; Goleman & Boyatzis, 2008; Goleman et al., 2013; Krén & Séllei, 2021); and seminal research on process work and deep democracy, where all voices in the system need to be heard (Mindell, 2012, 2014, 2015, 2019a, 2019b, 2019c). Arnold and Amy Mindell's work through the Deep Democracy Institute (2009) has created a worldwide think tank for the development of leadership that emphasizes the dynamic interplay between individual and collective transformations, and the seminal and empirical research conducted on relationships (Gottman, 2007, 2011; Gottman & Silver, 2015). These new approaches focus on connections between and among members of a system, and recognizing that people are in relationships at all times, starting with themselves. In 2011, Gottman wrote on the science of trust and asserted that trust is a cornerstone of relationships and an essential component of negotiation, as will be explored later in the chapter. Gottman and Gottman have been groundbreakers in bringing an evidence-based approach to couples and family therapy (2018).

Since 2007 and now entering its 26th year, CRR Global has created a ground-breaking and now sustained international model for coaching that is used for coaching within organizations and groups to unfold the power and potential of relationship systems. This methodology for facilitating human relationships is inspired by and combines concepts from coaching, psychology, organizational development, mediation, quantum physics, process work, and general systems theory, all of which are directly applicable to the DNP's role in negotiation. In effect, the negotiation role includes managing and leading relationship systems.

CRR Global's approach is founded on the following principles, which DNPs can use to create desired outcomes rather than focus on solving a problem. The first principle is creating a shift from "who is doing what to whom" to "what is happening here?" It creates a climate of being in the right relationship with oneself, others, and the larger organization or system in which the DNP is functioning. In this view, all parties have a voice that needs to be heard and acknowledged before a successful conclusion to any negotiation can occur. Every relationship system is characterized by various dynamic and evolving situations and human interactions. The DNP needs to be prepared to assess what is happening in the situation that creates the need for negotiation. Sometimes what is needed is to reveal that there is a system breakdown that is essential to address to move forward.

The second principle is that the relationship system is naturally creative and whole. In this view, there is no "they"; rather, there is "I, you, and we." Whenever one falls into a "they" view of a situation, the individual risks putting themselves in the place of the victim, undermining their effectiveness and ability to resolve the situation. Assuming that all parties in the relationship form something larger than the whole, this change empowers members of the system to negotiate new ways of working together effectively.

A third principle is that the DNP works with the whole system within a larger context, not just what appears on the surface. It is taking a meta-view of the larger picture that is important here, much like an orchestra conductor. Think of a gestalt where the whole is greater than the sum of its parts. For example, Dr. Schmidt needs to acknowledge that all opinions need to be voiced to uncover the real issues under the resistance to change. She can then articulate what is going on that may be negatively impacting optimal patient outcomes and use the collective knowledge and wisdom of the group to create better solutions for ensuring that a holistic framework is used. This means that the old way of working the system needs to yield to one that is more empowered toward collective interest versus individual self-interest.

In summary, the role of the DNP in a system's context is essential to reveal the system to itself. In contrast to "fixing" what appears on the surface (a common, perhaps default response), the nurse can hold up a mirror to what seems to be happening so that others may be able to respond in ways that better meet the needs of the larger system. The metaphor for the principle is "the view of the eagle looking at the system versus the ant on the floor."

POLITICAL, CULTURAL, AND GENDER CONTEXTS WITHIN THE SYSTEM

Organizations may be viewed through various perspectives through which the DNP must practice. Bolman and Deal (2013) describe the four frames of an organization from a system's perspective, which include the structural, human, political, and symbolic/cultural frames. The structure includes buildings, departments, technology, and equipment. Human resources include the people and hierarchy within the system. However, negotiation mostly takes place within the context of the political and symbolic frames. Bolman and Deal use the metaphor of a jungle to view the political frame. This is where the intersection of power, conflict, and coalitions takes place. A critical lens through which one views negotiation recognizes that the system is composed of various political arenas, including administration, governing bodies, medical groups, ancillary personnel, and nurses at all levels of education and experience. Therefore, individuals could argue that one dimension of the DNP role is that of a politician, but not in the traditional sense. For example, titles connote power in society and organizations. The title "doctor" has historically been seen as belonging to a physician or perhaps to a university professor. The title "doctor" when describing a nurse creates both confusion and conflict related to the power and political meaning of the term. The DNP needs to be prepared to respond to this issue. Bolman and Deal also describe a symbolic frame, which includes the organizational culture and its symbols. A metaphor here is the system as theater and includes many cues, symbols, and stories that create system norms that often resist challenge or change. A recent review of the literature (Hobson & van Nieuwerburgh, 2022; Zuñiga-Collazos et al., 2020) supports the positive impact of a coach approach to organizational change and is consistent with the model developed by CRR Global.

Thus, the DNP role includes viewing the system from the meta-view of both political and symbolic or cultural frames. Combining an acute understanding of these frames along with skill in being in the right relationship with self and others distinguishes the role of the DNP from others. For example, DNPs who are using evidence-based practice may challenge organizational ways of practice (as will be seen in the following case example).

Gender Effects in Negotiation

An examination of context would not be complete without including thoughts on the effect of gender and other measures of equity on the system and the ability of the DNP to negotiate effectively. According to the National Council of State Boards of Nursing (NCSBN), their 2020 National Nursing Workforce Survey reported that 88.4% of RNs were female and 11.6% male. This represents a slight increase of 3% in male nurses from

2017 (2022). The issues of gender also apply to issues of race, ethnicity, and considerations of equity and social justice (Valderama-Wallace & Apesoa-Varano, 2020; van der Heever et al., 2019).

In several studies on gender differences in negotiation strategies, it was found that men tend to view bargaining situations as short-term and episodic, whereas women tend to view transactions with others as part of a long-term relationship (Babcock & Laschever, 2008). Consequently, saying that women adopt more flexible bargaining stances than their male counterparts can be explained by their attitude toward the length of the relationship. But this difference in negotiating behavior can also be explained as women's concern for the equity of interpersonal relationships. In another gender-related study, the results suggested that women report having obtained a good outcome when they felt they had a pleasant interaction with the other party, even though they did not resolve or even discuss the conflict between them (Donaldson & Frohnmayer, 2007). The results of these studies suggest that women need to learn that it is legitimate to say what they want, even if it conflicts with what they think the other person wants.

Another gender difference Babcock and Laschever (2008) report is that men are significantly more likely to use negotiation to promote their interests than women. The accumulation of this disadvantage is sharply seen in salary negotiation, where women are leaving thousands of dollars, potentially millions by the time they retire, on the table (Hess, 2020). They also sacrifice visibility, training, and career growth because they also do not seek opportunities or rewards as men do. However, in Finland, there is an opposite finding where women are better at financial and retirement planning than men (Kalmi & Ruuskanen, 2018).

Holt (2010) is a seasoned executive and an executive coach, whose key focus is helping women move forward. She believes women have to break some rules and deep-seated assumptions, such as that self-promotion and a will to win are wrong. She learned that expecting to be treated fairly if you do a great job was a myth and that she needed to ask for interesting projects, promotional opportunities, and a higher salary. Gallo (2015) interviewed two experts on their perspectives on negotiating salary—myth versus reality. This article shatters some myths and provides women with six important strategies for negotiating salary. For example, the "play hardball" myth is shattered by advising them to focus on the overall package and be prepared to justify the amount requested.

Sheryl Sandberg (2013), COO of Facebook (rebranded Meta), popularized the "Lean In" movement to put women in top spots across the organizational terrain. Her book and directive to women that they should "lean in" had many supporters and critics, but the encouragement she gives women wins out (Adams, 2013; Alkon, 2015). The most controversial part of the book, which stirred feminist ire, is her discussion on the internal obstacles that hold women back. She struggled with the need to be liked, which she believes interferes with women's ability to take a competing versus compromising style. She scrutinizes why women's progress in succeeding at leadership roles has stalled, enlightens them on the root causes, and proposes convincing, commonsense solutions that can enable women to attain their full potential. She cautions women not to be relentlessly pleasant in negotiation and to take their rightful seat at the uneven negotiation table. So, was Sandberg's concept of "lean in sustainable?" Phipps and Prieto write 7 years later:

> Therefore, Sandberg's book is insightful in terms of making many women aware of how they can strive to empower themselves more by leaning in to lead, and can serve as a motivational tool, but moving forward, organizations and society at large must also be accountable, acknowledging responsibility for structures and systems that create obstacles for women to lean in to lead. (2020, p. 227)

In summary, the leadership needed for successful negotiation requires the DNP to assess and balance the principles of the structural, human, political, and symbolic frames of the organization. This means going beyond the organizational structure, staff-reporting lines, and job descriptions to develop skills in the political dynamics and understand cultural norms that have an often unseen but huge impact on negotiation outcomes. The four frames also need to be balanced with an understanding of the impact of gender and diversity on the issue at hand.

Rank and Privilege

To delve deeper into the concept of rank and privilege requires distinguishing among rank, power, and privilege. Mindell (2012) describes rank as a way of indicating a level of status and the amount of power that a person has relative to others in a given situation. Privilege and power can be derived from different bases or sources, such as educational, social, economic, or cultural. Therefore, a nurse with a doctoral degree has greater inherent privilege and implied power than a nurse with a baccalaureate degree. At present, society and organizational structures grant physicians greater rank and privilege than nurses, regardless of education or other forms of standing. It will be interesting to see if this will change when there are increased numbers of DNPs, especially those functioning autonomously or specifically in clinical settings.

> Dr. Bowman completed her DNP degree, where she also received a certificate in clinical research for the four courses she completed in research. She was interested in researching the "Role Strain in Family Caregivers of Persons Diagnosed with Alzheimer's Dementia," as her clinical focus was on patients with Alzheimer's disease. Up to this point, she had been the nurse collecting information for many physician-led studies. After conducting this study, she was now ready to be the primary or co-investigator of studies. She put forth research ideas and possible funding sources but met with resistance. Members of her interdisciplinary team were having difficulty seeing her as the primary researcher and as a leader. What ideas and skills can we offer Dr. Bowman in negotiation?

The DNP needs to stand in her integrity and awareness that she now has the experience and skills to be an effective co-investigator. Kay and Shipman (2014) speak on the importance of confidence and the self-assurance needed to be a successful negotiator. Their book on the neuroscience of confidence states that visits with high-powered women across the globe could give Dr. Bowman a different perspective in her approach. But is this a mirage? Khan and colleagues (2019) from the United States, Europe, and Canada studied the career progression of female academics from the 15 leading universities in this geographic study in the fields of public health and social sciences. Using a mixed methods methodology with 619 participants they reported the following:

- Non-ethnic-minority women represent the highest proportion of junior staff (37%), but the proportion declined from mid to senior levels in 11 (73%) of the 15 universities.
- Similarly, the proportion of ethnic-minority women declined from mid to senior levels in all 15 universities.
- Ethnic-minority women comprised a smaller proportion of the total cohort at the junior level (19%) and, coupled with the downward trajectory moving along the seniority pathway, this resulted in less than 9% of senior positions being held by women of ethnic minorities.

- Non-ethnic-minority men comprised 25% of the faculty at the junior level overall and showed a sharp increase across seniority categories, particularly between mid and senior levels, surpassing the proportion of non-ethnic-minority women at the mid-to-senior level.
- Although there were initiatives to increase the percentage of women (the article did not outline any specific initiatives geared toward ethnic-minority women), monitoring and evaluation activities were poorly reported and, among those that were presented, they lacked detail and tended to focus on process indicators such as identifying implemented actions without associating outcomes.

In this study, it is evident that gender discrimination is significant, as academic women were marginalized in the promotion to senior academic leadership roles as compared to men, and the differences were more pronounced for ethnic-minority women. These findings have enormous implications for women in the junior academic leadership role being weakened in their ability to negotiate for themselves in an unequal environment with gender bias. This is compounded, and even more so, when accompanied by ethnic-minority bias, whether explicit or not.

Mindell (2014) further describes low rank as being devalued, disrespected, and excluded from influence, decision-making, and other benefits that come from having a high rank. Because of this norm, nurses have historically been impacted in areas of self-esteem and self-worth. A source of conflict can be the unconscious use of rank. For example, a person in a higher position, confronted with "pulling rank" or dismissing the concerns or needs of others, often becomes angry or uses denial as a defense mechanism. The DNP has two critical roles here: the first is to know and effectively use skills and strategies for negotiation; the second is to use a systems approach in resolving issues involving negotiation strategies. In the case example, Dr. Bowman was seen by her colleagues as having neither the rank nor the privilege to warrant being the primary investigator of the study. One successful outcome of her negotiation is acknowledging the contributions of her colleagues, choosing to take the first step as a co-investigator of the study, and demonstrating how research builds evidence-based practice and the importance of implementing it to improve patient outcomes.

THE ROLE OF THE DNP IN NEGOTIATION—THE TACTICAL VIEW

Dr. Land is a recent DNP graduate and he is negotiating for a promotion to a chief nursing officer position in an academic medical center, where he has been a director of cardiovascular services for 10 years. He knows his competition and all have either an MSN in nursing administration or an MBA and they are from out of the state. He decides to leverage his DNP degree and his understanding of the organization's culture and goals, which will allow him to hit the ground running. Since many on the search committee do not understand what knowledge and skills a DNP degree can bring, he decides to provide them with two brief articles outlining the MSN and DNP curriculum differences. He also plans to use his organizational power by having one of his recommendations come from the chairperson of surgery. He knows all his years as a critical care nurse will help him think clearly under the stress of the interview. His reputation as a person of integrity and his willingness to be assertive in conflict situations, with a focus on problem resolution, will stand well for him. What ideas and skills can we offer Dr. Land in negotiation?

The next section focuses on the specific tactics and strategies used in negotiation, which fit within the strategic thinking or systems framework where the DNP functions. The literature describes the traits of successful negotiators and the strategies for a win-win outcome (Hennig, 2008; Lewicki et al., 2015). Dr. Land is already applying some of the crucial traits and elements for successful negotiation, and the following section should prove helpful as he plans his next steps.

Traits of Successful Negotiators

When we study the diplomatic styles of individuals, we can identify seven traits in individuals that we would rate as key to their success (Malhotra & Bazerman, 2007; Raiffa et al., 2007). The first trait is having strong planning skills. Successful negotiators often state that they spend 50% or more of their time planning what will be said in their interactions. Such planning includes not only the content, but where they will meet, who else should be present, whether information should be sent before the meeting, and even what time of the day the meeting should occur. Successful negotiators want to maximize their opportunities for success; therefore, they recognize that the process and place are as important as the meeting's discussion.

The "ability to think clearly under stress" is the second trait of successful negotiators. Being prepared is one way to reduce the stress in any negotiation process. Two other ways are staying focused on problem-solving, not on individual personalities, and recognizing at any point you can back away from the negotiation and come back at a later time. Diplomats tend to project an air of confidence; therefore, when an attack occurs, their positive self-regard holds them in good stead.

A third trait, and often an undervalued trait, is the "ability to use common sense." The most common meaning of this phrase is good sense and sound judgment in practical matters. Taking the time to establish rapport, providing sufficient information on which to base a decision, and remembering the basics of positive interpersonal relationships are all utilizing common sense.

The individual's "verbal ability" is the fourth trait. This is the ability to state one's ideas and opinions assertively, as well as to clarify the other party's ideas and opinions (Awate & Rukumani, 2021; Bishop, 2013; McClure, 2007; Murphy, 2011). The ability to manage other people's defensiveness, side-stepping issues as well as overt hostility in a nondefensive manner, is also a key verbal skill. An example of persuasion skill is that agreement is facilitated when the desirability of the agreement is stressed.

"Content knowledge" is the fifth trait found in successful negotiators. For example, if Dr. Land was going to negotiate a union contract that involves changing the role of the nurse aides in the institution, he would certainly come to the table having already investigated licensure laws, how other institutions have handled such a change, and the current attitude of the staff.

The sixth trait is "personal integrity." In truth, if one is not perceived as trustworthy and credible, the person will not be seen as an individual with integrity. Being seen as trustworthy requires that the person be honest, open instead of defensive, consistent in standards and approach, and someone who treats individuals with the respect that they deserve. Gottman (2011) cites the difficulty in specifically defining trust and uses the mathematics of game theory to help us understand that trust goes beyond a cognitive definition. It entails observable behavior represented by a trust matrix that accepts each partner will bargain for their interests and will do so employing a "nice-nice" exchange in contrast to a "nasty-nasty" exchange.

The final and seventh trait of successful negotiators is "the ability to perceive and use power." Power is the ability and willingness to affect the outcome (Wareham &

Overbeck, 2020). Multiple sources of power are available for use in negotiation. For now, suffice it to say that successful negotiators keep their eye on the outcome that they desire and use multiple sources of power to move the negotiation to the conclusion they desire (Aquilar & Galluccio, 2007).

In the case example, Dr. Land needed to be consciously aware of and apply the traits or skills of planning, thinking clearly under stress, using his common sense and verbal skills, and having strong knowledge of the content or information required in the situation. To this, he needed to balance his sense of personal integrity to create a positive trusting environment with his ability to perceive and use power effectively. This is not "power over" but the courage and willingness to step forth and do what is needed in the situation.

Three Crucial Elements for Successful Negotiation

Power, time, and information are the three interrelated variables in any negotiation process (Cohen, 2007; Guo, 2023; Thompson, 2007). Power is the capacity to get things done, and to exercise control over people, events, or situations. Usually when knowledgeable people complain about power, it is for one of two reasons: (a) they do not like the way power is being used—it is often power over an individual and (b) they do not approve of the goal of the person exerting control—power should never be a goal in and of itself, but should be a means of transport to a desired outcome.

In any negotiation, the second variable of time needs consideration. Expect the most significant concession behavior in any settlement action to occur close to the deadline. Both parties must know the deadline. However, deadlines are more flexible than most people realize. DNP clinicians need to use this misunderstanding of the time dimension to negotiate for outcomes that support excellence in patient care, quality education, or crucial changes in organizational effectiveness.

Information is the third crucial element in the negotiation process. During the actual negotiating event, it is often a common strategy for one or both sides to conceal their true interests, needs, and priorities. The rationale is that information is power, particularly in situations where one cannot trust the other side fully.

It is important to gain information by asking questions every time you are given answers. A way to test the credibility of the other side is to ask questions, the answers to which are already known. The more information one has about the other person's priorities, deadlines, and real needs, the better one can bargain. A key piece of information that all negotiators want to know is: "What are the real limits of the other party?" or "How much will they sacrifice to make a deal?" Very often this can be ascertained by observing the pattern of concession behavior on the part of the other side.

Turning back to the case of Dr. Land, one can see how he has used the aforementioned principles. He established his background and credentials early in a negotiation. He demonstrated the kind of expertise that is required for most negotiations by asking intelligent questions to know whether the responses are accurate. Dr. Land needs to remember that he brings to the table clinical and managerial expertise in the negotiation process.

For example, the search committee may state that they want their candidate to have had previous experience as a chief nursing officer, whereas their real need is that the candidate knows how to work effectively in a complex academic medical center. The more Dr. Land can acquaint himself with the committee's needs, the better will be his position to negotiate a possible resolution for their real need. An example of using the power of identification is when Dr. Land mentions that a well-respected academic medical center had just hired their internal candidate last year and he has been very

TABLE 15.1 Five Steps in the Negotiation Process

The Negotiation Process Steps	Key Points to Include
1. Prepare	Know the facts Know what self and others want Develop the strategy Identify the "must-have"
2. Develop Objective Criteria	Includes laws, policies, precedence, moral standards, and community norms as possible criteria Consider accreditation standards Seek benchmark models for comparison
3. Communicate Interests and Needs	Communication includes both clear dialog and a connection to others Body language sends messages that others will see
4. Search for Mutually Acceptable Solutions	Look for areas of agreement and common ground Be willing to accept mutually accepted options, not previously considered
5. Finalize the Agreement	Ensure clear agreement on the details Who will do what and in what time frame Distribute a summary with the agreed-upon outcomes Identify areas for future discussion

Sources: Cohen, H. (2007). *Negotiate this! By caring, But not T-H-A-T much*. Business Plus; Fisher, R., Ury, W., & Patton, B. (2011). *Getting to yes: Negotiating agreement without giving in*. Penguin Books; and Raiffa, H., Richardson, J., & Metcalfe, D. (2007). *Negotiation analysis: The science and art of collaborative decision making*. Belknap Press.

successful. If the organization has had a precedent of promoting from within, Dr. Land can use the power of precedent.

The best outcomes employ a systems approach where the parties rise above individual interests to view the greater good. While holding the strategic view, it is also important to use the tactical skills needed in a negotiation process (see Table 15.1).

BARRIERS TO SUCCESSFUL NEGOTIATION

Barriers to successful negotiation are multidimensional and involve behaviors that people use, often at an unconscious level, to thwart resolution. This section also includes descriptions of the "Four Horsemen of the Apocalypse" (Gottman, 2011; Gottman & Silver, 2015) and individual common mistakes (Changing Minds.org) that the DNP needs to understand to be successful in negotiating. Individuals like Dr. Ross need to overcome these barriers for successful negotiation.

> Dr. Ross began her academic teaching career after she completed her DNP degree last year. Before this, she had been a women's health nurse practitioner in a busy practice connected to the academic medical center for 10 years. It became quickly apparent that several of the other professors with a background in women's health were unhappy with her appointment as a track coordinator. Her initial efforts at inclusion in curriculum planning were met with stonewalling and disrespect. It appeared her questions about the present curriculum were taken as criticism, rather than her effort to understand the rationale used for the inclusion of the courses. The nonverbal responses included eye-rolling, silence, or looks of shock when she suggested changes. What ideas and strategies could we offer Dr. Ross in negotiation?

The "Four Horsemen of the Apocalypse"

Dr. John Gottman (Gottman, 2007, 2011; Gottman et al., 2020; Gottman & Silver, 2015) has mostly conducted empirical research on healthy and unhealthy marriages (including homosexual couples) throughout his career. His work has also been extrapolated and further validated for use in organizations (Gottman, 2007). Four toxic behaviors doom relationships, regardless of the setting, and are called the "Four Horsemen of the Apocalypse." (Gottman, 2007; Gottman et al., 2019). These behaviors include:

1. Blame/criticism, consisting of attacking or blaming others instead of their own behavior
2. Defensiveness in response to being criticized, which is another way of blaming
3. Contempt, which is the use of sarcasm, belittling, cynicism, hostile humor, and belligerence
4. Stonewalling, which includes cutting off communication, silent treatments, refusals to engage, withdrawal, or in some cases just not directly expressing what you are thinking

Gottman (2011) found that 69% of all problems are perpetual, meaning that they can be managed through dialog, but resist ultimate resolution. Therefore, the role of the DNP is not to "fix" the issue but to engage in negotiation strategies that will increase positive dialogue, reduce the negative effect during the conflict, particularly the difficult challenge of working with contempt, and increase the positive effect during and after a conflict resolution. Figure 15.1 includes some antidotes that are effective in working with the Four Horsemen.

The "Four Horseman of the Apocalypse" can lead negotiators to make common mistakes (see Table 15.2). Of the 15 mistakes listed (Changing Minds.org), the most

Toxic Behaviors	Strategies to Deal With Them
General Behaviors	• Name the behavior and educate the parties on the negative impact/destructiveness. • Review what happened and discuss alternative behaviors/strategies. • Increase positive behaviors and attitudes where possible with a soft approach, accepting influence, and noticing efforts to "repair" what has happened. • Encourage that there are alternative ways to negotiate through a situation or conflict.
Blame/Criticism	• Ask are you willing to resolve this without blame? • Address the behavior, not the person. • Try a soft start up to lessen the impact. • Look for the request behind the criticism. • Encourage the use of "I want..., I feel..." statements.
Defensiveness	• Actively listen and clarify what the other person is hearing. • Assume that 2% of what you or the other person is saying is true. Look for areas of truth behind the complaint.
Contempt	• Ask are you willing to resolve this without sarcasm or name calling? • Allow the parties to ventilate to you. • Check for emotional flooding and soothe. • Encourage the use of "I want..., I feel..." statements.
Stonewalling	• Check for emotional flooding and soothe. • Address fears of what will happen if the person speaks what is being thought or felt. • Encourage moving beyond the edge that is keeping the person back and support the effort.

FIGURE 15.1 The "Four Horsemen of the Apocalypse" Behaviors

Source: Adapted from Gottman, J. M., & Silver, N. (2015). *The seven principles for making marriage work.* Penguin Random House.

TABLE 15.2 Common Mistakes That Negotiators Make

1. *Accepting positions*: Assuming the other person won't change their position
2. *Accepting statements*: Assuming what the other person says is wholly true
3. *Cornering*: Giving the person no alternative but to fight
4. *Hurrying*: Negotiating in haste (and repenting at leisure)
5. *Hurting the relationship*: Getting what you want but making an enemy
6. *Issue fixation*: Getting stuck on one issue and missing greater possibilities
7. *Missing strengths*: Not realizing the strengths that you actually have
8. *Misunderstanding authority*: Assuming that authority and power are synonymous
9. *Misunderstanding power*: Thinking one person has all the power
10. *One solution*: Thinking there is only one possible solution
11. *Over-wanting*: Wanting something too much
12. *Squeezing too much*: Trying to gain every last advantage
13. *Talking too much*: Not gaining the power of information from others
14. *Thinking in absolutes*: Assuming that there are only a few possibilities
15. *Win-lose*: Assuming a fixed-pie, win-lose scenario

Source: Adapted from Changing Minds.org. *Negotiation mistakes.* http://changingminds.org/disciplines/negotiation/mistakes/mistakes.htm.

recurrent ones are accepting positions, hurrying, issue fixation, and missing strengths. Creative thinking needed for win-win solutions will not occur if others do not change their positions and do not look for innovative solutions, but remain fixated on their chosen solutions. Many beginning negotiators fail to see the strengths they have, often because they are hurrying to a solution to please others.

An important role of the DNP is to first assess what is going on within the system that requires negotiation. Taking a systems view, understanding issues of rank and privilege, using the skills needed to negotiate effectively, and having a clear understanding of what gets in the way of resolution—all of these approaches arm the practitioner with the background to be an effective negotiator. It is also important to be grounded in a strong sense of self and know what values one brings to the situation. Using the approaches delineated in Table 15.2 enables the DNP to be effective in dealing with toxic behaviors.

Based on the work of CRR Global (2011), overcoming the barriers is predicated on the principle of finding a common interest. The following questions are useful: (a) Are you willing to resolve this without blame? (b) Why is it important to resolve this? (c) What do you agree on? A caveat: if the parties are unwilling to resolve the issue without blame, there is no point in proceeding further. One needs to develop another strategy for resolution.

SUMMARY

Negotiation is a complex process where individuals are seeking an agreement that all parties can commit to follow through to completion. In this context, the role of the DNP includes holding a strategic or systems view of the negotiation process. How to negotiate and with whom one can negotiate is largely determined by the organizational culture in which negotiators find themselves. There are cultural and gender variables to be aware of in the process. CRR Global speaks directly to possible strategies to right the system.

The role of the DNP also requires skillful and effective use of tactical strategies for negotiation. Critical is creating a climate of trust. The five steps in the negotiation process are fraught with possible complications from the "Four Horsemen of the Apocalypse" and the common errors in negotiation. It is an act of inner courage and conviction that allows the DNP in their leadership role to be authentic in any situation that requires the use of negotiation skills. Essential inner qualities include increasing inner awareness, being a truth-teller, and standing by your integrity.

CRITICAL THINKING QUESTIONS

1. How do you assess or evaluate your current negotiation skills as you approach applying for your first job as a newlyminted DNP graduate or as an experienced new DNP seeking a promotion?
2. Why is it important to focus first on common versus conflicting ideas in the negotiation process?
3. What are the three principles designed to resolve conflict in a system put forward by CRR Global?
4. Compare your present skills to the six skills of successful negotiators. What are your strengths and areas for development?
5. Gottman describes the "Four Horsemen of the Apocalypse." What is necessary to resolve conflicts utilizing this model?
6. There are five steps in the negotiation process. Why is the first step, preparation, described as the most important step?
7. Common mistakes in the negotiation process involve cognitive and affective errors. Of this list, where are your vulnerabilities in negotiation in your workplace?
8. Due to the gender differences discussed, what are the vulnerabilities of women negotiating?
9. What personal values are important to bring to situations requiring negotiation for successful resolution?
10. Review the case examples included in this chapter. Based on your experience, what are other effective strategies?

NOTE

1. The use of the quadrant word "four" from "The Four Horsemen of the Apocalypse" has been used as an analogy in many fields –

    - *Medicine*: Inflammation, oxidative stress, apoptosis, and autophagy in diabetes mellitus and diabetic kidney disease: The Four Horsemen of the Apocalypse,

    Journal of International Urology and Nephrology (Turkmen, 2016)

    - *Sociology*: The Four Horsemen of the Fair Housing Apocalypse: A Critique of Fair Housing Policy in the USA: 1) The Fair Housing Assistance Program, Underfunding and Inconsistent Implementation; 2) The Fair Housing Initiatives Program, Underfunding and Inconsistent Implementation; 3) The US Department of Justice (DOJ), a Lack of Continuity in Fair Housing Enforcement and 4) The Neoliberal Harbinger of Death,

    Critical Sociology (Silverman & Patterson, 2011)

    - And many others.

    Feser, C. (2016). *When execution isn't enough: Decoding inspirational leadership*. Wiley.

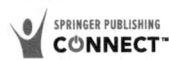

A robust set of instructor resources designed to supplement this text is located at http://connect.springerpub.com/content/book/978-0-8261-8137-4. Qualifying instructors may request access by emailing textbook@springerpub.com.

REFERENCES

Adams, S. (2013). 10 Things Sheryl Sandberg gets exactly right in 'lean in.' *Forbes*. http://www.forbes.com/sites/susanadams/2013/03/04/10-things-sheryl-sandberg-gets-exactly-right-in-lean-in/#3e148675466f

Alkon, A. (2015). Science says 'lean in' is filled with flawed advice, likely to hurt women. *Observer*. http://observer.com/2015/05/science-says-lean-in-is-filled-with-flawed-advice-likely-to-hurt-women

Aquilar, F., & Galluccio, M. (2007). *Psychological processes in international negotiations: Theoretical and practical perspectives*. Springer Nature.

Awate, S. J., & Rukumani, J. (2021). Assertiveness in nursing. *International Journal of AdvancedPsychiatric Nursing*, 3(2), 20–22.

Babcock, L., & Laschever, S. (2008). *Asking for it: How women can use the power of negotiation*. Bantam.

Berdahl, J. L., Cooper, M., Glick, P., Livingston, R. W., & Williams, J. C. (2018). Work as a masculinity contest. *Journal of Social Issues*, 74(3), 442–448.

Berman, R. A., & Gottlieb, A. S. (2019). Job negotiations in academic medicine: Building a competency-based roadmap for residents and fellows. *Journal of General Internal Medicine*, 34, 146–149.

Bishop, S. (2013). *Develop your assertiveness* (3rd ed.). Kogan Page.

Bolman, L. G., & Deal, T. E. (2013). *Reframing organizations: Artistry, choice and leadership*. Jossey-Bass.

Chang, H., & Milkman, K. L. (2020). Improving decisions that affect gender equality in the workplace. *Organizational Dynamics*, 49(1), 100709.

Changing Minds.org. *Negotiation mistakes*. https://changingminds.org/disciplines/negotiation/mistakes/mistakes.html

Chambers, R. (2023). Transforming power: From zero-sum to win-win? *Open Docs, Institute of Development Studies*, 37(6). https://doi.org/10.1111/j.1759-5436.2006.tb00327.x

Cohen, H. (2007). *Negotiate this! By caring, but not T-H-A-T much*. Business Plus.

CRR Global. (2011). *Organization and relationship systems coaching manual*. Author.

Deep Democracy Institute. (2009). http://deepdemocracyexchange.com

Donaldson, M. C., & Frohnmayer, D. (2007). *Negotiating for dummies* (2nd ed.). Wiley.

Feser, C. (2016). *When execution isn't enough: Decoding inspirational leadership*. Wiley.

Fisher, R., Ury, W., & Patton, B. (2011). *Getting to yes: Negotiating agreement without giving in*. Penguin Books.

Gallo, A. (2015). Setting the record straight on negotiating your salary. *Harvard Business Review*. https://hbr.org/2015/03/setting-the-record-straight-on-negotiating-your-salary&cm_sp=Article

Gates, S. (2022). *The negotiation book: Your definitive guide to successful negotiating* (3rd ed.). A Wiley Brand.

Goleman, D. (2012). *Emotional intelligence*. Random House.

Goleman, D., & Boyatzis, R. (2008). Social intelligence and the biology of leadership. *Harvard Business Review*, 86(9), 74–81.

Goleman, D., Boyatzis, R., & McKee, A. (2013). *Primal leadership: Unleashing the power of emotional intelligence*. Harvard Business Review Press.

Gottman, J. M. (2007). Making relationships work. *Harvard Business Review*, 85(12), 45–50.

Gottman, J. M. (2011). *The science of trust*. W. W. Norton.

Gottman, J. M., & Gottman, J. S. (2018). *The science of couples and family therapy: Behind the scenes at the "Love Lab."* W. W. Norton & Company.

Gottman, J. M., & Silver, N. (2015). *The seven principles for making marriage work*. Penguin Random House.

Gottman, J. M., Cole, C., & Cole, D. L. (2019). Four horsemen in couple and family therapy. In J. Lebow, A. Chambers, & D. C. Breunlin (Eds.), *Encyclopedia of couple and family therapy* (19th ed., pp. 1212–1216). Springer.

Gottman, J. M., Gottman, J. S., Cole, C., & Preciado, M. (2020). Gay, lesbian, and heterosexual couples about to begin couples therapy: An online relationship assessment of 40,681 couples. *Journal of Marital and Family Therapy, 46*(2), 218–239.

Guo, L. (2023). Gathering information before negotiation. *Management Science, 69*(1), 200–219, Retrieved Gathering Information Before Negotiation (informs.org)

Hennig, J. (2008). *How to say it: Negotiating too win: Key words, phrases, and strategies to close the deal and build lasting relationships*. Prentice Hall.

Hess, B. (Ed.). (2020). *Growing old in America: New perspectives on old age*. Routledge.

Hobson, A. J., & van Nieuwerburgh, C. J. (2022). Extending the research agenda on (ethical) coaching and mentoring in education: Embracing mutuality and prioritising well-being. *International Journal of Mentoring and Coaching in Education, 11*(1), 1–13.

Holt, J. L., & DeVore, C. J. (2005). Culture, gender, organizational role, and styles of conflict resolution: A meta-analysis. *International Journal of Intercultural Relations, 29*(2), 165–196.

Holt, M. D. (2010). Overcoming the mental barriers to equal pay. *Harvard Business Review*. https://hbr.org/2010/04/overcoming-the-mental-barriers

Kalmi, P., & Ruuskanen, O. P. (2018). Financial literacy and retirement planning in Finland. *Journal of Pension, Economics & Finance, 17*(3), 335–362.

Katz, N. H., & Pattarini, N. M. (2008). Interest-based negotiation: An essential business and communications tool for the public relations counselor. *Journal of Communication Management, 12*(1), 88–97.

Kay, K., & Shipman, C. (2014). *The confidence code: The science and art of self-assurance—What women should know*. Harper Business.

Khan, M. S., Lakha, F., Tan, M. M. J., Singh, S. R., Quek, Y. C., Han, E., Tan, S. M., Haldane, V., Gea-Sánchez, M., & Legido-Quigley, H. (2019). More talk than action: Gender and ethnic diversity in leading public health universities, *The Lancet, 393*(10171), 594–600.

Krén, H., & Séllei, B. (2021). The role of emotional intelligence in organizational performance, *Periodica Polytechnica Social and Management Sciences, 29*(1), 1–9.

Lewicki, R. J., Barry, B., & Saunders, D. M. (2015). *Essentials of negotiation* (6th ed.). McGraw-Hill.

Malhotra, D., & Bazerman, M. (2007). *Negotiation genius: How to overcome obstacles and achieve brilliant results at the bargaining table and beyond*. Bantam.

McClure, J. S. (2007). *Civilized assertiveness for women: Communication with backbone . . . not bite*. Albion Street Press.

Mindell, A. (2012). *Bringing deep democracy to life: An awareness paradigm for deepening political dialog, personal relationships, and community interactions*. Process Work Institute. https://www.aamindell.net

Mindell, A. (2014). *The leader as martial artist*. Deep Democracy Exchange.

Mindell, A. (2015). *Sitting in the fire: Large group transformation using conflict and diversity*. Deep Democracy Exchange.

Mindell, A. (2019a). *The dreambody in relationships*. Gatekeeper Press.

Mindell, A. (2019b). *The year 1: Global process work: Community creation from global problems, tensions and myths*. Gatekeeper Press.

Mindell, A. (2019c). *The leader's 2nd training: For your life and our world*. Gatekeeper Press.

Murphy, J. (2011). *Assertiveness: How to stand up for yourself and still win the respect of others*. CreateSpace.

National Council of State Boards Nursing. (2022). *2020 National nursing workforce survey*. Retrieved The 2020 National Nursing Workforce Survey (ncsbn.org)

Phipps, S. T. A., & Prieto, L. C. (2020). Leaning in: A historical perspective on influencing women's leadership. *Journal of Business Ethics, 173*(2), 245–259.

Raiffa, H., Richardson, J., & Metcalfe, D. (2007). *Negotiation analysis: The science and art of collaborative decision making*. Belknap Press.

Sandberg, S. (2013). *Lean in: Women, work, and the will to lead*. Knopf.

Shapiro, R. M. (2015). *The power of nice: How to negotiate so everyone wins—especially you!* John Wiley & Sons.

Silverman, R. M., & Patterson, K. L. (2011). The four horsemen of the fair housing apocalypse: A critique of fair housing policy in the USA. *Critical Sociology, 38*(10), https://doi.org/10.1177/0896920510396385

Thomas, K. W., Thomas, G. F., & Schaubhut, N. (2008). Conflict styles of men and women at six organizational levels. *International Journal of Conflict Management, 14*(2), 1–38.

Thompson, L. (2007). *The truth about negotiations*. FT Press.

Turkmen, K. (2016). Inflammation, oxidative stress, apoptosis, and autophagy in diabetes mellitus and diabetic kidney disease: The four horsemen of the apocalypse. *International Urology and Nrphrology, 49*, 837–844.

Valderama-Wallace, C. P., & Apesoa-Varano, E. C. (2020). The problem of the 'color line': Faculty approaches to teaching social justice in baccalaureate nursing programs. *Nursing Inquiry, 27*(3), e12349.

van der Heever, M. M., van der Merwe, A. S., & Crowley, T. (2019). Nurses' views on promotion and the influence of race, class and gender in relation to the Employment Equity Act. *SA Journal of Industrial Psychology, 45*(1),1—13. Retrieved Nurses' views on promotion and the influence of race, class and gender in relation to the Employment Equity Act (scielo.org.za)

Wareham, D. J., & Overbeck, J. E. (2020). The unspoken language of power: Interpersonal dynamics of nonverbal behavior in mixed-gender negotiations. In M. Olekains & J. A. Kennedy (Eds.), *Research handbook on gender and negotiation: Research handbooks in business and management,* (pp.207–242), EE Elgar Online

Zuñiga-Collazos, A., Castillo-Palacio, M., Montaña-Narváez, E., & Castillo-Arévalo., G. (2020). Influence of managerial coaching on organisational performance. *Coaching: An International Journal of Theory, Research and Practice, 13*(1), 30–44.

CHAPTER FIFTEEN

Reflective Response 1

TINA MERTEL

Creating a climate of trust to increase favorable negotiations is also well served by having a strategy and tactics. In my work with individual leaders and leadership groups, being clear on the difference between strategy and tactics helps keep one aligned toward the goal.

Strategy is one level below purpose. The first building block of trust is having trust in oneself. Considering one's purpose in becoming a DNP heightens self-regard and builds confidence for the negotiation process. Access to one's purpose is often found in one's values. Values that are most helpful are often expressed in active phrases, such as developing others, creating policy, helping youth, navigating change, and researching data. Knowing one's purpose builds trust in oneself.

I see two paths to having a strategy for building a climate of trust. One path is to become an expert in something, through first-hand experience, academic study, or both. An interviewer is looking to fill a gap or an opportunity. As the negotiation unfolds, the interviewer is mentally checking off a list, answering the question, "Can I see this person in the role?" If there is alignment between the DNP's experience and the needs of the interviewer, the value increases as more is said. The expertise starts to win over the interviewer as a picture of the DNP in the role.

The other path is having a positive mindset. Often, the behaviors at the start of a relationship are behaviors that continue throughout the relationship. The opportunity to offer a win-win, positive mindset at the onset helps the interviewer see the "being" of the individual rather than only the "doing" of the individual. The field of nursing is a relational field. Tasks are crucial, but how a task is delivered is also important. Relationships are key and are created, built, and maintained with many stakeholders. A win-win framework has been shown to decrease the probability of conflict as well as better navigate conflict when it occurs.

Moving now into tasks that build trust, looking at both a framework for communicating your value and individual techniques of communication can be advantageous. Interviewers want to remember their top candidates. Thinking about how to be remembered is worth some preparation. An interviewer will have a hard time remembering more than three attributes or reasons for their top candidates. Creating a framework for being remembered may take some time. Narrowing down the reasons one should be hired may start out as stories or a narrative until clarity rises to the surface. Thinking chronologically may be helpful to keep the reasons easy to remember, like developing a picture of a three-wedged pie, or describing them as one's pillars.

When in negotiation, basic communication theory gives us a good reminder of what is occurring. The sender is delivering a message that is encoded (created), and the receiver is to decode (understand) the message as intended. The sender has options for how to create the communication. The receiver has options for how to listen to the communication. Practice in both makes for a savvy communicator.

Techniques when sending include:

- Using relational presence to create space and clarity in delivering the message. This form of communication stresses the importance of using breath and one's eyes to build trust and psychological safety from the sender to the receiver.
- Summarizing for the receiver, which may be content just heard from the other, or summarizing one's own messaging.
- Using statements of win-win, such as "I trust we can come to a solution"; "With you and me leading, I don't see how we can't do well"; or "Our team has what it takes."
- Let them know what's about to be said, say it, and ask for understanding. Examples of starting this include "I have three reasons you should consider me..."; "Hearing that this role requires technical expertise, I'd like to outline my work at the university..."

Techniques when receiving include:

- Listening for the meaning behind the words, and reflecting it back, such as, "I can hear how this hospital values quality..." or "It sounds like that's been a real issue for the staff..."
- Listening for one or more of the following areas of focus: people, results, or process. Through personality studies, often a sender leans toward one or more of these areas of focus. Is the communication about people? Getting results? Or processes? Hearing this will help in receiving the message so one can communicate back the framework the sender is using.
- Paraphrasing what is heard. Trust is built by paraphrasing, showing that the receiver is present with the sender and values their thoughts.

In addition to the content listed in Chapter 15, having a strategy to build trust and using tactics for effective communication are worth investing in. Know that each and every negotiation will build upon the last in terms of what was learned and can be used in the future. Commending yourself for showing up and being in the game continues to reinforce the positive mindset that will carry into the next negotiation.

CHAPTER FIFTEEN | # Reflective Response 2

CATHERINE PARADISO

■ THE NEW SKILL OF NEGOTIATION: SOME HELPFUL ADVICE

Negotiating for Yourself: Some Pearls

My career in nursing took me throughout the full continuum of care: acute care, community health, home care, and ambulatory care, with positions in executive leadership, government, and academia. Along the way, I learned a lot about how to negotiate. I found myself transitioning from seeking the job to hiring professionals. The most valuable lesson is that we negotiate with people, not jobs. People have different perspectives, understandings, and sensitivities. The DNP is a fairly new role/title in the confusing lexicon of nursing roles. Not everyone in the larger system of healthcare understands what a DNP is versus a master's-prepared nurse practitioner or even a PhD (McCauley et al., 2020). This is a chronic imperfection in our profession. As a new DNP, you must be prepared for this. The employer is often asking the basics: Can you take care of my patients or not? Can you do this job or not? It is up to all of us in nursing to communicate our roles not only through our words but also through our actions. Let's start with negotiating for a job.

    Negotiation is a process. The intent is to resolve an issue so that both parties are satisfied with the result. Compromise is at the center of *negotiation*. In a career such as nursing, where patients come first and self-care is secondary, negotiating can be counterintuitive. Feeling fulfilled, energized, and overall excited about where we work—or not—impacts every aspect of life. Therefore, negotiating throughout the hiring process is central to your future quality of life. Negotiation is often thought about with regard to salary. Expectations, hours, days, assignments, and many other things may be more important for work-life balance. To negotiate for yourself, inventory your personal skill set. Necessary skills for a good negotiator include preparedness, being a good listener, and being a good communicator. Flexibility, likability, critical thinking, patience, open-mindedness, and quick thinking are advantages.

    Since negotiation ends with compromise, there are some steps to take before starting. Using the steps nurses are familiar with and that are the foundation of our critical thinking, assess, plan, implement, and evaluate (yes, the nursing process again!). Before even thinking about negotiating, understand the details of what is and is not feasible.

■ ASSESSMENT: KNOWLEDGE IS POWER

Assessment Starts with Self

Expectations must be managed, so an accurate assessment is vital. First, assess yourself. Know your desires and priorities. Assessing your own value relative to the position you seek is the first step. As best as possible, know the employer's perspective. In some cases, the interviewer may not know what a DNP is, what their competencies are, or what sets a DNP apart from another nurse. While a DNP degree is valuable, the interviewer and employer may value experience more, and you may not know what they value. Ask *Do I actually have the experience required?* Here are a few examples of situations where a DNP may have very valuable experience, but the interviewer may not see their value:

- A nurse practitioner (NP) with years of critical care experience applies to a medical office seeking a position as a primary care provider. The DNP believes they are prepared and qualified; after all, they just completed a rigorous program and 750 clinical hours. The intensive care unit experience is very valuable but also very different from primary care. The NP may be an expert ICU nurse, but a novice primary care provider. If the medical practice wants an experienced provider, the interviewer may not see a new DNP with ICU experience as adequate. In this case, the DNP can discuss what they did by describing their hours, what they treated, and how they worked with the preceptor. This highlights the experience and matches it to the job requirements.
- A new DNP in any specialty may be applying for an academic position where publications and scholarship are priorities. A doctorate is valuable, but experience in teaching methods and strategies is also prioritized, so experience in an academic environment in education may be valued over clinical practice. In this case, it may be better to admit that teaching experience is limited and highlight transferrable skills, such as family teaching or professional presentations. Then, highlight your willingness, motivation, and reasons for seeking the position that portray you as an asset.
- A DNP applying for a senior leadership position without a background in progressive management or experience managing large budgets with financial accountability must prove why the doctoral degree prepares them for such a role. In reality, a DNP in anything other than leadership does not!

Often, the DNP must secure the position before negotiating the employment package. Look closely at the position, the organization, or the medical practice, and know what you bring before negotiating. Do not dwell on your deficiencies for the job, but have awareness of them. Do not try to "build" relevance between your work experience and the position, and at all times be truthful. Approach negotiations after assessment; know your priorities, and be sure that these priorities are possible with this position.

Assess the Community

When determining your leverage in negotiations, know the community. Are you unique or presenting with the same credentials as everyone else? Is this market saturated with DNPs? Are others seeking these positions? Are there many others who can do this job? Are NPs competing for jobs exclusively with other NPs exclusively, or are physician assistants competing for the same jobs? Some possibilities vary with each community and state.

    Assess the scope of practice in your state. Do NPs have full practice authority? If not, to what degree are they reliant on the physician? This is important. Are you a candidate who can generate income? Will you use resources? Last, what is the average salary in your community for the position you seek?

Vignette

Upon completing my first graduate degree, I was the only nurse in the hospital with a master's. My supervisors had not yet completed the BSN. None of my supervisors, physicians, or even colleagues understood the rigor of my program or where I studied, and for sure, they did not know (or care) what clinical nurse specialists were. Discussions about continuing for a doctorate were met with comments like, "You mean a doctorate in nursing? I don't get that. Why don't you just go to medical school?" Frustrated with the narrow environment, I left and sought employment in a larger medical center where colleagues shared my values and the progress of the profession. This was my personal problem, but it stemmed from the profession not messaging the broader healthcare community about advanced practice and its role in patient care. Neither the clinical, quality, or economic benefits were communicated to others, so no wonder. Not much has changed. Many administrators believe the DNP in a medical practice is valuable because they can bill and support the physician.

Assess Compensation Possibilities

This is the hardest, but often the most important. Salary and money do not necessarily mean the same thing to all people. Your expectations must be reasonable and based on what the organization can pay, so do your financial homework. Research what you can bill and use that as a gauge for compensation possibilities. Generally, a specialty practice will generate more revenue than a primary care practice. Know the answers to more details.

- Is the salary in a "box" as in a union environment? If so, salaries are most likely published or posted on the initial offering.
- Organizations generally have salary ranges for various position titles, and in many cases, these salaries are published.
- Compensation may be based on relative value units (RVUs). A compensation package may be partially or completely based on RVUs. RVU-based compensation requires paying a provider based on the type and amount of work they do treating a patient.
- The RVU may not be negotiable. For example, if one joins a group practice, one cannot expect a better RVU formula than that in place for existing providers. If an RVU compensation system is not for you, this may not be the right job.

Before starting any discussion about salary, know what is and is not possible. Avoid statements such as "I am worth it" or "I deserve it." Statements such as "I am asking" or "Can you do a bit more?" are softer. Assess if there are other trade-offs. For example, if the person cannot bend on the salary, maybe they can yield on time off or work-from-home possibilities.

Vignette

I once interviewed a nurse practitioner whom I intended to hire. Once the subject turned to salary, she asked for an amount I could not possibly secure. Her posture and facial expressions were very firm as she said, "I am worth (she stated an amount more than the senior medical officer was making) and will not take less." I felt as though I had a gun pointed at me! Not only did she not get the job, but much time was wasted.

Assess the Negotiator

Know exactly who is on the other side of the table. Is the person across the table a hiring manager? A physician? A human resource director? How well do they know the job they are interviewing you for? Do they know what a DNP is? Will you be the direct report to the person you are negotiating with? This is especially important in clinical positions, where a human resources representative may be hiring in accordance with policies and procedures, but a physician, senior NP, or any person with clinical expertise prioritizes values differently. Negotiation with a "boss" is different than with an HR representative. The HR representative can speak about the offer, benefits, and maybe negotiate. However, you need to be sure the potential boss does not get the impression, either directly from you or indirectly from HR, that you have a "demands" list.

Plan

Before even thinking about negotiating, understand the details of what is and is not feasible. When negotiating, it is always better to have the upper hand. One can easily imagine the questions that will be asked, and the answers set up the candidate for a position of strength or weakness in negotiations.

- What do you bring to this position?
- Examples of how you managed situations relevant to this position
- Why did you apply for this position?
- Identify your strengths and weaknesses
- Questions about the DNP itself

Energy is contagious; be positive! Nobody wants to leave an interview feeling negative. Likability is very important. An old wives tale, "You catch more flies with sugar than you do with vinegar," is true. Do your best to make the person like you. Employers are more likely to extend themselves and/or advocate for those they like. Remember that the person hiring must consider the entire organization, and how you "fit" in. The employer must also know that you really want the job, and not feel like you are doing them a favor by allowing the interview. Avoid mentioning any other offers you may have or giving the impression that "everyone wants me." Discuss how you will enhance *their* organization without overdoing it. Self-aggrandizement is a definite turn-off.

Vignette

As a candidate, a mistake I made once was allowing the interview process to extend for a very long time. Interviewing from one person to another before knowing the salary. When I arrived at the final person, the salary was too low to accept the position. The position was unionized, so there was little flexibility, and I had invested considerable time and emotional energy. Another time, I was interviewing for a position that was a unique opportunity. The interview process dragged on for 6 months. I really wanted the job, so I was encouraged each time I was called back to meet another person. I did not care a bit about the salary.

Practice Makes Perfect

Some stress during negotiations is expected. Sensitize yourself by practicing with a friend or colleague, preferably with someone experienced in negotiations. Practicing with another allows for valuable feedback. You can learn how your responses make the other person feel. This helps you avoid feeling flustered at a critical moment later on. Avoid being perceived as unreasonable, greedy, or petty. Anticipate and plan for hard questions, and never appear awkward or defensive.

Language and Attitude

When an offer is extended and you want to negotiate, a few things are asked all at once. The ideal is if the interviewer makes the offer and then asks something like, "Is this acceptable?" A response could be, "There are a few areas I would like to discuss." Then, present all the issues at once. Under no circumstances should you wait to acquire one thing, then ask for another. You will appear as someone who is never satisfied, and few people will be inclined to help someone with this characteristic.

If there is more than one thing you wish to change, emphasize the importance of each. Words like "deal breaker" or "hardball" can be a turnoff. It may land better by saying, for example, "One thing that is very important is conference tuition reimbursement." Negotiations can mean meeting people halfway, but some things may be so important to you or the employer that there is no "halfway." Professional demeanor is very important, and never use ultimatums.

Implementation

Once you have your plan in place, you should feel more comfortable. There is only one chance to make a first impression. Remember how first impressions have impacted you in the past? Dress for success is an old-fashioned statement, but it still applies. Enter negotiations as a top-notch professional. Energy is contagious, so be sure to project positivity in your verbal and nonverbal language. You may find yourself negotiating for a site, a role, salary, hours, tuition reimbursement, and a variety of other things, so the preparedness will pay off. Timing is everything, so be sure to read the room accurately and not raise certain subjects until the negotiator is ready. Be aware of nonverbal communication in yourself and note the same in others.

Vignette

I once saw an RN arrive to an interview in scrubs because she had come right from work! That individual was hired by the hiring manager and turned out to be a stellar employee, but she did not want the manager to hire another nurse because she works in open-toed shoes! A professional appearance is an indicator, fairly or unfairly, of the professional behavior that can be expected.

Patience is a virtue. What is not negotiable today may be tomorrow. Be willing to continue the conversation. There was a time when working part of a week from home could never be considered; now it is commonplace. I hope you find the information in this section helpful.

Evaluation

The final step in the nursing process is evaluation. If you get the things you want and the job, your outcome is achieved. If not, learn from the experience. Do not take anything personally. Use the experience to learn and move on.

■ REFERENCE

McCauley, L. A., Broome, M. E., Frazier, L., Hayes, R., Kurth, A., Musil, C. M., Norman, L. D., & Villarruel, A. M. (2020). Doctor of Nursing Practice (DNP) degree in the United States: Reflecting, readjusting, and getting back on track. *Nursing Outlook, 68*(4), 494–503.

CHAPTER FIFTEEN | Reflective Response 3
==

ROSEMARY KUNAZCUK

I started my path to midwifery by accident. I began school as a chemistry major but quickly decided to get married. I was considering going to Germany with my husband, so I thought instead that I would become a nurse and work overseas. At that time, the community college had a two-year associate degree program for registered nurses. I completed that program, had a baby, and, life being what it is, I ended up taking a job in a private psychiatric hospital for 2 years. I had another baby! Feeling that I needed more nursing skills, I took a med-surg position near my house. Another 2 years passed, and needing a change, I made the most significant decision of my life. I took a job at a big city hospital in labor and delivery, at Hahnemann University Hospital. The experience totally changed my life. I loved every second of being with women while they were giving birth. Being in a university hospital, I was exposed to a full OB-GYN residency program and was privy to all of their teaching. As the years flew by, I finished my BSN and was considered a senior labor and delivery nurse. I did my share of births when the unit was busy and often, the medical staff let me deliver the patient under their supervision. I wanted more. More of the labor management and more in the relationships with the women giving birth.

Looking into midwifery programs, I found Frontier School of Midwifery and Family Nursing, now known as Frontier University, in Hyden, Kentucky. It was online and worked well with my family's needs. I graduated in 1995. It was life-changing, and I have worked as a midwife since graduating. My first job as a midwife was in a small town in Leighton, Pennsylvania, after a coworker of mine saw an advertisement in the local paper. This was the big step in my career. I sent my resume, interviewed, and was offered the job. It was 57 miles from my house! I started there and commuted there for 3 years. It was the best time. It was a small hospital with only three labor rooms. There were only two physicians there, and I would sleep in a hospital room when I worked overnight. There were no obstetricians in-house. I had an office practice there and relied on my former colleagues and physicians to provide guidance and advice. Some of those patients still keep in touch with me to this day!

I left there to change my commute to Cape May County in New Jersey (I live outside of Philadelphia). I still remember driving there after the second plane hit the World Trade Center on September 11, 2001. The roads were deserted and eerie. There were three physicians at that hospital, and again, I was the first midwife there. Some fireworks ensued at the way I did things. The episiotomy rate fell (hooray!) as the doctors felt pressured by my lack of use of that procedure. Again, there were neither obstetricians nor anesthesiologists in house, so I had to manage my patients carefully. The physician I worked for decided to close the practice, and so I moved on.

After leaving Cape May County, I continued to seek employment in New Jersey. Pennsylvania laws were more restrictive for midwives at that time. I took a position in Voorhees, New Jersey, at a private practice. The hospital had only two other midwives there, one an older and very established certified nurse-midwife (CNM) who worked with a private physician and did both home and hospital births. The second midwife worked for the hospital practice. This practice was very busy, and I worked hard. I was in the office 28 hours per week and 24 hours in labor and delivery. I really enjoyed this job and had so much satisfaction in my practice. I was there for 5 years and entered the Doctor of Nursing Practice (DrNP) program while working there.

After Voorhees, I took a position in Plainfield, New Jersey, at a Federally Qualified Health Center (FQHC). In 2009, I graduated from the DrNP program at Drexel University. I don't regret one minute of the time and hard work that took. And I made lifelong friends in that program!

In 2015, I decided to stop commuting all over the place and open my own practice where I lived. I obtained privileges at the local hospital with my backup doctor, whom I met while working during his residency at Hahnemann. I learned that while I am a great midwife, I am not so great as a small business owner. My next move was working at a doctor's practice and as a hospitalist midwife, where I continue to work to this day. Luckily for me, the hospital is only eight miles from my house, and I absolutely love it there. I work three 12-hour shifts a week. In 2022, I had the privilege of helping 186 babies (10% of all hospital births!) enter this world.

So, that's my story. Now, what do I have to say to you?

Be passionate about your career. Expect to work hard. Take the first offer and establish yourself as a hardworking and devoted midwife. Learn from others. Some will teach you how to be a great midwife, and others will teach you how not to be. We are not all equal! Commit to your first job for at least 2 years, as that will demonstrate your stability, and if you don't like a job, you will quickly quit. In that first job, find what is important to you. Don't agree to 10-minute patient slots; it is absolutely never enough time. Be willing and excited to learn from the established midwives. Take suggestions nicely from the physicians and nurses, especially when they are seasoned practitioners.

As you mature in your practice, look around and evaluate what you like and don't like, and search for the positions and places that appeal to you. Try per-diem positions while maintaining your main job, and compare them to each other. Some midwives have hospital-only positions, and some have only office positions. I believe a mix of office and hospital care is best, taking care of the whole woman.

Midwifery is not just about delivering babies. Women's care and family planning are important roles for midwives to embrace. Helping women navigate contraceptive options. Helping women deal with abusive situations. Helping women deal with mental illness in their own lives, whether it's themselves or a member of their family. Knowing when to make referrals to other healthcare professionals.

Postmenopausal women need care and advice regarding sexual comfort, menopausal symptoms, and breast health. I get immense satisfaction from caring for non-childbearing women. They will often open up to a caring nurse-midwife, and many feel a physician is too hurried for these types of discussions. These are all part of a holistic, care-for-the-whole-person nurse-midwifery practice.

But the joy of handing that baby to their parents is immeasurable. Embrace your soul when dealing with intrauterine fetal demise. Your care in this situation can make all the difference in how the parents deal with loss. The postmenopausal woman who returns year after year for a PAP smear no longer needs just to see and check in with you. We just chat and do a general exam. Gather the teenagers around you. They will often take your advice but not their parents', even if it's the exact same!

It takes time and a lot of energy to be a great midwife. Embrace the pain and the love. There will be laughter and tears, sore feet and sore backs. But oh, so worth it. Good luck and have fun, whether you are a new DNP urse-midwife or a seasoned CNM with a new DNP degree and embarking on the next step of your journey.

CHAPTER FIFTEEN Reflective Response 4

DIANE MAYDICK

My Story and Trajectory as a Clinical Nurse Specialist
   First, Job Interview Inviolable Strategies
   Know everything about the organization.
   Do not negotiate anything in the first interview.
   Maybe avoid asking about salaries, a necessary second interview question.
   Establish good eye contact.
   Listen actively.
   Ask three smart questions.
   End with, "Thank you very much. I am very interested in this position. I will be in touch quickly." TRUE
   OR
   "Thank you very much. I am interested in this position. I will be in touch quickly." True, but decline politely. Don't burn bridges that may reflect negatively on your previous Alma Mater(s)!
   Before you agree to sign, ask for a tour of your unit and meet some staff.
   Now is the time to negotiate.
   If you had a lot of experience before your DNP degree, you will have more leverage to negotiate from a position of some degree of strength.
   Second, My Story
   A career has many "first jobs," and most clinicians can look back and realize each job is a stepping stone. My career spans almost half a century, with each role building upon prior experience. Continuous learning enhanced my ability to develop knowledge and a set of skills to positively influence patients and their families, nurses, and the healthcare system. Each role afforded me opportunities for growth and development, during which I developed skills as an expert collaborative clinician, ethical decision-maker, manager, consultant, educator, researcher, coach, and mentor. My first job as a clinical nurse specialist (CNS) was preceded by clinical experience and specialty certifications prior to having the master's degree conferred.
      Upon graduating from a diploma school of nursing in New York City in 1972, my dream job was at an urban, academic medical center where "team nursing" was practiced. This exposed me to a baccalaureate-prepared specialty nurse, who was called an "enterostomal therapist (ET)" and served as an expert for individuals who had surgery resulting in an ostomy. The ET would perform patient assessments, develop a plan of care, and provide demonstrations of skills needed for the care of individuals who had surgery resulting in a colostomy, ileostomy, or urostomy. The ET nurse provided care, education, and discharge planning for this population of patients. The role quickly caught my attention and sparked my desire to pursue this specialty. At the time, admission to specialty programs for ET training required that an employer commit (in writing on the application), that they planned to use the employee as an ET. Since my employer already had an ET, I began to explore ET specialty education programs

while convincing local hospitals about the importance of the role. Unfortunately, it would take several years and changes in employment to realize this goal. Meanwhile, in 1980, I was finally able to attend an educational program for enterostomal therapy and became certified as an enterostomal therapist. Eventually, the specialty evolved into a trifold specialty known as wound, ostomy, and continence (WOC) nursing, with opportunities to become certified in all three specialty areas. Despite this professional education program and certification in a specialty, it became clear that advanced education was needed to improve care at the bedside. In 1985, while pursuing a bachelor of science degree at Rutgers, The State University of New Jersey, I learned about the role of a clinical nurse specialist (CNS). Thus, the trajectory of my career pointed toward an advanced practice CNS role with a focus on becoming an expert collaborative clinician, ethical decision-maker, manager, consultant, educator, researcher, coach, and mentor.

CLINICAL NURSE SPECIALIST IN HOME HEALTH CARE (FIRST CNS ROLE)

Upon completion of the master of science degree at the City University of New York Hunter College, I was offered a role as a CNS in my specialty area of WOC nursing in 1995. This was prior to the National Association of Clinical Nurse Specialists (NACNS) engagement in discussions in 1995 to articulate CNS practice competencies, educational guidelines, and requirements for credentialing; in fact, certification as a CNS was not yet available. It was not an advanced practice role.

Providing direct care in the practice environment with patients and families leads to using knowledge for improved health outcomes in larger populations. Expert clinical skills, knowledge, complex decision-making, and competency form the basis for expanding practice to influence care not only for individuals but for groups, healthcare organizations, and communities too.

Changes in healthcare delivery in the United States and changes in reimbursement are challenges for home healthcare agencies. My first formal CNS role was in a system-wide home health agency that provided patients, families, and communities access to nursing services, and more specifically, a CNS with wound, ostomy, and continence specialist expertise. The role involved working with nurses, patients, families, and other professionals within the system to provide education, mentorship, and system-level change based on the needs of the population served by the agency to deliver evidence-based healthcare.

The CNS role in home health care afforded the opportunity to expand the practice boundaries of my nursing practice, provide essential direct care, support and advance the practice of professional colleagues, and develop system changes to improve patient outcomes and nursing practice. From a patient/system perspective, access to a CNS addresses the need for quality healthcare for persons who are diverse and culturally different, those who live in rural and underserved areas, those who are aging and disabled, and those with acute and/or chronic conditions, specifically those with wounds, ostomies, and incontinence.

CLINICAL NURSE SPECIALIST IN ACUTE CARE (SECOND CNS ROLE)

In 1997, I assumed the role of clinical nurse specialist with wound, ostomy, and continence certification in an academic medical center. The CNS's primary role is to improve patient care and patient care outcomes. The CNS has skills that overlap those of other advanced practice colleagues but also has distinct characteristics differentiating them from the nurse practitioner, nurse anesthetist, and nurse-midwife. What distinguishes a CNS from other colleagues includes performing a higher level of analysis, implementing newly emergent nursing science, initiating evidence-based practice (EBP) to facilitate health maintenance, preventive care, early diagnosis and treatment of acute and chronic illness, and optimizing the transition of care from one care setting to another.

In the acute care environment, the CNS must be prepared to encounter complex scenarios with vulnerable patient populations. A consultation with an experienced CNS in WOC nursing will be focused on a multifocused plan of care with the patient/family, nurse, and other professional colleagues to ensure implementation of a plan of care and to set goals for care leading to safe and effective care delivery, allowing patients to reach their healthcare goals. Over time, the experience of a CNS in home health care or acute care serves as a framework for future practice.

The CNS role in acute care afforded me the opportunity to expand the boundaries of my nursing practice, provide essential direct care, support and advance the practice of professional colleagues, and develop system changes to improve patient outcomes and nursing practice. From a patient/system perspective, access to a CNS addresses the need for quality healthcare for persons who are hospitalized with acute and/or chronic conditions, specifically those with wounds, ostomies, and incontinence. Monitoring trends in adverse outcomes such as hospital-acquired conditions or post-discharge problems led to interprofessional collaboration for addressing system changes. Some examples include:

1. Monitoring pressure injury prevalence and incidence, which were found to be rising; plan: designing programs of continuous quality improvement within the acute care setting.
2. Self-report of discharged individuals with a new ostomy experiencing leakage and peristomal skin complications after discharge to home; plan: development of an ostomy support group and outpatient ostomy service.

In 2008, during my years in acute care, there was a release of the Consensus Model of advanced practice registered nurse (APRN) licensure, accreditation, certification, and education (APRN Consensus Model; APRN Joint Dialogue Group, 2008), and subsequently, the title of *clinical nurse specialist* became a "protected title" for CNSs, which is elucidated in the law and scope of practice as outlined in regulations. Eventually, the American Nurses Credentialing Center developed the Adult Health Clinical Nurse Specialist Certification, adding further credibility to the CNS role.

THIRD, ARTICULATING FOR THE DNP CLINICAL NURSE SPECIALIST ROLE

The ability to assess, diagnose, develop a plan, initiate the plan, and reevaluate actual changes made by individuals and systems addresses the need for safe, high-quality, cost-effective care, which we all strive to achieve. Most employers do not fully understand the role and benefits of a CNS. How do we better articulate what a CNS brings to the table?

1. Know your value: Inform administrators of the value of a DNP/CNS. Articulate your ideal job as a DNP/CNS and create a job description including:
    a. A short summary of the role (what is a clinical nurse specialist?)
    b. Education and certification(s) required (master's/DNP and specialty certifications)

c. Knowledge, skills, and experience required for the role (prior applicable experience)
   d. Goals for the role (improved outcomes, decreased costs, etc.)
   e. Clarify the reporting structure (who has the power to help you be successful?)
2. Showcase yourself with your curriculum vitae:
   a. Include a short executive summary about yourself
   b. Showcase your education (school, program, degree)
   c. Highlight employment history/outcomes (organization, job title, summary of role)
   d. List publications/presentations (journals, posters, podiums); become a clinical scholar at your healthcare agency
   e. Include current specialty certifications
   f. Lessons learned; often, the employer does not fully understand what a CNS does—we have to educate them!
   g. Keep a running list of accomplishments (successful projects, evidence of supporting staff in quality improvement and projects, demonstration of collaboration across multiple healthcare disciplines
   h. Maintain a log of your activities (direct and indirect patient care, administrative tasks, daily, weekly, and monthly)
   i. Showcase outcomes for administration
   j. Define the identified problems, desired outcomes, action steps, and results you want to accomplish in your job search
   k. Don't settle immediately
   l. Be sure to understand the expectations of your job (e.g., reporting structure, salary, time for research, conferences, presentations to the organization, and professional colleagues)
   m. Recommendations for the DNP CNS
   n. Publish your work; don't minimize the importance of the publishing "process" or quality improvement papers (many colleagues want to know how you achieve outcomes)
   o. Join the ethics committee
   p. Collaborate with interprofessional teams at all times, avoid working in "silo"

The successful CNS is a very visible APRN. You really create your career role every day. With a DPN degree, you will be in a special class of DNP CNSs. Go forth, negotiate your career trajectory. Go forth and succeed!

CHAPTER FIFTEEN

Reflective Response 5

MICHAEL CONTI

Typical "first jobs" as a staff certified registered nurse anesthetist (CRNA) are package- and seniority-dependent. For example, compensation (salary, paid time off) is based on years as a CRNA: 0 to 2 years, 2 to 5 years, etc., and is not usually negotiated. One potential area for negotiation is scope of practice, where depending on the practice environment, one may negotiate whether they can practice in any of the subspecialty areas: obstetric anesthesia, pediatric anesthesia, and if they can place invasive lines and perform neuraxial and regional anesthesia. Scheduling usually depends on departmental needs, but there may be opportunities for self-scheduling or providing input regarding your own scheduling. Negotiation may occur in the setting of a 1099 employee or locum tenens provider (independent contractor), where you may have more opportunity to negotiate salary and benefits.

Lessons learned:

1. Spend some time in the department to assess the culture.
2. Ask current staff what they like, dislike, and would change in the department.
3. Inquire about compensation time for nonclinical responsibilities or projects.
4. Ask about nonclinical opportunities: leadership, research, and representing the department at institutional meetings and committees.
5. If there is a student registered nurse training program (SRNA) at the institution, inquire about potential teaching opportunities within the program.
6. Are there anesthesia assistants (AAs)? If so, what is the relationship between the members of the department?
7. Is there an AA training program? If so, is there a teaching requirement for the CRNAs to teach AA students?

The only possibility for salary or benefits negotiation is if the experienced CRNA with a master's degree obtains a DNP or DNAP and attempts to negotiate work terms after achieving the doctoral degree.

CHAPTER SIXTEEN

Three Real Career Role Trajectories From a Bedside Registered Nurse to a DNP-Prepared Family Nurse Practitioner

VERONICA QUATTRINI, COURTNEY HICKS,
MARY GRACE RENFROW, MARY MARASA RADCLIFF,
AND VALERIE T. COTTER

COURTNEY HICKS

Nursing is a unique field that is vast and ever changing. Many of us got into the field because we wanted to help others. I always knew I wanted to work in the medical field so that I could help others. Where or in what capacity has been a journey that I am still on. I chose a magnet high school outside of my home district that allowed me to take extra health science classes within their Allied Health program. After high school I went on to the University of Maryland College Park and graduated with a bachelor of science in community health and a minor in human development. While in college I worked as a student athletic trainer and after graduation I worked within the public health arena for a government contracting company in their child welfare division. Feeling unsatisfied and wanting to do more direct, hands-on care, I applied to nursing school.

I attended nursing school at the University of Maryland School of Nursing. While in school, I worked at the University of Maryland Medical Center as a patient care technician and a student nurse. I graduated with my BSN and was able to secure a job in the Surgical Intensive Care Unit (SICU), where I completed a semester of clinicals as a student. After a few years in the SICU, I transferred to working as a bedside nurse in multi-trauma critical care within the Shock Trauma Center. This was among one of the units I worked in as a student nurse. While on each unit I was able to serve on several committees, help implement evidence-based projects, and precept new employees.

While working and completing school I got to experience firsthand the variety that the nursing field has to offer. There are so many areas, specialties, subspecialties, and diverse roles we can transition to and from. I was given the opportunity to learn a variety of skills, procedures, and knowledge sets. In addition to the professional growth nursing provides, it also provides the opportunity to meet people. From coworkers, patients, to members of different disciplines the ability to meet and collaborate with others is unlike any other field.

After working as a bedside nurse for several years, I knew I wanted more. I went back to the University of Maryland School of Nursing to obtain my doctor of nursing practice (DNP) degree. At the time I went back to school, DNP programs were just starting to pop up, and there were still many MSN programs to choose from. I did apply and was accepted to several MSN programs, but ultimately chose to pursue my DNP. I knew this would entail more schooling and more debt, but I felt it was worth it. I always worked within a large academic institution, so staying on top of best practice measures and implementation of evidence-based practice was something I was not only very familiar with, but it was something I was and remain passionate about. To me, obtaining my DNP was what made the most sense in order to keep in tune with my practice.

I graduated from the University of Maryland School of Nursing DNP/family nurse practitioner (FNP) program after 4 years. During my schooling, I was fortunate to be assigned (I know not everyone is) some amazing clinical experiences. Not only did they serve as great learning opportunities, but my preceptors were fantastic mentors and many of them I still keep in contact with. When I graduated school, I was offered jobs at two of my previous clinical sites.

One of my favorite activities in my DNP program was slightly unconventional. In my diagnosis and management course, my professor challenged us each week to write down three interesting facts or cases we dealt with during clinicals. Of course, at the time she introduced this idea, many of us were a little apprehensive knowing we already had so much to log for clinical time. It felt like this was just something extra and irrelevant. While yes, this activity did take some extra time, it quickly became my favorite. It was a fun way to learn about other students' experiences while also getting to hear about different conditions/diagnoses and learn tips/tricks/nuances for evaluating and treating patients. It was also a challenge for many of us to really learn our own patients and their conditions prior to presenting them as we quickly learned in class that many of us would have questions. I found that I still remember my fellow classmates' unique clinical experiences and found their perspectives and thought processes helpful in my learning as well.

I have worked as a DNP/FNP for 3 years. My first nurse practitioner job was through the University of Maryland Medical Center in the Emergency Department (ED). As I mentioned above, I had the opportunity to complete a semester of clinicals in this department and really fell in love with the variety the ED has to offer. I was able to work in the adult ED, Urgent Care, and even pick up some shifts in the pediatric ED. After 3 years in the ED, my personal life changed with the expansion of my family and the rotating shifts, on call, and weekend requirements no longer fit well with my personal needs. I left the ED and am currently working for another health agency within its ENT/plastic surgery department. I still enjoy the ED setting so I do maintain PRN status there.

My role as a DNP/FNP is still evolving. When I first started out after graduation, I mentally separated these roles. I focused on the FNP role for the first 2 years of practice. I focused on honing my clinical skills, improving my knowledge base as a new practitioner, and getting comfortable and confident in my new role. As my comfort level grew as an FNP, I began to let my DNP shine. I joined committees that focused on practice change and improving patient care. I helped start a task force to improve patient flow. I coauthored research papers and presented in our journal club. In my current role, I didn't feel the need to separate the FNP and DNP roles this go-round. I find that as I am learning new skills and processes, I am not only just learning them, but I am asking myself is this best practice, can this be improved upon, or is there a way to improve patient flow? I am not only learning a new specialty, but I am also learning a new environment and am approaching each new experience as a cohesive DNP/FNP.

My education as a DNP has given me a stronger clinical knowledge set. The "why" and "how" are always thoughts in my clinical practice. "Why" am I ordering or doing this for my patient? Is it best practice? Or "How" can we improve this, whether it's a policy, practice guideline, or patient experience, etc. When the answers to those questions are unsatisfactory, I dig to find additional answers or spark a need for change. The ability to think beyond not only helps current patients, but hopefully improves outcomes for future patients. As I mentioned before, nursing is an ever-changing field, so I am unsure what my future will hold. I currently still thoroughly love direct patient care, so I imagine myself continuing patient care while working on committees and task forces to improve patient outcomes and experiences. I hope in the future many more nurse practitioners gain their DNP to continue to help evolve our practice and improve outcomes for our patients.

MARY GRACE RENFROW

Having been tasked with brutal honesty and transparency: I do not think I can authentically discuss my DNP/FNP work without first touching on my undergraduate nursing career, and my long path to the DNP. When I really think about my why, I was a ship lost at sea. I have always been semi-talented at so many things, a Jill of all trades—sports, academics, music—but an expert at none. After college, I was working in this high-level corporate job, making plenty of money, and even though I had a lot of responsibility, I felt no purpose. I had it all—the cute apartment in Dupont Circle, a crew of young professionals to do dinner with, expendable cash for vacations. But I felt very empty inside—no anchor. It was during this time that both of my grandfathers died within a few months of each other. During my final conversations with them, both said the same thing: "Molly, you deserve to be happy." It was as though they could both sense how empty I felt inside—yes, I had the trappings of a successful corporate career, but they knew I was longing for meaning. As my grandfathers passed on, I watched my mother and aunts provide hospice care. Want to hear an anomaly? Both of my grandfathers were able to die in their sunrooms, being cared for by family. I wanted so badly to offer the same service to my loved ones. I decided right then and there: time to go back to school and become a nurse.

I started my journey at the Community College of Baltimore County, where I earned my ASN. I will say this: that associates degree program was the scariest thing I have ever done! Shortly thereafter, I earned my BSN and master's in nursing education at Towson University. The first few years of bedside nursing were wild, and I remember feeling incredibly overwhelmed but intellectually stifled at the same time. Then a good friend of mine suggested we start applying to nurse practitioner schools. The theory was: you get rejected the first two times you apply, then you might get in the third time. Ha! To my surprise, I was offered seats at multiple brick-and-mortar programs in the Baltimore-DC-Metro area. When I was looking over my options, I decided that going to a DNP program made more sense than an MSN program, but I was not exactly sure why. I was casually thinking, hey: if you are going to do it anyway, why not get a terminal degree and get it over with? In my naivete, I had no idea how much my DNP would serve me, and I am so very glad I chose the DNP path—more about this later.

As a member of the inaugural DNP/FNP cohort, I graduated from the University of Maryland School of Nursing (UMSON) in 2018. During my schooling, I was blessed with a wide variety of clinical experiences: emergency departments, urgent care, primary care, outpatient specialty clinics, and the governor's well-mobile. One of my most memorable clinical experiences was in the President's Clinic, which is an outpatient pediatric gastroenterology interdisciplinary clinic at the University of Maryland Medical Center (UMMS). The University of Maryland, Baltimore values interdisciplinary professional education and devotes many resources to the mission of promoting teamwork in healthcare—they really put their money where their mouth is. In the President's Clinic, I was paired with other healthcare professionals (GI fellows, social workers, pharmacists). We would all see the patients together, we would devise a plan, and then we would all meet afterward over lunch to discuss the experience. I learned how to effectively communicate with professionals outside my area of study and began to realize how strongly interprofessional communication can affect the quality of care of our patients. I carry these skills with me today. There is so much tribalism in healthcare, and it is so important to remember that we are all on the same team.

After three hectic years, a few months prior to graduation, I began receiving recruiting calls and emails. One of the most memorable positions was in a rural community health clinic which offered primary care, dental, optical, and behavioral health services. The integrated care model was incredibly appealing to me, as was the salary—$160,000! Meanwhile, I continued to work as a bedside RN and when the head hospitalist learned I was nearing graduation, she encouraged me to apply to the gastroenterology service. After working over a decade in the same hospital, I was familiar with the gastroenterology attendings and I was keenly aware of their expertise and bedside manner. To say I was conflicted is an understatement. On the one hand, I could earn a lot more money doing exactly what I went to FNP school for: primary care. I would likely be more comfortable doing the work for which I had been trained. But, I would not know much about my colleagues and mentorship at the rural clinic. On the other hand, I could accept a lower salary, but would know exactly the quality of the people who would be training me. The one small problem being that I knew next-to-nothing about gastroenterology!

In the end, I chose the position with the gastroenterology service and 5 years later, I continue to work with the same providers. I cannot more strongly advise new graduate nurse practitioners (NPs) regarding the importance of good mentorship! It is so important to work with people—whether they be MDs, DOs, NPs, or PAs—who want you to be successful. For the first year or two, my days were very long. At the start, I was never made to feel rushed to complete consult notes and was encouraged to take my time and dive deep into UpToDate. I remember the chief saying, "read, read, read." Each physician rounded with me on every patient, every day, and looked over my consult notes with a fine-toothed comb. This level of detailed tutelage translated to adding 2 to 3 hours of work each day after my on-call shift was over, but I appreciate that this also meant my attendings were staying late in order to train me. The gastroenterology practice paid for, and I attended, two conferences within 6 months of hire. Later, I earned an advanced practice provider scholarship to attend the GUILD conference in Maui, Hawaii. As my learning progressed, I developed more confidence and depth of knowledge. I now see patients independently. My attendings trust my clinical judgment. When I see a patient who I believe requires urgent oversight on the part of an attending, they appreciate my recommendations and back me up.

During the initial pandemic years of 2019 to 2020, the job became dismal and depressing; five days a week of inpatient GI consulting service began to wear on me. Then one day, as fate would have it, I was assigned a DNP student. The act of teaching again breathed life into me! I had forgotten how much I loved teaching students (prior to obtaining my DNP/FNP, I was an undergraduate clinical instructor for many years). As the months progressed, I began seeing more and more students reemerging in the halls throughout the hospital. I jumped right in anytime I had an opportunity to teach at the bedside, whether it was graduate or undergraduate students. Through much self-reflection, I decided to switch gears and apply for faculty positions at all of my alma maters. I wanted to give back to the very institutions that had brought me so much personal fulfillment. As luck would have it, I was offered a position in the DNP/FNP program at UMSON. Getting back to my comments on the MSN versus the DNP, I am so glad I earned my DNP or my wonderful FNP faculty position would never have been attainable. I love teaching at the DNP-FNP level, and I love that my institution requires all FNP faculty to maintain clinical practice. I love bringing my students with me to GI clinical practice. Most of all, I love supervising students who are completing DNP quality improvement projects in my beloved home hospital. I truly feel that, as an FNP, I can make a difference to one patient at a time, but as a DNP/FNP, I am casting a wider net and making positive changes on the organizational and population-based levels. The DNP has truly opened doors for me.

When I think about my future as a DNP/FNP, my mind goes blank. I am in such a state of satisfaction, I cannot imagine wanting more or something different. I have the best of both worlds: maintaining clinical practice and teaching FNP students at the DNP level. My students are making so much positive change with their quality improvement projects and without having my DNP, I would never have the benefit of this bird's eye view. I feel comfortable guiding students in leadership roles in my hospital which I also attribute to my DNP education.

When I think about the future of nursing and careers in nursing, I feel both heartbroken and full of hope. Nurses, like all healthcare workers, have been through so much these last few years. I feel sad for people who feel stuck. Stuck because they are making too much money to try something new? Stuck because their level of education keeps them tethered? Stuck because they are brilliant and smart but cut off at the knees? I read forums online about nurse practitioners, and specifically DNP-prepared nurse practitioners. There are a lot of naysayers out there. I am here to proclaim one thing: hopelessness is the worst diagnosis of all. Having my DNP/FNP has enabled me to achieve joy. For me it is not about the money, it is about loving what I will be doing 40 hours a week for the next 20+ years. It is about feeling proud of my hardworking and bright students. It is about feeling proud of my brave and strong patients. It is about feeling proud of myself. I am hopeful and proud, all around, to the fullest of my ability—and that is a wonderful feeling. I am so glad I earned my DNP/FNP.

MARY MARASA RADCLIFF

Being a part of the nursing profession never felt like a choice to me. It always felt like it was something I was drawn to and was the only career option that genuinely felt right. Yet, when I started my nursing career in 2013, I had no idea where it would lead me. It started with an unexpected interest in oncology care, then on to the University of Maryland, Baltimore's DNP/FNP program, and then moving across the country for a nurse practitioner fellowship. I graduated from the DNP/FNP program in May 2021 and pursued a fellowship in oncology at Fred Hutchinson Cancer Center in Seattle, Washington. This path led me to where I am now, working at Johns Hopkins Hospital in a nurse practitioner–led oncology urgent care clinic.

I attended Towson University for my undergraduate nursing degree and graduated in May 2013. As my final semester approached it was time to make requests for my final clinical rotation. When I started nursing school, I thought I wanted to be in pediatrics or women's health. So, when we were asked to pick three specialties for potential placement, I put labor and delivery and the neonatal intensive care unit. For the third, I was not sure what to request. Around that time a family member was diagnosed with leukemia, and I saw the impact their care team had on their life. Inspired by the team, I decided to put oncology as the third option. I was then placed at Mercy Medical Center's inpatient oncology unit for my final clinical rotation. I was amazed by the resilience and hope in each of the oncology patients, and when graduation came, I was thrilled to be offered a position on the unit.

The first 4 years of my bedside nursing career were filled with learning curves, involvement in unit and hospital-wide councils, and clinical advancement projects. Through those professional and leadership developing opportunities, I started to feel drawn to pursue the University of Maryland, Baltimore's DNP/FNP program. I felt I was coming to a crossroads in my career, and it was time to take the next steps to become more involved in making decisions about patient care and system-wide change.

After getting accepted into the University of Maryland, Baltimore's DNP/FNP program, I was looking forward to starting the next chapter of my career in primary care where I could help facilitate healthy lifestyles and promote well-being. After working with patients admitted to the hospital with multiple comorbidities, I hoped to be involved in preventative care. Though that is not where I ended up working, my clinical experiences and DNP project during that time helped prepare me for my current role as an oncology nurse practitioner.

During my DNP/FNP program, I had clinical rotations in various outpatient settings. In the Spring 2020 semester, my clinical placement was at a local urgent care clinic. My preceptor was a wonderful clinician and teacher, who had a passion for medical care that was contagious. I did not expect that this placement would spark so much interest in urgent care practice. This was also the start of the COVID-19 pandemic, which impacted my ability to go into certain clinical settings. Luckily, I was able to continue working in the urgent care clinic during that semester and picked up extra clinical hours in future semesters. It turns out that spending extra time in the urgent care clinic would be extremely beneficial to my current job in an oncology urgent care clinic.

Throughout my time in the DNP/FNP program, I continued to work as a bedside nurse on an inpatient oncology unit. Although I enjoyed each clinical experience I had in school, there was something about working with the oncology population that I was not ready to give up. As I approached graduation, I was at a crux between my knowledge of being an inpatient oncology nurse and my training to be a primary care nurse practitioner. Then I saw a post about an oncology fellowship for nurse practitioners that sparked my interest and thought this could be the perfect opportunity to bridge the gap between my two knowledge sets. I was on a nationwide search for the program that was the best fit to foster my career passions.

It wasn't long before I found Fred Hutchinson Cancer Center's Advanced Practice Provider Fellowship program. They were offering a yearlong fellowship for nurse practitioners and physician assistants in Hematology/Oncology or Bone Marrow Transplant. I pursued the Hematology/Oncology track with the goal to get as much exposure as possible to different aspects of oncology care. I was fortunate to be one of three people offered a position in the program and prepared to move to Seattle, Washington, following my graduation in May 2021. The fellowship consisted of clinical rotations, structured learning, and professional development opportunities. It was the perfect transition from being a bedside nurse to an oncology nurse practitioner.

The fellowship was made up of clinical rotations in solid tumors, hematologic disorders, and supportive care subspecialties. It provided valuable experience and foundational knowledge about oncology care that I use daily in my current role. It also provided me with clinical experiences in both outpatient and inpatient settings. Training as a family nurse practitioner focused my clinical expertise in the outpatient setting. However, when working in oncology, I found the clinical experience in acute care settings very beneficial. During that time, I was able to see how issues were managed in an inpatient setting and developed a better understanding of what issues required admission and what could be managed outpatient.

One of the most directly transferable learning experiences during the fellowship to my current role was my time in the Acute Care Evaluation Clinic. This clinic receives referrals from a patient's longitudinal oncology team to evaluate urgent concerns. They assess for signs of oncologic emergencies, provide symptom management, evaluate the need for inpatient admission, and more. I really enjoyed the time I spent in this clinic and elected to spend additional time there during an elective rotation. As the end of the fellowship approached, I began pursuing job opportunities closer to home. Feeling prepared and motivated to apply my sharpened expertise, I applied to an opening at Johns Hopkins Oncology Urgent Care Clinic, where I currently work. In this role, we support oncology patients within the Hopkins system to evaluate concerning symptoms, provide symptom control, and help decrease emergency room visits. This felt like the perfect position to utilize the knowledge I had gained in my DNP/FNP clinical rotations and throughout the fellowship. I was thrilled when offered the position and prepared to start there following the completion of the fellowship program.

In addition to clinical experience, the fellowship had structured learning activities. Every Thursday and Friday we had didactic lectures about different topics in oncology care. There were also conferences and continued learning medical education events that we attended throughout the year. The program offered dynamic and diverse presentations on a wide variety of topics that I could then apply to my patients at Johns Hopkins. Our schedules also included dedicated academic time for review of different topics or preparing for clinical rotations. This independent study and structured learning time allowed me to prepare for and ultimately obtain my certification as an advanced oncology certified nurse practitioner by the end of the fellowship.

The third component of the fellowship was professional development. This included an opportunity to collaborate with other members of the team to write an article titled "Considerations and Evaluation of Early Onset Colorectal Cancer" which was submitted and published in the *Journal of Nurse Practitioners*. Each fellow also did an end-of-the-year presentation on a topic of interest. I reviewed available evidence on psilocybin therapy for anxiety and depression in oncology patients. My experience with my DNP project, "Implementing a Mobility Scale for Gynecologic Oncology Patients to Increase Postoperative Mobility Levels," proved valuable for these activities. I felt confident in my ability to search literature, review high-quality evidence, and find ways to apply it to current practice.

Each experience and opportunity throughout my nursing career has led me to my current role as a nurse practitioner in the Johns Hopkins Oncology Urgent Care Clinic. I started this position in January 2023 and look forward to continuing to learn and grow as a nurse practitioner. As a DNP/FNP, an important responsibility is providing high-quality clinical care. My training in school and during the fellowship prepared me to be a competent and safe provider. Most importantly, it also taught me that to be a high-quality provider, you must be dedicated to lifelong learning and continue to seek knowledge in the constantly changing world of medicine. The role of a DNP/FNP also involves questioning the status quo and continuing to look for ways to improve care delivery. As DNPs we have the unique perspective and experience of being involved in patient care and implementing change to improve patient outcomes.

As I continue my DNP/FNP career I hope to continue to make a positive impact on the lives of the patients I am privileged to work with and grow as a leader in the healthcare system. Remaining open to opportunities and adaptable to change has led me to where I am in my career. I plan to continue with this agile mindset as I move forward and seize opportunities that can make meaningful impacts. At the Fred Hutchinson Cancer Center and during my DNP/FNP training I had the privilege to work with DNPs who were practicing at the top of their licensure, involved in management, and led independent clinics. This has helped prepare me and inspired me to be a part of a nurse practitioner–led clinic at Johns Hopkins Hospital.

My DNP education has shown me the immense impact that nurses have on the healthcare system. Nurses have a role in direct patient care, workflow, safety, implementing change, and organizational growth. This provides endless career opportunities and I look forward to each step in my career. I am immensely grateful for the wonderful educators, clinicians, and leaders I have learned from so far in my career. Each experience has led me to where I am today and will continue to shape the trajectory of my career. As a DNP/FNP, I know that I can have a meaningful impact and look forward to what the future will bring.

CRITICAL THINKING QUESTIONS

1. Do you think RN clinical experience is helpful to prepare for DNP education and practice? Why or why not?
2. Currently, 47 states have NP and NP/PA postgraduate residency and fellowship training programs to help prepare new NPs/PAs for primary care. Discuss issues/barriers in NP postgraduate training programs.
3. Explain how leadership activities could be achieved by the DNP graduate.

CHAPTER SIXTEEN Reflective Response

VERONICA QUATTRINI AND VALERIE T. COTTER

There are several common themes discussed in the three career stories. First, they all knew that they wanted to be nurses and had an underlying desire to help and care for others. These choices were often precipitated and inspired by family experiences. There was a stated need for fulfillment in their chosen profession with a calling to satisfy the feeling of emptiness with the "right" feeling. They also remarked on the flexibility associated with nursing opportunities, as well as the ability for growth in clinical practice and academia.

After several years of bedside nursing, they all felt the need to take the next step in their careers, and wanted to continue with patient care. There was a strong focus on mastering their clinical skills as a nurse practitioner before engaging in other DNP roles. There was also a common struggle associated with the learning curve in their first nurse practitioner position.

They thoughtfully chose to pursue a DNP versus a master's degree and realized the importance of a terminal degree. These DNP/FNP graduates considered the importance of being proficient with literature searches, reviewing high quality evidence, and applying it to clinical practice. There was a strong connection with improving patient care through policy, practice guidelines, patient experience, and overall patient outcomes through implementation of quality improvement change.

They pursued the DNP degree not only to practice as a nurse practitioner, but also for leadership opportunities and the ability to make change at a higher level. They all discussed the importance of involvement on committees and task forces to improve overall patient outcomes and patient care delivery, as well as collaboration on research, manuscripts, and professional presentations. There was a larger calling noted to create positive change in organizations and population-based health, and lifelong learning to maintain current evidence-based practice.

There are some unique differences in each of the career stories. One DNP/FNP pursued a formal fellowship program in oncology after graduation. This preparation is consistent with the Advanced Practice Registered Nurse (APRN) Consensus Model (Institute of Medicine, 2011) that regulates specialty practice as a much more focused area of preparation and practice than does the APRN role/population focus level. The additional clinical training prepared her for specialty certification as an advanced oncology certified nurse practitioner.

Another DNP/FNP had an informal mentorship with specialists who she had practiced with as a registered nurse for years. Her informal mentorship was unique to her needs and required that she spend additional time in the practice. The formal mentorship was structured, and all mentees received the same training. There are few fellowships for gastroenterology nurse practitioners and no national certification, so this informal mentorship was key to her success (NPS, 2023).

One DNP/FNP graduate discussed the importance of educating DNP students in her clinical practice. She described the fulfillment that she felt while educating DNP students at the bedside. With that she felt the need to change her professional trajectory and pursued academia as a full-time profession. Once again, this confirms the flexibility and opportunities that all three graduates stated about nursing. She highlighted the importance of a DNP to educate students at this higher level. She also called attention to the importance of all faculty maintaining clinical practice to stay current with evidence-based guidelines but also to educate students.

REFERENCES

Institute of Medicine (US) Committee on the Robert Wood Johnson Foundation Initiative on the Future of Nursing, at the Institute of Medicine. (2011). *The future of nursing: Leading change, advancing health*. National Academies Press (US); 2011. D, APRN Consensus Model. https://www.ncbi.nlm.nih.gov/books/NBK209870

NPS. (2023). *A Bona Fide Guide to Life as a Gastroenterology NP: Three Experts Weigh In*. https://www.npschools.com/blog/guide-to-becoming-a-gastroenterology-np

CHAPTER SEVENTEEN

Interprofessional and Interdisciplinary Collaboration: Essential for the Doctoral Advanced Practice Nurse

JIHANE HAJJ, KRISTEN NOBLES, AND MARY FRANCIS

INTRODUCTION

The U.S. healthcare system continues to face numerous systemic challenges at various levels. The coronavirus pandemic highlighted the issues of racial/ethnic health disparities in the delivery and receipt of quality care, now commonly referred to as "systemic racism in healthcare" (Gravlee, 2020; Johnson-Agbakwu et al., 2022). Black and Hispanic persons, who constitute 13% and 18% of the U.S. population, were disproportionately affected by COVID-19, resulting in 33% of new cases nationally and 22% of COVID-19-related deaths (Blumenthal et al., 2020). In addition, the effect of poverty and disadvantaged neighborhoods dominated by non-White persons contributed to higher disease incidence and mortality compared to White neighborhoods less affected by poverty (Adhikari et al., 2020). These unfortunate realities, reflecting a healthcare system in great need of an overhaul, are among many issues that need to be addressed by implementing health policy, federal policy, and public health reforms. Realizing the need to improve healthcare quality, patient safety, patient satisfaction, and access to cost-effective healthcare delivery, the Institute of Medicine (IOM) Future of Nursing report 2010 called for the generation of doctorally prepared nurses (i.e., doctor of nursing practice [DNP]) to help transform and "reengineer" the unstructured healthcare system. Similarly, the American Association of Colleges of Nursing (AACN, 2006) released the eight DNP Essentials competencies for advanced nursing practice, which are transformational to the education of doctorally prepared advanced practice nurses. These Essentials spoke of the crucial role DNP graduates play in the area of advancing "Scientific Underpinning for Practice" (Essential I), "Organizational and Systems Leadership" (Essential II), "Evidence-Based Practice" (Essential III), "Information System/Technology" (Essential IV), "Health Policy" (Essential V), "Interprofessional Collaboration for Improving Patient and Population Outcomes" (Essential VI), "Clinical Prevention and Population Health" (Essential VII), and "Advanced Nursing Practice" (Essential VIII). The purpose of this chapter is to discuss the role future DNP graduates play in leading interdisciplinary and interprofessional collaboration, which supports all the AACN Essentials described above. This chapter's authors believe that interdisciplinary collaboration "live" in all these Essentials. Therefore, this chapter will elaborate on the DNP graduate's interprofessional and interdisciplinary collaboration potential in the areas of scholarship, academia, clinical practice, and leadership.

INTERDISCIPLINARY/INTERPROFESSIONAL COLLABORATION AMONG DNP GRADUATES: AN INTEGRATED MODEL OF PRACTICE

While there are clear delineations of the DNP graduate roles in the academic setting, their roles outside academia remain unclear. Clarifying the interdisciplinary and interprofessional collaboration endeavors of DNP graduates at all levels may render a much clearer picture, which is needed to address the many gaps in our current state of an ill-structured healthcare system. Using a systems thinking approach and guided by the AACN DNP Essentials, the model described in this chapter is an envisioned representation of the DNP's roles across all layers of the healthcare system. We believe, like many scholars, that the complex American healthcare system requires a systems-thinking approach to realize needed improvement and equity. Following this approach, the ideal DNP professional should learn how to "act over broader spaces and dimensions" using a "high leverage" thinking approach. In other words, the DNP should ask how to improve the system's performance with the least unintended negative consequences. In fact, we posit that collaboration among healthcare stakeholders is a key tool to transform the fragmented "parts" of the healthcare system into a more "stable" one, a system less prone to "rupture" (CDC, 2017).

This envisioned model of practice has multiple layers and is metaphorically similar to the earth's structures. In this model, the DNP graduate has a prominent role at every single "layer," where their functions and roles have a stronger impact when steered by collaboration with colleagues in the field.

At the inner, strongest core of this model is the individual's health, which is impacted by various healthcare organizations, social determinants of health, and the patient's personal belief system. The outer core represents the healthcare governing bodies—this is where the DNP should advocate and serve the patient by informing public policies—feeding back to the inner core. The "crust" represents the population health, which is indicative of the performance of the healthcare system. In this model, the DNP is present throughout all layers and should use collaboration with other disciplines and professionals as a tool to help improve individuals' and health system's performance.

INTERPROFESSIONAL AND INTERDISCIPLINARY COLLABORATION IN DNP EDUCATION

It is nearly impossible to translate existing research, produce evidence, advance health policy initiatives, and improve health outcomes by working in silos. If we step away from healthcare and dive into the aviation world, we quickly learn the strict rules of teamwork and leadership within the teams, both of which are required for safe flying practices. In fact, errors and accidents were found to be associated with failure to perform within teams (Aviation safety, human error, human factors, 2022). Collaboration within teams, disciplines, and professions is at the core of and makes up one of the main infrastructures of a healthy healthcare system. Within the context of DNP education, as guided by the AACN Essentials, the National Organization of Nurse Practitioner

Faculties (NONPF), and the IOM, this chapter details the role of DNP-prepared nurses in leading interprofessional and interdisciplinary collaboration in four distinct areas. These are scholarship, academia, clinical practice, and leadership.

SCHOLARSHIP: EVIDENCE GENERATION USING AN INTERPROFESSIONAL AND INTERDISCIPLINARY COLLABORATIVE APPROACH

Evidence-Based Practice

In their final report, Crossing the Quality Chasm: A New Health System for the 21st Century, the IOM (2001) stressed the importance of evidence-based practice (EBP) to guide practice guidelines. In their report, the IOM discussed the importance of an "ongoing analysis and synthesis of the medical evidence," as well as "enhanced dissemination efforts to communicate evidence and guidelines to the general public and professional communities" (IOM, 2001, p. 146). The AACN Essentials I and III (2006) called on DNPs to create an innovative clinical practice that is based on evidence and generated through proper evaluation and critical appraisal of research findings (i.e., EBP). In that context, the nursing curriculum aims at preparing future DNPs to follow the steps of EBP, which most importantly include asking the right and relevant clinical questions (i.e., PICO), properly evaluating the soundness of the scientific research designs and using the various critical appraisal techniques taught within the program. Achieving this goal of advancing scholarship within clinical practice requires the DNP nursing scholar to actively engage with various teams using collaborative skills. How is this translated into reality? DNPs, being immersed in the clinical world, may partner with physicians, PhD-prepared nurses, and statisticians to address medical dilemmas or change the nature of a medical or a nursing practice by engaging in projects such as systematic reviews or meta-analyses. In fact, in an editorial in the Joana Briggs Institute Database of Systematic Reviews and Implementation Reports, Christian and Palokas (2018) called for collaboration and sharing of knowledge and resources between PhD and DNP-prepared nurses. They believed that such collaboration would "further a unique but necessary dimension to nursing education" (p. 587).

Quality Improvement (QI)

Performing a quality improvement (QI) project is at the core of DNP practice. To realize this goal, the DNP must lead and collaborate. In fact, AACN Essentials II and VI highlight the importance of leadership and collaboration within institutions to promote patient safety, address health disparities, and improve patient outcomes. The DNP curriculum aims to provide students with tools to create change in any area (hospital, community, government). For example, QI projects in a hospital setting are performed to improve patient health outcomes. Let us take this hypothetical clinical question of a QI project. "How does enhancing the advanced practice nurse's ultrasound skills improve patient outcomes in a given intensive care unit?" Answering this question, which evidently aims at improving outcomes of critically ill patients, requires not only the possession of technical skills needed to perform a QI project but a creative interprofessional and interdisciplinary collaboration with several entities such as nursing leadership, physician colleagues, and diagnostic technology representatives, among others. As well, the success of the project greatly depends on the nature of that collaboration. In fact, proper collaboration requires relationship building which is essential in determining the success potential of a project. Some of the main features of relationship building are clinical competence and trust (Chism, 2021). Would it be realistic for a large company such as Siemens to partner with a DNP scholar who is not competent in using the company's ultrasound technology? Not possessing clinical competence automatically terminates any potential for relationship building. However, a competent and experienced DNP scholar can use these two features to bargain on a grant to initiate a QI project. Relationship building starts with a given reputation, which is determined by clinical competence and based on trust.

In summary, this section emphasizes the crucial role of interdisciplinary and interprofessional collaboration in advancing the DNP's scholarship agenda. Whether it is creating evidence from systematic reviews, meta-analyses, or QI projects, working in teams and building healthy strong professional relationships based on trust are at the heart of this collaboration. Finally, scholarship projects that inform practice and improve outcomes are best realized within strong, efficient, competent, collaborative teams.

ACADEMIA

Nursing professionals must be prepared academically to address the challenges of an expensive healthcare system that has not succeeded yet in addressing the nationwide health inequalities. They are key component of the matrix of providers caring for patients in a vast array of settings both inpatient and outpatient. They practice in diverse settings, for example, hospitals, homes, schools, primary care clinics, outpatient surgical centers, mental health agencies. To accomplish the varying roles of care giver, researcher, faculty, and leader, nurses must have adequate knowledge that encompasses business, statistics, medicine, and leadership. The education pathway for academic preparation for nursing can begin at a diploma level, and progresses to associate, bachelor's, master's, and doctorate degrees. Students can enter the DNP track as a bachelor's or master's prepared nurse. At either educational level, the DNP student must accomplish the same program competencies to earn the doctorate degree and be a DNP or PhD. A PhD in nursing is traditionally a research-oriented degree designed to prepare nurses for opportunities to conduct research in nursing education, clinical trials, and social sciences. The DNP is the accompaniment of other practice doctorates, such as the MD, PharmD, and doctorate of physical therapy. The DNP was designed to prepare nurses to be clinical scholars who have the ability to interpret research and develop effective healthcare systems for individuals and populations (Trautman et al., 2018). The DNP-prepared nurse will seek out the answers to clinical issues and translate the findings into practice. The DNP- or PhD-prepared nurse has the knowledge and ability to occupy various positions in leadership, quality improvement, health policy, and clinical faculty as practice scholars. The IOM recommends that all advanced practice nurses be prepared at the doctoral level and possess a blend of clinical, organizational, economic, and leadership skills (IOM, 2011). The unique blend of nursing, clinical inquiry, and leadership adds an insightful vision to the delivery of healthcare.

In 2004, the member schools associated with the AACN endorsed moving the level of preparation for advanced nursing practice from master's degree to the doctorate level (AACN, 2004). The rationale for endorsing a doctorate degree is the tremendous growth of knowledge acquired to be a competent provider and the increase of the acuity of the patients. DNP programs are now available in all 50 states and the District of Columbia. Doctoral coursework should incorporate interdisciplinary collaboration, knowledge that will position the advanced practice nurse to be adept at navigating the healthcare environment and collaborating effectively with health team members. Schools of nursing should create opportunities within their curriculum for students to engage in interdisciplinary collaboration. The following is a case study that incorporates multiple aspects of care that could be utilized as a multidiscipline care rounds.

A male patient has been admitted for cerebrovascular accident and is presenting with right-sided weakness and dysphagia. He has a past medical history of hypertension (HTN), coronary artery disease (CAD), hyperlipidemia (HLD), and type II diabetes. The patient has been admitted to the neurology service, and physical therapy, speech therapy, and occupational therapy have been consulted. Pharmacy is following to reconcile medications for this admission and cardiovascular service has been consulted for ongoing management of the patient's CAD. The classroom assignment would have representatives of each team discuss the clinical aspects and design a comprehensive medical plan. It is helpful for DNP students to participate in a multidisciplinary round to appreciate other teams' concerns and challenges. It provides the opportunity for DNP students to be aware of various aspects that each service examines for a patient plan. DNP projects may need to incorporate interdisciplinary collaboration, creating opportunities to impact healthcare delivery systems and change healthcare policies. The practice doctorate has a focus on translating research and bringing the findings to the providers (Giardino & Hickey, 2020). DNP programs prepare clinicians who can strengthen the healthcare system. Curricula with collaborative learning opportunities instill in nurses the ability to advocate for the patient's perspective when practice decisions are being made. The collaborative learning experience provides the DNP student the opportunity to be cognizant of the information for which they should have prepared to assist the patient in their transition through their healthcare trajectory. DNP programs prepare clinicians who can be strong advocates for their patients during interdisciplinary discussions.

To improve the safety and efficiency of practice, the IOM (2000) highly recommended a focus on interdisciplinary collaboration. Competencies include a focus on quality, safety, and education of nurses, and teamwork and collaboration must be woven into the curriculum. A team of clinicians from different disciplines, together with the patient, undertake the care for the patient. This approach allows for collaboration of care from multiple disciplines and the utilization of resources efficiently considering the multiple variables that impact healthcare. DNP projects focusing on the competencies of quality, safety, and education could incorporate interprofessional collaboration for medication education and protocols with pharmacy; mobility with physical therapy; activities of daily living with occupational therapy. There are infinite opportunities for DNP scholars to incorporate other disciplines and discover interventions that would improve the health of many individuals and improve healthcare systems.

The Essentials: Core Competencies for Professional Nursing Education (AACN) are the educational framework for future nursing professionals. The Essentials of Doctoral Education for Advanced Nursing Practice provide guidance for nursing curricula. Nursing in the 21st century has many challenges and opportunities to shape the future workforce. The AACN Essentials are organized in Domains. Domain number six focuses on Interprofessional Partnerships. The description is stated as intentional collaboration with other professionals, families, and patients to improve the healthcare experience for individuals and communities. The institution of interprofessional partnerships is dependent upon effective intentional conversation. The doctoral-prepared nurse is equipped to facilitate improved communication and provide expert consultation for other members of the healthcare team. Additionally, the DNP nurse has the ability to facilitate team dynamics by role modeling the ability to navigate disagreements and conflicts. Interprofessional collaboration provides opportunities for learning by constructive sharing of multiple perspectives. The DNP can be the leader within the interprofessional team possessing the unique relationship with the patient and team members to provide optimal care and address health inequities.

CLINICAL PRACTICE

The DNP-prepared clinician is able to provide leadership, comprehensive care, and education to patients, families, and nurses. The DNP clinician can bring together clinicians from multiple disciplines, hospital administration, policymakers, and leaders in insurance to be advocates for patients. The unique skills the DNP possesses as researcher coupled with clinical care and collaborating with multiple disciplines allows for the opportunity to apply knowledge from technology, science, medicine, and fiscal awareness to solve the challenges many patients face. An interdisciplinary focus has been recommended to improve the safety and efficiency of practice (IOM, 2000). The DNP curriculum incorporates interdisciplinary work at a variety of levels and provides knowledge to solve complex clinical problems. DNP providers will utilize technology and analysis of best practice to translate to practice. DNP will collaborate with families, communities, and individuals within healthcare systems and assist in navigating the changing environments of care from home to hospital and then transitioning to rehabs or home again. The focus of care should include a rural and global perspective. Through interdisciplinary collaboration, the DNP clinician integrates advanced practice skills with an understanding of systems management for best practice, health policy on information technology, and the evaluation and implementation of evidence into practice.

Many individuals today have multiple diagnoses along with multiple complex healthcare needs. The best possible health outcome will be achieved through a collaborative approach with patient, family/caregivers, and an interdisciplinary team. An interdisciplinary approach can improve patient outcomes by reducing the length of stay, avoiding duplication of medical tests and assessments, leading to a more comprehensive care of the patients. The sharing of information has become more convenient with the use of technology to share confidential medical information with the patient. The DNP-prepared nurse, who is prepared as an expert clinician with a business and technology background, has the ability to coordinate the data from various patient sources and institute a plan of care that is efficient and thorough, yielding the best patient outcome at the most economical cost.

Effective communication and collaboration are crucial in the increasingly complex healthcare system in which the DNP-prepared nurse can play a key role. Communication is a vital component to building a successful team. The DNP nurse possesses the ability to understand clinical perspectives from various levels. They have the capability to assess the patient's concerns, understand the pathology that is occurring, and share that vital information with all team members. The DNP is the link in the chain of communication that is indispensable. Effective communication between the patient and team members can decrease adverse consequences from unnecessary healthcare procedures and improve on missed opportunities for better healthcare management. The opportunity to share crucial data can be lost if the parties involved do not value the information. The DNP is situated to be the patient advocate by understanding the patient's concerns and collaborating with the team to strive for optimal health outcomes.

The AACN Essentials call for interprofessional relationships that demonstrate shared accountability. It should be a coordinated effort with mutual respect within the teams and displayed to patients, families, and all community members involved in the care. Effective collaboration requires an understanding of team dynamics and an ability to work within a team. The DNP-prepared nurse has the ability to be the liaison for team members and demonstrate leadership in coordinating the team's actions with the individual, community, and healthcare personnel.

LEADERSHIP

Nurses must assume leadership roles in healthcare. Nurses comprise the largest group of healthcare professionals, numbering approximately 4.2 million (AACN, 2022). The daily assessment and administration of care that nurses provide are crucial to the healthcare system. The DNP- or PhD-prepared nurse has the knowledge and ability to occupy various positions in leadership, quality improvement, health policy, and clinical faculty as practice scholars. The unique blend of nursing, clinical inquiry, and leadership adds an insightful vision to the delivery of healthcare. Additionally, as the national shortage of nurses increases the strain for patient management, nursing leaders must be able to optimize resources and design safe, quality care. Doctoral-prepared leaders possess the knowledge of health systems and quality patient outcomes to provide management of resources to ensure high quality care.

In their 2001 report, *Crossing the Quality Chasm – A New Health System for the 21st Century*, the IOM urges nursing professionals to design new healthcare delivery models with increased emphasis on safety and quality improvement (IOM, 2001). In addition, the AACN highlighted in their Essentials the importance of DNPs in organizational leadership for quality improvement with a focus on systems thinking. As a result, the DNP curriculum now encompasses leadership development to meet competency requirements established by the AACN Essentials (2006, 2020) and NONPF NP Role Competency 10.3: Articulate the complex leadership role of the NP (NONPF, 2022). Thus, in the following section we will consider DNP-prepared nurses' roles in leadership development within the healthcare system. A particular emphasis is on the DNP's crucial role in high-reliability organizations (HROs).

DNP Leadership Development: Closing the Quality Gap

Medical errors and quality shortcomings affecting patient safety and, ultimately, clinical health outcomes are still infecting the American healthcare system. Fatality due to medical errors are estimated to be the country's third leading cause of death (Veazie et al., 2019). Unfortunately, a high level of performance, which includes eliminating major quality failures, does not exist in healthcare today. There is a marked difference between expectation and reality. For example, there are discrepancies between what is expected to work well for patients based on available evidence and what is implemented in clinical practice. The doctoral-prepared nurse is poised to partner with physicians and other leaders to close this quality gap by implementing fundamental HRO principles. In this section we briefly discuss an historical overview of HROs, then address the crucial roles of DNP leaders within HROs.

HROs are organizations that run high-risk, complex, and hazardous systems and dependably operate them error-free (i.e., air traffic control system, nuclear power operation; Weick & Roberts, 1993). The research in this field started with the Berkley group, which examined organizations whose errors had catastrophic consequences, such as U.S. Navy Aircraft Carriers and commercial nuclear power plants. Researchers stressed the importance of decision processes to avoid catastrophes, which involved all members of the organization, including those at the "lowest levels" (Roberts et al., 1994). A prominent example is the *USS Greenville* accident. This historical event is believed to have occurred as a result of the accumulation of a few small errors without proper corrective actions, one being the failure in communication of the operating technician to question the orders of the commanding officers (Roberts & Tadmore, 2002). Researchers, as a result, shared key features of HROs that make them reliable, successful, and error-free. HROs were built on three pillars: (a) leadership commitment, (b) culture of safety, and (b) a focus on continual process improvement. HROs should be able to reinvent themselves by adapting and making changes in their decision-making tree based on any complex situations that arise. Historical experiences in high-risk industries led to the infiltration of high-reliability operations into healthcare systems beginning in the 1990s. Discussions around the integration of early HRO principles in healthcare led to the formation of the National Patient Safety Foundation of the American Medical Association. Ultimately, HRO constructs designed to eliminate catastrophic errors have become pillars for success in healthcare systems. However, success requires efficient translation of evidence and adoption of processes by all entities within healthcare organizations. An otherwise challenging feat. From their vantage point, DNP-prepared professionals can evaluate, empathize, and ideate. They can also design, test, and implement practice changes. Therefore, the DNP-prepared nurse is at the heart of these HROs.

The DNP curriculum is designed to enhance knowledge in organizational and systems leadership, which ultimately helps strengthen practice and healthcare delivery (AACN, 2006). The DNP graduate is also prepared to conceptualize new care delivery models based on current nursing science that aligns with organizational, political, cultural, and economic perspectives (AACN, 2006). Organizations can contribute significantly to preventing accidents when all system components work together cohesively. DNP-prepared nurses help to prevent accidents by collaborating with interdisciplinary professionals and adhering to key HRO principles. For example, the DNP may collaborate with informatics specialists to implement "hard stops" or clinical decision supports prior to ordering high-stakes medications. Incorporating human factors engineering to avoid medical errors within the electronic medical record has reduced prescribing errors thereby improving patient safety (Taheri Moghadam et al., 2021).

Several interventions have been defined in HROs, including education on error prevention, implementation of standardized root cause analysis processes, leadership training in quality improvement, and universal promotion of a just culture (Veazie et al., 2019). In that context, with the collaboration of professionals from various disciplines, DNPs may play prominent roles in overseeing these HRO interventions within various healthcare organizations and settings. The question remains, how does the DNP use the HRO principles to enhance excellence within the HROs and address the challenges that continue to threaten patient safety and care quality within HROs? In fact, it is not enough to perform within the scope of practice clinically; DNP leaders must expand further by using research skills acquired within the DNP curriculum. Doctoral-level knowledge in organizational and systems leadership strengthens practice and healthcare delivery (AACN, 2006). DNPs are naturally adaptive leaders who can innovate and engage stakeholders in meaningful system improvement (Kendall-Gallagher & Breslin, 2013). The DNP can conceptualize new care delivery models based on current nursing science that align with organizational, political, cultural, and economic perspectives (AACN, 2006). A thorough examination of research and efficient translation into practice is required to deliver high-quality care. Healthcare transformation demands on strong leadership. DNP leaders can establish organization and departmental practice standards while simultaneously setting strategic goals for the corporation.

In conclusion, in a world that is overwhelmed with health inequalities, in order to contribute to quality, safe healthcare, DNP graduates' real option is to collaborate.

Starting with the academic teaching and extending into real-world applications, interdisciplinary and interprofessional collaboration are skills that must be learned. These skills are at the heart of DNP practice and pave the way to establishing relationships based on trust and respect. Most importantly, DNP graduates possess strong clinical insights and have the potential to advance many valuable projects within healthcare organizations, community, academic settings, and public health arenas.

CRITICAL THINKING QUESTIONS

1. Consider your own organization. Can you describe any training or education programs implemented to enhance staff's understanding of HRO principles and their role in promoting reliability and safety?
2. What steps has your organization taken to promote a culture of safety and resilience?
3. Consider your DNP education. Did the curriculum contain education on HRO principles?
4. What specific competencies and skills does doctoral-level knowledge in organizational and systems leadership bring to practice and healthcare delivery?
5. The American Association of Colleges of Nursing (AACN) Essentials for Doctoral Education for Advanced Practice identifies Domain Six as Interprofessional Partnerships. One key element is an understanding of team dynamics and an ability to collaborate with others. What strategies and skills would a doctorally prepared advanced practice nurse utilize to resolve interprofessional conflict and manage disagreements?
6. How would a DNP-prepared advanced practice nurse integrate diversity, equity, and inclusion into interdisciplinary practice?
7. In what ways could a DNP-prepared advanced practice nurse practice self-assessment to develop an awareness of one's biases and how that could impact mutual respect and communication with fellow team members?
8. Within your capacity as a doctorally prepared advanced practice professional, discuss how generating evidence impacts health policy changes.
9. As a future clinical scholar, discuss ways social determinants of health impact health status and outcomes and what projects do you envision implementing to address these goals.
10. Discuss your vision for how interdisciplinary collaboration advances quality improvement projects in hospital settings.

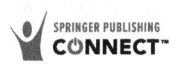

A robust set of instructor resources designed to supplement this text is located at http://connect.springerpub.com/content/book/978-0-8261-8137-4. Qualifying instructors may request access by emailing textbook@springerpub.com.

REFERENCES

Adhikari, S., Pantaleo, N. P., Feldman, J. M., Ogedegbe, O., Thorpe, L., & Troxel, A. B. (2020). Assessment of community-level disparities in coronavirus disease 2019 (COVID-19) infections and deaths in large US metropolitan areas. *JAMA Network Open*, 3(7), e2016938. https://doi.org/10.1001/jamanetworkopen.2020.16938

American Association of Colleges of Nursing (AACN). (2004). *AACN position statement on the practice doctorate in nursing October 2004*. Repot of the Task Force on the Clinical Doctorate (aacnnursing.org)

American Association of Colleges of Nursing. (2006). *Essentials of doctoral education for advanced nursing practice*. https://www.aacnnursing.org/portals/42/publications/dnpessentials.pdf

American Association of Colleges of Nursing. (2021). *The essentials of doctoral education for advanced nursing practice*. https://www.aacnnursing.org/DNP/DNP-Essentials

Aviation safety, human error, human factors. (2022). *Teamwork: The essence of safe operations*. Teamwork – The essence of Safe Operations | Aviation Medicine :: Aerospace Medicine (avmed.in)

Blumenthal, D., Fowler, E. J., Abrams, M., & Collins, S. R. (2020). Covid-19—Implications for the health care system. *New England Journal of Medicine, 383*, 1483–1488.

Chism, L. A. (2021). Leadership, Collaboration and the DNP Graduate. *The doctor of nursing practice: A guidebook for role development and professional issues*. Jones & Barlett Learning, (5th ed., pp. 35–64).

Christian, R., & Palokas, M. (2018). Systematic review methodology in graduate nursing education. *JBI Database of Systematic Reviews and Implementation Reports. 16*(3), 587–588. https://doi.org/10.11124/JBISRIR-2017-003704

Center for Disease Control and Prevention (CDC). (2017). The Systems thinking mindset: Finding leverage by becoming less and less wrong. Retrieved from: (80) The Value of Systems Thinking - YouTube

Giardino, E., & Hickey, J. (2020). Doctor of nursing practice students' perceptions of professional change through the DNP program. *Journal of Professional Nursing, 36*(6), 595–603. https://doi.org/10.1016/j.profnurs.2020.08.012

Gravlee, C. C. (2020). Systemic racism, chronic health inequities, and COVID-19: A syndemic in the making? *American Journal of Human Biology, 32*(5), e32482.

Institute of Medicine. (2000). *America's health care safety net: Intact but endangered*, National Academies Press

Institute of Medicine. (IOM). (2001). *Crossing the quality chasm: A new health system for the 21st century*. National Academy Press

Institute of Medicine. (2011). *The future of nursing leading the change, advancing health*. The National Academies of Press. https://www.nap.edu/read/12956/chapter/1https://www.nap.edu/read/12956/chapter/1

Johnson-Agbakwu, C. E., Ali, N. S., Oxford, C. M., Wingo, S., Manin, E., & Coonrod, D. V. (2022). Racism, COVID-19, and health inequity in the USA: A call to action. *Journal of Racial and Ethnic Health Disparities, 9*(1), 52–58.

Kendall-Gallagher, D., & Breslin, E. (2013). Developing DNP students as adaptive leaders: A key strategy in transforming health care. *Journal of Professional Nursing, 29*(5), 259–263. https://doi.org/10.1016/j.profnurs.2013.06.009

National Organization of Nurse Practitioner Faculty (NONPF). (2022). *NONPF's NP role core competencies*. https://www.nonpf.org/page/NP_Role_Core_Competencies

Roberts, K. H., Stout, S. K., & Halpern, J. J. (1994). Decision dynamics in two high reliability military organizations. *Management Science, 40*(5), 614–624. https://doi.org/10.1287/mnsc.40.5.614

Roberts, K. H., & Tadmore, C. T. (2002). Lessons learned from non-medical industries: The tragedy of the USS Greenville. *Quality Safety Health Care, 11*(4), 355–357. https://doi.org/10.1136/qhc.11.4.355

Taheri Moghadam, S., Sadoughi, F., Velayati, F., Ehsanzadeh, S. J., & Poursharif, S. (2021). The effects of clinical decision support system for prescribing medication on patient outcomes and physician practice performance: A systematic review and meta-analysis. *BMC Medical Informatics and Decision Making, 21*(1), 1–26. https://doi.org/10.1186/s12911-020-01376-8

Trautman, D. E., Idzik, S., Hammersla, M., & Rosseter, R. (2018). Advancing scholarship through translational research: The role of PhD and DNP prepared nurses. *The Online Journal of Issues in Nursing, 23*(2), 1–8. https://doi.org/10.3912/OJIN.Vol23No02Man02

Veazie, S., Peterson, K., & Bourne, D. (2019). *Evidence brief: Implementation of high reliability organization principles*. Department of Veterans Affairs (US)

Weick, K. E., & Roberts, K. H. (1993). Collective minds in organizations: Heedful interrelating on flight decks. *Administrative Science Quarterly, 38*, 357–381. https://doi.org/10.2307/2393372

CHAPTER SEVENTEEN Reflective Response

BRIDGETTE GOURLEY

In this chapter, the authors urge us to explore the myriad ways in which the DNP-prepared nurse is poised to lead in this moment in healthcare. The confluence of health disparities, poverty, and structural inequities experienced prior to and exacerbated during the COVID-19 pandemic have reinforced the need for thorough examination of the healthcare system to reimagine an equitable environment of care. This call for improvement is not new. The American Association of Colleges of Nursing (AACN) in 2004 identified the eight doctor of nursing practice (DNP) Essentials as the key mechanisms for the newly described DNP to affect change. The Institute of Medicine (IOM) report in 2010 supported the vision of the clinical doctorate to aid in the transformation of healthcare (AACN, 2004; IOM, 2011). In this postpandemic healthcare haze, it is clear DNP's are uniquely prepared to lead the changes necessary to invigorate our health system. The interprofessional and interdisciplinary lens the DNP applies across and within systems may best be understood when categorized into the domains of scholarship, academia, clinical practice, and leadership, as noted by the authors.

A new DNP may wonder, is it truly possible or even necessary to practice interprofessionally within each of these domains? The scope seems tremendous, and that is exactly the point! Each domain presents an opportunity to partner with professionals and experts within and outside of nursing. Imagine the impact on the health of populations and the healthcare system if each of the 40,000 DNP students enrolled nationally in 2021 accepts the challenge to collaborate intentionally upon graduation (AACN, 2022).

To realize this charge, the DNP must remember their foundation as a nurse that has prepared them to navigate the complexities of the healthcare silos and to work with the diverse professionals and collaborators within this system. Nationally, 55% of 875 DNP respondents indicated they were employed in clinical care as nurse practitioners, nurse-midwives, and nurse anesthetists (AACN, 2022). For the practicing DNP, clinical excellence in their specialty can provide entry to interprofessional partnerships to advance care, patient outcomes, and systems change. However, let us not be limited to interprofessional partnerships that fall only inside the hospital—let's explore what partnerships can occur where patients live, work, and learn. In the community there may be additional care providers: dentist, substance use counselor, outreach worker, pharmacist, or minister to create innovative partnerships for care. Interprofessional care may be traditionally implemented within a hospital or large healthcare system, but it is not necessary to limit the location or the providers of care who participate in these models as long as patients remain the central focus. Healthcare is moving beyond the boundaries of a hospital or campus. This presents DNP-prepared nurses a canvas for innovation in care delivery models and the interprofessional teams that will expand access to care in the community.

Beyond the clinical area, rich opportunities exist for collaboration in the domains of scholarship, academia, and leadership. With the implementation of the Nursing

Essentials, doctorally prepared faculty with PhDs and DNPs are challenged with how to best develop content to meet Domains I and II competencies for nursing students of all levels (AACN, 2021). Working together, doctorally prepared nurses can develop, implement, and evaluate the pedagogies most effective for students to be practice ready. Best practices in the classroom or simulation setting can further be adapted to improve onboarding, mentorship, and transition to practice roles postgraduation in the clinical setting, reducing burnout and improving retention. Further examination of successful onboarding and transition to practice can help faculty prepare students better for the realities that await them in the clinical environment. Partnering schools and health systems can bring mutual benefit in nurse-led initiatives, and this is possible when the operational and implementation skills of a DNP are paired with the research skills of a PhD to capture the evidence.

Together, nurse academic and practice leaders can build this environment of care with the patient in the center. Forward thinking at the intersections of nursing scholarship, academia, clinical practice, and leadership, combined with operational best practices and quality improvement, can be the foundation for the best of interprofessional care. It simply cannot wait another decade to happen.

REFERENCES

AACN. (2021). *The essentials: Core competencies for professional nursing education.* https://www.aacnnursing.org/Portals/0/PDFs/Publications/Essentials-2021.pdf

AACN. (2022). *The state of doctor nursing practice education in 2022.* https://www.aacnnursing.org/Portals/0/PDFs/Data/State-of-the-DNP-Summary-Report-June-2022.pdf#:~:text=Since%20the%20completion%20of%20this%20study%2C%20new%20data,enrollees%20in%202021%20at%2040%2C834%20students%20%28AACN%2C%202022%29.

CHAPTER EIGHTEEN

The DNP Graduate's Role in Health Policy and Advocacy

SR. ROSEMARY DONLEY

This chapter discusses the unique role that nurses who hold the doctor of nursing practice (DNP) play in health policy and advocacy. Since 2006 when the members of the American Association of Colleges of Nursing (AACN) adopted the Essentials of Doctoral Education for Advanced Nursing Practice (AACN, 2006), nursing has emphasized higher education of clinically oriented nurse leaders (AACN's Position Statement on the Practice Doctorate in Nursing, 2004).

THE EVOLUTION OF THE PRACTICE DOCTORATES

Achieving higher education of professional nurses has been a struggle since nursing's humble beginnings in hospitals. Scheckel (2009) provides a time-oriented context for the emergence of the DNP degree, describing four phases in the development of doctoral education in nursing: the doctor of education (EdD; 1900–1940), a PhD degree in the basic or social sciences (PhD: 1940–1960), a PhD in the basic or social sciences with a minor in nursing (PhD: 1960–1970), and the development of two pathways, research and practice (PhD and DNP: 1970–present). This chapter discusses advanced clinical education as the newest pathway in nurses' long journey toward academic and health professional recognition.

The AACN (2016) document, *Advancing Health Care Transformation: A New Era for Academic Nursing*, reports that most leaders in academia and in practice do not hold influential positions in academic health centers. Absent from the policy tables, they are not in a position to inform or direct healthcare transformation. However, because about 55% of 2.8 million registered nurses (RNs) work in the nation's hospitals in both inpatient and outpatient settings, nursing is on the agenda of academic health centers and community hospitals and clinics, even when their leaders are not visible in health institutions' circles of power (Bureau of Labor Statistics, 2021; AACN, 2022a, 2020b).

Ironically, the initiative to develop professional or practice doctoral degrees comes at a time when traditional PhD programs are being challenged as irrelevant, costly, time consuming, and too narrowly focused on scholarly research (Nyquist, 2002). In describing the Re-visioning PhD Education Project funded by the Pew Foundation and carried out at the University of Washington, Edwardson (2004) compares their findings to the state of doctoral education in nursing in the early years of the 21st century. The Re-visioning Project described the over-production of PhDs in traditional fields, ritualistic degree requirements, overuse of doctoral students in undergraduate education, low program completion rates, long periods of doctoral and postdoctoral training, limited job availability in universities and colleges, and lack of a diverse student body. In her thesis, Edwardson stated that PhD programs in nursing lacked diversity and that some students spend a longtime completing degree requirements (Edwardson, 2004). Nursing recognizes the gap in diversity among nurses, other healthcare professionals, and their patients and has worked to enhance it.

The U.S. Census Bureau (2020) found that 40% of the people who participated in their census were people of color (Budden et al., 2013). The 2009 survey of the National Council of State Boards of Nursing and The Forum of the State Nursing Workforce Centers reported that 19.4 % of RNs who completed the survey (39%) came from diverse racial backgrounds: 39% White, 28% African American, 32% Asian, and 30% Hispanic. While these studies represent different years and different populations, they show that professional nursing recognizes the diversity gap between them and their patients. There are other differences between White and minority nurses. The 2008 National Sample Survey of RNs found that RNs from minority backgrounds were more likely than White nurses to seek baccalaureate and higher degrees (USDHRSA, 2010)

Although doctoral programs in nursing were not included in the Re-visioning Project, nurse educators are considering how this report and the loss of faith in traditional PhD education affect their discipline. Nurse leaders are very aware that less than 1% of the nursing workforce (0.67%) holds a PhD in nursing or in a related field (AACN, 2022a, 2020b). This percentage is not expected to increase in the near future. Since 2012 enrollment in PhD nursing programs has declined by 12% (AACN, 2022a, 2020b). There is improvement in the diversity and the age of nurses enrolled in nursing's a PhD programs. The number of schools of nursing that offer a PhD in nursing has also increased by 14% (AACN Trends, 2022).

Prior to the COVID-19 pandemic the length of time for master's-prepared nurses to complete a PhD was 4 to 6 years. The theoretical component of the program for full-time students is usually 2 years. Completion of the dissertation depends on many factors, methodology, subject recruitment, good health for the student and their loved ones, director availability, and writing skills. Some of these factors are outside the student's control. Nurses who elect or have to work during their program of studies take longer to complete their dissertations. Unlike students in liberal arts or science programs, who receive scholarships or are funded by grants or the university, most nurses pay for their doctoral education.

Some schools have accepted the challenge of the Robert Wood Johnson Foundation (RWJF) to shorten the length of their PhD programs and admit younger students. The RWJF's Focus on Scholars program seeks to decrease the age of new PhD nursing graduates by offering significant grants to nurses who enroll in 3-year PhD programs (RWJF, 2013). Other schools have adopted the AACN's proposal to develop a bachelor of science in nursing (BSN) to PhD program as another way of shortening the time that nurses spend in post-baccalaureate studies (Loomis et al., 2006). Equally significant as the age of new PhD graduates and the small percentage of nurses with PhDs is the lack of a robust PhD pipeline, a factor frequently emphasized in policy statements about nurse faculty shortages and the rise of DNP education (AACN, 2015b; Berlin & Seachrist, 2002; Martsolf et al., 2015).

It is also interesting that more than 10 years after the AACN's proclamation on DNP education, nurses who evaluate DNS programs continue to compare practice-oriented doctorates to research doctorates (AACN, 2015c; Fulton & Lyon, 2005; Loomis et al., 2006). Sometimes, the comparisons are critical (Meleis & Dracup, 2005), usually they are descriptive efforts to differentiate the purpose, the educational and/or clinical content, and the intended outcomes of each program (AACN, 2014, 2015a). The 2015 report from the AACN's task force on the implementation of the DNP program is the AACN's latest effort to restate the intent of the DNP degree: emphasize the incorporation of *The Essentials of Doctoral Education for Advanced Nursing Practice* into curriculum and outcome assessments and restate its position that the DNP degree is the educational pathway to the advanced practice of nursing (AACN, 2015a).

Martsolf et al. (2015) note that although many schools have developed and value DNP education as the route to advanced practice, only about 30% of the schools offer the BSN to DNP program as the entry level into advanced practice. Their data also suggest that the master of science in nursing (MSN) remains a viable and perhaps preferred option for advanced practice education. There are no published studies that link patient outcomes to the educational pathway of the DNP-prepared advanced practice nurse (APN). Outcome studies support the quality of care provided by MSN-prepared APNs (Cronenwett et al., 2010; Stanik-Hutt et al. (2013).

Although the DNP is relatively new, it is being embraced by the nursing community. Early objectors to the DNP program saw this new degree as adding another dimension to the confusing educational preparation for entry into practice (Meleis & Dracup, 2005). Others acknowledge that nurses aspiring for clinical or administrative careers would select DNP programs because they are shorter and are more appropriate for their future roles (Loomis et al., 2006).

There is also strong support for DNP education from national organizations, notably the AACN, the American Association of Nurse Practitioners (AANP), the American Academy of Nurse Practitioners (AANP), the National Association of Pediatric Nurse Practitioners (NAPNAP), and the National Organization of Nurse Practitioner Faculties (NONPF, 2015). Their websites actively market the significance and the importance of the practice doctorate. The literature also presents opinion articles, survey data, and reports of interviews and studies of nursing schools' approaches to the BSN to DNP or the post-master's DNP (Martsolf et al., 2015). Almost 40 years ago, Downs (1989) observed that educators have debated the differences surrounding doctoral education since it began in the United States. It seems that nursing has now found a way to extend the entry into practice debates at the doctoral level.

THE DNP DEGREE

What can be said about the state of the DNP? There has been an amazing response from schools of nursing to the AACN's 2004 statement on practice doctorates. Reviewing the AACN's (2016) website, the month after the 2015 transition deadline for recognizing the DNP degree as the entry level into advanced nursing practice had passed, 271 schools of nursing offered DNP programs and another 100 programs were said to be in planning stages. The AACN (2015a) notes, however, that the variability among existing DNP programs transcends the different entry pathways: the BSN to DNP or post-master's DNP. Institutional, academic, regulatory, professional, and economic factors influence how each dean and faculty plan, implement, evaluate, and fund the DNP program of studies and establish admission standards (AACN, 2014).

The drafters of the 2004 position statement envisioned that the competencies and scope of practice of DNP graduates would transcend the institutional walls of the Academy (AACN, 2015a). Citing the Institute of Medicine's (IOM's) classic studies on medication errors and patient safety, *To Err Is Human* (1999) and *Crossing the Quality*

Chasm (2001), the authors argued that a new type of APN was needed if this country were to improve the quality of healthcare. Guided by the proposal *Health Professions Education: A Bridge to Quality* (2003), the IOM spoke of a new care delivery system that was patient centered, evidence based, interdisciplinary, informed by informational technology, and oriented to improve quality of care. In proposing practice doctorates in nursing, the AACN (2004) increased the educational competencies of master's-prepared APNs, slightly lengthened advanced practice programs to establish educational parity with other health professionals, sought to improve practice and patient care outcomes, and increased the supply of clinical faculty.

Essential V, Health Policy for Advocacy in Health Care identified health policy as a core concept in doctoral education for advanced nursing practice (AACN, 2004). Although the language of the Essentials document has become more complex, reflecting the rapidly changing healthcare system and the centrality of the social determinants of health, health policy remains an essential concept in DNP education (AACN, 2021; Keller & Ridenhauer, 2021). Any nurse who aspires to a position of leadership in nursing or healthcare needs to be grounded in health policy.

HEALTH POLICY COMPETENCE AND THE ADVANCED PRACTICE NURSE

While there are many definitions of health policy, most authors purport that policies are decisions about the allocation of resources made by persons with authority (Longest, 2016; Mason et al., 2016; Meacham, 2021). In the United States, healthcare decision-making resides in both the public and private sectors. This public/private engagement is unique among developed countries; in other developed countries healthcare is considered to be a benefit of citizenship. DeLeire et al. (2014) reported that USDHHS data showed that 4 years after the Patient Protection and Affordable Care Act (ACA) was enacted, the number of uninsured adults decreased by 10.3 million. Five years later, the employer-based commercial health plans remained the major source of health insurance for the majority of American workers and their families (Kaiser Family Foundation [KFF], 2014a). The aged, the poor, the totally and permanently disabled, and special populations such as active duty military and their dependents, and veterans participate in health insurance programs supported by federal and state governments. At the time of the enactment of the ACA, it was estimated that approximately 47 million Americans (18% of the population) remained underinsured (KFF, 2014b). In 2021, 8.6% of the population remained uninsured (kff.org, 2021).

Despite its complexity and the engagement of the government and the private sector, American healthcare faces three persistent policy challenges: the iron-triangle of access, cost, and quality (McClellan & Rivlin, 2014).

Access

Without health insurance there is limited access to healthcare services unless a person has the ability to pay their own healthcare bill. For the majority of Americans, health insurance is obtained through enrollment in employer-supported health insurance plans, plans purchased from private sector insurance brokers, the ACA's health exchange, or government-sponsored health plans such as Medicare and Medicaid. Each option requires that enrollees and their dependents meet eligibility requirements, adhere to enrollment timelines, and pay required premiums and fees.

The major purpose of the ACA (2010) was to reduce the number of uninsured Americans. As a means to this end, the law included a mandate that all American citizens would have health insurance. This mandate affected employees, insurance providers, employers that offer insurance plans, and all under- or uninsured citizens. Those who failed to comply with the mandate paid fines. The mandate was not popular; efforts to rescind it or challenge its constitutionality engaged all levels of government.

The ACA was an issue in the 2016 presidential election. Republican members of Congress introduced repeated bills to rescind the ACA and/or change some of its provisions. The Supreme Court ruled on its constitutionality in *The National Federation of American Business (NIFIB) v. Sebelius, 2012* and in *King v. Burwell, 2015* (Center for Health Law, 2012; Scotus Blog, 2015). Education in health policy is required to actualize nursing leadership and participation in health policy deliberations. The mandate provision in the ACA was repealed in December 2017 when President Trump signed the Tax Cut and Jobs bill into law (Davis, 2022).

Essential V and VI urge nurses, especially DNP nurse leaders, to actively participate in health policy development and evaluation.

Cost

Another important goal of the ACA is the reduction in the growth of healthcare costs. Although the United States has the highest healthcare costs in the world and invests 19% of its gross domestic product (GDP) in healthcare (Wagner et al., 2021) cost control is challenging. McClellan and Rivlin (2014) suggest three complementary strategies to slow cost escalation: avoid wasteful spending, especially waste linked to inefficiencies; increase market competition; and improve population health.

Waste reduction is a popular political theme, because waste accounts for about 30% of healthcare expenditures. Authors delineate seven categories of wasteful behavior: overtreatment, lack of care coordination, failure in care delivery processes, administrative complexity, pricing failures, errors, and fraud and abuse (Wagner et al., 2021). Another common theme in post-ACA discussions is the cost of medication errors in acute care settings. While most patients have not read the IOM's trilogy on patient safety, they know that medication errors are more than costly; they can cause death (IOM, 1999). Nationally, there are many efforts within the healthcare, medical, nursing, pharmacological, technological, and accreditation communities to improve medication practices and make hospitals safer places. At the governmental level, beginning in 2009, Medicare changed its payment system and withheld payments to hospitals when patients acquired pressure ulcers or injuries from falls during their hospital stays (Watcher et al., 2008).

Insurance plans compete on product design and price. Healthcare is a lucrative business; capitalism rewards the most successful health entrepreneurs. Market forces are influenced by supply and demand, not human vulnerability, poor health status, need, or poverty. Cost plays an important role in the American healthcare establishment because healthcare affects all sectors of the economy. Berwick and Hackbarth (2012) were not alone in thinking that competition among healthcare providers will bring down costs (Porter & Lee, 2013). However, the American healthcare marketplace is yet to produce a delivery system that improves health status, enhances the quality of care, and lowers costs.

Population Health and Building a Culture of Healthcare

Although population health has been a mantra in public health circles for years, it is now identified as an Essential (Essential VI) in the AACN's Essentials of Doctoral Education for Advanced Nursing Practice (AACN, 2006; Marmot, 2005). Population health addresses a global awareness that the treatment of illness provides only a partial answer to improving the health status of individuals and populations (Starfield & Shi, 2002). The social, environmental, and living situations that determine health are increasingly linked to improved health status, reduced health disparities, and cost control (Centers for Disease Control [CDC], 2015). The IOM (2016) recently published a high-level framework to educate future health providers about the importance of the social determinants of health. In 2013, the RWJF, working with the RAND Corporation, embarked on an ambitious project, a *Culture of Health Initiative* (Acousta et al., 2016). Their vision was expressed as six priorities: bridging health and healthcare, building demand for healthy places and practices, eliminating health disparities, engaging business for health, strengthening vulnerable children and families, and leadership (RWJF, 2015). Plough (2015) challenges the public health workforce to initiate these analyses.

Essential VII, Clinical Prevention and Population Health for Improving the Nation's Health, promotes DNP-prepared nurses as leaders in population health (AACN, 2004). Although the DNP nurse leaders' role in promoting and transforming healthcare into a culture of health is yet to be clearly articulated by the AACN (2004; 2022a, 2022b), the Essentials documents or the newly released AACN (2016) report on *Escalating Academic Nursing's Impact on Transforming Health and Health Care,* the documents are compatible with this vision. Plough's (2015) related call to learn how to use big data sets is also very relevant to any DNP nurse leader who aspires to analyze patterns of population health.

Quality of Care

Quality of care is the most elusive and difficult concept to define and measure within the access, cost, and quality triad. Quality of care is increasingly linked to achieving successful outcomes rather than describing and measuring structures, processes, or patient satisfaction (Mitchell et al., 1998).

For many years, patient satisfaction was associated with quality of care. If patients liked the medical and nursing teams, the cleanliness and convenience of the hospital, and sometimes the food that was served, it was considered to be a good hospital. Patients also liked seeing "their doctor." Some thought that a particular hospital was their family's hospital. These views have not disappeared. If you or someone that you know has recently been hospitalized, the evaluation forms sent to patients after discharge still reflect an interest in measuring satisfaction.

However, since the implementation of the ACA, attention has focused on the relation between outcomes and quality. Value-based incentives are thought to improve outcomes. The Centers for Medicare and Medicaid Services (CMS) argues that the best way to improve outcomes is to change providers' practice patterns and reframe payment strategies (CMS, 2016).

If CMS is successful, new payment systems will replace the old fee-for-service payment models. This has been a long-term goal of those who want to lower healthcare costs. It remains to be seen if other payment models replace the fee-for-service system. We do know that efforts to move away from fee-for-service payment creates management and political challenges (Miller, 2012). However, there is growing traction among policymakers around strategies that link value-based payments and care management practices to patient outcomes (McClellan & Rivlin, 2014).

These alternate payment methods (APMs) are designed to lower costs and enhance quality of care. APMs vary in design. Some, such as accountable care organizations, target total population spending, while others focus on creating incentives for providers to limit spending by accepting bundles, case rates, evidence-based case rates, and global bundled payments. Bundling compresses all possible charges for an episode of care and provides a single payment for a defined treatment.

Patients know what a hip replacement will cost them or their insurance company. Because bundling is used for common and predictable procedures, such as knee replacements, providers and insurers can estimate and manage the risks of accepting bundled payments rather than fees for service (Delbanco, 2014). Bundling is designed to reduce waste and overtreatment. Alternate payment models go by many names, including episode-based payment, episode payment, episode-of-care payment, case rate, evidence-based case rate, and global bundled payment. What they have in common is a shift of financial and clinical risk from payers to providers. Payment models capitalize on the providers' need to manage a budget and ensure quality. The provider who accepts a bundled payment earns higher margin if a patient utilizes less care.

However, the bundled payment must also cover the cost of unexpected utilization and complications. Public and private payors in many countries are implementing APMs that work on the theory that if care providers have a financial stake in their patients' outcomes, it will be more effective than asking patients to assume financial risk through deductibles, co-payments, and out-of-pocket payments (AMA, 2022).

The American healthcare establishment also relies on technology to deliver and advance patient care. Initially, the technology was medically oriented. Now, high-technology medicine competes with sophisticated informational technology in institutional and community-based centers and group practices. These include the electronic medical record (EMR) and telehealth. The EMR is very helpful because of a compelling need to access timely, accurate, and secure data by patients, clinicians, insurance companies, and the government.

Telehealth is also a technological assisted delivery system that came into its own during the pandemic. Robeznieks (2017) reports that specialists, especially radiologists (39.5%), psychiatrists (27.8%), and cardiologists (24.1%) use telehealth the most. Prior to the COVID-19 public health emergency, telehealth linked primary care doctors in rural parts of the United States to specialists. The Veterans Administration (VA) medical centers are major users of telehealth. People who live a distance from specialized VA hospitals can avoid cumbersome day trips by using telehealth. For example, the VA in Pittsburgh provides specialized care to veterans in the mountain cities of Altoona and Johnstown. Before telehealth, veterans who needed to see specialists, traveled by car or a VA bus to Pittsburgh; in good weather a round trip takes more than 4 hours. If several veterans traveled in the same van, their appointment times were usually different. It was a long day for these elderly and chronicallyill veterans. The VA found that many patients who lived at a distance from the VA medical centers did not schedule or keep their appointments in the winter. This affected their health outcomes and wasted the time and resources of the health team in Pittsburgh. Telehealth has overcome this barrier to care.

Most specialists practice in large urban settings close to academic health centers. As noted earlier in this chapter, psychiatrists have become leaders in the use of telehealth. Psychiatrists see one patient for an extended period of time. Assessment and treatment do not require that the psychiatrist or mental health therapist touch the patient. Because mental illness knows no geographic boundaries, tele-mental-health has improved care outcomes for psychiatric patients who do not live in urban areas.

Protecting the right to patient privacy is a major concern about the use of healthcare technology. Competing concerns about privacy and appropriate access to health data challenge the healthcare establishment to rethink how it spends its $3 trillion budget.

Health Policy Competence

When Longest (2016) speaks of policy competence, he notes that anyone who wants to influence health policy must understand the policy process and comprehend how health policies are made. This knowledge gives leaders the skill in scanning policy and political environments, and identifying the threats and opportunities on the horizon. These insights help leaders shape the policy environment for the benefit of their group's interest. Longest is speaking of federal and state health policy, but his advice also applies to nongovernmental sectors, because U.S. health policy arises from the private as well as the public sector. Advocacy is ineffective if the person or group desiring change does not grasp the workings of extant systems and the powerful forces that sustain them.

Longest (2016) also proposes that successful policy advocates possess two skill sets: the ability to gain access to policy environments and the organizational acumen to build consensus around their agenda. In this context, access means that nurses know their elected representatives and can get their attention; they have the power to bring their issues or problems to government. That nurses can have access to political power brokers is not surprising. American nurses (2.8 million RNs and 690,000 licensed practical nurses [LPNs]) are a large, geographically distributed group of healthcare providers. Approximately 55% of the 2.8 million RNs hold BSN degrees; approximately 11% have master's or doctoral degrees. While the majority of nurses live in urban areas, about 445,000 RNs and 166,000 LPNs live in rural communities where 52 million people also reside (HRSA, 2013). The number and the geographical locations of nurses give them natural access to members of Congress, especially members of the House of Representatives. Four large nursing organizations that represent practicing nurses, educators, researchers, accreditors, and administrators, the American Nurses Association (ANA), the National League for Nursing (NLN), the American Association of Colleges of Nursing (AACN), and the American Organization for Nursing Leadership (AONL), form the Tri-Council for Nursing. This alliance of autonomous nursing organizations periodically issues policy and position papers that represent the view of its member organizations. The Tri-Council for Nursing (n.d.) also discusses and advocates for policies that cross and occasionally unite the special interests in nursing.

What constitutes the policy agenda of organized nursing? The best clues are found on the websites of the four Tri-Council organizations and that of the American Academy of Nursing and the many specialty organizations.

The ANA (n.d.), the official spokesperson for nursing, lists 10 position statements on nursing practice: drugs and alcohol, the electronic health record, ethics and human rights, HIV and viral hepatitis, nursing practice, patient safety, privacy and confidentiality and social causes, health care, role of the registered nurse, and workplace advocacy. Their website also publishes information about the ANA-PAC (political action committee), the fundraising and political support arm of the ANA. The NLN (2021–2022), the voice of nursing education, affirms its role as accreditor of all pre-professional programs that lead to licensure and graduate programs at the master's and DNP levels, lists its 2015–2016 governmental affairs agenda as: access, education, diversity, and the workforce. The AACN's (2020) Pathway for Excellence speaks to five standards: Leadership, Patient and Nurse Safety, Quality of Care, Wellbeing and Workplace Culture, and Professional Development. The AONL (n.d.—formerly the AONE), identifies Identification and Support of Nurse Leaders, Advocacy, Work to Have Nurse Leaders at Policy Tables and Oversight of State and Federal Legislation and Regulation. The American Association of Critical-Care Nurses (AACCN, n.d.), the largest of the specialty organizations, updates its members about Equity, Diversity, and Inclusion, Legislation and Regulatory Issues, Healthy Workplaces for Nurses, Scope of Practice, and Clinical Advocacy.

The ANA is the only nursing organization that is officially registered as a lobbyist. Many nursing groups hire Washington-based lobbying firms to advise them about issues in Congress or the executive agencies. The Tri-Council and a large number of specialty nursing organizations employ policy experts on their staffs. These individuals frequently visit the Hill and bring their organizations elected and appointed leaders to meet with members of Congress, its committees, and office staffs. If one aspires to leadership in nursing or healthcare, competence in health policy is a necessity. Advocacy must be balanced and informed.

Organization

Then, there is the question of organization. Nurses do not agree or rally around a common agenda. At the state level, nurses and their organizations engage in power battles with organized medicine and hospital and nursing home associations over access to care, cost, and quality.

Abood (2007) makes an important contribution when she observes that bedside nurses know that cost containment and lack of coordination can affect their patients' quality of care. She also insists that if nurses are to address access, cost, and quality of care in meaningful ways, they must move out of their comfort zones. Although Abood is examining policy or practice change at the micro level, she affirms that if nurses are to bring about changes in policy, they need the access to power, the will to carry their activities forward, the time, and the energy. Her observations about the level of commitment that policy change requires can be generalized to state and federal policy work.

SUMMARY

As has been stated frequently in this chapter, AACN's Essentials V and VI challenge DNP nurse leaders to engage in health policy. Nursing's engagement at federal and state levels will not create a common voice for nursing in policy arenas or break down the silos that limit interdisciplinary collaboration. However, nursing's engagement will bring firsthand observations of patient care experiences to federal and state policy tables. It is well recognized that unidentified problems cannot be solved. Because nurse leaders work in institutions, primary practices, urgent clinics, and in communities, they can inform systems thinking, decision-making, and innovative, evidenced-based practice. In discussing what leadership means for DNP-educated APNs, Walker and Polancich (2015) posit that contemporary practice requires the application of specialized knowledge, clinical expertise, and the capacity to discern appropriate interventions and policy changes that will improve care. Leadership requires a mix of cognitive, clinical, and interpersonal skills.

Years ago, Hildegarde Peplau said that nurses can win the battle for quality of care at the bedside but lose it at the policy table. Essentials V and VI challenge DNP graduates to advocate for quality of care, not only at unit and service centers in institutions, but also in board rooms, in the literature, and in public forums. DNP nurse leaders' voices must be heard in the places where decisions that affect practice, patient care, and health outcomes are made. As the largest group of health professionals in the world, there is a great potential for nurses to create forward movement regarding a healthy society. DNPs must come to see political engagement as a professional obligation and health policy as something that they can shape rather than something that happens to them.

In conclusion, it is essential for DNPs to stay abreast of current population health issues and to fully engage in health policy development. This engagement is inherently multilayered and complex, from the education and representation of clients at the individual and community levels to the representation of nursing issues at the local, state, and national levels. The ultimate goal is a safe, equitable, and affordable healthcare system, ensuring improved health and well-being of the population (RAND Corporation, 2014).

CRITICAL THINKING QUESTIONS

1. Discuss the engagement of DNP nurse leaders in creating health policy changes?
2. How can DNP nurse leaders improve the quality of community-based care?
3. Describe the differences between MSN and DNP nurse leaders' engagement in health policy.
4. How can DNP-prepared nurse leaders impact the healthcare policy challenges known as the iron-triangle: access, cost, and quality?
5. Describe how a DNP-prepared nurse leader can reduce healthcare disparities at the population level?
6. To what do you attribute the increasing number of DNP graduates versus PhD graduates?
7. What are some policy areas where DNP-nurse leaders can have a critical impact?
8. Describe how you might individually impact local, regional, national, or global health policy.

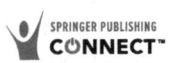

A robust set of instructor resources designed to supplement this text is located at http://connect.springerpub.com/content/book/978-0-8261-8137-4. Qualifying instructors may request access by emailing textbook@springerpub.com.

REFERENCES

Abood, S. (2007). Influencing health care in the legislative area. *The Online Journal of Issues in Nursing*, 12(1). https://www.nursingworld.org/MainMenuCategories/ANAMarketplace/ANAPeriodicals/OJIN/TableofContents/Volume122007/No1Jan07/tpc32_216091.html

Acousta, J. D., Whitley, M. D., May, L. W., Dubowitz, T., Williams, M. V., & Chandra, A. (2016). *Perspectives on a culture of health*. RAND Corporation.

American Association of Colleges of Nursing. (2004). *Position statement on the Doctor of Nursing Practice (DNP)*. https://www.aacn.nche.edu/publications/position/DNPpositionstatement.pdf

American Association of Colleges of Nursing. (2006). *The essentials of doctoral education for advanced nursing practice*. https://www.aacn.nche.edu/publications/position/DNPEssentials.pdf

American Association of Colleges of Nursing. (2015a). *The doctor of nursing practice: Current issues and clarifying recommendations*, 1–23. https://www.aacn.nche.edu/aacn-publications/white-papers/DNP-Implementation-TF-Report-8-15.pdf

American Association of Colleges of Nursing. (2015b). *Nursing faculty shortage*. https://www.aacn.nche.edu/media-relations/fact-sheets/nursing-faculty-shortage

American Association of Colleges of Nursing. (2015c). *The Doctor of Nursing Practice: Current issues and clarifying recommendations*. https://www.pncb.org/sites/default/files/2017-02/AACN_DNP_Recommendations.pdf

American Association of Colleges of Nursing. (2016). *Advancing healthcare transformation: A new era for academic nursing*. Author.

The AACN's. (2020). Pathways to Excellence. nursingworld.org

American Association of Colleges of Nursing. (2021). *Fact sheets*. aacnnursing.org.

American Association of Colleges of Nursing. (22 March 2022a). *Trends in nursing's PhD programs*. aacnnursing.org.

American Association of Colleges of Nursing. (16 November 2022b). *The Essentials Core Competencies for Professional Practice*. Author.

American Association of Critical Care Nurses. (n.d.). *History of health policy at AACN*. http://www.aacn.org/wd/practice/content/publicpolicy/publicpolicyhistory.pcms?menu=practice

American Medical Association.(10 August, 2022). *Medicare alternative payment models*. ama,assn.org

American Nurses Association. (n.d.). *ANA official position statements*. https://www.nursingwork

American Organization for Nursing Leadership (AONL). (n.d.). *Promoting professional development for nurse leaders*. aonl,org

Berlin, L. E., & Sechrist, K. R. (2002). The shortage of doctorally prepared nursing faculty: A dire situation. *Nursing Outlook, 50*(2), 50–56. https://doi.org/10.1067/mno.2002.124270

Berwick, D. M., & Hackbarth, A. D. (2012). Eliminating waste in U.S. healthcare. *Journal of the American Medical Association, 307*(14), 1513–1516.

Budden, J. S., Zhong, E. H., Moultos, P., & Cimiotti, T. P. (22 July 2013). *Highlights of the National Workforce Survey of Registered Nurses*. Researchgate.net

Centers for Disease Control. (2015). *Social determinants of health*. https://www.cdc.gov/socialdeterminants

Centers for Medicare & Medicaid Services. (2016). *Value-based payment modifier*. https://www.cms.gov/medicare/medicare-fee-for-service-payment/physicianfeedbackprogram/valuebasedpaymentmodifier.html

Cronenwatt, L., Dracup, K., Grey, M., McCauley, L., Meleis, A., & Salmon, M. (2010). The Doctor of Nursing Practice: A national workforce perspective. *Nursing Outlook, 59*(1), 9–17. https://doi.org/10.1016/j.outlook.2010.11.003.

Davis, E. (2022, April 17). *What is the individual mandate?* Verywellhealth.com

Delbanco, S. (2014). *The payment reform landscape: Bundled payment*. http://healthaffairs.org/blog/2014/07/02/the-payment-reform-landscape-bundled-payment

DeLiere, T., Joynt, K., & McDonald, R. (2014, August 31). *Impact of insurance expansion on hospitals' uncompensated care costs in 2014*. https://hhs.gov.reports.imp

Downs, F. S. (1989). Differences between the professional doctorate and the academic/research doctorate. *Journal of Professional Nursing, 5*(5), 261–265. https://doi.org/10.1016/8755-7223(89)90036-7

Edwardson, S. R. (2004). Matching standards and needs in doctoral education in nursing. *Journal of Professional Nursing, 20*(1), 40–46. https://doi.org/10.1016/j.profnurs.2003.12.006

Fulton, J. S., & Lyon, B. L. (2005). The need for some sense making: Doctor of Nursing Practice. *The Online Journal of Issues in Nursing, 10*(3). https://www.nursingworld.org/MainMenuCategories/ANAMarketplace/ANAPeriodicals/OJIN/TableofContents/Volume102005/No3Sept05/tpc28_316027.html

Health Resources and Services Administration (HRSA). (2013). *The U.S. nursing workforce: Trends in supply and education*. https://bhpr.hrsa.gov/healthworkforce/reports/nursingworkforce/nursingworkforcefullreport.pdf

Institute of Medicine. (1999). *To err is human*. National Academies Press.

Institute of Medicine. (2016). *Assessing progress on the Institute of Medicine report on the Future of Nursing*. National Academies Press.

Kaiser Family Foundation. (2014a). *Health insurance coverage of the total population*. http://kff.org/other/state-indicator/total-population

Kaiser Family Foundation. (2014b). *The uninsured at the starting line: Findings from the 2013 Kaiser survey of low-income Americans and the ACA*. http://kff.org/uninsured/report/the-uninsured-at-the-starting-line-findings-from-the-2013-kaiser-survey-of-low-income-americans-and-the-aca

Kaiser Family Foundation. (2021). *Insurance coverage of the total population*. kff.org

Keller, T., & Redenour, N. (2021). The essential core competencies for Professional nursing practice ethics. In J. Giddens (Ed.), *Concepts for nursing practice*. St. Louis Elsevier.

Longest, B. B. (2016). *Health policymaking in the United States*. Health Administrative Press.

Loomis, J. A., Willard, B., & Cohen, J. (2006). Difficult professional choices: Deciding between the PhD and DNP in nursing. *The Online Journal of Issues in Nursing, 12*(1).

Marmot, M. (2005). Social determinants of health inequalities. *Lancet, 364*(9464), 1099–1104. http://www.thelancet.com/action/showAbstract?pii=S0140673605742343

Martsolf, G. R., Auerbach, D. I., Spetz, J., Pearson, M. L., & Muchow, A. N. (2015). Doctor of nursing practice by 2015: An examination of nursing schools' decisions to offer a doctor of nursing practice degree. *Nursing Outlook, 63*(2), 219–226. https://doi.org/10.1016/j.outlook.2015.01.002

Mason, D. J., Gardner, D. B., Outlaw, F. H., & O'Grady, E. T. (2016). *Policy and politics in nursing and health care*. Elsevier.

McClellan, M., & Rivlin, A. (2014). *Health policy issue brief: Improving health while reducing growth: What is possible?* The Brookings Institution.

Meacham, M. (2021). *Longest's Health policy making in the United States*, Health administrative Press.

Meleis, A., & Dracup, K. (2005). The case against the DNP: History, timing, substance, and marginalization. *Online Journal Issues in Nursing, 10*(3). Nursingworld.com

Miller, H. D. (2012). Ten barriers to healthcare payment reform and how to overcome them. Center for HealthCare Quality and Patient Reform. http://www.chqpr.org/downloads/overcomingbarrierstopaymentreform.pdf

Mitchell P. H., Ferketich S., & Jennings B. M. (1998). Quality health outcomes model. American academy of nursing expert panel on quality health care. *Image Journal of Nursing Scholarship, 30*(1), 43–6. https://doi.org/10.1111/j.1547-5069.1998.tb01234.x. PMID: 9549940.

National Organization of Nurse Practitioner Faculties. (2015). *The doctorate of nursing practice NP preparation: NONPF perspective*. http://c.ymcdn.com/sites/www.nonpf.org/resource/resmgr/DNP/NONPFDNPStatementSept2015.pdf

Nyquist, J. (2002). The PhD: A tapestry of change for the 21st century. *Change, 34*(6), 12–20.

Plough, A. L. (2015). Building a culture of health: A critical role for Public Health Services Research. *American Journal of Public Health, 105* (Suppl. 2), S150–S152.

Porter, M., & Lee, T. H. (2013). The strategy that will fix health care. *Harvard Business Review, 91*(10), 50–70.

RAND Corporation. (2014). *The DNP by 2015: A study of the institutional, political, and professional issues that facilitate or impede establishing a post-baccalaureate Doctor of Nursing Practice program*. https://www.aacnnursing.org/Portals/0/PDFs/Data/DNP-Study.pdf

Robert Wood Johnson Foundation. (2013). *Focus on nursing scholars*. http://futureofnursingscholars.org

Robert Wood Johnson Foundation. (2015). *Our areas of focus*. http://www.rwjf.org/en/our-focus-areas.html

Robeznieks, A. (2017, January 11). *What medical specialists use tele-medicine the most?* https://www.ama-assn.org/practice-management/digital/which-medical-specialties-use-telemedicine-most

Scheckel, M. (2009). Nursing education: Past, present, future. In G. Roux & J. Halstead (Eds.). *Issues and trends in nursing education: Knowledge for today and tomorrow* (pp. 27–55). Jones & Bartlett.

Scotus Blog. (2015). *King v. Burwell*. http://www.scotusblog.com/case-files/cases/king-v-burwell

Stanik-Hutt, J., Newhouse, R. P., White, K. M., Johantgen, M., Bass, E. B., Zangaro, G., & Weiner, J. P. (2013). The quality and effectiveness of care provided by nurse practitioners. *Journal of Nurse Practitioners, 9*(8), 492–500. https://doi.org/10.1016/j.nurpra.2013.07.004

Starfield, B., & Shi, L. (2002). Policy relevant determinants of health: An international perspective. *Health Policy, 60*(3), 201–218. https://doi.org/10.1016/s0168-8510(01)00208-1

Tri-Council for Nursing. (n.d.). *Joint statement from the Tri-Council for Nursing on recent registered nurse supply and demand projections*. https://www.google.com/?gws_rd=ssl#q=what+is+the+Tri+Council+in+nursing

U.S. Census Bureau. (2020). *The chance that two people chosen at random are of different race or ethnicity groups has increased since 2010*. https://www.census.gov/library/stories/2021/08/2020-united-states-population-more-racially-ethnically-diverse-than-2010.html

U.S. Bureau of Labor Statistics. (2021). *Occupational outlook handbook: Registered Nurse*. https://www.bls.gov/ooh/healthcare/registered-nurses.htm

Wagner A. K., Ubel P. A., & Wharam J. F. (2021). Financial pollution in the US health care system. *JAMA Health Forum, 2*(3), e210195. https://doi.org/10.1001/jamahealthforum.2021.0195

Walker, D. K., & Polancich, S. (2015). Doctor of nursing practice: The role of the advanced practice nurse. *Seminars in Oncology Nursing, 31*(4), 263–272. https://doi.org/10.1016/j.soncn.2015.08.002

Watcher, R. M., Foster, N. E., & Dudley, R. A. (2008). Medicare's decision to withhold payment for hospital errors: The devil is in the details. *The Joint Commission Journal on Quality and Patient Safety, 34*(2), 116–123. https://doi.org/10.1016/s1553-7250(08)34014-8

CHAPTER EIGHTEEN Reflective Response

DEBORAH DILLON

Health Policy for Advocacy in Health Care, Essential V, is a core concept in doctoral education for advanced nursing practice (AACN, 2004). Advocating for healthcare policy is a responsibility of all nurses, but one especially to be embraced by the doctor of nursing practice (DNP)-prepared nurse. Imagine if all the voices of the 4.2 million registered nurses (Smiley et al., 2021) could be heard—what could be accomplished in the political arena? In the 17 years since the American Association of Colleges of Nursing (AACN) endorsed the Position Statement on the Practice Doctorate in Nursing, more than 60,500 have graduated with a DNP (AACN, 2022a, 2022b). These graduates are our clinical practice leaders and are prepared to be our advocates and voices in healthcare policy.

As a DNP-prepared advanced practice registered nurse (APRN), I sought opportunities to address healthcare issues at the state and local levels. My first experiences in healthcare policy were at the institutional level. Despite an expanded scope of practice (SOP), there are institutional barriers that exist for APRNs. As a volunteer member of the hospital's Allied Health Committee, I was the only acute care APRN representative. Using my intellectual capital, my "voice" advocated for implementation of the Consensus Model for Nursing (NCSBN, 2008).

The Consensus Model represents the four APRN roles: certified registered nurse anesthetist (CRNA), certified nurse-midwife (CNM), clinical nurse specialist (CNS), and certified nurse practitioner (CNP). The six population foci for APRNs were also identified. The population foci within the APRN role include family/individual across lifespan, adult-gerontology, neonatal, pediatrics, women's health/gender related and psychiatric/mental health. Within the pediatric and adult-gerontology population foci there are both a primary care and acute care population (Dillon, 2021). Clinical practice should be in alignment with the APRN's licensure, accreditation, certification, and education or LACE.

Newly hired family nurse practitioners (FNPs) were applying for positions that were not in alignment with the Consensus Model. An FNP applicant was requesting privileges to be on the acute stroke management team and her practice would include managing patients in the neurological intensive care unit. Per the Consensus Model this SOP would be within the adult-gerontology acute care nurse practitioner's SOP in managing patients who are hemodynamically unstable.

Having a voice and a vote at the table enabled me to educate other committee members (predominantly physicians) on SOP and the Consensus Model. Despite multiple meetings in which documentation was presented supporting implementation of the model, I was continually beaten down by physicians who did not understand the SOP differences between RNs and APRNs let alone the differences in APRN SOP. I used my political capital and met with the hospital attorney to discuss the legal implications to garner support. Every month when the vote was held to approve the APRN's privileges, my nursing colleagues and I denied the privilege request. After three meetings, the chief medical officer said to me, "I finally get this. I'll take care of it today." On this date after his presentation, in which he summarized everything stated in the prior meetings, all members voted not to approve the FNP privileges as requested. I felt a sense of vindication, that I had successfully advocated for the APRN role and for patient safety.

The next step in the credentialing process is the Medical Executive Committee. The chief nursing officer, who also was on the Credentialing Committee, has a seat at the table on the Medical Executive Committee, but not a vote. The Medical Executive Committee (predominantly physicians) overruled the decision of the Credentialing Committee. As a member of the Credentialing Committee you can be held liable for privileging decisions. In view of the overruling by the Medical Executive Committee, I submitted my resignation from the committee—after 10 years of voluntary service. Ironically, simultaneously, I received my "thank you for your service" letter from the physician chair of the Credentialing Committee.

My next exposure to healthcare policy was again for APRNs, but at the state level. At that time, there was a movement in Virginia toward full practice authority (FPA) for APRNs. As a member of the Governance Council of the local chapter of the Virginia Council for Nurse Practitioners we had opportunities to attend State Day where you can meet with your state and local representatives to discuss healthcare issues. I also participated in local activities where we invited members of Congress to listen to our practice and healthcare concerns. They do want to hear from their constituents.

My "big voice" came at our statewide educational conference. Members were discussing the current lack of support for the "rural approach" to achieving FPA. FPA is APRN practice without physician collaboration. FPA allows the APRN to practice to the full extent of their education and licensure and is supported by many organizations, including the Institute of Medicine (IOM, 2010). The "rural approach" to FPA supports APRN care for the underserved in rural areas where patients often have a shortage of healthcare providers. On that day I felt my "voice" was strong. I approached the microphone in the crowded conference room and discussed considering taking a different approach, FPA using the transition to practice model. In this model, APRNs are granted FPA after a designated number of transition to practice hours. The lobbyists changed their approach. In 2018, Virginia joined more than 20 other states to become an FPA state—with third party administrator (TPA).

Advocating for policy at the local or institutional level requires having intellectual and political capital. It requires knowing policy and being the topic expert. DNP-prepared nurses are educationally and clinically prepared for making changes in healthcare policy. You may not feel like you know a lot about policy, but you are the expert in your area of practice. Use that voice to communicate healthcare issues and advocate for your patients. Utilize your DNP leadership skills to include RNs in your advocacy role. Take advantage of or make opportunities to call, email, write, or visit your local representatives. Publish on healthcare policy and nursing's role in op-eds and journals. Let your voice be heard.

Unfortunately, the policy change that I described earlier at the institutional level did not occur at that time. Move forward 2 years—job postings for these NP positions were specified as for "acute care nurse practitioners." Even policy change at the local level requires moving mountains. As described by Longest (2016), If the individual or group advocating for changes does not understand how the current systems operate and the strong forces that maintain them, then advocacy will be ineffective. Policy change at the state level can take years. DNPs can also impact healthcare policy at the federal level and, if you are fortunate enough, the global level. Find your political voice.

"Success is not achieved by winning all the time. Real success comes when we rise after we fall. Some mountains are higher than others. Some roads are steeper than the next. There are hardships and setbacks, but you cannot let them stop you. Even on the steepest road you must not turn back." Muhammad Ali

REFERENCES

AACN. (2004). *Position statement on the Doctor of Nursing Practice (DNP)*. https://www.aacn.nche.edu/publications/position/DNPEssentials.pdf

AACN. (2022). *AACN. DNP Fact Sheet*. https://www.aacnnursing.org/News-Information/Fact-Sheets/DNP-Fact-Sheet

Dillon, D. L. (2021). *Successful transition to practice: A guide for the new nurse practitioner*. McGraw-Hill.

IOM. (2010). *The future of nursing: Leading change, advancing health*. https://www.iom.edu.Reports/2010/The-Future-of-Nursing-Leading-Change-Advancing-Health.aspx

Longest, B. B. (2016). *Health policy making in the United States*. Health Administrative Press.

NCSBN. (2008). *APRN consensus model*. https://www.ncsbn.org/nursing-regulation/practice/aprn/aprn-consensus.page

Smiley, R. A., Ruttinger, C., Oliveira, C. M., Hudson, L. R., Lauer, A. R., Reneau, K. A., & Alexander, M. (2021). The 2020 National Nursing Workforce Survey. *Journal of Nursing Regulation, 12*(1), Supplement. S1–S48. AACN Nursing Fact Sheet.

CHAPTER NINETEEN

The Role of the Doctoral-Prepared Nurse Leader During the COVID-19 Pandemic: Lessons Learned in Disruptive Times

MARY BETH KINGSTON AND CLAIRE ZANGERLE

Nursing leadership in any situation presents challenges, but none more so than during a once in a lifetime pandemic. When the first cases of COVID-19 were reported in China in December 2019, the world had very little understanding of what was ahead. Then, when on March 11, 2020, the World Health Organization declared a global pandemic, it was evident healthcare resources were soon to be strained as alternative care sites were created, elective surgeries and procedures were cancelled, and full-on disaster protocols were enacted (Cucinotta & Vanelli, 2020). It was also evident that doctor of nursing practice (DNP)-prepared leaders would have to employ all their skills and creativity to ensure adequate response to the seismic shifts in multiple care settings.

In this chapter the authors share lessons learned from the COVID-19 pandemic through the lens of the DNP leader and will examine the practice of the DNP leader operationally, clinically, and educationally. With the knowledge and experience that DNP leaders possess, they are equipped to manage complexities within the healthcare delivery system. This chapter presents examples of that influential role, including the impact of the pandemic on care disparities in multiple settings, its effect on the workforce, and system-level dyad leadership. The authors highlight leadership of operational and clinical initiatives, the transition of roles within the health system to meet patient needs, and the contribution of DNP-prepared educators. In addition, the authors share insights on managing clinical practice changes and creating and implementing new care models.

FOUNDATIONAL SKILLS OF THE DNP NURSE DURING THE COVID-19 PANDEMIC

The pandemic demonstrated without question that all nurses, no matter the level of education or position within the healthcare system, are leaders. All nurses were thrust into situations that required a wider skill set that was, at times, new to them. While the authors do not suggest that DNP leaders were the sole nurse leaders during this crisis, there are increasing numbers in key leadership positions—operational, clinical, and educational. They played a significant role in healthcare organizations' ability to respond quickly and effectively to the challenges of the pandemic. Because the DNP focuses on improving patient outcomes by advancing healthcare for the general population via policy change, clinical practice, and education, their unique skill set was a valuable contribution in these uncertain times. The DNP leader served as a subject matter expert in these areas and demonstrated robust capabilities of leading, innovating, and communicating within their sphere of influence and beyond. The American Association of Colleges of Nursing (AACN) created the DNP Essentials document initially in 2006, outlining and defining skill sets that create a DNP-prepared nurse. Later, the Essentials: Core Competencies for Professional Nursing Education was revised and provides a framework for preparing individuals as members of the nursing discipline, reflecting expectations across the trajectory of nursing education and applied experience. *Competency-based education* is a process whereby students are held accountable for the mastery of competencies deemed critical for an area of study (AACN, 2021). *The Domains* constitute a descriptive framework for the practice of nursing. These Essentials include 10 domains that were tailored to reflect the discipline of nursing. The domains used in the Essentials are:

- Domain 1: Knowledge for Nursing Practice
- Domain 2: Person-Centered Care
- Domain 3: Population Health
- Domain 4: Scholarship for Nursing Discipline
- Domain 5: Quality and Safety
- Domain 6: Interprofessional Partnerships
- Domain 7: Systems-Based Practice
- Domain 8: Informatics and Healthcare Technologies
- Domain 9: Professionalism
- Domain 10: Personal, Professional, and Leadership Development

In addition to domains, there are featured *concepts* associated with professional nursing practice that are integrated within the Essentials. A concept is an organizing idea that represents important areas of knowledge. The concepts are (a) clinical judgment; (b) communication; (c) compassionate care; (d) diversity, equity, and inclusion; (e) ethics; (f) evidence-based practice; (g) health policy; and (h) social determinants of health.

These skills are practice-focused and identify the value of developing advanced competencies and knowledge to improve nursing practice and outcomes- (AACN, 2021). Utilizing these skills during the pandemic became core to practice at such a critical time. Throughout this chapter, the authors demonstrate how the DNP essentials, regardless of the DNP role, served as a basis of practice at this critical time. Foundational is Domain 1, *Knowledge for Nursing Practice,* as it guides all those in DNP roles in navigating new knowledge and nimbly responding to changing practice environments.

LEADING HEALTHCARE SYSTEM INITIATIVES

Throughout the country, we witnessed nurse leaders stepping into significant hospital and system roles during the pandemic. Elevating nurses to lead system and site initiatives early in the pandemic had a major impact on an organization's ability to respond to the many challenges of the pandemic (Retzlaff, 2020). Nurses' existing knowledge of and experience with clinical operations, person/family-centered care, workforce challenges, and leading across boundaries positioned them to provide logistical, clinical, and communication leadership, particularly at the beginning of the pandemic. All of these skill sets are competencies the DNP leader possesses and are critical to improving patient care and health outcomes. These elements are noted in Domain 7, *Systems-Based Practice*. DNPs respond to and lead within complex systems of healthcare. Nurses effectively and proactively coordinate resources to provide safe, quality, equitable care to diverse populations.

The chief nursing officer often partnered with their chief medical officer counterpart to lead the clinical crisis response, with operational leaders serving in lead roles in the incident command structure (Stamps et al., 2021). These roles required a system perspective, understanding the impact of decisions on patients and families and the healthcare team in every setting. At New York-Presbyterian Hospital in Bronxville, New York, DNP leaders served as clinical advisors in an interprofessional COVID-19 Crisis Command Center. Using existing infrastructure within nursing, they were fully empowered, down to the front line, to offer solutions on command center decisions that impacted patient care and safety. Clinical advisors provided valuable updates to all levels of leadership, while ensuring time-sensitive information provided to all caregivers was accurate and efficient. The most valuable lesson learned was that a systematic approach to the command center model created calm during the crisis and had a positive impact on outcomes (Sansolo et al., 2022).

In addition to the critical role in crisis response leadership, many led other broad system or site projects and initiatives essential in the response to COVID-19. As the pandemic progressed, healthcare organizations led and assisted in the public health response, collaborating with community and local health department colleagues (Grimm, 2021). Nursing leadership demonstrated significant competencies in interprofessional leadership, ethical decision-making, problem-solving, and project management as they spearheaded COVID-19 testing capabilities in both healthcare settings and the community; coordinated vaccine policies, programs, and distribution in the face of initial shortages (Chan et al., 2021); and designed and reviewed key care provider and external messages.

The visibility and impact of DNP leaders in system and site leadership roles was a significant lesson learned during the pandemic. The value of the nursing voice at the executive leadership level in healthcare organizations was clearly evident in all areas of the prolonged crisis response. It is critical moving forward to ensure that the visibility and inclusion of nurse leaders in these broad-based roles and forums continues.

CLINICAL PRACTICE CHANGES

The pandemic required nurses and the healthcare team to quickly implement and/or change policies, procedures, and care delivery. For example, at Advocate Aurora Health, a 27-hospital integrated healthcare system in the Midwest, there were 115 nursing practice and policy changes within the first 5 months of the pandemic. DNP leaders in many roles were integral in working with teams to identify the challenges, adapt or change practice as needed, and evaluate clinical outcomes. Communication occurred frequently as recommendations for COVID-19 clinical care changed over the course of the pandemic. Demonstrative of this work are Domain 4, *Scholarship for the Nursing Discipline* and Domain 5, *Quality and Safety*, including concepts of health policy and evidence-based practice or in the case of new COVID policies and treatments, practice-based evidence. DNP leaders were called upon to utilize research and scholarly findings to integrate knowledge from a variety of sources, across disciplines, to solve practice problems that would lead to improved health outcomes (AACN, 2006).

Relative to policy and advocacy, DNP leaders provided guidance at the local, state, and federal levels on waivers, licensures, and regulatory matters that affected practice and, ultimately, patient outcomes during the COVID-19 crisis. The onset of the pandemic required state and federal waivers to improve access to care in the face of increased need. For the DNP advanced practice registered nurse (APRN), this resulted in state waivers that suspended restrictive physician practice agreements. Additionally, specific licensure requirements were waived to decrease barriers allowing out-of-state providers to perform telehealth services (CMS, 2022). The Coronavirus Aid, Recovery, and Economic Security (CARES) Act also permitted APRNs and other advanced practice clinicians to certify eligibility for home care services for patients covered by Medicare (HUD, 2020).

As information evolved and practice-based evidence emerged, DNP leaders worked with the clinical team to clarify and implement changing guidelines regarding appropriate use of personal protective equipment, ventilator versus high flow oxygen utilization, and implications for proning. Innovative work around such practices as implementing proning teams (Cotton et al., 2020) and stationing intravenous pumps outside of the patient room (Blake et al., 2021) are illustrations of rapid responses to innovation and timely evaluation of outcomes. For example, the clinical team quickly recognized that the additional length tubing posed fall risks and potential medication delivery impacts and steps were taken to mitigate those effects. Staffing challenges and increased patient volume necessitated changes to standard nursing practices, such as decreasing formalized rounding programs and documentation standards. Various changes to reduce the burden of nursing documentation were initiated, including waiving nursing care plan requirements for patients. Navigating these changes to workflow, small and large, required additional education and oversight. DNP leaders assisted in implementing and evaluating the impact of practice and policy changes, setting the stage for reevaluation of documentation practices in the postpandemic period (Moy et al., 2021).

Collaboration at all levels during the pandemic was essential. Once such partnership, previously mentioned, was that of the chief nursing officer and the chief medical officer. This dyad leadership model provided structure associated with improved clinician engagement and team results. Working together, this dyad team proved to be well-suited to lead teams through challenging times. Whether in-person or virtually, the value of this partnership in uncertain times provided stability to clinical teams. Most valuable was the collective messaging from the dyad and consistent communication through virtual meeting platforms, in-person huddles, and virtual town halls. This increased frequency of communication from the dyad partners appeared to reduce the level of anxiety among the healthcare team (Joslin & Joslin, 2020).

NEW CARE DELIVERY MODELS

The delivery of healthcare changed dramatically during the pandemic and required nurses to adapt accordingly. Most notable was the reexamination of the role of technology in providing care to patients. The pandemic forced closer evaluation of telemedicine as a clinical tool with the government and payors following suit. Shifting to technology-enabled care delivery required nurses to possess new technological skills and to be able to communicate care to/with the patients via different media, that is, by videoconferencinga and telephone. Further, nurses became aware of the risk of this technology to older patients who may not be adept at such media and continued to advocate for them (Barrett & Heale, 2021). Learnings from Domain 8, *Informatics and Healthcare Technologies,* informed information and communication technologies and informatics processes to provide care, gather data, form information to drive decision-making, and support nurses as they expand knowledge and wisdom for practice for improvement and transformation of healthcare. Additionally, it provided DNP leaders with the foundational principles to apply new knowledge in this space to ensure appropriate development, refinement, and execution of technology-based care models (AACN, 2006, 2021).

One of the most immediate and effective strategies was the shift to telehealth to maintain and improve access for primary care, chronic disease management, and behavioral health. Telehealth, telemedicine, and virtual care are often used interchangeably, with telehealth encompassing the use of telecommunications technology, audio and/or video, in healthcare delivery, information, and education (Rutledge et al., 2017). DNP leaders impacted the expansion of telehealth services through their direct clinical practice, as well as in leadership roles expanding registered nurses' capabilities. APRNs were instrumental in the training of DNP leaders who were able to demonstrate various competencies to execute telehealth strategies. In a recent review of nurse-led telehealth interventions during the COVID-19 crisis (Joo, 2022), the following strengths were identified:

- Care was provided without transmitting COVID-19.
- Access to care was increased during a time of stress and anxiety for patients and nurses.
- Patient-centered care and continuity of care were preserved.
- Satisfaction with the process was high for both patients and nurses.

Weaknesses were identified as well, including a lack of evidence-based telehealth guidelines, technical issues, and challenges in providing physical and psychological care (Dhaliwal et al., 2022; Joo, 2022). Telehealth services increased dramatically throughout the United States during the pandemic and are predicted to continue to be utilized in many care settings. Clearly, there is an ongoing role for the DNP leader to spearhead the development of guidelines, team roles, and patient experience improvement strategies. The rapid adoption and expansion of telehealth and the need to fully integrate this technology into care delivery was one of the earliest lessons learned during the pandemic.

Another creative care model in the technology space was the development of the infrastructure for the "hospital at home," which DNP leaders were essential in creating. Elements included remote monitoring, providing direct care, and leading and serving on interprofessional care teams. Providing acute care services in the home is not a new innovation and research has demonstrated these programs result in a better patient experience, lower readmission rates, and lower cost of care (Caplan et al., 2012). However, in an effort to expand surge capacity, the Centers for Medicare and Medicaid Services (CMS) initiated an "Acute Care Hospital at Home" waiver program providing payment and flexibility to treat patients in the home. As a result of strained bed capacity and the CMS waiver, healthcare systems accelerated partnerships, programs, and processes to provide acute care in the home during the pandemic. The initial program encompassed more than 60 acute conditions, including heart failure and pneumonia, typically identified in the emergency care setting. An added benefit of acute care in the home has been an increased ability for nurses to identify the social drivers that impact health and connect patients to community services. In the future, there is significant opportunity to expand home services and include longitudinal care programs and wrap-around services for episodic care, though barriers, including reimbursement issues, may persist (Ritchie & Leff, 2022).

WORKFORCE CHALLENGES: STAFFING, CONTINGENT LABOR, AND REDEPLOYMENT TRAINING

The COVID-19 pandemic and the subsequent effects have, undoubtedly, changed the nursing workforce. Increasingly and consistently, nurses are reporting their intent to leave the workforce, either in their current role in direct care or the profession all together. This widens the already massive gap between supply and demand of nurses to care for the patients who are in need. The gap existed pre-pandemic, but has worsened since. It is predicted that by 2025, the United States will have a gap of between 200,000 and 450,000 nurses available in direct care settings. To meet the demand, the United States would need to double the number of new graduates entering the workforce and staying in direct care, consistently, for the next 3 years (United States Bureau of Labor Statistics, 2020).

While the future is concerning, and must be aggressively addressed, it is the immediate workforce challenges that DNP leaders face that require attention. During the pandemic, direct care nurses encountered an unknown adversary, a virus that was highly contagious and deadly. Even as the virus surged and retreated, the instability of the workforce remained. Nurses who aspired to retire in the near future accelerated those plans. Nurses with young children were without daycare and were unable to work their scheduled hours. Nurses with school-aged children were faced with remote schooling. Nurses with aging parents were reticent to be exposed to a deadly virus, and potentially expose their loved ones. All of these factors led to a reduced number in the nursing workforce, limiting care capacity and leading to burnout of those nurses who were able to maintain their regular work schedules while picking up the slack for those who weren't. Demand for care continued and in some instances became more urgent as the virus surged (Yang & Mason, 2022).

To fill the staffing gaps, DNP leaders turned to contingent labor to staff open shifts. Utilization of agency nurses is a general practice in many organizations, but the number of nurses was generally controllable. The pandemic changed that practice. In a survey conducted by the American Association of Critical Care Nurses of more than 6,500 critical care nurses, 92% of respondents reported their staff numbers had been depleted as a result of the pandemic and mitigating the staffing shortage had, by 2021, already cost hospitals an estimated $24 billion dollars above and beyond scheduled labor costs. In 2020, travel nursing grew by 35%, with the practice expected to grow another 40% in the future (Yang & Mason, 2022). DNP leaders found themselves in a moral dilemm—filling open shifts to ensure care could be delivered and reducing the burden on hospital-employed nurses by increasing the number of agency nurses at a cost that, at times, was four to five times above a standard hourly rate (Evans & Carlton, 2021). To respond to the increased utilization of contingent labor and address the issue in their own way, many health systems created their own internal staffing agencies. With this internal flexibility, they were able to fill open shifts and avoid adding excessive numbers of agency nurses. All DNP leaders were faced with flexing up staffing to address volume and acuity surges (Joslin & Joslin, 2020). DNP leaders relied on their training related to Domain 5, Quality and Safety, and Domain 7, Systems-Based Practice, developing and refining systems for quality improvement and systems-based thinking, to address the staffing challenges and to manage the effects of the influx of contingent labor into the existing workforce.

Redeployment of existing staff became common during the pandemic, especially during times of surge. At Allegheny Health Network, a 14-hospital integrated system in Pittsburgh, engaging nurses from non-inpatient areas and those down-sized due to volume impacts (suspended operating room cases) quickly became valuable resources. Those nurses were able to fill gaps in the surge model to provide inpatient nursing care. Preparing nurses to deploy to a new practice area required rapid assessment of training needs and was fully coordinated by DNP-prepared educators. A redeployment algorithm was created to ensure consistency in structure and process (Coe Paula et al., 2020).

THE IMPACT OF COVID-19 ON THE WELL-BEING OF THE REMAINING WORKFORCE

The global COVID-19 pandemic was like nothing any practicing nurse had experienced in their lifetime. Regardless of their area of practice—direct care, education, research, or leadership—nurses across the globe were faced with unprecedented challenges in their work and personal lives. And for some, there was very little differentiation between the two. The DNP leader utilized their holistic knowledge and skills to address the various elements of workforce challenges as the pandemic emerged, peaked, and abated and the workforce was left with what many call the "new normal."

The importance of both a healthy nursing workforce (ANA, 2016) and a healthy work environment (American Association of Critical Care Nurses, 2005) had been identified long before the pandemic. Pre-pandemic, 35% to 45% of nurses reported symptoms of work-related distress (Madara et al., 2021). However, the stresses associated with the COVID-19 crisis intensified challenges to physical and psychological health and workplace safety. One of the most important lessons learned is that healthcare organizations must prioritize the health and well-being of those engaged in providing care to others (Rosa et al., 2020). DNP nurses in leadership, practice, and education roles led initiatives, practices, and policies that addressed the stresses faced by nurses in all practice settings. Considering the many challenges posed by the pandemic, nurse leaders noted they struggled the most with responding to the emotional health and well-being of the nursing teams (Joslin & Joslin, 2020).

At the beginning of the pandemic, the risk of exposure to COVID-19 was a pervasive fear for all frontline healthcare workers, particularly nurses. Additionally, shortages of personal protective equipment (PPE) and testing supplies, along with changing guidelines, created a pervasive sense of anxiety and distrust. Many nurses felt isolated as they feared exposing their families and friends to the coronavirus. Increasing numbers of patients and healthcare team members with COVID-19 contributed to staffing issues in the inpatient setting, with resulting fatigue and potential cognitive issues from long hours and an unrelenting pace of care. As the pandemic progressed, there was an increase in depression, burnout, and worsening of existing mental health issues exacerbated by sleep disturbances, disruptions in traditional social and collegial supports, and ongoing workplace hazards (McGaffigan et al., 2021). Nurses were also facing the same issues as the general public with child and elder care concerns and general interruptions to routine activities, such as seeking their own healthcare. The stress intensified as the pandemic became politicized with divergent views on PPE requirements, vaccinations, and even the existence of COVID-19 (Chen et al., 2021).

DNP leaders responded by leading and participating in interventions based on feedback from clinical nurses providing direct care. Many system interventions—virtual support groups and educational sessions—required time away from work, either during the workday or at home. To supplement these offerings, interventions were initiated that brought support to the nurses in the care setting. Sharing healthy habits at huddles, providing nourishment on the unit, rounding and listening to concerns and developing peer support programs were implemented to lessen the stress experienced at the point of care. The Well-Being Initiative was created to provide resources to support the mental health and resilience of nurses during and after the COVID-19 pandemic. Organizations contributing to and distributing the valuable information included the American Nurses Foundation, the American Nurses Association, the American Association of Critical Care Nurses, the American Psychiatric Nurses Association, and the Emergency Nurses Association (American Psychiatric Nurses Association, 2022).

MORAL DISTRESS

The pandemic presented situations that were unfamiliar, uncertain, and uncomfortable and caused moral distress for nurses and other healthcare providers. Moral distress was defined by Jameton (1984) as a phenomenon that occurs when someone knows the right thing to do but cannot pursue that action due to organizational constraints. In the nursing literature, moral distress also reflects a violation of professional versus personal values (Epstein et al., 2019; Hamric & Epstein, 2017). In a recent study, Silverman et al. (2021) identified the following themes and subthemes relating to major causes of moral distress in nurses caring for patients with COVID-19:

1. Lack of knowledge and uncertainty regarding how to treat COVID-19
2. Being overwhelmed by the depth and breadth of the COVID-19 illness
3. Fear of exposure to the virus leading to less-than-optimal care
4. Adopting a team model of nursing care that caused intraprofessional tensions and miscommunications
5. Organizational policies to reduce viral transmission, specifically visitation and PPE policies, that prevented nurses from assuming their caring role
6. Practicing within a crisis standard of care
7. Dealing with medical resource scarcity (Silverman et al., 2021)

DNP leaders were instrumental in implementing strategies to mitigate the impact of these causative factors. The lack of resources and changing guidelines regarding PPE influenced clinical nurses' trust of administrative leaders in their organizations (Sperling, 2021) and clinical leaders and educators were present at the point of care to assist in communicating updates and demonstrate clinical changes. One of the frequently cited causes of moral distress during the pandemic were visitation restriction protocols (Silverman et al., 2021). Patient-centered care, including the support and engagement of loved ones, is central to professional nursing practice, and visitor restriction policies implemented to reduce COVID-19 transmission conflicted with nursing values. In some instances, nurses reported an improvement in workflow and ability to provide care with visitor restrictions but universally experienced distress at end-of-life situations where they were often the sole support for the patient (Wendlandt et al., 2022). Knowing the rationale for restricting visitors did little to ease the grief of patients, families, and nurses. DNP leaders, notably those in practice and education roles, worked with clinical nurses to utilize technology to bring the presence of families to the bedside. Continued work is needed to identify how to safely provide the presence of family and loved ones in the event of another pandemic.

Moral Injury

Exposure to repeated instances of morally distressing events as seen during the pandemic can result in moral injury. Moral injury has been defined as the "deleterious long-term emotional, psychological, behavioral, spiritual, and social effects" related to situations that cause moral distress (Litz et al., 2009). Initial studies have focused on war veterans' experiences (Shay, 1995) and have been recently examined in nursing and healthcare overall (Cartolovni et al., 2021; Lake et al., 2022) for psychiatric symptoms, such as depression, anxiety, and post-traumatic stress disorder (PTSD).

While not all nurses and healthcare team members experienced long-term effects of morally distressing events and moral injury, it is essential that DNP leaders recognize the feelings and behaviors that can result. Feelings of guilt, shame, self-blame, or anger may result in changes in sleep, withdrawal or isolation, errors, and changes in empathetic responses (Watson et al., 2020). Symptoms of PTSD similar to those experienced in post-battle situations can also occur, including persistent memories, difficulty concentrating, changes in mood, and avoidance of people or places.

There is a lack of research focused on prevention and mitigation of moral distress and moral injury (Riedel et al., 2022). Promising interventions include increasing training in psychological first aid, encouraging nurses to seek assistance with available resources, decreasing mental health stigma, and frequent and intentional leader check-ins (Watson et al., 2020; Williams et al., 2020). DNP leaders can provide forums for nurses to discuss their experiences, either in group settings or individually, and share available organizational resources, such as counseling and behavioral health support, as well as services that address financial, child care, and other personal needs. The pandemic has provided an opportunity to better understand the long-term impact of morally distressing events and DNP leaders can be actively involved in both qualitative and quantitative studies. Additionally, continued clear, honest, open, and frequent communication is essential in beginning to build back trust and confidence in organizational leadership that may have been lost during this period of uncertainty.

HEALTHCARE DISPARITIES

The tremendous stress of the COVID-19 pandemic has shone a bright light on long-standing healthcare disparities (Brownson et al., 2020). Defined by the Centers for Disease Control (2020) as preventable differences in the burden of disease, injury, violence, or opportunities to achieve optimal health, these elements became most evident relative to people of color. During the initial surge, Black, Hispanic, and American Indian and Alaskan Native (AIAN) people had higher death rates than White people. When compared to White people, Hispanic people were five times and Black and AIAN people three and four times, respectively, more likely to die (Hill & Artiga, 2022). There are many factors that explain the higher rates of mortality among people of color, including increased risk of exposure related to working and living situations and increased risk of serious illness when infected due to underlying comorbid health conditions. Additionally, testing and treatment barriers as a result of existing issues in access to care contributed to the disparities highlighted during the pandemic (Lopez et al., 2021). Addressing healthcare disparities requires a multitude of strategies. DNP leaders are positioned well to address the "social determinants of health" and structural racism and bias from their training in Domain 6, Interprofessional Partnerships promoting interprofessional collaboration for improving patient and population health outcomes and for improving the nation's health, respectively (AACN, 2006).

There is widespread recognition that nurses, in every care setting, are called to play a role in addressing disparities and achieving health equity. One need to look no further than the National Academies of Science, Engineering and Medicine (NAM) and the Robert Wood Johnson Foundation report "The Future of Nursing 2020–2030: Charting a Path to Achieve Health Equity, that clearly describes the essential role of nurses in addressing this issue (Wakefield et al., 2021).

In the post-pandemic world, DNP leaders in healthcare systems are redoubling efforts to fully integrate the social determinants of health using the electronic health record to assess, intervene, and refer based on patient needs in all healthcare settings (Azar, 2021). Additional strategies include incorporating health equity measures into organizational goals and using a diversity, equity, and inclusion lens when evaluating programs, strategies, and outcomes. While these are important components to improve care, a robust public health system is required to achieve significant progress (Brownson et al., 2020). Efforts in this area necessitate advocacy at the local, state, and federal levels and DNP leaders can influence both policy and practice. Bekemeier et al. (2021) identify the need for more DNP-prepared advanced practice nurses who are skilled in population health and the care of marginalized communities and DNP programs that prepare nurses for public health specialty practice.

During the first year of the pandemic, the entire country was also wrestling with issues of equity and civil unrest following the death of George Floyd and attacks on members of racial and religious communities. Understanding existing bias in nursing is essential and DNP leaders have developed programs to assist in this effort. However, there is much work to be done in this area (Stamps, 2021). In addition to a focus on health equity, DNP nurse leaders increasingly recognized the importance of an inclusive work environment and diverse nursing workforce in achieving health equity and creating a positive work environment and are committed to implementing programs, such as leader mentorship programs (Brown-Deveaux et al., 2021) and academic-practice partnerships (Morrison et al., 2021), to achieve these goals.

EMERGENCY PREPAREDNESS

As COVID-19 moves to an endemic stage, it is important to not lose sight of the need to be prepared for future public health emergencies and other crises, such as mass trauma events and natural disasters. The strain on resources and the healthcare system was apparent from the beginning of the pandemic, evidenced by lack of PPE, lack of coordination between federal and state agencies, changing guidelines, and workforce issues. At the local level, many hospitals and healthcare systems were simply not prepared for a prolonged event with increased patient volume, acuity and mortality, capacity constraints, staffing challenges and workforce issues, ethical dilemmas, and testing/immunization needs in the community. DNP leaders can increase their own crisis response skills (Cariaso-Sugay et al., 2021) and influence emergency preparedness at their organizations and in advocacy efforts at the local, state, and federal levels. Specific local measures include incorporating lessons learned from COVID-19 and engaging the entire organization, as well as the community, in routine drills and preparedness activities.

POSTPANDEMIC ERA

The postpandemic era presents additional challenges for DNP leaders. Issues in the work environment, including an increase in workplace violence and a staffing shortage that may take years to recover, will continue to affect the health and well-being of the workforce. In 2022, the combination of inflation, workforce shortages, and reimbursement issues resulted in significant financial pressures on hospitals and healthcare systems (AHA, 2022) and the DNP leader will be called on to lead and participate in advocacy, efficiency innovations, and care model development. The interconnectedness of the healthcare system continuum and transitions of care have long been known to be crucial elements in care, yet significant breakdowns were blatantly obvious during the pandemic. Strengthening community, ambulatory and postacute partnerships, and preparing nurses to practice in these settings will inform the work of the DNP leader moving forward. From a clinical perspective, "long COVID" is just beginning to be understood and there is a role for the DNP APRN in providing expert care for this unique population.

It is most likely too soon to understand the full impact of the COVID-19 pandemic on healthcare and nursing. However, if we don't learn and change because of this experience, we will not be prepared for the next crisis and will have missed an opportunity to improve care now and in the future. The list of lessons learned is long, some of which will serve us well and others that point out what might be done differently. DNP leaders contributed to system leadership efforts, provided clinical expertise, helped to develop and expand telehealth and hospital at home, and developed solutions for workforce shortages and challenges to health and well-being. They will bring these lessons to bear as they strengthen the nursing workforce, continue to develop innovative models of care, expand clinical skills and advocacy skills to promote health equity, and prepare for future crises.

CRITICAL THINKING QUESTIONS

1. What are the essential leadership qualities and behaviors exhibited by nurses that were effective during the COVID-19 pandemic?
2. What was the DNP-prepared nurse's greatest lesson from the COVID-19 pandemic?
3. What have we learned from the COVID-19 pandemic with respect to nurse wellness and healthy work environments?
4. What are examples of clinical practice changes that occurred as a result of practice-based evidence during the pandemic?
5. How can ethical training and ethical debriefing impact moral injury and moral distress?
6. What structural issues need to change to view nurses as revenue generators and leaders in quality and safety rather than an expense in healthcare organizations?
7. The Great Resignation, following COVID, has placed additional staffing burdens on nursing and healthcare. What strategies can assist with encouraging individuals to enter the profession or return to the profession?
8. As a result of the pandemic, what curricular changes need to be made in DNP academic programs to prepare future nurses and nurse leaders for crisis situations?

CASE STUDY

An area that has not been discussed is ethical triage during COVID-19. Critical care units' triage is the process of examining incoming patients to quickly identify those patients needing immediate intensive care and treatment, and to make efficient use of resources (ICU beds, ventilators, etc.) in cases of emergency. The recent coronavirus disease 2019 pandemic (COVID-19) has placed triaging and the allocation of scarce health resources more broadly at the center of ethical and policy discussions. Triage protocols and guidelines have been developed by different individuals in the healthcare system and have led to controversy over which clinical criteria should be used and who should receive care if there are limited ICU beds or equipment. As a DNP-prepared nurse in health policy, the question at which level triage protocols should be developed (e.g., in local hospitals, or on a state or national level), which system should be designed, and who is authorized to pass and enforce such protocols are necessary (Vinay et al., 2021). Rather than focus on an individual patients' medical criterion, and who does or who does not have access to an ICU bed or ventilator based on that criterion, a state or regional approach is necessary. If there are no ICU beds in Hospital A, there should be a state-wide or regional system monitoring ICU bed usage to determine which healthcare facilities have ICU beds available. The DNP-prepared nurse in health policy can lead initiatives to create a state-wide or regional ethical triage system for COVID-19 or other disasters.

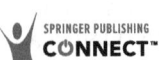

A robust set of instructor resources designed to supplement this text is located at http://connect.springerpub.com/content/book/978-0-8261-8137-4. Qualifying instructors may request access by emailing textbook@springerpub.com.

REFERENCES

AHA. (2022). *Data brief: Financial challenges for hospitals persist through 2022.* https://www.aha.org/system/files/media/file/2022/10/data-brief-financial-challenges-for-hospitals-persist-through-2022.pdf

American Association of Colleges of Nursing (AACN). (2006). *The essentials of doctoral education for advanced nursing practice.* https://www.aacnnursing.org/Portals/42/Publications/DNPEssentials.pdf

American Association of Critical-Care Nurses. (2005). AACN standards for establishing and sustaining healthy work environments: A journey to excellence. *American Journal of Critical Care, 14*(3), 187.

American Nurses Association. (2016). *Healthy nurse, healthy nation.* https://www.nursingworld.org/practice-policy/hnhn

American Association of Colleges of Nursing. (2021). *The essentials: Core competencies for professional nursing education.* https://www.aacnnursing.org/Portals/42/AcademicNursing/pdf/Essentials-2021.pdf

American Psychiatric Nurses Association. (2022). *Well-being initiative.* https://www.nursingworld.org/~49d911/globalassets/covid19/nurses-guide-pdf-003.pdf

Azar, K. M. (2021). The evolving role of nurse leadership in the fight for health equity. *Nurse Leader, 19*(6), 571–575. https://doi.org/10.1016/j.mnl.2021.08.006

Barrett, D., & Heale, R. (2021). COVID-19: Reflections on its impact on nursing. *Evidenced Based Nursing, 24*(4), 112–113. https://doi.org/10.1136/ebnurs-2021-103464

Bekemeier, B., Kuehnert, P., Zahner, S. J., Johnson, K. H., Kaneshiro, J., & Swider, S. M. (2021). A critical gap: Advanced practice nurses focused on the public's health. *Nursing Outlook, 69*(5), 865–874.

Blake, J. W., Giuliano, K. K., Butterfield, R. D., Vanderveen, T., & Sims, N. M. (2021). Extending tubing to place intravenous smart pumps outside of patient rooms during COVID-19: an innovation that increases medication dead volume and risk to patients. *BMJ Innovations, 7*(2). https://doi.org/10.1136/bmjinnov-2020-000653

Brown-DeVeaux, D., Jean-Louis, K., Glassman, K., & Kunisch, J. (2021). Using a mentorship approach to address the underrepresentation of ethnic minorities in senior nursing leadership. *JONA: The Journal of Nursing Administration, 51*(3), 149–155. https://doi.org/10.1097/NNA.0000000000000986

Brownson, R. C., Burke, T. A., Colditz, G. A., & Samet, J. M. (2020). Reimagining public health in the aftermath of a pandemic. *American Journal of Public Health, 110*(11), 1605–1610. https://doi.org/10.2105/AJPH.2020.305861

Caplan, G. A., Sulaiman, N. S., Mangin, D. A., Aimonino Ricauda, N., Wilson, A. D., & Barclay, L. (2012). A meta-analysis of "hospital in the home." *Medical Journal of Australia, 197*(9), 512–519. https://doi.org/10.5694/mja12.10480

Cariaso-Sugay, J., Hultgren, M., Browder, B. A., & Chen, J. L. (2021). Nurse leaders' knowledge and confidence managing disasters in the acute care setting. *Nursing Administration Quarterly, 45*(2), 142–151. https://doi.org/10.1097/NAQ.0000000000000468

Cartolovni, A., Stolt, M., Scott, P. A., & Suhonen, R. (2021). Moral injury in healthcare professionals: A scoping review and discussion. *Nursing Ethics, 28*(5), 590–602. https://doi.org/10.1177/0969733020966776

Centers for Disease Control and Prevention. (2020). *Health disparities.* https://www.cdc.gov/healthy youth/disparities/index.html

Centers for Medicare and Medicaid Services. (2022). *COVID-19 Emergency declaration blanket waivers for healthcare providers.* https://www.cms.gov/files/document/covid-19-emergency-declaration-waivers.pdf

Chan, G. K., Waxman, K. T., Baggett, M., Bakerjian, D., Dickow, M., Grimley, K. A., & Kiger, A. J. (2021). The importance and impact of nurse leader engagement with state nursing workforce centers: Lessons from the COVID-19 pandemic. *Nurse Leader, 19*(6), 576–580. https://doi.org/10.1016/j.mnl.2021.08.014

Chen, E., Chang, H., Rao, A., Lerman, K., Cowan, G., & Ferrara, E. (2021). COVID-19 misinformation and the 2020 US presidential election. *The Harvard Kennedy School Misinformation Review.*

Coe Paula, F., Graper Lisa, L., & Zangerle Claire, M. (2020). Leading through the unknown: A network perspective of the COVID-19 pandemic. *Critical Care Nursing Quarterly, 43*(4), 451–467.

Cotton, S., Zawaydeh, Q., LeBlanc, S., Husain, A., & Malhotra, A. (2020). Proning during covid-19: Challenges and solutions. *Heart & Lung, 49*(6), 686–687. https://doi.org/10.1016/j.hrtlng.2020.08.006

Cucinotta, D., & Vanelli, M. (2020). WHO declares COVID-19 a pandemic. *Acta Biomedica, 91*(1), 157–160. https://doi.org/10.23750/abm.v91i1.9397

Dhaliwal, J. K., Hall, T. D., LaRue, J. L., Maynard, S. E., Pierre, P. E., & Bransby, K. A. (2022). Expansion of telehealth in primary care during the COVID-19 pandemic: Benefits and barriers. *Journal of the American Association of Nurse Practitioners, 34*(2), 224–229. https://doi.org/10.1097/JXX.0000000000000626

Epstein, E. G., Whitehead, P. B., Prompahakul, C., Thacker, L. R., & Hamric, A. B. (2019) Enhancing understanding of moral distress: The measure of moral distress for health care professionals. *AJOB Empirical Bioethics, 10*(2), 113–124. https://doi.org/10.1080/23294515.2019.1586008

Evans, M., & Carlton, J. (2021, April 8). Soaring costs of nurses during COVID-19 pandemic are at center of lawsuits. *Wall Street Journal.* https://www.wsj.com/articles/soaring-costs-of-nurses-during-covid-19-pandemic-are-at-center-of-lawsuits-11617914600

Grimm, C. A. (2021). *Hospitals reported that the COVID-19 pandemic has significantly strained health care delivery.* U.S. Department of Health and Human Services.

Hamric, A. B., & Epstein, E. G. (2017). A health system-wide moral distress consultation service: Development and evaluation. *Hec Forum, 29*(2), 127–143. https://doi.org/10.1007/s10730-016-9315-y

Hill, L., & Artiga, S. (2022). *COVID-19 cases by race/ethnicity: Current data and changes over time.* https://www.kff.org/coronavirus-covid-19/issue-brief/covid-19-cases-and-deaths-by-race-ethnicity-current-data-and-changes-over-time Accessed: November 26, 2022.

Housing and Urban Development. (2020). *Flexibilities/waivers granted by the CARES Act + Mega waiver and guidance.* https://www.hud.gov/sites/dfiles/CPD/documents/Flexibilities_Waivers_Guidance_for_CARE_Act_CPD_Funds_062320.pdf

Jameton, A. (1984). *Nursing practice: The ethical issues.* Prentice-Hall.

Joslin, D., & Joslin, H. (2020). Nursing leadership COVID-19 insight survey: Key concerns, primary challenges, and expectations for the future. *Nurse Leader, 18*(6), 527–531.

Joo, J. Y. (2022). Nurse-led telehealth interventions during COVID-19: A scoping review. *CIN: Computers, Informatics, Nursing, 40*(12), 804–813. https://doi.org/10.1097/CIN.0000000000000962

Lake, E. T., Narva, A. M., Holland, S., Smith, J. G., Cramer, E., Rosenbaum, K. E. F., & Rogowski, J. A. (2022). Hospital nurses' moral distress and mental health during COVID-19. *Journal of Advanced Nursing, 78*(3), 799–809. https://doi.org/10.1111/jan.15013

Litz, B. T., Stein, N., Delaney, E., Lebowitz, L., Nash, W. P., Silva, C., & Maguen, S. (2009). Moral injury and moral repair in war veterans: A preliminary model and intervention strategy. *Clinical Psychology Review, 29,* 695–706. https://doi.org/10.1016/j.cpr.2009.07.003

Lopez, L., Hart, L. H., & Katz, M. H. (2021). Racial and ethnic health disparities related to COVID-19. *Journal of the American Medical Association, 325*(8), 719–720. https://doi.org/10.1001/jama.2020.26443

Madara, J., Miyamoto, S., Farley, J. E., Gong, M., Gorham, M., Humphrey, H., Irons, M., Mehrotra, A., Resneck, J., Jr., Rushton, C., & Shanafelt, T. (2021). Clinicians and professional societies COVID-19 impact assessment: Lessons learned and compelling needs, *NAM Perspectives, National Academy of Medicine*. https://doi.org/10.31478/202105b

McGaffigan, P., Kingston, M. B., & Bender Schwich, K. (2021). Tackling the healthcare acquired condition (HAC) of workforce harm: Lessons learned from COVID-19. *Management in Healthcare, 6*(2), 142–154.

Morrison, V., Hauch, R. R., Perez, E., Bates, M., Sepe, P., & Dans, M. (2021). Diversity, equity, and inclusion in nursing: the pathway to excellence framework alignment. *Nursing Administration Quarterly, 45*(4), 311–323. https://doi.org/10.1097/NAQ.0000000000000494

Moy, A. J., Schwartz, J. M., Withall, J., Lucas, E., Cato, K. D., Rosenbloom, S. T., Johnson, K., Murphy, J., Detmer, D. E., & Rossetti, S. C. (2021). Clinician and health care leaders' experiences with—and perceptions of—COVID-19 documentation reduction policies and practices. *Applied Clinical Informatics, 12*(5), 1061–1073. https://doi.org/10.1016/j.cpr.2009.07.003

Retzlaff, K. J. (2020). COVID-19 emergency management structure and protocols. *AORN Journal, 112*(3), 197. https://doi.org/10.1002/aorn.13149

Riedel, P. L., Kreh, A., Kulcar, V., Lieber, A., & Juen, B. (2022). A scoping review of moral stressors, moral distress and moral injury in healthcare workers during COVID-19. *International Journal of Environmental Research and Public Health, 19*(3), 1666. https://doi.org/10.3390/ijerph19031666

Ritchie, C., & Leff, B. (2022). Home-based care reimagined: A full-fledged health care delivery ecosystem without walls: Commentary reimagines home-based care. *Health Affairs, 41*(5), 689–695. https://doi.org/10.1377/hlthaff.2021.01011

Rosa, W. E., Schlak, A. E., & Rushton, C. H. (2020). A blueprint for leadership during COVID-19: Minimizing burnout and moral distress among the nursing workforce. *Nursing Management, 51*(8), 28–34. https://doi.org/10.1097/01.NUMA.0000688940.29231.6f

Rutledge, C. M., Kott, K., Schweickert, P. A., Poston, R., Fowler, C., & Haney, T. S. (2017) Telehealth and eHealth in nurse practitioner training: Current perspectives. *Advances in Medical Education Practice, 8*, 399–409. https://doi.org/10.2147/AMEP.S116071.

Sansolo, H., Wuerz, L., Grandstaff, K., Schwartz, T., & Peres-Mir, E. (2022). Nurses as Clinical Advisors in an interprofessional COVID-19 crisis command center. *The Journal of Nursing Administration. 52*(9), 486–490. https://doi.org/10.1097/NNA.0000000000001187

Shay, J. (1995). *Achilles in Vietnam: Combat trauma and the undoing of character*. Simon & Schuster.

Silverman, H. J., Kheirbek, R. E., Moscou-Jackson, G., & Day, J. (2021). Moral distress in nurses caring for patients with COVID-19. *Nursing Ethics, 28*(7–8), 1137–1164. https://doi.org/10.1177/09697330211003217

Sperling, D. (2021). Ethical dilemmas, perceived risk, and motivation among nurses during the COVID-19 pandemic. *Nursing Ethics, 28*(1), 9–22. https://doi.org/10.1177/0969733020956376

Stamps, D. C. (2021). Nursing leadership must confront implicit bias as a barrier to diversity in health care today. *Nurse Leader, 19*(6), 630–638. https://doi.org/10.1016/j.mnl.2021.02.004

Stamps, D. C., Foley, S. M., Gales, J., Lovetro, C., Alley, R., Opett, K., Glessner, T., & Faggiano, S. (2021). Nurse leaders advocate for nurses across a health care system: COVID-19. *Nurse Leader, 19*(2), 159–164. https://doi.org/10.1016/j.mnl.2020.07.011

United States Bureau of Labor Statistics. (2020). *Labor force statistics from the current labor statistics survey*. https://www.bls.gov/cps/cpsaat11.html

Wakefield, M., Williams, D. R., & Le Menestrel, S. (2021). *The future of nursing 2020–2030: Charting a path to achieve health equity*. National Academy of Sciences.

Watson, P., Norman, S. B., Maguen, S., & Hamblen, J. L. (2020). *Moral injury in healthcare workers*. National Center for PTSD. https://www.ptsd.va.gov/professional/treat/cooccurring/moral_injury_hcw.asp. Accessed November 24, 2022.

Wendlandt, B., Kime, M., & Carson, S. (2022). The impact of family visitor restrictions on healthcare workers in the ICU during the COVID-19 pandemic. *Intensive and Critical Care Nursing, 68*, 103123.

Williams, R. D., Brundage, J. A., & Williams, E. B. (2020). Moral injury in times of COVID-19. *Journal of Health Service Psychology, 46*(2), 65–69. https://doi.org/10.1007/s42843-020-00011-4

Vinay, R., Baumann, H., & Biller-Andorno, N. (2021). Ethics of ICU triage during COVID-19. *British Medical Bulletin, 138*(1), 5–15. https://doi.org/10.1093/bmb/ldab009

Yang, Y. T., & Mason, D. J. (2022). COVID-19's impact on nursing shortages, the rise of travel nurses, and price gouging. *Health Affairs Forefront*. https://www.healthaffairs.org/do/10.1377/forefront.20220125.695159

CHAPTER NINTEEN **Reflective Response**

CYNTHIA ROST

While we are very early in the postpandemic phase of COVID-19, we look toward a future of endemic seasonal COVID outbreaks globally. This leads us to the question, how has the doctor of nursing practice (DNP)-prepared nurse assisted in the fight against COVID during the pandemic, and how will that morph into permanent practice models for future outbreaks? DNPs use their clinical skills and the study of nursing research to gather and analyze data related to the impact of COVID on the global patient population. We are trained to use evidence-based practice and research to inform decision-making and develop innovative solutions to complex health problems.

Chapter 19 reflects on the work of DNP-prepared nurse leaders but with particular emphasis on inpatients, while only briefly discussing the DNP's community and public health nursing roles. It is my opinion that the role of the DNP-prepared nurse specifically related to the postpandemic COVID era will focus more now on community, public health, primary care, health promotion, and mental health components of COVID with an emphasis on outpatient or post-hospitalized (recovered or long-haul) patient populations.

The pandemic has highlighted the need for healthcare professionals to play a more active role in public health initiatives, especially in the community setting. DNP specialty preparation in public/population health can advance the overall effectiveness of the nation's most trusted profession (Reinhart, 2020), by educating nurses prepared to promote health among underserved populations, and to work to effectively change the systems that undermine health equity (Bekemeier et al., 2021, p.871).

As advanced practice nurses, DNPs have the knowledge and skills to contribute to the overall well-being of community health efforts in a multitude of ways, both in leadership and clinical roles. These roles can be categorized as follows:

1. Health education and promotion. DNPs provide health education and promotion to individuals and groups within the community setting. This includes dissemination of current (and ever-changing) information regarding COVID-19 prevention, the importance of vaccination as a method to prevent severe disease if infected, and the healthy lifestyle choices that are responsible for maintaining a healthy immune system.
2. Chronic disease management. It is well known that those persons with chronic diseases such as asthma, heart disease, diabetes, obesity, and autoimmune disorders have a higher likelihood of hospitalization and/or death if infected with COVID-19. DNPs have the clinical expertise to use the most current research to design practice models that assist community health professionals to develop and implement personalized plans of care and provide ongoing support for such individuals. There is also a growing understanding that COVID itself may become a chronic illness for many, and thus, we must have a proactive and nimble response to the needs of that population.

3. Telehealth services. The pandemic has accelerated the adoption of telehealth services, and the DNP-prepared nurse plays a critical role in providing virtual care to patients within the community. This issue is especially true of nurse practitioners who have gone on to earn a DNP and have the leadership skills to play a critical role in the design of virtual care models for those in the community without the means to be seen in an office environment. During the pandemic, this was especially necessary for primary and mental health virtual consultations, follow-up visits, and remote monitoring of the chronically ill. Nurses should also be prepared to act in an advocacy role, as third-party payers and health systems debate this new delivery model. The system must be designed with the needs and preferences of the communities we are serving as the highest priority.
4. Community outreach. DNPs have the knowledge and clinical background needed to work with community organizations to identify health needs and develop prevention programs to address them in an upstream manner. As part of their education, they are taught to serve as advocates for underserved populations and promote health equity and social justice. This also includes managing effective communication efforts that combat misinformation, promote accurate and evidence-based guidelines, and provide individuals, families, and communities the opportunity to make truly informed decisions about care.
5. Policy development. The DNP-prepared nurse contributes to, and advocates for, policy development and implementation at the local, state, and national levels. This includes face-to-face meetings with legislators and other government officials to promote funding for public health initiatives and the expansion of community healthcare services.

The above priorities, like most of healthcare today, focus on the response to COVID as it evolves. However, the most critical role of the community and public health DNP is prevention and emergency preparedness. We must invest now in the preparation of a highly specialized public health workforce that has the required skills and abilities to navigate future outbreaks. We also need to ensure that the hard lessons we learned, described so well in Chapter 19, are not wasted. The knowledge we gained must be used to inform our planning and preparation for next time. And, by all accounts, there will be a next time.

In conclusion, while I agree with the role of the DNP-prepared nurse as viewed in Chapter 19, the future of a world with global COVID as an expectation among community and public health nurses will need the advanced education of the nurse with a terminal practice degree to lead them forward in preventing a repeat of the overwhelming protection failures seen in the original pandemic.

REFERENCES

Bekemeier, B., Kuchnert, P., Zahner, S. J., Johnson, K. H., & Swider, S. M. (2021). A critical gap: Advanced practice nurses focused on the public's health. *Nursing Outlook, 69*(5), 865–874. https://doi.org/10.10166/joutlook.2021.03.023

Reinhart, R. (2020). *Nurses continue to rate highest in honesty, ethics*. Politics. https://news.gallup.com/poll/274673/nurses-continue-rate-highest-honesty-ethics.aspx

CHAPTER TWENTY

Enhancing the Role of a Doctor of Nursing Practice Graduate: Two Models for Global Studies Experiences

MELANIE T. TURK, H. MICHAEL DREHER, RICK ZOUCHA, MANJULATA EVATT, AND MELISSA A. KALARCHIAN

With the sudden global onset of the COVID-19 pandemic in February 2020, the Centers for Disease Control and Prevention (CDC) recommended that colleges and universities consider postponing or canceling foreign exchange programs and asking students on study-abroad programs to return to the United States (Redden, 2020). Students in Italy and South Korea were among the first to return to the United States (Svluga, 2020). Accordingly, study-abroad programs were canceled, most students were sent home from colleges and universities, and some were stranded overseas as countries quickly went into lockdown and limited or ceased international travel (Moody, 2020).

With global COVID-19 rates declining, educational institutions are now evaluating how to restart their programs and provide their students with the kinds of study-abroad experiences they offered prepandemic. Many colleges and universities will struggle as they assess the risk to students and faculty and face new challenges with our students entering a new reality of living around COVID-19 (Redden, 2021). It has not disappeared, and new antiviral boosters will likely need to be developed. This has affected not only undergraduates, but also graduate students.

The focus of this chapter is to describe two formal doctor of nursing practice programs where a short-term global experience was designed to enhance nursing students' education and positively impact their future practice as DNP graduates. We could not find any others. The first was at Drexel University in Philadelphia and the second at Duquesne University in Pittsburgh, which later expanded to include students in their PhD program. Each model is and was unique and often changed the lives of participating students.

In 2006, Drexel University started what was the first mandatory study-abroad program for any nursing program in the United States. Drexel developed a two-week study-abroad experience as part of its DNP program. It should be noted that Columbia University and Drexel used the degree initials DrNP until they both later changed them to DNP. For simplicity this chapter will use the initials DNP except where it may be important to refer to it being a DrNP degree. Duquesne University initiated its DNP study-abroad program in 2008, and although the course in which the global experience occurs is required, attending the global experience is not. This chapter describes the experiences of Drexel students and faculty who participated in programs in London and Dublin (although students did attend programs in Edinburgh, Florence, and Ontario, not described in this chapter) and Duquesne students and faculty who have an annual program in Rome and had one global experience in Singapore.

WHY STUDY ABROAD FOR DOCTORAL NURSING STUDENTS?

In an increasingly geopolitical, global-oriented world, it is incumbent that the most educated health professionals, including doctorallyprepared clinicians, scientists, and scholars, have the kinds of real-world experiences that will give them the best context for discussing the international implications of health issues and in making informed decisions about health policy and practice. The 2003 severe acute respiratory syndrome (SARS) virus, 2009 H1N1 flu virus, the 2014 to 2016 ebola virus, and now the global COVID-19 pandemic, which has killed 6.6 million people (World Health Organization, 2022), are vivid examples of why nurses, now more than ever, know that the health of someone in a bordering country or on another continent may have a direct impact on the health of citizens wherever they live. Now, we likely await the next global virus. Speaking at Germany's annual Munich Security Conference in February 2022, Bill Gates stated, "We'll have another pandemic. It will be a different pathogen next time" (Gilchrist, 2022).

International higher education is a big business, and although it has been stalled by COVID-19, it will return. However, it will look different as students want different things such as more flexibility, and many now want access to online courses and programs (Nestor, 2022). Will COVID-19 permanently impact study-abroad travel? Probably. Will there be increased institutional insurance costs with specific riders? Of course. Our United States global study programs are now slowly reemerging and will face these and other transitional issues (Kremer, 2021; Redden, 2021).

In 2006, the forward-thinking doctoral nursing faculty (in the Doctoral Nursing Department) at Drexel University was convinced that a short-term formal study-abroad experience would be an innovative enhancement to its DrNP program. It would ideally prepare the students to better face the contemporary global problems that highly educated nursing and other health professionals are increasingly being challenged to solve. Similarly, the Duquesne School of Nursing faculty thought about the importance of an international education component in their DNP program. This chapter provides practical information related to the approval and funding process necessary to implement these types of programs and, given the lack of doctoral nursing study-abroad programs described in the literature, highlights the perspectives of both faculty and students who have participated in programs at both institutions.

DREXEL UNIVERSITY'S DNP INTERNATIONAL STUDY-ABROAD PROGRAM

Why Was the Program Created?

The Drexel DNP[1] program's international study-abroad program was first conceived in early 2006. It grew from the university's desire to invest more resources to promote the Drexel brand more internationally, and with a renewed focus on encouraging international programs for both undergraduate and graduate students. The first doctoral nursing students and faculty participated in the inaugural program in London in April 2007. The DNP International Study Abroad Program was designed as a two-week intensive program that was offered in the second year of study. It took place during the student's last quarter of study (spring quarter) before completing all the formal doctoral coursework. Because the DNP program was designed for working adults, with classes one day a week, a two-week program was deemed the most feasible. Although a two-week study-abroad program may not seem like a long time, short-term study-abroad programs (2–8 weeks in duration) predominated then, attracting approximately 57% of all study-abroad students in 2011 (Chow & Villarreal, 2011). The organization Forum on Education Abroad in their 6th edition 2020 text on *Leading Short-Term Study Abroad Programs: Know the Standards* states these programs are 8 weeks or less.

In retrospect, the new DNP curriculum was wellpositioned both to integrate and accommodate a short-term study-abroad program. The first course in the 3-year part-time doctoral program was the *Politics of Health: Implications for Nursing Practice*, and there was a desire by the doctoral faculty to include the content on how doctorallyprepared nurses should and could participate more fully in a dialogue and in the activism regarding international health issues (Dreher et al., 2008). This idea of a 2-week program seemed ideal and feasible, and in consultation with the MBA program (which had a required one-week international experience as part of their program), the chair and teaching faculty and had a precedent campus-based graduate program model that provided design guidance.

Why Was the Program Mandatory?

One of the very first decisions the Drexel faculty made was that if the experience would be embedded in the program, it would be mandatory, not optional. This view was rooted in egalitarian ideals. At the undergraduate level, too often study-abroad becomes an "elite" activity for privileged students. This view of study abroad as a sign of prestige and social status was identified almost 30 years ago by Fry in 1984. Moreover, this sense of "access for the few" continues with articles like "*5 Reasons Why You Should Study Abroad if You Have the Privilege to Do So*" (Maslow, 2020). Diversity data on study-abroad participation is hard to discern as there are so many difficulties in collecting it, using the best metrics, and being inclusive in their definition of diversity. However, there is some positive trend data. The U.S. Department of State's USA Study Abroad website (U.S. Department of State, n.d.) posts the most current available from the opendoors website, a portal for national study-abroad data also endorsed by the Institute of International Education and other organizations interested in data collection on this topic (2015). From 2005–2006 and 2016–2017, the percentage of individuals from racial and ethnic minority groups studying abroad rose from 7% to 29.2% (opendoors, 2018).

Although the first 11 doctoral students all worked full-time, they certainly had financial obligations beyond the typical undergraduate, and some even had children in college (the mean age of the first class was 43 years). Yet, it was calculated that an affordable program could be created; however, the concern was that if the activity were optional, it likely would not have full participation. Thus, the goal of making the DNP program more innovative with one emphasis on global learning would not be complete. Further, the department chair did not see administratively how the DNP program could be operated effectively with some students going abroad and others not. As this program was conceived after the first class matriculated in September 2005, the 11 enrolled students were approached in January 2006 about their willingness to participate. The program proposal would only move forward if all of them agreed to participate. Initially, only 10 of 11 students were willing, but with some coaxing, the one recalcitrant student agreed. Thus began what turned into a full year of planning to get the graduate study abroad program designed, approved, funded, and then scheduled to be implemented in year three.

How Was the Program Funded?

The germination of this idea came at an opportune time for the DNP program. The Drexel annual budget planning process for the following academic year usually began each February and this allowed strategic time to create and submit a proposal to the associate dean for doctoral education and research, to the college dean, and the university provost. There were two strategies taken that were critical for the rapid and ultimate approval in the first cycle submission. First, this new graduate study abroad program closely matched the evolving mission of the university to enhance its international image and reputation; one way was by increasing study-abroad offerings to students. This program's particular emphasis on graduate students, specifically doctoral students, was deemed highly innovative in the approval process. Second, the department chair proposed using a creative financing procedure that would make the offering more palatable to prospective students, who might initially think they could never afford to attend both a 3-year doctoral nursing program and participate in a 14-day study-abroad program, which would certainly require them to take time off from work. The faculty believed the idea of a mandatory study program would be attractive to students who were looking for a distinctive DNP doctoral program, but in the end, the idea had to become "real" to the prospective student. Since funding the doctoral study abroad program involved funding both student and faculty travel, each will be discussed separately.

FUNDING DOCTORAL STUDENTS STUDYING ABROAD

To make the program both attractive and "doable" for prospective students, the decision was made to take the full cost of the program (airfare, housing, events, health insurance, and administrative costs) and divide the total cost of the program to each student into a DNP International Study Fee paid in eight separate quarterly payments. Because Drexel was on quarters, this allowed the first-year students to make a payment of some $450 over four quarters in years one and two and thus attend the global study program in their seventh quarter (spring quarter) in year two.[2] On their return, they did make one final payment in the summer quarter. If the students were on graduate financial aid (and some of them were), their international study fee was considered part of their financial aid package as the program was mandatory. This was a very critical point. If it were optional, financial aid would not cover it. This procedure was followed for years and was very effective. Even students who were not on financial aid did not view the quarterly charge as excessive. Later, with new billing procedures, the program billed students over 12 quarters (the full 3-year program of study), but in an attempt to simplify billing, the intra-college budgetary implications were impacted, especially if a student later went to a one course per semester program of study. This approach was withdrawn.

Certainly, the international study fee was a creative way to provide for the financing of doctoral students to attend the program. Their eight-quarter (or 12-quarter) fee went into a designated college account whereby the department chair could then annually fund the group airfares, the shared apartment accommodations abroad (two students share one apartment and single upgrades at the individual student's expense were usually available), the costs for all tours, the events, the additional local guest scholars for the two courses that were offered abroad each year, and the administrative fee charges by the study abroad company partner, the London-based Foundation for International Education (FIE). Because Drexel University was one of the founding schools to participate in FIE's London program, they had experience with Drexel University and the quarter system. However, the Drexel DNP program was not only FIE's first short-term study abroad program they sponsored, but also the first graduate and first doctoral program they hosted.

FUNDING DOCTORAL FACULTY ACCOMPANYING DNP STUDENTS ABROAD

Although the quarterly international study fee covered the expenses of the participating doctoral students, it did not cover the expenses of the participating faculty. Doctoral global study programs are inherently different from undergraduate global study programs. It would be inconceivable to simply place a full cohort of doctoral students in another institution abroad and have them taught completely by external faculty. However, this is the model for most undergraduate study-abroad programs, especially language study-abroad programs. The doctoral students followed a certain prescribed curriculum; its departmental teaching faculty (by rotating which courses were scheduled to be taught abroad) rotated going abroad. Indeed, this study-abroad program was not exclusively designed for the students, but its mission was also designed to benefit the program's doctoral nursing faculty scholars as well. By also including a faculty objective for this program, traveling teaching faculty were then able to make international contacts that could lead to global collaborations, which in turn, could further enhance Drexel's international image and reputation. In preparation for each year's program, the selected teaching faculty secured local scholars to come into the classroom as guest speakers to enhance each course's content.

The Drexel program's emphasis on the international benefits to the doctoral teaching faculty was one real difference in undergraduate versus graduate study abroad. Second, securing guest scholars for rotating different doctoral-level courses is an activity that cannot easily be outsourced to another host school or institution. Recruiting scholars with a very specific type of expertise or area of scholarship requires that the traveling faculty (who know a year in advance what courses are going to be offered abroad and who will be teaching them) make international connections, and through their network of referrals, approach the best local or regional university scholars to invite them to speak. Because the 2-week program was structured with one course offered usually from 9 a.m. to 12 noon Monday through Thursday, and the second class from 1:30 p.m. to 4:30 p.m.[3] (Fridays were reserved for class field trips, and the weekends were free for students and faculty), typically there were two guest speakers per class per week. Additionally, the program was successful at arranging a full day off campus at another host institution (Dublin Trinity College, Kingston University/St. George's of London, and the University of Brighton). As mentioned previously, since Drexel operated on a 10-week quarter system, students attended class on campus in weeks 1 and 10 only, and weeks 3 and 4 were entirely abroad. Thus, the students were not on campus in Philadelphia for the other 6 weeks, and all 30-class hours in the quarter were met using this model.

As Drexel's DNP program relied on its doctoral faculty traveling abroad to teach, network, and act as semiformal guides for student activities (undergraduate students must be chaperoned and supervised to a larger degree than graduate students to avoid risks to the university), there must be a separate budget for faculty expenses (housing, food, and travel). The Drexel DNP program typically sent two or three faculty abroad each year with each class of students. For the fourth annual program in London in 2010, there was a new day program at the University of Brighton with their professional doctoral students and faculty, and this was the program's first experience with Drexel DNP students networking with other international students in professional nursing and other health-related doctoral programs.[4]

The department chair selected courses taught abroad as part of the annual nursing teaching schedule procedures. Doctoral nursing courses were purposefully rotated so that a diverse set of faculty could take part in the global experience. However, there was no standard procedure for faculty selection (e.g., by seniority), the philosophy of the department chair was mostly to use the experience to reward highly productive faculty who had been awarded tenure, received a major grant, or had exceptionally high teaching evaluations in the doctoral program. If the international mission of a university or college is important, then annual requests to fund this particular faculty activity can become part of the normal budget process.

CASE STUDY I   A Doctoral Student's Perspective on the Drexel DNP-in-London Program

As I boarded the Virgin Atlantic Boeing 747 in the spring of 2008, I was filled with anticipation. For weeks leading up to our departure, I poured over the itinerary and gathered as much travel information as I could about London and the surrounding countryside. Despite my best intentions to sleep during the flight, I diligently read the course material while we flew over the Atlantic. But my eyes periodically drifted from my articles on ethics and pedagogy sitting on my tray table to the clouds out of my window, as I daydreamed about the time yet to be spent 5,700 km across the ocean. With an hour remaining in the flight, some skeptical thoughts also interrupted my pleasant escape. Although the required experience abroad was one of the intriguing elements of the Drexel University DNP degree, I harbored a small amount of doubt regarding the impact this experience was going to have in changing how I viewed the world around me. Our itinerary allowed for two full days of acclimation before the start of the class. I spent my first day familiarizing myself with the local surroundings. Nestled in west London, our accommodations off Gloucester Road in the Borough of Kensington were equal distance between Hyde Park and Kensington Palace, and the nearest tube stop and the building housing the classrooms. The neighborhood streets were lined with several foreign embassies and a variety of eclectic restaurants, including several "Gastro Pubs" which I frequented often during my 2-week stay. The next day, we took a walking tour of Kensington in the morning and a bus tour of London in the afternoon, which truly gave me the lay of the land. That evening, as I sat preparing for the following day's classes, I stared out my hotel window at the street lights below, once again daydreaming about the experiences yet to be had. I awoke the following morning to the start of a 2-week journey filled with discovery in and out of the classroom. In addition to the intellectual rigor fostered by the Drexel faculty and readily embraced by my peers, something I had grown to expect over the last year in the DNP program, I was challenged by several guest lecturers specializing in the field of nursing ethics. Dr. Wainwright provided a perspective on research ethics, not entirely unfamiliar, but still unique to the United Kingdom. Dr. Gallagher lectured on virtue ethics, inviting a dialogue impossible not to join. We also had the honor of having Dr. Dickenson, who spoke on reproductive ethics, and much of the concepts she presented that morning in late April were ideas shared from

(continued)

her soon-to-be-published book. Particularly memorable was a pleasant train ride to the University of Bedfordshire, north of London, to hear Professor Christopher Johns, author of several books including *Engaging Reflection in Practice: A Narrative Approach* (Johns, 2006), used the previous semester before our London experience. Dr. Johns lectured as if he was telling a story, a format many of the British lecturers seemed to follow. We were encouraged to discuss our own personal experiences, and by the end of our time together, a tapestry of our reflections had been woven together as a testament to the power of reflective practice. Hearing from, interacting with, and then being escorted through the reflective process was far more enriching than my previous attempt at reading his book and then attempting to synthesize reflective practice into my everyday life. A visit to the St. George's Healthcare National Health Service Trust main campus in Tooting, southwest London, one of the United Kingdom's largest teaching hospitals and associated with the renowned St. George's University of London, provided an opportunity to observe and compare a socialized healthcare system to our own capitalistic healthcare system in the United States. Perhaps the highlight of the visit for me was speaking with the nursing staff on their vascular unit. I was encouraged to find far more similarities than differences in the management of clients with vascular disease. It was also refreshing to see the importance placed on the nursing contribution to the care of the patient. By the completion of the visit I had a true appreciation for the National Health Services and the attempt to provide every citizen with availability and access to primary healthcare. The remainder of the time not taken up with academic and professional pursuits was spent with my classmates touring Cambridge, exploring the culture, people, and historical sites of London, including a fascinating medical walking tour and a visit to the Florence Nightingale Museum. On the last day of my London adventure, I took a walk into Hyde Park, a stroll I had become quite fond of over the previous 2 weeks. As I slowly walked along the edge of Round Pond, my mind was no longer consumed with daydreams of anticipated future experiences or skepticism. Instead, it was filled with the knowledge, experiences, and memories obtained from the past 2 weeks. Knowledge gleaned from the exceptional guest lecturers who so willingly shared their expertise. Experiences fostering an international perspective of nursing, and a realization of the responsibility I bear to my profession that goes beyond the door of my institution and is not limited by borders. And memories of people and places that I will carry with me for the rest of my life.

Scott Oldfield, DrNP Student, CRNP, Vascular Surgery Clinic, Geisinger Medical Center, Danville, Pennsylvania, Drexel University, Class of 2006

THE DREXEL DNP-IN-DUBLIN PROGRAM: A FACULTY PERSPECTIVE

In London, students learned to love the city. In Dublin, the Drexel students learned to love and appreciate the people of Ireland. Initially, many of the students were less than enthusiastic about having their study-abroad experience in Ireland. They wanted to go to a country that they perceived as culturally sophisticated and known for its theatre and museums. Instead, they were introduced to a country that had its own charm, unique culture, and rich history. The program's study tour guide in 2009 was an American graduate student from Chicago studying at the Dublin School of Business.

They helped students and faculty navigate the city as well as shared their experiences as an international student.

Again, after a short Saturday orientation, the second day in Ireland began with a medical walking tour conducted by a well-known Dublin historian, author, and artist who has developed a unique walking tour service for Dublin. Indeed, we were the first medical walking tour that our guide ever conducted. On this tour alone students learned about the Irish Healthcare System, the potato famine, religious oppression, women's healthcare, and the political and religious landscape's effect on childbearing rights, as well as had a visit to the Rotunda Hospital, which specializes in women's health and midwifery services. The hospital, founded in 1745, was the original Dublin Lying-In Hospital and maternity training hospital, the first of its kind in Europe. There the students had an opportunity to have a question and answer session with the nursing administrator on call, and began to get a glimpse of nursing education and nursing practice in Ireland.

Two doctoral courses were offered during the Drexel Dublin global study experience: Legal Issues Confronting Nursing Faculty and Administrators and Qualitative Methods for Clinical Nursing Inquiry. Irish guest lecturers were invited to the classes to present the "Irish Perspective" on assigned topics and readings. The legal issues course used a case-based approach to examine the multitude of legal and ethical issues that confront the contemporary nursing faculty member in the classroom, in clinical settings, or in situations in their professional role as a faculty member. A lecturer from the University of Limerick discussed basic Irish nursing education from both a historical and current perspective. Students and faculty learned that Ireland moved swiftly to the BSc in nursing studies entry only in the 1990s, and unlike the United States, undergraduate nursing students specialize early on in their education in one of five specialties: general population, intellectual disabilities, psychiatric mental health, midwifery, and child nursing.

The program also consisted of a day at Trinity College School of Nursing and Midwifery, which provided an opportunity to interact with their doctoral students and faculty, and also to hear a lecture on our host country's health system, always an integral part of our program. Drexel students attended a presentation on the PhD program in nursing and midwifery outlining the school's research resources, and they attended a PhD proposal defense. Trinity students heard a similar Drexel DNP program presentation. All students were then able to compare and contrast institutional research infrastructure, including release time, research support, and incentives, as well as the differences related to research start-up packages and salary incentives, which were greater for Drexel. Although doctoral nursing education was relatively new to Trinity College, the institution had a wide and historic international legacy, educating both Oscar Wilde and James Joyce, among others.

Trinity College provided a wealth of guest scholars for our qualitative methods course and a wider discussion of graduate nursing education in Ireland. Guest lecture topics included:

- *Ethical considerations in qualitative research*—using a study on women's experiences of carrying a fetus with an abnormality as an exemplar
- *Qualitative research data collection strategies*—using a study on women's experiences of myocardial infarction as an exemplar
- *Mixing data, design and analysis: Triangulation as a qualitative research strategy*—using examples from studies on student midwives' views of their education and quality of life at end-of-life care
- *Qualitative sampling issues*—using field notes, memoing, and interviewing, focusing on a grounded theory approach and using a study on sexuality in mental health nursing as an exemplar

Unlike the prevailing paradigm in the United States, Trinity College of Nursing and Midwifery faculty are trying to hone their quantitative research program, while American nursing faculty are still grappling with balancing qualitative and quantitative research as equal partners. These presentations provided valuable opportunities for discussion, as the Drexel DNP program is a hybrid nursing doctorate, and all doctoral candidates complete a clinical dissertation. Thus, the PhD students at Trinity and the DNP students from Drexel appreciated and benefited from exploration of each other's research projects during our day visit.

In the context of their multicultural global study education, students and faculty experienced such activities as the Unmanageable Revolutionaries: Women in Irish History Walking Tour, a Dublin Literary Pub Crawl, and an incredible night of tragic drama attending Arthur Miller's *All My Sons* at the famed Gate Theater in Dublin. During the Irish women's history tour, it was startlingly apparent to us that the accomplishments of Irish women were sadly missing as a major aspect of Irish history. Foreign domination, a historically patriarchal society, religious oppression, and lack of childbearing rights appear to have largely contributed to Irish women's invisibility in Irish history. This walking tour alone led to a great discussion about the Irish role of women and of women's right globally that permeated the classroom. As a faculty member having attended the London program once and now the Dublin program, each was uniquely different, and both were incredibly rewarding for students and faculty.

CASE STUDY II   A Doctoral Student's Perspective on the DREXEL DNP-in-Dublin Program

As an adult doctoral student with multiple responsibilities, including a full-time career and family, the thought of adding an international study-abroad program seemed daunting. As the time neared, however, with all the planning and packing upon us, the excitement grew. Spending 2 weeks in Ireland with my 11 peers, learning about healthcare and healthcare education, as well as taking two courses, would soon be a reality, and not just a paragraph on paper, or as a small blurb describing the DNP program. The courses selected to be taken in Ireland were oriented to qualitative research methods and legal issues in nursing academia, both very appropriate for study abroad. I do not think we could have experienced and learned more about qualitative research in any better way than with the opportunities we were given in Ireland. We had multiple qualitative researchers, all well established in their fields, coming to the Dublin School of Business and giving us lectures about their own research, as well as various methods used in their research. Each lecturer was well prepared and willing to entertain questions from each of us. Also, after the lectures, our professor from Drexel would summarize and clarify any questions raised during the morning's session and prepare us for the next day. I think we were each impressed how each lecturer brought to us a living classroom from which we were able to absorb much more than if we had just read their articles and discussed them in class in Philadelphia. We also spent a day at Trinity College with the doctoral nursing students in the morning and in the afternoon learned about their educational system, types of research being pursued by the students, and strengths of their program. During lunch, there were informal opportunities to share personal experiences of doctoral education and our own research interests with the Trinity students and faculty. We discussed the differences between the United States and Ireland, as well as the differences between Drexel University and Trinity College.

(continued)

> Many of us also visited the *Book of Kells* and Trinity Library that same day. In our time off, we enjoyed taking in the sights and tastes of Ireland. Each of us wandered in our own directions, some of us taking in Howth, Belfast, Galway, the Cliffs of Moher, and Cork, to name a few. We enjoyed watching football and rugby from the local taverns, and of course had to spend some time in the Temple Bar Area listening to Irish music and enjoying the Guinness (we were doctoral students!). As a group, we visited Glendalough and the Wicklow mountains on our last day in Ireland. We even got used to the rainy damp weather and appreciated the beautiful days we had, as well. The country of Ireland is beautiful, and the people could not have been more welcoming. The camaraderie among many of us was enhanced significantly, and was a bonus to everything else we experienced and learned on this short but expansive learning experience. Many other programs *encourage* their students to study abroad, but we were privileged that this was a mandatory part of our curriculum. I know some of my classmates clearly underestimated the impact this trip would have on our lives. I am sure if it were only optional, our chief nursing officer colleague, for example, would have said she could not afford to leave her high-powered position for 2 weeks. Instead, she had to go and, indeed, had a ball. For any doctoral students studying abroad, it will most likely be an unforgettable, life-altering experience, well worth the inconveniences it may have caused in the life of a doctoral student.
>
> Cynthia Gifford-Hollingsworth, DrNP, CRNP, CPNP, Surgical Research Nurse Supervisor, Department of Surgery, College of Medicine, Drexel University, Class of 2007

WHAT DREXEL LEARNED FROM BOTH EXPERIENCES

When Drexel planned and implemented the mandatory 2-week global study experience, the faculty was not clear on the direct impact that such an experience would have on the overall student's global and doctoral educational experience. In year one, faculty were immediately and pleasantly surprised by how deep an impression the study abroad experience had on the students, both personally and professionally. Simply based on assessments from first-year faculty, students, and FIE partners in London, the study program became a standard part of the DNP curriculum, and it was advertised as "mandatory" for the second class of 2007.

During the first 4 years of this program, it was evident that many of the students had never been abroad, and others who had traveled abroad had not visited London or Dublin. A few had no passports! Although some students were reticent about going abroad due to family responsibilities, most adapted quite well and enjoyed the experience immensely. However, this program was not designed to be a cultural immersion experience. These were doctoral students with a specific curriculum and our goal was to match our content by inviting local scholars as guest speakers. As nurses and doctoral students, we always learned about the nursing education system and healthcare system of each country. We tried to match our cultural tours with the same learning objective. In Ireland, students were quite interested to learn about the religious oppression of the Irish people and its effects even today. Many modern Irish who had not experienced oppression still spoke about the psychological pain of oppression in their normal dialogue with the students. Many of the students identified with these feelings and their pain resonated with them. In London, students were able to experience an incredibly massive, cosmopolitan city that probably provided a more diverse cultural experience, but certainly less intimate and personal, than Dublin. The faculty was particularly observant of the impact Ireland had on many of our students who were of Irish descent and in the country for the first time.

Overall, the DNP global study experience provided students with an opportunity to experience another country and learn another culture while maintaining full-time or part-time employment in the United States. These doctoral students, all studying part-time, had an opportunity to immerse themselves in their studies for a 2-week period and also bond as a group, becoming familiar with each other as individuals, students, and professionals. Students also learned about London or Dublin in the classroom and out in the field without the immediate pressures of family and work. They learned that largely Anglophilic London and Dublin are indeed very different from their own American culture and that despite having an accent or having a different educational system or healthcare system, we are still at the core more alike than different.

DREXEL PROGRAM SUMMARY

From 2007 to 2010 and the fifth, sixth, and seventh global study programs (which added a 4-day experience in Edinburgh, Scotland, when DNP students attended the Second International Conference on the Professional Doctorate in 2011 as part of their London program; in 2012, the program returned to Dublin; and in 2013, the students split time with one week in London and then to Florence for a second week for the Third International Conference on the Professional Doctorate), it became clear that this innovation had become an integral part of the curriculum. Even with the downturn in the economy with the global recession in 2007, the program was sustainable and able to only modestly increase the quarterly fee each year (e.g., one year due to increased fuel charges and another due to fluctuating currency exchange rates). The initial intention was never to be based solely in London, although partnering with the London-based FIE made the job of planning such a short-term study abroad program much easier. It should be noted that despite the trend toward globalism and outreach to new international locations like China and India, almost 40% of current United States students in 2019–2020 completed their study-abroad experience in just four countries (ranked by order), Spain, Italy, the United Kingdom, and France (Nietzel, 2019).

Still, it takes an incredible amount of planning to put a high-level, scholarly program together. The Drexel faculty were adamant to communicate that this program was not a "vacation" but truly a study-abroad experience. Families were not permitted (of course as far as that could be enforced, but the families did "lay low"), until week two of the program, so students could at least have one week where they could concentrate on themselves and this formative experience without the distractions of family obligations. A doctoral study-abroad program requires meticulous planning to secure scholars to come to a new, foreign-based doctoral seminar classroom. It requires months of networking and, indeed, the program compensated the visiting classroom scholars with modest honoraria. The faculty continuously debated to what extent this should be a "cultural immersion" experience. The department chair tried to take the program to Madrid one year, but unfortunately, there was a scarcity of scholars fluent in English who could guest lecture on the focused topics. A faculty scout (who was traveling nearby in Spain at the early planning stages of the program for the following year) found the accommodations and suburban location of the host school unacceptable. Indeed, graduate students, and particularly doctoral students, will not want to be treated as undergraduates or mixed in with them in the same type of accommodations. The majority of the Drexel students worked full-time, so they did typically have discretionary income that would allow them to pay a little more for more upscale accommodations and amenities. Before Dublin was selected as the second site, the department chair flew to Dublin to inspect the facilities (again, he was traveling nearby). It was foreseen that having satisfactory accommodations for graduate students, not the "Spartan" ones that undergraduates may not flinch at, became critically important when returning students discussed their study-abroad program with new students in the program.

Finally, it was discerned that the amount of time necessary to plan such a program required more time for graduate students than undergraduates. The Drexel MBA colleagues had also confirmed this. Therefore, one of the doctoral nursing faculty later served as a global study facilitator and worked in concert with the chair each year to plan the micro details of the program. The department chair went in the first year and in the second year with the new venue so the program could be fine-tuned to enact a planning process for wherever we went. When a department chair is walking in Dublin with a fellow faculty member who says, "Wow, I am so privileged to be here," then the expectations that these faculty will use their new international experiences to network, collaborate, and ultimately increase their global scholarly reputations (and hence to the college and university) become realized (and well worth the investment).

After many successful program years, the overall evaluation was that this mandatory international experience became an important and distinctive part of the DrNP program. If this model was used for PhD in nursing programs, PhD students could perhaps be matched up with an international faculty mentor in the host city and have DNP and PhD students share one course and take another separately. London and Dublin became excellent alternating sites, but in 2014 and 2015, students were sent to Ontario, Canada. The students did not deem Canada an "international destination, " and subsequently the study-abroad program was terminated.

With the rise of globalization, it is critical that nursing students, particularly doctoral-educated clinical nursing scholars, have an enhanced understanding of international health issues. Participation in a mandatory study-abroad program for doctoral nursing students is one way to accomplish this. So when the article "So What Did You Learn in London?" was republished on the internet (Redden, 2007), it caught both the students' and faculty's eyes, and the answer is, "a lot."

THE ADVENT OF THE GLOBAL STUDIES OPPORTUNITIES FOR DNP STUDENTS AT DUQUESNE UNIVERSITY

Duquesne University is a private Catholic University founded by the Spiritan Congregation of Priests in 1878 in Pittsburgh, Pennsylvania. The university was founded on the values of serving God through serving students, so that, in turn, they can go and serve others. The mission of the university is rooted in these values through an ecumenical atmosphere open to diversity that includes service to the Church, the community, the nation, and the world. It is in this long history, tradition, and philosophy that the School of Nursing embarked on this opportunity to learn beyond the confines of the campus located in Pittsburgh.

The School of Nursing has a long history of global studies that started in the early 1990s with the development of The Center for International Nursing. Through the center, relationships were formed and a formal sister school relationship between *Universidad Politecnica de Nicaragua* (UPOLI) in Managua, Nicaragua, and Duquesne University School of Nursing (DUSON) was established. The sister school relationship resulted in many opportunities for student and faculty exchanges, clinical experiences, and collaborative research. In the early 2000s the Center for International Nursing was dissolved, but the spirit and intention of the center remained. Student and faculty exchanges, clinical experiences, and collaborative research continued beyond Nicaragua.

Once the DNP program at Duquesne University started in 2008, it seemed appropriate in the historical spirit of the efforts of the university and school of nursing to consider a global studies opportunity for students in the new program. Two faculty in the school conceived the idea of offering students the opportunity to engage in global studies in Guanajuato, Mexico, in the context of the required course Transcultural and Global Health Perspectives. One of the faculty did a sabbatical in Guanajuato from January to August 2008 focusing on research and grant writing. During his time in this city, they were able to make many connections with healthcare institutions and professionals, as well as locals who knew the city and its people.

Two faculty from the school of nursing wrote, planned, and secured approval for a global studies experience for the DNP students in the summer of 2009. It is important to note that Duquesne University offers a creative incentive for its students to engage in global studies. If a global-studies proposal is written and approved for the summer semester as a short-term experience, the planners are able to use a portion of the course tuition to fund aspects of the global experience. This is usually sufficient to cover housing, airfare, some excursions, and some meals. There are additional costs for students, but the major items mentioned are covered. Every aspect of the global studies experience was planned, including housing and flights. Unfortunately, the novel influenza A (H1N1) emerged in the United States and Mexico, and the university canceled the planned global studies experience. Not to be deterred, the pair of faculty acted quickly and were able to connect with colleagues and peers in Toronto and Montreal and created a global studies experience in Canada. It was imperative that the students be immersed in a non-English-speaking environment, at least for part of the experience. Montreal served this purpose and offered students the insight into the potential experiences of their future patients who may not speak English. The global experience was a success, and it provided encouragement to plan for the next year.

In the summer of 2010, the same two faculty wrote, planned, and received approval for a global studies experience to Guanajuato, Mexico. Every aspect of the experience was again set, including housing, excursions, and flights. Unfortunately, due to violence in some cities along the U.S./Mexican border, the university canceled the global studies experience to Mexico. Remaining undeterred and based on the previous year, the pair contacted their colleagues from Canada and were able to switch the experience back to Toronto and Montreal. Again, the experience was a success. However, it was becoming more apparent that another attempt to plan a global studies experience in Mexico might not be successful.

In planning for the summer of 2011, two faculty began to explore other global studies options. In the early 2000s Duquesne University opened the Duquesne University Rome campus. The pair began to explore this opportunity. At this time, undergraduate students typically engaged in semester-long studies at the Rome campus, including in a variety of majors. However, nursing students were not able to attend the semester-long opportunities due to the intensity of the nursing curriculum in the United States. At this time, there were no graduate nursing or other graduate students participating in global studies at the Rome campus during the summer semester. With the assistance of the staff at the Rome campus, two faculty were able to successfully write, plan, and implement a global studies experience with 30 DNP students in the summer of 2011 for 2 weeks at the Rome campus. The School of Nursing has successfully engaged in meaningful annual global studies experiences at the Rome campus for the DNP students from 2011 to the present.

THE DUQUESNE DNP-IN-ITALY GLOBAL IMMERSION OPPORTUNITY: A FACULTY PERSPECTIVE

During the summer term, DNP students and PhD students have an opportunity to participate in a 10- to 12-day global immersion experience as part of the course Transcultural and Global Health Perspectives. The immersion time frame was shortened from the original 2-week experiences to make it more manageable for the students, most of whom worked full-time. This is a required course in the DNP curriculum, and PhD students may choose to take it as a cognate to support their dissertation work. Although Duquesne's School of Nursing has a long history of participation in study-abroad programs with undergraduate students, graduate student involvement in global initiatives was not a focus until the DNP program began in 2008. To assist DNP students' thinking about health and illness from a perspective other than that of the U.S. healthcare system, the program has included a global immersion experience in Canada (as mentioned earlier), Italy, and Singapore (to be discussed later in this chapter); most trips have been to Italy. The global immersion experience is not a required part of the course, but it is strongly encouraged, and most students choose to participate. Because Duquesne University permits faculty to use summer tuition money to fund study-abroad experiences as described above, students pay full tuition for the three-credit course, and their tuition dollars cover most of the expenses associated with air travel, lodging, meals, cultural immersion experiences, and guest speakers/lecturers. This course and global immersion help increase doctoral students' capacity to design culturallysensitive healthcare systems that facilitate positive health outcomes within the cultural context.

The global immersion experience began in summer 2009, and the Italy experience has been taking place annually since 2011, except during the COVID-19 pandemic in 2020 and 2021. Duquesne University has an Italian campus in Rome located just outside the city that serves as the hub for the experience. The location of the campus requires that students take a bus and the metro to get to the city-center of Rome. Riding public transportation is an intentional component of the experience because students must travel throughout the city as Roman citizens often do and prepare for common occurrences, such as pickpocketing. Two faculty members work closely with the assistant director of the Italian campus to plan the activities for 10 to 12 days, which have also included trips to Florence, Pompeii, Naples, Capri, and Palermo. Because all graduate courses at the School of Nursing are online, students can complete some requirements of the 12-week summer course before and after the global immersion period. This allows Italy to become the classroom, where students engage in fieldwork to document their observations about the influence of culture on health and the healthcare system. Activities and excursions are designed to immerse students in the Italian culture and expose them to the social, religious, political, and economic influences on individual health and global health systems. So that students may focus on the global immersion experience with their peers and faculty, family members are only permitted to join students after the designated time frame for the immersion.

Students engage in a variety of experiences that highlight the importance of historical and contemporary culture as well as religion and family on individuals and the Italian healthcare system. Students learn about the special value placed on food and the camaraderie of enjoying a meal during extended Italian dinners, a cooking class, and a traditional Sunday Sicilian lunch at an Agriturismo, or farm-to-table restaurant. The importance of high quality, fresh foods purchased daily and shared with family and friends is soon recognized by the students. Other cultural activities include attending the Papal Audience at St. Peter's Square, where students hear biblical readings and receive a blessing from the pope in several languages, including Arabic, English, French,

German, Portuguese, and Spanish, for example. Some visiting groups are announced as attendees of the Papal Audience, and Duquesne's student group is announced as "pilgrims from Duquesne University in Pennsylvania." Students tour the Vatican Museums and Sistine Chapel with a professor of art history and Vatican art historian to learn about the influence of Rome's emperors and the Catholic Church from ancient Rome to modern day, including how a new pope is elected within the Sistine Chapel. These are some of the many experiences that emphasize the impact of religion on the Italian culture. Special visits in Florence include the Santa Maria Novella pharmacy, the oldest pharmacy in the world, where medicines and herbal products have been made since 1221, and the Museo degli Innocenti. This museum was created to exhibit the works of art of the ancient hospital, the Istituto degli Innocenti, a large institution that housed and cared for children without families for six centuries. Visits to these cultural places are led by art historians with specialized knowledge to highlight the rich, extensive history of Italy and the influence on its citizens.

One objective of the course is for students to compare systems of health through immersion in a cultural context with a nontraditional or non-Western health system. Thus, several immersion activities focus on health and healthcare settings within the Italian culture. Examples of such activities include tours of private hospitals, such as Salvator Mundi International Hospital in Rome and UPMC ISMETT, a United States–run hospital in Palermo, Sicily, that began as an organ transplant hospital in 1997. Students also tour public hospitals such as the Policlinico Tor Vergata, a public teaching hospital of the University of Rome, and Ospedale San Giovanni Calibita Fatebenefratelli, founded on the Tiber Island in 1585 and known for sheltering Jews during the holocaust by diagnosing them with a fabricated, contagious disease. During these experiences, students learn about the public healthcare system of Italy, how it is funded through regional taxation in the country, and how it can be supplemented with private insurance. Students meet with directors of nursing, physicians, nurses, nurse researchers, and other hospital personnel to learn about the inner workings and procedures of these healthcare institutions. As students conduct their observational fieldwork, they often ask questions about the standard Italian practices in their individual areas of interest to compare them to the United States, such as neonatal care, infectious disease prevention, mental health care, and disability accommodations, to name a few. Students are sometimes surprised to hear the Italian healthcare practices are the same or similar to the United States. Other highlights of the immersion experience include a conference day with invited speakers. Topics have included the life of a registered nurse in Italy, nursing research and scholarship in Italy, and intercultural sensitivity in healthcare, presented by a practicing nurse, the director of the Center of Excellence for Nursing Culture and Research, and a professor from the University of Milano Bicocca, respectively.

Another focus of the course is on approaches for influencing public health policy for vulnerable and immigrant populations. Therefore, global immersion planning has included experiences with facilities and organizations whose missions are to assist marginalized individuals in Rome, such as older adults who are sick and shut-in, individuals experiencing homelessness, and refugees and asylum seekers. Specifically, students attend a prayer service held by the Community of Sant'Egidio in the Trastevere neighborhood of Rome. This prayer service is often dedicated to praying for resolution of global issues, such as peace in countries affected by war, for example, Ukraine. After the prayer service, students meet with a leader of the community for a discussion about this lay community's outreach and programs for disadvantaged people living in Rome. One of these initiatives includes a partnership with Trattoria de Gli Amici (Trattoria of Friends). This restaurant offers classes for individuals with disabilities on how to work in a restaurant and employs individuals with mental and physical disabilities, accompanied by medical professionals and adult volunteers. During a visit to the Joel Nafuma Refugee Center, students meet with refugees at this day center to hear about their daily life in Rome and experiences as refugees. The center operates from the basement of St. Paul's Within the Walls Episcopal Church and offers as many as 250 people a day a safe space for rest and recuperation. Students learn about the various services offered at the center, such as basic supplies for those in immediate need and employment clinics for individuals wishing to make plans for long-term settlement.

Learning outcomes of this global immersion experience have been profound from both an academic and personal perspective. Over 150 doctoral students have participated in the Italian global immersion component of the course, and, although these students are all adults with years of professional and life experience, many have discussed the experience as transformational. Students have described the experience as having a life-changing impact on their personal life, education at Duquesne, and implementation of their doctoral projects. They have described how learning about vulnerable populations during the immersive experience was humbling and will change how they work in clinical practice. Many have described a newfound appreciation for the impact of culture on the physical, psychological, and social components of health. The final writing assignment of the course requires that students generate and discuss a case study for providing care to a patient from the health system in which they were immersed, but students are also offered the choice to be creative and write the paper as a publishable manuscript. Three student groups have published papers about their immersion experience in peer-reviewed journals as it relates to implications for nursing education (Easterby et al., 2012), fieldwork as a way of knowing (Gregg et al., 2013), and nursing faculty's cultural competence (Montenery et al., 2013). The global immersion experience in Italy helps doctoral students apply their unique cultural experiences to patients and families from diverse cultures when designing and implementing care within the United States healthcare system.

CASE STUDY III   Doctoral Students' Perspectives on the Duquesne Global Immersion Experience in Italy

Students found the global study in Italy quite beneficial, as described in the words of participants:

DNP students at Duquesne University were offered an opportunity to travel and study abroad in Italy during the summer semester of 2022. Leaving work and family behind amid an ongoing pandemic would bring doubts and fear. When we arrived at our rooms at Duquesne University Italian Campus, my weary mind wondered how I could sleep in such a bare and simple dorm room for 10 days with a classmate I had only met through Zoom meetings. These would be the last of my negative thoughts as we stepped back in time to ancient grounds, art, religion, and history. Our professors and guides were experts and historians, enabling us to experience and explore Italian culture. A pivotal moment came in Florence as we visited the Istituto Degli Innocenti and learned that the most vulnerable children who lost their mothers during childbirth were taken in and cared for six centuries ago. There were breathtaking paintings of Mary, mother of Jesus, with children nestled under her cloak. The commitment to children's rights continues there today. Through national health insurance, all people have access to care. The Italian people welcomed us with hospitality, making me yearn for the human connection we are

(continued)

losing in the United States. Our DNP cohort grew close to one another in a short time. We enjoyed whole foods and paused for hours at mealtime to connect and discuss our experiences. I am deeply grateful as this experience served as a life pivot. I returned with an awareness of our interconnectedness as humans and a desire to seek our similarities rather than differences. Through this experience, I also believe we are responsible for understanding one another's culture and expanding our time and talents globally. Looking back, I would not change a thing.

Donna Durant, CRNP, FNP, MSN, Nurse Practitioner, UPP/UPMC General Medicine, Division of Palliative and Supportive Care, DNP Student, Duquesne University School of Nursing

A global journey over 4,500 miles to Rome, Italy, was a life-changing experience, both professionally and personally. The opportunity to talk with the nurses and staff was exceptional at the Universita Tor Vegata, Policlinico, a hospital in Rome. We had the pleasure of attending a fascinating medical conference highlighting the hospital's recent research on the well-being of nurses and the contributions from advanced nursing professionals. The master's- and doctoral-prepared nurses specialized in specific areas of research to advance patient care outcomes. While touring the hospital the environment was filled with fresh air flowing through the wide and tall hallways. During my time in Florence and Rome, I realized that there was so much that heightened my senses. While trying to take it all in, the experience was more meaningful when I stopped to admire and appreciate being in the presence of the simple things. For example, our visit to the Santa Maria Novella Pharmacy, the oldest pharmacy in Italy, displayed historical backgrounds of healing, offered natural products for supporting good health, and was beautified by simply hanging sweet and inviting scented dried flowers at its entrance. Another meaningful experience was the appreciation of statuary of intricate details of the human body. The sculpture of Laocoön and the Sons with the serpent represented their intricate musculature used during the attempt to escape the serpent among them. In Rome, the statuary was magnificent and historically profound. The experience was overwhelming and finding peace in the presence of the La Pieta was so emotional as the Blessed Virgin Mary looks at her lifeless son's body. Details of Jesus's body were remarkable, especially his dropped left foot and right arm from his malnourished body. These details never entered my mind when I began planning the travel to the Rome campus of Duquesne University, and I am so humbled by the entire experience.

Diann S. Schmitt MSN, FNP, BC, RN, Graduate Nursing Instructor, Franciscan University of Steubenville, DNP Student, Duquesne University School of Nursing

As a Duquesne University DNP student, I was privileged to spend 10 days in Rome and Florence, Italy- as part of a Transcultural Care and Global Health Perspectives course. It was clear to me that this cross-cultural field immersion was intentionally planned by Duquesne faculty and staff to target not only knowledge, but also individual skills and attitudes. Each day was saturated with unique learning that filled mind, body, and soul with experiences that sparked curiosity and enthusiasm for more. This began in Florence, where we were met at the train station by a charismatic art historian who spent 3 days teaching us art, history, culture, and their impact

(continued)

on population health and healthcare. The remainder of our trip was spent at the Duquesne campus in Rome. The campus is a busy and energetic place filled with undergraduate and graduate students, faculty, and staff, as well as a convent with nuns. Throughout these 10 days, we toured special places and shared unique experiences where all of my senses were assaulted with learning. A partial list included tours of Italy's private and public hospital systems, museums, religious charities, historical sites, lectures, presentations by Italy's nursing leaders, a traditional Italian dinner in Tuscany, a cooking class, and papal audience. This list of formal experiences only represents the intentional aspect of this cultural immersion. Throughout my 10 days, Italian culture, as well as simply being in an unfamiliar environment with a diverse group of people, were equally important to my transformation. Traveling, sleeping, and eating meals while conversing with new people, while experiencing new foods and cultural practices, meant I was inhaling and exhaling cultural learning with each breath. These experiences helped me to grow personally and professionally and were central to my understanding of how culture affects the priorities and practices that govern health. I was challenged each day to examine my own cultural practices, assumptions, and biases and to understand global healthcare system approaches more fully. Living within another culture helped me to move from a position of ethnocentrism to ethnorelativism in a way that reading a textbook never could. At the beginning of the trip, I felt frustrated by the slower pace of meals when I wanted to go see a new site. As this scenario was repeated throughout our stay, I began to appreciate these moments as they allowed me to not simply see new things, but experience them, through deeper conversations with Italians and my colleagues, and to savor the sights, sounds, and smells of Italy. I developed cultural humility and learned that maybe "When in Rome ..." is not just a trite expression. I felt this course, and specifically this immersion, helped my evolution from viewing nursing and healthcare at the individual to the global level. This course instilled confidence in my knowledge and skills as a nursing leader to advocate for improvements to public healthcare policies. My time in Italy was life altering and the beginning of a deeper cultural self-reflection and exploration.

Tammy Schwaab BA, DNP, RN, CHSE, Professor of Nursing and Simulation Specialist, Carroll Community College, Westminster, Maryland

THE DUQUESNE DNP-IN-SINGAPORE OPPORTUNITY: A FACULTY PERSPECTIVE

The global immersion experience at Duquesne has extended beyond Rome to other countries that host the International Council of Nurses (ICN) Congress. Within the context of two online courses, Transcultural Care and Global Health Perspectives and Foundations of Transformation: Translating Evidence into Practice, graduate students were provided an opportunity to study abroad in both Rome and Singapore. Eight DNP and four PhD students chose to travel to Singapore in 2019 for 10 days. During the program, students participated in the ICN Congress; visited communities and public/private hospitals within the country; and explored places that exhibit its cultural diversity, such as temples and mosques, and ethnic food restaurants.

The theme of the ICN Congress was "Beyond Healthcare to Health," hosted by the Singapore Nurses Association. This international gathering of roughly 10,000 nurses from around the globe explored the many ways in which nurses work to achieve universal access to health. The focus was on addressing the social determinants of health, such as safety, education, gender equality, poverty, etc. The congress provided opportunities for nurses to build relationships and to disseminate nursing and health-related knowledge.

The Duquesne students were involved in fieldwork/immersion experiences in order to understand Singapore's heathcare system, which differs from their own. The fieldwork findings were then synthesized with the literature to compare their own health system and its impact on individuals and communities with the observed health system. In addition, students learned through formal presentations at the ICN Congress from experts in intercultural care, bioethics in healthcare, and other global issues in healthcare, such as staffing ratio issues, retention, and job burnout. During their stay, students got an opportunity to meet with nurses from around the world to discuss their personal experiences and further understand how culture can influence healthcare; the international nurses' experiences include the lack of professional development, an absence of involvement from nurses in quality improvement projects, shortages of nursing leaders in higher roles, and physician-dominated hospital structures. Many international nurses were unaware of the shared governance model, which addresses inadequate collaboration in quality care.

The DNP courses for the global immersion were culturally focused, with the first course aptly named Transcultural Care and Global Health Perspectives. This course explored the impact of globalization on healthcare delivery and the need to design healthcare systems that are responsive to diverse cultural needs. The global health problems were assessed in a multidisciplinary manner to assure attention to the underserved and their complex cultural needs. The objective of this course was to increase the capability of nurses in advanced practice to develop culturally sensitive healthcare ethics in their respective practices. The course was taught online, and the fieldwork/immersion portion occurred in Singapore. For the online portion, students were engaged in readings and other learning activities in preparation for their fieldwork and cultural immersion experiences. The students then connected with professionals, healthcare systems, and both public and private institutions in Singapore during their visit.

The PhD students worked on their independent study (cognate) while they were in Singapore, and the DNP students took another course paired with the global immersion, Foundations of Transformation: Translating Evidence into Practice. This course built on the foundational principles of evidence-based practice to enhance the comprehension and practice of quality care, analyzing existing healthcare programs and policy through translational research at an advanced level. The DNP students learned to contribute to the expansion of knowledge underlying advanced professional nursing through the translation of research into practice.

CASE STUDY IV Doctoral Students' Perspectives on the Duquesne Global Immersion Experience in Singapore

Students found the global immersion in Singapore beneficial, as described in the words of participants:

While in Singapore, we were privileged to have the opportunity to tour Raffles Hospital, the top private hospital in Singapore. This multidisciplinary health system offers a wide range of care, from the typical specialties such as orthopedics and rehabilitation to other more specific specialties such as entire departments just for Chinese medicine and Japanese medicine. The students would have benefited more

---

(continued)

with more time to tour the hospital or the opportunity to tour other hospitals, including a public hospital system.

The experience in Singapore was an eye-opening, phenomenal experience. It has allowed most of us to meditate on what nursing means to us, what our purpose is in nursing, how we can influence nursing, and what we can do to make a change in this profession. We were fortunate to be the first cohort to complete our study-abroad experience in Singapore, as well as attend the biannual International Council of Nurses (ICN) Congress. Our interactions and conversations with international nurses were eye-opening and gave us much "food for thought." Each of us brought something different back from the Congress that was meaningful personally.

We all thoroughly enjoyed the interaction with the nurses from various countries as well as the plenary sessions during the Congress. We found the plenary sessions to be the most valuable. While the breakout sessions were interesting, the downside to that was that they were provided in 10-minute increments and did not allow time for great detail to be provided regarding the topic nor for discussion following the presentations. One highlight for all of us, however, was attending the Tri-Council meeting where many of us were able to network with other nurse leaders from all over the country.

Jewel L. Tartt, DNP, FNP-C, MSN SANE, Primary Care Provider, Southeast family Health Care Center, MCR

The culture in Singapore is highly influenced by Malay, South Asian, and East Asian cultures, as apparent by the residents living and working here, and the food served in most of the eating venues, although there seemed to be a moderate number of eastern Europeans out and about in Singapore. Although Singlish is the colloquial dialect spoken by Singaporeans, English seemed the most common language spoken in Singapore, next to Malaysian, Mandarin, and different dialects of South Asian Indian during my encounters with Singaporean residents. The tourist industry seems to be huge in this country. In most parts of the country I visited, there were many banks, shopping centers, boutiques, and tourist shops. Additionally, restaurants and eating venues are also prevalent throughout. During our time here, most of what I witnessed were the upper-class sectors of Singapore. I would have liked to have had more time spent in the more suburban areas and meeting and speaking with the local residents to understand their culture better. From a cultural immersion perspective, it is challenging to achieve given that our time was prioritized with the ICN Congress. Nevertheless, this was still a great learning opportunity.

Last but by no means least, I truly enjoyed getting to know my DNP classmates and the PhD students who attended this study-abroad experience. I would also like to commend Dr. Evatt for doing a wonderful job in facilitating and coordinating a great study-abroad experience.

Lester Lledo, DNP, RN, CRNP, Director of Clinical Research Operations, Penn Medicine-Center for Cellular Immunotherapies Clinical Trials Unit; Graduate of Duquesne University School of Nursing DNP Program

We are writing to express our profound gratitude for your support of study-abroad experiences for doctoral students. We recently traveled to Singapore and the ICN conference with Dr. Manjulata Evatt and a group of DNP students.

> Singapore was beautiful and its people were welcoming! Although we wish we would have had more time to deepen our cultural knowledge of the people of Singapore, the opportunity to travel to a part of the world we had never visited and attend the ICN conference was invaluable. It was inspiring to see thousands of nurses who arrived from around the world to learn about the impact of the nursing profession at the global health level. We had the great opportunity to interact with nurses from different countries and hear about their professional roles and/or research focus. We were able to have contact with nursing leaders such as Dr. Ernest Grant, Dr. Beverly Malone, Dr. Pam Cipriano, and Dr. Marion Broome. We learned about tools, programs, and studies that related to our research focus. The conference served to underline the role of nurses as leaders and change agents who can use their voice to influence global healthcare, policy, and professional practice.
>
> We felt honored and blessed to be able to travel to Singapore and participate in an experience that will shape our personal and professional lives. We extend our sincere appreciation to you, Dr. Evatt, Dr. Turk, Dr. Zoucha, the School of Nursing, and Duquesne University for your commitment to and investment in study-abroad learning for PhD students.
>
> Griselle B. Estrada, MSN, RN Clinical Assistant Professor Baylor University
Louise Herrington School of Nursing PhD candidate,
Duquesne University School of Nursing
>
> Jennifer Stephen PhD, RN, CPN Clinical Practice &
Advanced Education Specialist
Cook Children's Health Care System
>
> Kimberli I. Roberts PhD (c), RN, PMC-NE, CNL, Interim Program Director,
ASN program and Across Curriculum Courses Coordinator, Chattahoochee Technical College, PhD Student, Duquesne School of Nursing.
>
> Francesca C. Ezeokonkwo, PhD, RN, Assistant Professor,
James Madison University School of Nursing

Although challenging for the single faculty member in charge of the 12 students in a new country, it was a rewarding experience for the instructor. They noted, "Graduate students were able to demonstrate their leadership skills in engaging undergraduate nursing students during the excursions in Singapore, community partners and healthcare stakeholders of the private and public hospitals." The expectations for moving forward with global immersion were there, but COVID-19 hit and suspended the program until 2022.

SUMMARY AND WHAT DUQUESNE LEARNED FROM BOTH EXPERIENCES

According to Morrison and colleagues (2019), graduate professional students accounted for 11% of the total number of students studying abroad in 2013. This figure has been severely impacted by the COVID-19 pandemic. However, as the world is moving on with COVID-19, the students' enthusiasm about the global immersion experience has increased. A recent orientation program in August 2022 conducted for the DNP students at Duquesne validated the enthusiasm for a global immersion experience. As a global partner, Duquesne University has been perceived as a culturally sensitive and globally focused institution. The faculty has been innovative and creative in developing the global immersion courses for over a decade, including our newest offering in Singapore. Providing the global immersion experience to graduate students is an opportunity for them to experience different cultural norms and perspectives from various parts of the world and to broaden their understanding of the influence of culture on health and health systems. As DNP professionals, they must be prepared to be global citizens not only internationally but also in the United States. Recognizing the need to accommodate cultural differences in healthcare values, beliefs, and customs is essential for designing and implementing culturally congruent systems of health in their country as well.

Wolf and colleagues (2020) noted that students are highly motivated to experience cultures different from their own and explore healthcare settings in developing countries. It is critically important that schools of nursing provide opportunities for students to have that experience, especially at the doctoral level. The DNP Essential VII specifically states the need for cultural diversity and sensitivity that guide the practice of DNP graduates. As evidenced by the student perspectives provided, students who have engaged in a global studies experience are better able to integrate essential concepts related to cultural diversity into their thinking about methods of improving health for individuals and culturally diverse populations. Thus, Duquesne's DNP curriculum with these global studies experiences uniquely facilitates our graduates' attainment of DNP Essential VII: Clinical Prevention and Population Health for Improving the Nation's Health (American Association of Colleges of Nursing [AACN], 2006).

Global immersion helps doctoral students to develop the ability to understand how institutions, markets, or healthcare delivery systems shape symptom presentations and to mobilize for the correction of health and wealth inequalities in society. This ability further helps these future leaders to be responsive to the attitudes, feelings, and circumstances of various people around the globe that share a common and distinctive racial, national, international, religious, linguistic, and cultural heritage (AACN, 2021).

CONCLUSION AND FUTURE DIRECTIONS

Descriptions of DNP global study programs are lacking in the literature. This chapter highlights the perspectives of both faculty and DNP students who have participated in programs in London and Dublin at Drexel University and Rome and Singapore at Duquesne University. We hope that the practical information provided on the approval and funding process necessary to implement these types of programs, as well as the detailed information on the didactic and experiential aspects of these programs, will stimulate other DNP programs to consider enhancing the role preparation of their DNP graduates with global studies experiences.

It is widely recognized that the number of PhD nursing students has declined while enrollments of DNP students has risen. These DNP students will benefit from enhanced skills to help them develop as practice scholars and research team members, especially as tenured faculty retire. In a creative approach to addressing this need, at the University of Northern Colorado, a hybrid elective course, Global Health and Disaster Preparedness in the West Indies was held in the summer of 2018 (Snyder et al., 2021). Five DNP and PhD students conducted a mixed-methods needs assessment on the islands of St. Kitts and Nevis in the Caribbean, providing the opportunity for a hands-on approach for a mentored international research experience. The in-person experience also complemented the curriculum in two almost-exclusively online programs, allowing students and faculty to build relationships and collaborate in analyzing and disseminating their findings. Doctoral students at Drexel and Duquesne have repeatedly expressed the same appreciation for connecting, collaborating, and bonding with fellow classmates during their global studies experience.

In addition to DNP students studying abroad with PhD students, study abroad with DNP and undergraduate nursing students has been underutilized. In a novel approach to DNP curriculum development, an international school experience in Ireland was offered to DNP students as an elective study-abroad credit. Seven DNP students travelled with 11 undergraduate students from three universities in the United States to complete an intensive 2-week program of classes, clinical visits, Irish lifestyle workshops, historical and contemporary science gallery visits, and cultural immersion (Elliott et al., 2016). A key pedagogical strategy involved the use of an Oxford-style team debate as a means of stimulating critical inquiry into different healthcare structures and contemporary global health issues. Content analysis revealed that team debate fostered critical thinking and critical appraisal skills; encouraged teamwork; providing opportunities for mentoring, relationship building, and socialization into the profession; and, from the DNP student perspective, increased knowledge and global understanding of healthcare. Other DNP programs could readily adapt this type of approach.

Online learning also opens possibilities for "virtual" global studies experiences that do not include travel, but rather virtual interactions, or a combination of both. This was particularly useful in the context of COVID-19 as a second-degree nursing program developed an educational experience pairing students in the United States (17 in person; 64 through web conference) and Norwegian students (50 in person; 3 for web conference) in population health experiences (King et al., 2021). Integration of nontraveling DNP students in joint virtual global experiences related to practice, research, leadership, or policy warrants exploration. Online and in-person coursework can also help students adopt a global perspective in preparation for, or independent of, study abroad.

Innovation, extensive planning, and creativity are required to create meaningful learning opportunities for doctoral-level nurses in an increasingly complex and changing global healthcare environment. Extending global studies to nursing students at all levels and incorporating online learning will open new possibilities for optimizing the global study experience for DNP students.

ACKNOWLEDGMENTS

This chapter is dedicated to the faculty, students, and international partners that have contributed to global study experiences at Drexel University and Duquesne University.

CRITICAL THINKING QUESTIONS

1. How important is it for you to be educated with a "global nursing scholar framework?"
2. Describe an international nursing/health-related issue that you think you would have a better comprehension of if only you had more lived experience/experiential exposure to it.
3. Have you had international travel experiences? How has international travel helped your global IQ?
4. Undergraduate study-abroad models have proliferated. Should graduate study abroad be as prevalent? Why or why not?
5. Research indicates there is a shortage of global study opportunities in nursing. Why might this be, and what could be done about it?

6. If you had to design a global clinical practicum in your DNP degree, what would it entail?
7. Americans, even highly educated individuals, are notoriously monolingual. Do you speak a second language? What value would being proficient in a second language be to global health in the context of your career trajectory?
8. Describe how a lack of study-abroad opportunities for nurses, particularly doctoral-level nursing students, affects the health of the average global citizen. Or does it?
9. What did you learn from the case study narratives of the DNP students who described their study-abroad program in London, Dublin, Rome, and Singapore?
10. How would you go about helping to implement a novel global study offering in your own DNP program?

NOTES

1. The Drexel DrNP was a hybrid professional doctorate combining advanced nursing practice with the conduct of clinical research, and all students completed a clinical dissertation. The DrNP changed to a DNP with minor curriculum changes in 2015 (Dreher et al., 2005).
2. For the first class, the students were simply required to make eight quarterly payments that began the subsequent quarter after the program was approved. Starting with the second class in 2006, students began making quarterly payments immediately on matriculation.
3. The students were given a lunch break of 1.5 hours between classes to reflect the U.K./European culture, which takes a more leisurely attitude toward gastronomy. Predictably, the first class asked to decrease the mealtime to get out of the class early and the faculty politely refused. In the end, the longer lunch mealtimes were evaluated favorably.
4. Much to our dismay, the active volcanoes in Iceland in April 2010 delayed the global study program by a week, and so the decision was made to Skype in most of all the planned speakers as the students completed week 1 on campus. Students did attend week 2 in London and many stayed abroad longer after the formal program ended.

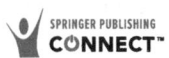

A robust set of instructor resources designed to supplement this text is located at http://connect.springerpub.com/content/book/978-0-8261-8137-4. Qualifying instructors may request access by emailing textbook@springerpub.com.

REFERENCES

American Association of Colleges of Nursing. (2006). *The essentials of doctoral education for advanced nursing practice*. https://www.aacnnursing.org/Portals/42/Publications/DNPEssentials.pdf

American Association of Colleges of Nursing. (2021). *The essentials: Core competencies for professional nursing education*. https://www.aacnnursing.org/Portals/42/AcademicNursing/pdf/Essentials-2021.pdf

Chow, P., & Villarreal, A. (2011). *Open doors: Report on international educational exchange*. Institute of International Education. https://www.iie.org/en/Research-and-Publications/Publications-and-Reports/IIEBookstore/Open-Doors-2011

Dreher, H. M., Donnelly, G., & Naremore, R. (2005). Reflections on the DNP and an alternate practice doctorate model: The Drexel DrNP. *The Online Journal of Issues in Nursing, 11*, 1. https://

www.nursingworld.org/MainMenuCategories/ANAMarketplace/ANAPeriodicals/OJIN/TableofContents/Volume112006/No1Jan06/ArticlePreviousTopic/tpc28_716031.aspx

Dreher, H. M., Lachman, V. D., Smith Glasgow, M. E., & Ward, L. S. (2008). *Educating the global clinical scholar: The first doctoral nursing program to institute a mandatory study abroad program*. AACN Doctoral Education Conference, Captiva Island.

Easterby, L. M., Siebert, B., Woodfield, C. J., Holloway, K., Gilbert, P., Zoucha, R., & Turk, M. W. (2012). A transcultural immersion experience: Implications for nursing education. *The ABNF Journal, 23*(4), 81–84.

Elliott, N., Farnum, K., & Beauchesne, M. (2016). Utilizing team debate to increase student abilities for mentoring and critical appraisal of global health care in doctor of nursing practice programs. *Journal of Professional Nursing: Official Journal of the American Association of Colleges of Nursing, 32*(3), 224–234. https://doi.org/10.1016/j.profnurs.2015.10.009

Forum on Education Abroad. (2020). *Leading short-term study abroad programs: Know the standards*, (6th ed.), Retrieved from Standards-of-Good-Practice-for-Education-Abroad-6th-Edition-2020.pdf (forumea.org)

Fry, G. W. (1984). The economic and political impact of study abroad. *Comparative Education Review, 28*(2), 203–220.

Gilchrist, K. (2022, February 18). *Bill Gates says Covid risks have 'dramatically reduced' but another pandemic is coming*. cnbc.com. Retrieved from Bill Gates: Covid risks have reduced but another pandemic will come (cnbc.com)

Gregg, K., Irwin, R., Houck, N., Kramer, N., Zoucha, R., Kattan, M., Stayer, D., Turk, M., & Wills, J. (2013). Fieldwork as a way of knowing: An Italian immersion experience. *Online Journal of Cultural Competence in Nursing and Healthcare, 3*(2), 16–27. https://doi.org/10.9730/ojccnh.org/v3n2a2

Institute of International Education. (2015). *Special reports: Economic impact of international students*. https://www.iie.org/Research-and-Publications/Open-Doors/Data/Economic-Impact-of-International-Students#.V_Ksbb83K9Y

Johns, C. (2006). *Engaging reflection in practice: A narrative approach*. Wiley-Blackwell.

King, T. S., Bochenek, J., Jenssen, U., Bowles, W., & Morrison-Beedy, D. (2021). Virtual study-abroad through Web conferencing: Sharing knowledge and building cultural appreciation in nursing education and practice. *Journal of Transcultural Nursing; Official journal of the Transcultural Nursing Society, 32*(6), 790–798. https://doi.org/10.1177/10436596211009583

Kremer, R. (2021). *Study abroad is coming back, But with more hurdles*. npr.org, Retrieved from Study abroad is coming back. But with more hurdles : NPR

Maslow, J. (2020). 5 reasons why you should study abroad if you have the privilege to do so. *New Rationalist Magazine*. https://newrationalist.com

Montenery, S. M., Jones, A. D., Perry, N., Ross, D., & Zoucha, R. (2013). Cultural competence in nursing faculty: A journey, not a destination. *Journal of Professional Nursing, 29*(6), e51–e57. https://doi.org/10.1016/j.profnurs.2013.09.003

Moody, J. (2020, March 27). Study abroad programs and COVID-19: What to know. *US News and World Report*. https://www.usnews.com/education/best-colleges/articles/how-coronavirus-is-changing-course-of-study-abroad-programs

Morrison, K. A. (2019). Designing a study abroad program to include humanities graduate students: Institutional constraints and possibilities In K. A. Morrison (Ed.), *Study abroad pedagogy, dark tourism, and historical reenactment* (pp. 21–38). Springer International Publishing.

Nestor, G. (2022, January 14). *19 Higher Education Trends for 2022/2023: Latest Forecasts To Watch Out For Finances Online*. Retrieved from 19 Higher Education Trends for 2022/2023: Latest Forecasts To Watch Out For - Finance-sonline.com

Nietzel, T. (2019). More U.S. students need to study abroad: Here's how congress can act. *Forbes.com* retrieved from More American Students Need To Study Abroad: Here's How Congress Can Help (forbes.com)

opendoors. (2018). *Open Doors 2018*. Institute of International Education. IIE Open Doors (opendoorsdata.org)

Redden, E. (2007). *So what did you learn in London?* http://insidehighered.com/news/2007

Redden, R. (2020). *CDC to colleges: 'Consider' canceling exchange programs*. insidehighered.com. https://www.insidehighered.com/news/2020/03/03/cdc-tells-colleges-consider-canceling-foreign-exchange-programs-because-coronavirus

Redden, E. (2021). *Restarting study abroad*. insidehighered.com Retrieved from Colleges grapple with resuming study abroad (insidehighered.com)

Snyder, A., Milbrath, G., Hood, T., Gaul, R., Hijmans, K., Leahy, N., & Matthew, S. (2021). The perspective of doctoral nursing students engaged in mentored international research. *Journal of Nursing Education and Practice*, *11*(1), 19–25.

Svluga, S. (2000, February 26). *Universities pulling students from Italy and South Korea as coronavirus outbreak spreads*, Washingtonpost.com, Retrieved from Universities pulling students from Italy and South Korea as coronavirus outbreak spreads - *The Washington Post*

U.S. Department of State. (n.d.). *USA study abroad*. https://studyabroad.state.gov/

Wolf, D., Wu, H., Spadaro, K., & Hunker, D. (2020). Chinese nurses' perceived impact of international educational experiences and cultural beliefs following a 1-year study abroad program: An exploratory study. *Frontiers of Nursing*, *7*(1), 23–29. https://doi.org/10.2478/fon-2020-0007

World Health Organization. (2022, December 9). *WHO Coronavirus (COVID-19) dashboard*. Retrieved from covid19.who.int

CHAPTER TWENTY Reflective Response

MICHELE BEDNARZYK

After more than 15 years of participating in study-abroad trips with both graduate and undergraduate students, I have gained many insights regarding the importance of these experiences for the students. I started taking graduate students before we had a DNP program, mostly with MSN nursing students. Now that there is a requirement for the DNP programs to have global health within the curriculum, it has changed the landscape and what is available for the students. The new DNP Essentials have put increased emphasis on the importance of global health for the DNP student. The Essentials state, "The DNP graduate has the capacity to engage proactively in the development and implementation of health policy at all levels, including institutional, local, state, regional, federal, and international levels."

At our university, we have many international programs available. The nursing school generally works between two sites: London and Austria. The doctoral students are able to substitute their three-credit-hour Global Health class for one of the three-credit-hour Special Topics Study Abroad courses. This ensures that the faculty will have the qualifications and specific objectives to meet the requirements of the study-abroad courses that are in the Global Health class. The College of Health also has a 12-hour Global Health Graduate Certificate program that is available to anyone in the college. All students must adhere to the requirements set by the program.

Once the faculty identifies which areas they are going to focus on and emphasize, the next step is to identify a college or university to work with. In our case, until this year due to COVID-19, we set up all of the logistics for the study-abroad courses in nursing. The universities that we have worked with are able to give us access to facilities that others may not be able to. In London, we are able to take the graduate nurse practitioner students to outpatient facilities that utilize these services and spend time working with the advanced practice nurses. The U.K. has restrictions regarding legal and malpractice issues that prevent the students from working independently, but they are able to observe patient care.

Despite these restrictions, London has been a natural choice for a healthcare study-abroad program because of its rich history as the birthplace of medicine and nursing. It is a great place for first-time travelers outside of the United States because of the language and the many landmarks to see. The graduate study abroad in nursing in London is a unique opportunity for DNP students to gain a new perspective on nursing, compare the U.S. and U.K. healthcare systems, and explore questions of universal healthcare, including issues of inequality in accessing it.

Austria, on the other hand, has allowed students to work within their healthcare facilities after negotiations with contracts and liability issues were met. Studying abroad in Austria has exposed students to a country with a vast political, artistic, and educational history.

Our nurse anesthesia students spend up to 3 weeks in study-abroad programs to work within their operating suites. One of the main opportunities offered by working with a university is to have presentations within each facility. Professors Michele Bednarzyk, Judy M. Comeaux, and John P. McDonough chaperoned 27 graduate and undergraduate students from Jacksonville, Florida, who attended the symposium. Prof. Nadja Nestler chaired the meeting at the Paracelsus Medical University (PMU) in Salzburg.

The symposium examined nursing and midwifery developments, as well as challenges across the World Health Organization's (WHO's) European Region and in local settings. Gabrielle Jacob, the WHO programme manager, and Dr. Rita F. D'Aoust from Jacksonville, gave their input virtually. Other guests, as well as all colleagues from the PMU, engaged the international audience with provoking talks on-site. In all lectures, attention was given to empowering nurses and advancing the nursing profession via novel educational strategies, such as introducing nursing practice development units (NDU), PhD, and DNP programs. This is a way that DNP students can participate in seminars and projects that will allow them to identify how they can improve healthcare from a global perspective. Our university has made a strong effort to promote global health experiences across all healthcare majors and across the university.

We believe this has enhanced the education of our DNP students and connected their education to concern for the health of our global community.

WHAT IS A NURSING PRACTICE DEVELOPMENT UNIT?

Mission Statement

We are a group of nurses and midwives who work together each with our own individual knowledge and experiences. We believe the staff, students and patients in SUH are all individual with potential for development. We work in partnership, promoting democratic inclusive decision-making processes and we accept and value all contributions. We commit ourselves to facilitate the growth of the student nurse and student midwife on their journey to become qualified, competent, reflective practitioners. We promote lifelong learning. When required we lead, support, facilitate, enable, participate or co-ordinate the development of nursing practice in partnership with our clinical colleagues. We incorporate evaluation into our practice to enable us to continually improve the quality of our service.

Nurse Practice Development Unit | Saolta University Health Care Group

CHAPTER TWENTY-ONE

The Role of DNP-Prepared Nurses as Organizational and Clinical Preceptors

YAMINI TEEGALA, ZYRENE MARSH, AMANDA AMBROSIO, LAURA O'ROURKE, AND VALERIE T. COTTER

■ EXEMPLAR: ZYRENE, A DNP STUDENT

Zyrene worked as a family nurse practitioner at Rocking Horse Community Health Center (RHCHC) while she pursued her doctor of nursing practice (DNP) degree. RHCHC is a Federally Qualified Health Center (FQHC) that operates multiple sites in two medically underserved areas in southwest Ohio, Clark County and Madison County. RHCHC delivers care for at-risk, vulnerable populations who face greater health disparities due to systemic obstacles to health that are historically linked to discrimination or exclusion such as race or ethnicity, religion, socioeconomic status, gender, age, mental health, cognitive, sensory, or physical disability, sexual orientation or gender identity, and/or geographic location. RHCHC presents a unique learning opportunity to aspiring healthcare providers and leaders who aim to simultaneously achieve the Triple Aims outlined by the Institute of Medicine: improve the quality of patient care and satisfaction, promote population health, and lower healthcare cost (Institute for Healthcare Improvement, 2022).

After a year of serving the marginalized community, Zyrene realized that clinical expertise alone is insufficient to meet the unique needs of her patient population. She then decided to advance her doctoral study with the support of Dr. Yamini Teegala, her mentor and collaborating physician. Dr. Teegala has served as the chief medical officer at RHCHC for over a decade and oversees students in various disciplines and various stages of their education. She believes that students learn to address health disparities by allowing them to collaborare with interdisciplinary teams and providing them with opportunities to foster relationships in the community. As a physician leader who understands the shortage of primary care physicians and the ever-growing need of it, she values the role of advanced practice nurses in a care team. Dr. Teegala invests her time on mentoring healthcare providers and leaders who can pass on the culture of mentorship for future generations, including Zyrene.

Zyrene is passionate about addressing the social determinants of health that negatively impact her patients' health outcomes, including poverty, food insecurity, and poor health literacy among others. Her organizational mentor or practice preceptor (Dr. Teegala) and her project mentor (Dr. Valerie Cotter, a DrNP-prepared nurse and faculty from the Johns Hopkins School of Nursing) were instrumental in materializing her vision to address the unique health disparities faced by her patients. Dr. Cotter advised and guided Zyrene in the development, implementation, and evaluation of her DNP project. Dr. Teegala provided adequate operational resources and raised stakeholders' support to implement evidence-based quality improvement projects. For Zyrene's DNP project, she developed a program leveraging telemedicine and mobilizing community health workers to improve access to care and health outcomes of community-dwelling older adults with diabetes. Zyrene collaborated with multisectoral and interdisciplinary professionals to successfully implement her DNP project. During the process, her organizational preceptor and project mentor adjusted their mentorship style while enabling Zyrene to discover her own leadership style. Zyrene's DNP project resulted in improved patient outcomes and her final output was disseminated through journal publications and national conference podium presentations.

The transformative leadership of her mentors inspired Zyrene to seek evidence-based solutions alleviating the challenges that they experience within their practice. The deliberate and meaningful preceptorship inspired Zyrene, a novice healthcare leader and practitioner, to make a difference in the healthcare delivery system while translating evidence into practice. As Zyrene continues her journey as a DNP-prepared healthcare practitioner and leader, her preceptors and mentors remain her role models. She hopes to foster the same mentorship to aspiring healthcare providers and leaders wherever her profession leads her. This chapter aims to provide DNP students and preceptors a guide to successful mentorship, including preceptor requirements, desired traits or qualities, role expectations, and clinical preceptorship.

ORGANIZATIONAL MENTORSHIP AND PRECEPTORSHIP

The American Association of Colleges of Nursing (AACN, 2021) promotes effective, collaborative, and interdisciplinary mentorship and preceptorship among DNP students to ensure their success in their program and to prepare students in their role as healthcare leaders. Mentorship and preceptorship in healthcare settings involve matching a student or a novice individual with a more experienced clinician or healthcare leader who will guide, teach, advise, encourage, and foster professional and personal growth while the mentee transitions into new roles and responsibilities (Higgins & Newby, 2020; Sherrod et al., 2020). Nursing preceptors facilitate a safe learning environment for patients and preceptees while honing the critical thinking and problem-solving skills of the novice practitioners (Sherrod et al., 2020).

DNP students may opt to have two types of mentors or preceptors during their DNP program and throughout their career. One of them is a DNP project mentor who guides the DNP student in designing, implementing, and evaluating the DNP project (Heitzler & Fullbright, 2021). The practice mentor or preceptor, on the other hand, possesses an extensive knowledge about practice problems, offers organizational context, and influences the decision-making and advancement of the DNP project within the organization (Heitzler & Fullbright, 2021). Both the project mentors and practice preceptors play a vital role in the progress of future DNP-prepared nurses.

PRECEPTOR EXPECTATIONS

As DNP programs across the United States continue to grow, the need for highly-qualified preceptors also rises. The AACN Essentials of Doctoral Education for Advanced Nursing Practice require DNP students to complete a doctorate project prior to graduation for scholarship advancement and practice improvement (AACN, 2021). Deliberate mentorship and preceptorship influence the success of a DNP project (Aroke et al., 2021; Heitzler & Fullbright, 2021). DNP-prepared nurses' first-hand knowledge of the DNP educational requirements (Higgins & Newby, 2020) and their robust experiences in clinical practice, leadership, policy, advocacy, quality improvement process, and evidence-based practice (Edwards et al., 2018) position them to effectively mentor future advanced practice nurses. Heitzler and Fullbright (2021) listed several desirable traits and basic expectations from DNP preceptors so they can effectively guide the students, including:

- Effective verbal and written communication
- Extensive knowledge about the DNP project
- Adaptive leadership and teaching style based on students' needs
- Providing organizational context and influencing decision-making within the organization
- Developing rapport and obtaining stakeholder buy-in
- Providing honest and timely feedback to students
- Assisting the student in risk management and overcoming project challenges
- Valuing collaboration, mentorship, and professional development

PRECEPTEE EXPECTATIONS

The DNP Essentials outline the competencies that are required from DNP students prior to program completion. The Essentials encompass various areas of healthcare, including the scientific foundation of practice, systems and organizational leadership, translation of research into practice, health policy and advocacy, incorporation of technology, prevention and population health, interprofessional collaboration, and advanced nursing practice (AACN, 2021). DNP doctorate projects must meet the DNP Essentials, thus preparing the students to tackle healthcare system deficiencies and improve patient outcomes (AACN, 2021). The doctorate project provides an educational immersive experience that enhances the student's clinical knowledge and expertise through project planning, implementation, evaluation, and dissemination (AACN, 2021). It is important for students to maintain a good relationship with their preceptors during this process to maximize learning opportunities and to ensure the success of their DNP projects. According to Higgins and Newby (2020), preceptees or students must reciprocate the time and effort provided to them by their preceptors through their proactive engagement in the mentoring process. Other expectations from DNP students include to:

- Ensure the DNP project aligns with the organization's mission or priorities
- Organize the workflow and timeline
- Coordinate and communicate project development with mentors timely
- Seek help when necessary and accept feedback professionally

DNP-PREPARED NURSE AS CLINICAL PRECEPTOR

The clinical preceptor serves a central role in the clinical education of DNP students who are learning an advanced practice registered nurse (APRN) role (certified nurse practitioner, certified nurse-midwife, certified clinical nurse specialist, certified registered nurse anesthetist). They are responsible for supervising the students' clinical experiences and providing feedback about their educational progress. Each APRN role requires a minimum of 500 supervised practice hours in the discipline of nursing (AACN, 2021) and upwards of 2,604 hours for nurse anesthetist programs (American Association of Nurse Anesthesiology, 2022).

Since 2004 when the AACN released its position statement in support of the DNP, more than 60,500 have graduated with a DNP (AACN, 2022a). In 2018, 60% entered full-time positions in schools of nursing, rather than bedside or clinical positions (McCauley et al., 2020). Currently, only 14.7% of nurse practitioners hold a DNP as their highest degree (AANP, 2021). These data suggest that the majority of DNP students will not have DNP-prepared clinical preceptors. In addition, the majority of DNP programs (69%) do not maintain contractual clinical site partnerships with universities, clinics, or hospitals for guaranteed preceptorships or graduate placement (AACN, 2022b), creating challenges when placing students in clinical sites.

As we look to educating DNP students in the future, the demand for clinical preceptors will increase. We should remain flexible in policies regarding clinical preceptor criteria, for example, APRN, physician, physician assistant, and their highest degree. While DNP graduates report that the DNP improved their competencies in quality improvement, evidence-based practice, and leadership (Minnick et al., 2019), there is no evidence that the clinical competence of graduates is related to whether the clinical preceptor is DNP-prepared.

SUMMARY

DNP-prepared nurses are uniquely positioned to influence the future of the nursing workforce through deliberate mentorships and preceptorships in the clinical, academic, and administrative arenas. Their extensive education, clinical expertise, and leadership experience provide students with experiential learning opportunities that enable novice nurses and practitioners to provide safe, high-quality, and value-based care to their patients. The mentees should actively participate in the learning process and be receptive to feedback to advance their knowledge and skills. Ultimately, regardless of their educational degree or profession, nursing preceptors and DNP mentors should be capable of empowering clinicians and future healthcare leaders to achieve their potential and realize their vision within their own communities.

CRITICAL THINKING QUESTIONS

1. Reflect on your previous nursing experience and explain what mentorship qualities have helped you in your professional development.
2. What are the important attributes for clinical preceptors? Do you think it matters whether the clinician is a nurse with a DNP or PhD and explain why?
3. Discuss the challenges DNP students face when developing and implementing their doctoral project. How can DNP students and faculty support the process?

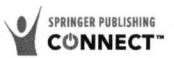 A robust set of instructor resources designed to supplement this text is located at http://connect.springerpub.com/content/book/978-0-8261-8137-4. Qualifying instructors may request access by emailing textbook@springerpub.com.

REFERENCES

American Association of Colleges of Nursing. (2021). *The essentials: Core competencies for professional nursing education*. https://www.aacnnursing.org/Portals/42/AcademicNursing/pdf/Essentials-2021.pdf

American Association of Colleges of Nursing. (2022a). *Fact sheet: The doctor of nursing practice (DNP)*. https://www.aacnnursing.org/Portals/42/News/Factsheets/DNP-Fact-Sheet.pdf

American Association of Colleges of Nursing. (2022b). *The state of doctor of nursing practice education in 2022*. https://www.aacnnursing.org/Portals/42/News/Surveys-Data/State-of-the-DNP-Summary-Report-June-2022.pdf

American Association of Nurse Anesthesiology. (2022). *Certified registered nurse anesthetists fact sheet*. https://www.aana.com/membership/become-a-crna/crna-fact-sheet

American Association of Nurse Practitioners. (2021). *The state of the nurse practitioner profession 2020: Results of the national nurse practitioner sample survey*. https://storage.aanp.org/www/documents/no-index/research/2020-NP-Sample-Survey-Report.pdf

Aroke, E. N., Wilbanks, B. A., Hicks, T. H., Thurston, K. L., & McMullan, S. P. (2021). Mentoring team projects for the doctor of nursing practice: Considerations for nurse anesthesia faculty. *AANA Journal, 89*(5), 435–442.

Edwards, N., Coddington, J., Erler, C., & Kirkpatrick, J. (2018). The impact of the role of doctor of nursing practice nurses on healthcare and leadership. *Medical Research Archives, 6*(4), 1–11. https://doi.org/10.18103/mra.v6i4.1734

Heitzler, E. T., & Fullbright, G. M. (2021). *The mentoring role for DNP projects*. https://www.npwomenshealthcare.com/the-mentoring-role-for-dnp-projects

Higgins. K., & Newby, O. (2020). DNP student mentorship: Empowering students and nurse practitioner organizations. *The Nurse Practitioner, 45*(4), 42–47. https://doi.org/10.1097/01.NPR.0000657320.35417.d2

Institute for Healthcare Improvement. (2022). *The IHI triple aim*. https://www.ihi.org/Engage/Initiatives/TripleAim/Pages/default.aspx

McCauley, L. A., Broome, M. E., Frazier, L., Hayes, R., Kurth, A., Musil, C. M., Norman, L. D., Rideout, K. H., Villarruel, A. M. (2020). Doctor of Nursing Practice (DNP) degree in the United States: Reflecting, readjusting, and getting back on track. *Nursing Outlook, 68*(4), 494–503. https://doi.org/10.1016/j.outlook.2020.03.008.

Minnick, A. F., Kleinpell, R., & Allison, T. L. (2019). DNPs' labor participation, activities, and reports of degree contributions. *Nursing Outlook, 67*(1), 89100. https://doi.org/10.1016/j.outlook.2018.10.008

Sherrod, D., Holland, C., & Battle, L. H. (2020). Nurse preceptors: A valuable resource for adapting staff to change. *Nursing Management, 51*(3), 50–53. https://doi.org/10.1097/01.NUMA.0000654876.89427.e0

CHAPTER TWENTY-ONE Reflective Response 1

AMANDA AMBROSIO

Mentors empower individuals to conceive the possibilities of a future and to believe it can be maintained. The role of mentorship manifests significantly in nursing, where new nurses and nursing students rely on experienced professionals to help them navigate the procedures, guidelines, and challenges of delivering quality care. Zyrene's example emphasizes the role of preceptorship in producing qualified nurses who can work in diverse settings; the mentorship and guidance from her mentors empowered her to develop evidence-based solutions to the challenges in nursing practice. Thus, she participated in converting evidence to practice through her project in leveraging telemedicine and using community health workers to increase to healthcare among older adults with diabetes.

There is an increasing need to raise up qualified professionals to serve in different practice settings and with patients of varying backgrounds. Notably, the DNP program is growing substantially, creating a demand for qualified preceptors to mentor learners into attaining optimal educational outcomes. DNP-qualified nurses have first-hand knowledge of the academic requirements of the DNP learners and the experiences in advocacy, leadership, and clinical practice that the students should attain through the program. While some preceptor skills are common in many nurse mentors, some are more prevalent in DNP preceptors. These include the ability to individualize learning and teaching styles based on learners' needs, conduct professional development and evidence-based research, and influence decision-making in organizations. While it may be unrealistic to expect all preceptors to be DNP- prepared nurses, learning institutions and healthcare organizations should work together toward linking DNP students to qualified preceptors of various educational backgrounds who can provide multidimensional mentorship.

CHAPTER TWENTY-ONE

Reflective Response 2

LAURA O'ROURKE

Doctor of nursing practice (DNP)-prepared nurses are perfectly poised to meet the ever-changing demands of the increasingly complex healthcare environment. Collaborating with interdisciplinary teams to translate research into practice, these terminallyeducated clinicians provide expertise and transformative leadership across all healthcare settings to tackle system- and organization-level deficiencies and improve patient outcomes. The authors of this chapter present an exemplar of one DNP student's passion for addressing health disparities through the development, implementation, and evaluation of an evidence-based quality improvement project. This community-based scholarly project's impact perfectly illustrates the profound effect organizational preceptors and faculty mentors extend to DNP students and the patients they serve. Moreover, it demonstrates DNP students' vital role in the symbiotic relationship between preceptor, mentor, and organization and the progress of future DNP-prepared nurses.

The authors highlight the necessity of a standardized guide, outlining preceptor requirements, desired characteristics, role definition, and clinical preceptorship. Particularly noteworthy is the assertion that the demand for clinical preceptors will continue to grow, underscoring the need for flexibility in policies surrounding clinical preceptor criteria. Higgins and Newby (2020) propose nurse practitioner professional organizations as a potential gap fill to provide DNP students with experiential learning and mentorship. This directly aligns with the American Association of Colleges of Nursing (AACN) Common Advanced Practice Registered Nurse Doctoral-Level Competencies and the American Nurses Association Code of Ethics for Nurses with Interpretive Statements, which encourage involvement in professional nursing organizations to advance both the profession and patient care (American Association of Colleges of Nursing, 2017; American Nurses Association, 2015). On the surface, it appears this novel approach to mentorship would be mutually beneficial, providing DNP students with valuable experiences while infusing innovative ideas and energy back into professional organizations.

This reflective author could not agree more with Anderson et al.'s (2019) suggestion that mentorship is a professional responsibility. Preceptorship and mentorship activities are undoubtedly time- and energy-intensive endeavors; fortunately, DNP projects deliver immense value back to the clinical practice site by positively impacting patient outcomes (Durham et al., 2019). The authors of this chapter have provided an expertly written guide to help ensure an interdependent relationship between DNP students, clinical preceptors, and faculty mentors that is enjoyable and fulfilling for all while maximizing learning opportunities and advancing the nursing profession.

REFERENCES

American Association of Colleges of Nursing. (2017). *Common advanced practice registered nurse doctoral-level competencies*. www.aacnnursing.org/Portals/42/AcademicNursing/pdf/Common-APRN-Doctroal-Competencies.pdf?ver=2018-01-25-133127-767.

American Nurses Association. (2015). Code of ethics with interpretive statements. www.nursingworld.org/coe-view-only.

Anderson, K. M., McLaughlin, M. K., Crowell, N. A., Fall-Dickson, J. M., White, K. A., Heitzler, E. T., Kesten, K. S., & Yearwood, E. L. (2019). Mentoring students engaging in scholarly projects and dissertations in doctoral nursing programs. *Nursing Outlook, 67*(6), 776–788. https://doi.org/10.1016/j.outlook.2019.06.021

Durham, M., Cotler, K., & Corbridge, S. (2019). Facilitating faculty knowledge of DNP quality improvement projects: Key elements to promote strong practice partnerships. *Journal of the American Association of Nurse Practitioners, 31*(11), 665–674. https://doi.org/10.1097/JXX.0000000000000308.

Higgins, K., & Newby, O. (2020). DNP student mentorship. *The Nurse Practitioner, 45*(4), 42–47. https://doi.org/10.1097/01.NPR.0000657320.35417.d2.

CHAPTER TWENTY-TWO

The Role of the DNP in Quality Improvement and Patient Safety Initiatives

CATHERINE JOHNSON AND ERIC VOGELSTEIN

HISTORY OF HEALTHCARE REFORM AND QUALITY IMPROVEMENT AND PATIENT SAFETY

It has been more than 20 years since the Institute of Medicine (2000) report was published with the call for all professionals in the U.S. health system to acknowledge its failure to provide high-quality and safe healthcare to their patients. This report called for a stronger safety culture in the healthcare system that would require a redesign of most of its patient care processes. In the second IOM report (2001), six aims for healthcare improvement were outlined that targeted key dimensions of the healthcare system and provided a framework for the healthcare reform efforts (Table 22.1).

Following this second report, an interdisciplinary summit was held to develop the next steps for the reform of education in the health professions that would enhance the achievement of improved patient outcomes and patient safety. Results from this summit were reported in the third IOM report (2003). The report described its goals as "an outcome-based education system that better-prepared clinicians to meet both the needs of the patients and the requirements of a changing health system" (p. 3). Table 22.2

TABLE 22.1 Six Aims for Healthcare Improvement

Safe: Avoiding injuries to patients from the care that is intended to help them.
Effective: Provide services based on scientific knowledge to all who could benefit and refrain from providing services to those not likely to benefit (avoiding underuse and overuse, respectively).
Patient-centered: Provide care that is respectful of and responsive to individual patient preferences, needs, and values and ensuring that patient values guide all clinical decisions.
Timely: Reduce waits and sometimes harmful delays for both those who receive and those who give care.
Efficient: Avoid waste, including waste of equipment, supplies, ideas, and energy.

Source: Institute of Medicine. (2001). *Crossing the quality chasm.* National Academies Press, p. 2.

TABLE 22.2 Health Professional Education: Interprofessional Core Competencies

Provide Patient-Centered Care:
• Identify, respect, and care about patients' differences, values, preferences, and expressed needs
• Relieve pain and suffering
• Coordinate continuous care
• Listen to, clearly inform, communicate with, and educate patients
• Share decision-making and management
• Continuously advocate disease prevention, wellness, and promotion of healthy lifestyles, including a focus on population health
Work in Interdisciplinary Teams:
• Cooperate, collaborate, communicate, and integrate care in teams to ensure that care is continuous and reliable
• Employ evidence-based practice by integrating best research with clinical expertise and patient values for optimum care and participate in learning and research activities to the extent feasible
Apply Quality Improvement:
• Identify errors and hazards in the provision of care
• Understand and implement basic safety design principles, such as standardization and simplification
• Continually understand and measure the quality of care in terms of structure, process, and outcomes in relation to patient and community needs
• Design and test interventions to change processes and systems of care, with the objective of improving quality
Utilize Informatics:
• Communicate, manage knowledge, mitigate error, and support decision-making using information technology

Source: Institute of Medicine. (2003). *Health professional education: A bridge to quality.* National Academies Press, p. 4.

describes the five core competencies for all healthcare professionals' education that included common quality improvement and patient safety core competencies.

Throughout the next decade, significant healthcare legislation funded the implementation of many of these strategies and recommendations, beginning with healthcare's entrance into the digital age. Through funding provided by the Health Information Technology for Economic and Clinical Health Act of 2009 (DHHS, 2009), the development of interoperable electronic health records connected hospitals, emergency services, ambulatory care centers, medical specialists, and primary care providers across the United States. This expansion stimulated the simultaneous development of a new health information infrastructure, as well as the creation of previously absent relationships between the multiple components of the healthcare systems. The creation of this new healthcare information system set the stage for the provision of better-coordinated and safer healthcare. Over the next 5 years, many points of the system and patient care vulnerability were identified, and important changes were put into place supporting the healthcare reform efforts (Gold & McLaughlin, 2016). Electronic health records (EHR) now exist in most healthcare practices and in all hospitals in the United States, resulting in massive amounts of patient care data being created and shared electronically. This innovation created the structure for monitoring, analyzing, and improving patient care processes, outcomes, and safety events within healthcare organizations (Gold & McLaughlin, 2016)

The primary legislation that would fund the next steps in the healthcare system redesign was the 2010 Patient Safety and Accountable Care Act (ACA). This massive legislation's primary goals were to make affordable health insurance available to more people, as well as address broad deficiencies in the current healthcare system (DHHS, 2010). The ACA supported the development of innovative medical care delivery methods designed to improve patient care, lower costs, and better align payment systems to promote patient-centered practices, through CMS Innovation Grants starting in 2012. The Centers for Medicare and Medicaid (CMS) Innovation Center (CMMI) was created as an interface between these new models and healthcare organizations and providers as a stimulus for innovation (CMS, 2022c).

The CMMI continues to provide access to these projects, which provide healthcare organizations and providers new approaches to the management of specific health conditions, care episodes, provider types, types of communities, and innovation to Medicare Parts C and D.

CMS published the report *Synthesis of Evaluation Results across 21 Medicare Models, 2012–2020* (CMMI, 2022), which summarized its evaluation of 21 Medicare models as "more than half (fourteen) demonstrated gross savings to Medicare. Changes in spending were driven by improvements in inpatient admissions (ten models) and/or post-acute care (fourteen models)" (CMMI, 2022, p. 1). These evaluation results will allow these new, tested models to be implemented with ongoing measurement of patient care outcomes and healthcare system costs.

Despite the massive redesign of many components of the healthcare system, recent reports have found that some parts of the country continue to struggle with poor patient outcomes and increased patient safety occurrences and have attributed this to "inadequate leadership preparation, system and process failures, poor communication and disempowerment of staff and patients" (Wong et al., 2020, p. 59). The role of the doctor of nursing practice (DNP) as a leader in implementing new approaches to healthcare delivery and healthcare quality will be determined by the expansion of the DNP's competencies and the creation of supportive DNP educational systems that support their achievement.

NURSING'S LEADERSHIP ROLE

The driving factors that led healthcare transformation over the past 20 years have been focused on improving quality, reducing errors, reducing fragmentation of care, inequitable access to healthcare, and reducing the cost of care. The HITECH Act of 2009 and the ACA of 2010 funded vital initiatives that redesigned health information technology, and developed new models of the healthcare organization and finance, resulting in increased expectations for improved performance in the delivery of healthcare and patient safety. These programs have been implemented relying heavily on the scope of practice of RNs and APRNs.

DNP programs focus on expanding nurse practitioners' and leaders' competencies in both clinical practice and administration in the expanded interprofessional team. These efforts and successes have realized the transformed role of nursing which was the focus of *The Future of Nursing: Leading Change, Advancing Health* (IOM, 2010) report which promoted this expectation for the nursing profession.

The *Future of Nursing* (IOM, 2010) report challenged nursing as a profession to realize the role of nurses as advocates and leaders in the healthcare reform process. It recognized that nurses are in the prime position, given their numbers and adaptability, to effect significant changes in the healthcare system's development and delivery. Through their experience in developing partnerships with both patients and other healthcare providers, nurses were thought to demonstrate skills and professional commitment to improving every environment in which they work.

Ten years after the first Future of Nursing report, the National Academies of Sciences, Engineering, and Medicine and the National Academy of Medicine published *The Future of Nursing 2020-2030: Charting a Path to Achieve Health Equity* (National Academies of Science 2021). This report focuses on the role of nurses in meeting the healthcare challenges of the 21st century. These included the aging population, access to primary care, mental and behavioral health problems, structural racism, high maternal mortality and morbidity, and elimination of the disproportionate disease burden carried by specific segments of the U.S. population (NAS, 2020). The report encourages nurses to become fully engaged in a partnership with other disciplines to address the underlying causes of these challenges. Nurses are encouraged to serve as leaders in the processes and their professional education must expand to include quality and patient safety competencies to meet this challenge. These competencies must also include interprofessional collaboration and the science of quality improvement and patient safety (NAS, 2020). The American Association of Colleges of Nursing (AACN, 2015a, 2015b) has consistently supported the development of the DNP to include these competencies, enabling the DNP to assume this healthcare leadership role.

DNP EDUCATION IN THE 21ST CENTURY

The AACN's 2015 DNP White Paper (AACN, 2015 a, 2015b) addressed the importance of the DNP's leadership, quality, and patient safety competencies and addressed inconsistencies in the implementation of the DNP curriculum throughout the United States. This white paper clarified the DNP role of healthcare system leaders in clinical practice, administration, quality improvement, and patient safety. Specific recommendations were made in the report regarding program refinements that would assure the achievement of DNP competencies and their application to the DNP role.

Faculty development in the areas of leadership, informatics, quality improvement, and patient safety science was encouraged due to the significant growth of these areas of healthcare. The report stressed the importance of assuring that all DNP programs' curriculum focuses on healthcare systems leadership, informatics, quality improvement and patient safety methods, evaluation of evidence-based practice in hospitals, and community-based clinical practices. They emphasized the use of the DNP residency and DNP project as the primary means to evaluate the student's attainment of the DNP competencies, which reflect nursing's collaboration and leadership in the implementation of all healthcare reform efforts. The DNP provides healthcare with a clinical expert with competencies in leading the development and implementation of needed healthcare change, based on effective evaluation of the quality and safety of patient care.

These changes have resulted in DNP programs proliferating throughout the United States and increasing numbers of DNP graduates, who are now finding healthcare system positions more readily and are leading these initiatives in healthcare centers across the country. Beeber et al. (2019) conducted an online survey of DNP program directors and graduates from 288 DNP programs across the United States. This survey provided descriptive information regarding the current programs, including location, modality, and profit status. The report found sharp increases in the number of DNP programs and graduates across the country. Employers reported that DNP-prepared nurses were assuming advanced practice and administrative nursing roles previously filled by MSN-prepared nurses. But employers admitted that they lacked a specific understanding of the difference between MSN and DNP competencies. They did, however, state that they are consistently seeking out DNP graduates to fill executive leadership and system-based quality improvement and patient safety roles (Beeber et al., 2019). This confusion could be due to the lack of acknowledgment of the DNP as the terminal degree for nursing advanced practice roles. There has been widespread debate about this professional designation, which persists today.

The DNP degree was originally established in 2004 by members of the AACN who voted to endorse the DNP as the "most appropriate degree for advanced-practice registered nurses to enter practice." In support of this, the AACN membership voted to approve the position that all master's degree programs that educate APRNs should transition to the DNP by 2015 (Auerbach et al., 2015). Despite widespread respect for the DNP role and significant increases in DNP program development, there was not enough momentum to make this transition happen. The AACN commissioned a report from RAND Health to survey DNP programs to investigate their progress, as well as evaluate the data obtained by an AACN online survey. Table 22.3 summarizes this important report's results (Auerbach et al., 2015).

The transition of nurse practitioner (NP) programs from MSN programs to DNP programs has continued to be a challenge into the second decade of the 21st century. The National Organization of Nurse Practitioners Faculties (NONPF) and the AACN continue to ask their members to support moving the entry level of preparation for NP education from the master's degree to the DNP degree by 2025. This recommendation is driven by several factors: (a) an increasingly complex healthcare system, (b) rapid expansion of knowledge underlying clinical practice, and (c) a desire for parity with other healthcare professions (NONPF DNP White Paper, 2022). The NONPF has stated its belief that the DNP NP curriculum should not be an add-on to the master's curriculum and instead, integrate objectives and learning opportunities for students to master the 2021 AACN Essentials for the advanced level of practice.

An infographic shared by the NONPF in late 2022 detailed the increase in the number of DNP NP graduates as 4,775 more in 2021 than in 2016, with 22,346 practicing NPs who are graduates of BSN-DNP programs. They also report that there are now 96 BSN-DNP NP programs across the United States (NONPF, 2022). The American Academy of Nurse Practitioners (AANP) shares that in 2021, 353,000 NPs were licensed in the United States, and more than 70% practice in primary care settings (AANP, 2022). The momentum to make the shift to BSN-DNP programs for NP education is increasing and the AACN and NONPF are increasing activities that are focused on convincing state boards of nursing and NP accrediting bodies to designate the DNP as the appropriate degree for nurse practitioner education by 2025.

TABLE 22.3 Summary of DNP Program Progress in 2015

- The DNP continues to expand steadily.
- The MSN remains the dominant pathway for APRN entry-into-practice education, though there is some limited movement toward replacement with the BSN-to-DNP.
- There will likely be two tracks toward the DNP for the near future (defined by schools' planning horizons): a single-step process (BSN-to-DNP) and a two-step process (BSN-to-MSN followed by an MSN-to-DNP at a later date).
- The value of the added content of the DNP education is almost universally agreed upon.
- Requirement of the DNP for certification and accreditation is an important factor in schools' decisions.
- Regarding the demand for DNP-educated nurse practitioners, employers are generally unable to differentiate between the MSN and the DNP, albeit with a few exceptions.

Source: Auerbach et al. (2015). The DNP by 2015: A study of the institutional, political, and professional issues that facilitate or impede establishing a post-baccalaureate doctor of nursing practice program. *Rand Health Q, 5*(1), 3.

AACN'S 2021 THE ESSENTIALS: CORE COMPETENCIES FOR PROFESSIONAL NURSING EDUCATION

In 2021, the AACN published The Essentials: Core Competencies for Professional Nursing Education (AACN, 2021), which defines the nursing role competencies for entry-level and advanced-level nursing education and practice. This edition of the Essentials document is a departure from the previous format that focused on the three educational levels of nursing education: baccalaureate, master's, and DNP degrees. This new Essentials document has introduced a new model focusing on two levels of professional nursing competencies: entry level and advanced level, and competencies within four spheres of care: disease prevention/promotion of health and well-being, chronic disease care, restorative care, and hospice/palliative/supportive care across the lifespan, with diverse populations (AACN, 2021).

The model employed in the development of the 2021 Essentials was built on the work of Englander et al. (2013), who developed a taxonomy of competency domains for the health professions. Carraccio et al. (2017) defined *entrustable professional activities* (EPAs) as milestones that defined the relationships between entry-level and advanced competencies. This model provides the framework for healthcare professionals to develop role-specific competencies at the entry and advanced levels that can be used to build better communication and collaboration, as well as improve healthcare team function.

Using this model, the AACN developed 10 Domains essential to nursing practice that included the definition of each domain, competencies that are central to that domain, and subcompetencies for each level of nursing (entry and advanced). These domains and competencies can be used to distinguish the unique role of nursing, as well as nursing's relationship with other health professions. Table 22.4 describes each of the 10 Domains of the Essentials.

TABLE 22.4 Ten Domains of the Essentials

Domain 1: Knowledge for Nursing Practice
Descriptor: Integration, translation, and application of established and evolving disciplinary nursing knowledge and ways of knowing, as well as knowledge from other disciplines, including a foundation in liberal arts and natural and social sciences. This distinguishes the practice of professional nursing and forms the basis for clinical judgment and innovation in nursing practice.
Domain 2: Person-Centered Care
Descriptor: Person-centered care focuses on the individual within multiple complicated contexts, including family and/or important others. Person-centered care is holistic, individualized, just, respectful, compassionate, coordinated, evidence-based, and developmentally appropriate. Person-centered care builds on a scientific body of knowledge that guides nursing practice regardless of specialty or functional area.
Domain 3: Population Health
Descriptor: Population health spans the healthcare delivery continuum from public health prevention to disease management of populations and describes collaborative activities with both traditional and non-traditional partnerships from affected communities, public health, industry, academia, health care, local government entities, and others for the improvement of equitable population health outcomes.
Domain 4: Scholarship for Nursing Discipline
Descriptor: The generation, synthesis, translation, application, and dissemination of nursing knowledge to improve health and transform health care.

(Continued)

TABLE 22.4 Ten Domains of the Essentials (*continued*)

Domain 5: Quality and Safety
Descriptor: Employment of established and emerging principles of safety and improvement science. Quality and safety, as core values of nursing practice, enhance quality and minimize the risk of harm to patients and providers through both system effectiveness and individual performance.

Domain 6: Interprofessional Partnerships
Descriptor: Intentional collaboration across professions and with care team members, patients, families, communities, and other stakeholders to optimize care, enhance the healthcare experience, and strengthen outcomes.

Domain 7: Systems-Based Practice
Descriptor: Responding to and leading within complex systems of health care. Nurses effectively and proactively coordinate resources to provide safe, quality, equitable care to diverse populations.

Domain 8: Informatics and Healthcare Technologies
Descriptor: Information and communication technologies and informatics processes are used to provide care, gather data, form information to drive decision-making, and support professionals as they expand knowledge and wisdom for practice. Informatics processes and technologies are used to manage and improve the delivery of safe, high-quality, and efficient healthcare services in accordance with best practices and professional and regulatory standards.

Domain 9: Professionalism
Descriptor: Formation and cultivation of a sustainable professional nursing identity, accountability, perspective, collaborative disposition, and comportment that reflects nursing's characteristics and values.

Domain 10: Personal, Professional, and Leadership Development
Descriptor: Participation in activities and self-reflection that foster personal health, resilience, well-being, lifelong learning, and support the acquisition of nursing expertise and assertion of leadership.

Source: AACN. (2021). *The essentials: Core competencies for professional nursing education.* https://www.aacnnursing.org/Essentials

DNP DOMAIN 5: QUALITY AND PATIENT SAFETY ROLE COMPETENCIES

The concept of quality care is associated with many aspects of professional role competencies as pointed out in the Essentials (AACN, 2021). Quality care is associated with critical aspects of the professional nursing role as described in the following:

- *Liberally educated graduates are well prepared to integrate knowledge, skills, and values from the arts, sciences, and humanities to provide safe, quality care; advocate for patients, families, communities, and populations; and promote health equity and social justice* (p. 5, the Essentials).

- *Diversity, equity, and inclusion, as a value, support nursing workforce development to prepare graduates who contribute to the improvement of access and care quality for underrepresented and medically underserved populations* (p. 6, the Essentials).

- Evidence-based, institution-wide approaches focused on equity in student learning and catalyzing culture shifts in the academy are fundamental to eliminating structural racism in higher education. Only through deconstructive processes can academic nursing prepare graduates who provide *high-quality, equitable, and culturally competent health care* (p. 7, the Essentials).

- Expanding primary care into communities will enable our healthcare delivery systems to achieve the Quadruple Aim of improving patient experiences (*quality and satisfaction*), improving the health of populations, decreasing per capita costs of healthcare, and improving care team well-being.

- Factors such as structural racism, cost containment, resource allocation, and interdisciplinary collaboration are considered and implemented to ensure *the delivery of high-quality, equitable, and safe patient care.*
- Health information technology is required for person-centered service across the continuum and requires consistency in user input, proper process, and *quality management* (p. 8, the Essentials).
- Thus, nurses need an understanding of consumer engagement and experience across all settings as an *essential component of person-centered, quality care* (p. 9, the Essentials).
- Effective individual/family involvement leads to *safer and higher quality care* (p. 9, the Essentials).

Providing quality care is one of the highest values of nursing, as well as all health professions. The act of assuring quality and safety of care has become one of the primary activities of the healthcare reform efforts of the past 20 years and will be used as the measure of its success. Each healthcare profession has established educational processes that include the basic components of care and quality improvement and patient safety. The AACN created these standards for the nursing profession in the Essentials for entry-level nurses and those practicing at advanced levels.

The DNP role competencies for quality and patient safety are described in the 3 competencies and 15 advanced level subcompetencies described in *Domain 5: Quality and Safety* (AACN, 2021). This domain describes quality and safety as core values of nursing practice and focuses on minimizing the risk of harm to both the patient and providers of care, due to the synergy between the two. The environment of care must be nonpunitive in its promotion of quality and safety through the empowerment of caregivers to act appropriately in the prevention and reporting of all adverse events and near misses. This is achieved through the employment of safety and improvement science impacting both the system's effectiveness and the nurse's individual performance. Evidence-based interventions and practice guidelines must systematize these actions, including addressing safety concerns such as environmental hazards, violence, burnout, ergonomics, and chemical and biological agents. These must be made available to all providers in the work environment and address both patient care recipients and providers of care. Domain 5: Quality and Safety Entry Level and Advanced Level Nursing Education competencies and subcompetencies for advanced nursing practice are listed in Table 22.5.

■ QUALITY IMPROVEMENT AND PATIENT SAFETY EDUCATIONAL STRATEGIES AND TOOLS

Specific quality improvement and patient safety strategies, approaches, and tools are now available to be incorporated into the DNP curriculum. Eliminating medical errors and improving patient safety are among the major drivers for healthcare transformation. Achieving a culture of patient safety requires understanding what values and beliefs are important in an organization and what attitudes and behaviors related to patient safety are supported, rewarded, and expected. Patient safety practices developed

TABLE 22.5 Domain 5: Quality and Safety

Entry Level Nursing Education	Advanced Level Nursing Education
5.1 Apply quality improvement principles in care delivery.	
5.1a Recognize nursing's essential role in improving healthcare quality and safety	5.1i Establish and incorporate data-driven benchmarks to monitor system performance
5.1b Identify sources and applications of national safety and quality standards to guide nursing practice	5.1j Use national safety resources to lead team-based change initiatives
5.1c Implement standardized, evidence-based processes for care delivery	5.1k Integrate outcome metrics to inform change and policy recommendations
5.1d Interpret benchmark and unit outcome data to inform individual and microsystem practice	5.1l Collaborate in analyzing organizational process improvement initiatives.
5.1e Compare quality improvement methods in the delivery of patient care	5.1m Lead the development of a business plan for quality improvement initiatives
5.1f Identify strategies to improve outcomes of patient care in practice	5.1n Advocate for change related to financial policies that impact the relationship between economics and quality care delivery
5.1g Participate in the implementation of a practice change	5.1o Advance quality improvement practices through dissemination of outcomes
5.1h Develop a plan for monitoring quality improvement change	
5.2 Contribute to a culture of patient safety.	
5.2a Describe the factors that create a culture of safety	5.2g Evaluate the alignment of system data and comparative patient safety benchmarks
5.2b Articulate the nurse's role within an interprofessional team in promoting safety and preventing errors and near misses	5.2h Lead analysis of actual errors, near misses, and potential situations that would impact safety
5.2c Examine basic safety design principles to reduce the risk of harm	5.2i Design evidence-based interventions to mitigate risk
5.2d Assume accountability for reporting unsafe conditions, near misses, and errors to reduce harm	5.2j Evaluate emergency preparedness system-level plans to protect safety
5.2e Describe processes used in understanding causes of error	
5.2f Use national patient safety resources, initiatives, and regulations at the point of care	
5.3 Contribute to a culture of provider and work environment safety.	
5.3a Identify actual and potential levels of risks to providers within the workplace	5.3e Advocate for structures, policies, and processes that promote a culture of safety and prevent workplace risks and injury
5.3b Recognize how to prevent workplace violence and injury	5.3f Foster a just culture reflecting civility and respect
5.3c Promote policies for the prevention of violence and risk mitigation	5.3g Create a safe and transparent culture for reporting incidents
5.3d Recognize one's role in sustaining a just culture reflecting civility and respect	5.3h Role model and lead well-being and resiliency for self and team

Source: AACN. (2021). *The essentials: Core competencies for professional nursing education.* https://www.aacnnursing.org/Essentials

within organizations are increasingly based on national standards related to accuracy in patient identification, communication systems among caregivers, and precautions for high-alert medications and procedures. Four organizations have created useful tools for faculty and practicing DNPs to build their knowledge of evidence-based quality improvement and patient safety approaches, tools, and data management strategies that will support the attainment of the advanced competencies to support the DNP's leadership role. These organizations are the American Academy of Colleges of Nursing (AACN), Quality & Safety Education in Nursing (QSEN), the Institute of Healthcare Improvement (IHI), and the Agency for Healthcare Research and Quality (AHRQ).

AMERICAN ACADEMY OF COLLEGES OF NURSING (AACN)

The AACN created a peer-reviewed Essentials Toolkit to provide nursing faculties classroom learning strategies, tools, and classroom assignments at the entry-level and advanced levels for each competency and subcompetency. Resources provided to assist faculty in preparing course materials and competency-based education evaluations can be found at the AACN website at https://www.aacnnursing.org/Essentials/Database/Kit/i/domain5_wg_xls.

One example of the resources available for quality improvement and safety education described in the toolkit for Competency 5.3 subcompetency 5.3.f is described in Table 22.6.

This availability of competency-based resources for each of the new competencies and subcompetencies of the 10 domains of the new essentials is vital to the development of new course content and evaluations. The AACN's commitment to supporting faculty

TABLE 22.6 The Essentials Toolkit: Domian 5, Quality and Safety

Competency: 5.3 Contribute to a culture of provider and work environment safety		
Subcompetency 5.3.f Foster a just culture reflecting civility and respect		
Learning Strategy	**Reference**	**Graduate Course and Student Population**
Invite your students to read Cynthia Clark's work on civility and respect in healthcare and nursing. Invite your students to reflect on their own experience of incivility in practice (between team members, between patients and nurses). Invite your students to reflect on what professional standards can they adopt in their own practice to support civility and respect.	Clark, C. M., & Dunham, M. (2020). Civility mentor: A virtual learning experience. *Nurse Educ*, 45(4), 189–192. Available at: https://www.ncbi.nlm.nih.gov/pmc/articles/PMC7329244 Clark, C. M. (2019). Fostering a culture of civility and respect in nursing. *Journal of Nursing Regulation*, 10(1), 44–52. Available at: https://www.sciencedirect.com/science/article/abs/pii/S2155825619300821	Professional Issues Course APRN MSN & DNP

Source: The AACN Essentials Toolkit: https://www.aacnnursing.org/Essentials/Tool-Kit

is clear, as well as their support of the healthcare reform efforts through the prompt implementation of the new Essentials in support of the expanded role of the DNP.

QUALITY AND SAFETY EDUCATION FOR NURSES (QSEN)

The Quality and Safety Education for Nurses (QSEN) project was funded by the Robert Wood Johnson Foundation, and the AACN led a national initiative to develop nursing competencies built on the IOM competencies (Table 22.2). QSEN's goal was to provide nurses with the knowledge, skills, and attitudes (KSAs) necessary to ensure continuous quality and safety improvement within healthcare systems (QSEN, 2014). Six competencies were developed that include patient-centered care, evidence-based practice, teamwork and collaboration, quality improvement, safety, and informatics. The AACN and the University of Minnesota developed interactive modules that are now available for undergraduate and graduate students for each competency. These learning modules are available at https://www.aacnnursing.org/Faculty/Teaching-Resources/QSEN/QSEN-Learning-Module-Series.

The QSEN Institute is one of the regional centers and is located within the Frances Payne Bolton School of Nursing, Case Western Reserve University. It is a collaboration of health professionals committed to the improvement of the quality and safety of healthcare systems through education, practice, and scholarship. The QSEN Institute serves as a central repository of information on the core QSEN competencies, KSAs, teaching strategies, and faculty development resources (QSEN Institute, 2022). Both graduate and undergraduate quality and safety competencies have been developed in six areas: patient-centered care, teamwork and collaboration, evidence-based practice, quality improvement, safety, and informatics. The graduate competencies can be found at www.qsen.org. QSEN has worked with the AACN and the Joint Commission (TJC) to develop a crosswalk between these six competencies and the new entry-level and advanced Essentials competencies and TJC requirements. These can be found on the QSEN Institute website: www.qsen.org. According to Sherwood (2021) patient safety is a shared responsibility between the healthcare organization and each nurse. Engaging in building a culture of safety through attainment of the QSEN competencies, the DNP can lead the efforts to build a safer and more effective healthcare system.

AGENCY FOR HEALTHCARE RESEARCH AND QUALITY (AHRQ)

The Agency for Healthcare Research and Quality's (AHRQ's) mission is to produce evidence to make healthcare safer, higher quality, more accessible, equitable, and affordable, and to work within the U.S. Department of Health and Human Services and with other partners to make sure that the evidence is understood and used (AHRQ, 2022). Through federal and national foundation grant support over the past 10 years, significant progress has been made in the development of evidence-based QI approaches.

Quality Indicators
AHRQ provides quality indicators (QI), at no charge, that can be used to assess healthcare quality by organizations and team members including DNPs (AHRQ, 2014). These measures of healthcare quality can be used by nurses, providers, program managers, researchers, and others at the federal, state, and local levels who are involved in healthcare quality measurement. These tools can assist in assessing clinical and program data,

highlighting potential quality concerns, identifying the need for further study and investigation, and tracking changes over time.

The QIs represent various aspects of quality: prevention quality indicators (PQIs), inpatient quality indicators (IQIs), patient safety indicators (PSIs), and pediatric quality indicators (PDIs). The AHRQ also provides free software and software programs that can be applied to administrative data to support healthcare organizations' quality improvement efforts as well as learning from others.

Care-Compare

The AHRQ shares quality information for select AHRQ quality indicators with the public, as well as with healthcare providers and administrators. CMS has made public quality indicators for hospitals and healthcare providers throughout the United States through their Care Compare program designed to assist people with Medicare to choose hospitals and providers who have the best quality of care and highest patient satisfaction based upon CMS required data, including selected quality indicators. This website can be found at https://www.medicare.gov/care-compare. The goal of Care Compare is to provide Medicare recipients with the quality of patient care, safety, and satisfaction data of healthcare providers in their region in order to make informed decisions regarding their own care (CMS, 2022a). This comparison data can also be used by healthcare organizations to evaluate the care provided by their competitors, which may generate improvement efforts of their own in order to meet community norms.

The AHRQ also provides quality data through a variety of informational materials posted on QualityNet. QualityNet is the only CMS-approved website for secure communications and healthcare quality data exchange between quality improvement organizations (QIOs), hospitals, physician offices, nursing homes, end-stage renal disease (ESRD) networks and facilities, and data vendors (CMS, 2022b). The goal of QualityNet is to help improve the quality of healthcare for Medicare beneficiaries by providing for the safe, efficient exchange of information regarding their care.

AHRQ's Hospital Quality Indicators Toolkits

The AHRQ built on the work of the Institute of Healthcare Improvement (IHI) and created the Hospital Quality Improvement Toolkit (AHRQ, 2022). This free, online resource for nursing and other professionals is used to assist in evaluating the quality of care provided and developing quality improvement programs in their hospitals. This QI toolkit is designed to support both nursing and hospital leadership, as well as quality improvement teams. The QI toolkit is divided into the six steps of the AHRQ's quality improvement process and includes tools and resources that support each step. Table 22.7 describes each step in the AHRQ quality improvement process and the tools provided to support each step within the QI toolkit (AHRQ, 2022).

One tool that is an important foundation for the implementation of the quality indicators in the quality improvement process in hospitals is detailed in the fourth step: Implementing Evidence-Based Strategies to Improve Clinical Care. In this step *25 indicator-specific best practices*, which are based on quality indicators, are presented (Box 22.1). These best practices have been developed by the AHRQ based on well-documented evidence. In addition to these best practices, the toolkit provides a gap analysis tool that assists healthcare team members in reviewing their current practice related to the QI and identifying gaps in their practice that decrease the quality of this practice as well as potentially increase risks to patients. The toolkit also provides the Project Charter tool, developed by the IHI, that supports the development of a quality improvement process

TABLE 22.7 AHRQ Quality Improvement (QI) Process and QI Toolkit Resources

1. Assessing Readiness to Change.
• Fact sheets on the Inpatient and Patient Safety Quality Indicators
• Board presentation template
• Survey to self-assess readiness to change
• Case studies of QI toolkit users
2. Applying QIs to Your Hospital's Data
• Software instructions to calculate the QI rates based on discharge data
• Tips for coding and documentation
3. Identifying Priorities for Quality Improvement.
• Prioritization worksheet and example of a completed worksheet
• Presentation template aimed at engaging staff in the improvement process
4. Implementing Evidence-Based Strategies to Improve Clinical Care
• 25 indicator-specific best practices based on quality indicators
• Project charter
• Gap analysis
• Implementation plan
5. Monitoring Progress and Sustainability of Improvements
• Guide to support staff in tracking trends and monitoring progress for sustainable improvement
6. Analyzing Return on Investment
• Step-by-step method for calculating the return on investment for an intervention implemented to improve performance on an AHRQ QI
• Case study of return on investment calculated by a hospital
7. Quality Improvement Resources
• Annotated list of related quality improvement guides and tools

Source: AHRQ's Quality Toolkit: https://www.ahrq.gov/patient-safety/settings/hospital/resource/qitool/index.html

to address these gaps within the hospital setting. The Implementation Planning tool is also provided that supports the implementation of needed changes in practice.

This toolkit can also be used by DNP students and educators to build their DNP projects using the AHRQ QI Toolkit focusing on practice improvement using the QI Specific Best Practices. Box 22.2 describes an example of a DNP project utilizing these steps, tools, and processes.

BOX 22.1   Quality Indicators Best Practices Tool (Step 4)

- *The purpose of this tool is to provide detailed descriptions of best practices as well as suggestions for improvement, prescribed process steps, and additional resources.*

- *Twenty-five QI-specific best practices have been developed that can be used to assess the quality of care within an organization and identify changes in practice that can improve practice and patient outcomes. Included in the QI Toolkit (step 4) is a Gap Analysis Tool (Tool D.5) that assists quality teams in identifying practices that are not meeting standards and developing plans for improvement.*

- *The AHRQ QI Toolkit also includes a Project Charter (Tool D.2) and Implementation Plan (Tool D.6) that can support quality improvement efforts and measure outcomes. These best practices were created in 2014 and updated based on feedback from evidence reviews evaluation.*

> **Box 22.2 Example of DNP Project Developed Using AHRQ Quality Indicators Toolkit**
>
> **Step 1: Diagnose the Problem**
> - Describe the improvement initiative using the Project Charter (Tool D.2) and convene an interdisciplinary team
> - Identify the patient safety problem as increased skin breakdown and pressure ulcers in patients by collecting ICD-10 dx data and determining adverse event rates against internal and external benchmarks
> - Select *PSI 03 Pressure Ulcer Rate* and review evidence-based recommendations for care
> - Complete Gap Analysis (Tool D.5) and compare the current hospital practices with the Best Practice Recommendations
>
> **Step 2: Plan and Implement Best Practice**
> - Develop an Implementation Plan including nursing and medical staff (Tool D6)
>
> **Step 3: Measure Results and Analyze**
> - Collect data on key process measures related to best practice
>   - Nursing documentation of turn schedule
>   - Daily Braden Scale skin assessment scores
> - Review data to determine the effectiveness
>
> **Step 4: Evaluate the Effectiveness of Actions Taken**
> - Determine if results are satisfactory:
>   - Continue implementation, data measurement, and analysis
>   - Integrate and standardize best practices throughout the facility
> - Determine if results are not satisfactory:
>   - Identify issues blocking success
> - Report results to facility leadership
>
> **Step 5 Evaluate, Standardize, and Communicate**
> - Utilize Project Evaluation (Tool D.8)
>   - Focus on lessons learned
>   - Future planning
>   - Standardization of best practices
>
> *Source:* Taken from AHRQ's Toolkit for Using the Quality Indicators: https://www.ahrq.gov/patient-safety/settings/hospital/resource/qitool/index.html

The AHRQ serves as a leader in the development of evidence-based practice guidelines that can guide nursing staff and interdisciplinary healthcare team members to evaluate the quality of the care they provide using QIs. QIs have been developed to address the highest-risk and most costly clinical problems encountered in hospitals. DNPs can utilize these tools as they build their competencies in quality and patient safety improvements as well as lead organizations in utilizing these beneficial approaches and resources.

INSTITUTE OF HEALTHCARE IMPROVEMENT (IHI)

IHI was founded in 1991 and is grounded in quality improvement science. Edward Deming (1990–1993) led the development of improvement science and focused on adherence to principles of management (IHI, 2022a, 2022b, 2022c). Deming focused on statistical process control methods and a technique known as "profound knowledge" that became the first step to examining a system in order to improve it. This involved starting with "appreciation of the system," which includes different methods of data collection such as the use of run charts and control charts to identify variation, which Deming felt was the cause of errors and reduced quality (Peden, 2013). Rapid cycle testing in practice sites was developed to support the generation of new knowledge regarding the change within the context of care. Foundational elements of this type of testing included expert subject knowledge drawing from science, theory, psychology, and statistics.

Building on this foundation, the Associates in Process Improvement developed the *Model for Improvement* (Langley et al., 2009). This simple model has led the IHI's work in creating practical quality improvement methods that have supported sustainable changes in healthcare for over 30 years. The IHI has provided quality improvement education for interdisciplinary teams of healthcare providers, as well as coaching these teams to achieve some of the most significant demonstration projects that have led to healthcare reforms' successes. Specific aspects of the Model of Improvement can be found at: https://www.ihi.org/resources/Pages/HowtoImprove/default.aspx.

IHI Open School

The IHI offers training modules for quality and safety education within their Open School. Thirty-three modules are offered in the Open School to interprofessional teams and individuals covering the concepts of quality improvement and patient safety, with 1.5 continuing education credits for each lesson. The Open School is free to students and faculty and charges an annual fee to healthcare organizations. Participants of the Open School can obtain a Basic Quality and Safety Certificate upon completion of 13 specific lessons, which signals achievement of basic quality and safety education.

These modules are appropriate for all levels of nursing education and can be spread across the curriculum as a quality and safety thread that runs throughout a DNP program. Table 22.8 describes the Open School courses focused on quality improvement and patient safety Initiatives. These courses are free to faculty and students at https://www.ihi.org/education/ihi-open-school/Pages/default.aspx.

DNP faculty and students can also interact with interprofessional groups through the IHI Forums and through special initiatives such as the IHI Leadership Alliance. This collaboration of healthcare executives and their teams share a goal to work with one another as well as in partnership with patients, workforces, and communities to deliver on aspects of the IHI Triple Aim. More information regarding these opportunities for collaboration can be found at https://www.ihi.org/Engage/collaboratives/LeadershipAlliance/Pages/default.aspx.

IHI Quality Improvement

The IHI has led the country in the development of a model that guides the improvement of healthcare systems and accelerates improvements. This model has been used successfully by healthcare organizations throughout the world and the model and its tools have been adopted by many U.S. governmental agencies including the AHRQ.

TABLE 22.8 IHI Quality Improvement and Patient Safety Courses

QI 101: Introduction to Health Care Improvement
QI 102: How to Improve with the Model for Improvement
QI 103: Testing and Measuring Changes with PDSA Cycles
QI 104: Interpreting Data: Run Charts, Control Charts, and Other Measurement Tools
QI 105: Leading Quality Improvement
QI 201: Planning for Spread: From Local Improvements to System-Wide Change
QI 202: Addressing Small Problems to Build Safer, More Reliable Systems
L 103: Making Publishable QI Projects Part of Everyday Work
IHI Patient Safety Courses
PS 101: Introduction to Patient Safety
PS 102: From Error to Harm
PS 103: Human Factors and Safety
PS 104: Teamwork and Communication
PS 105: Responding to Adverse Events
PS 201: Root Cause Analyses and Actions Courses
PS 202: Achieving Total Systems Safety
PS 203: Pursuing Professional Accountability and a Just Culture

Source: Taken from the IHI Open School: https://education.ihi.org/topclass/searchCatalog.do?catId=0

The Model for Improvement was developed by Associates in Process Improvement and is a simple yet powerful tool for accelerating improvement in healthcare (Langley et al., 2009). The model asks three foundational questions, which can be asked in any order. To answer each question a specific action must be taken to define the improvement process. Table 22.9 describes the questions and the actions required.

Deming (2000) described the Plan-Do-Study-Act (PDSA) cycle to test changes in real work settings and it continues to be used in the IHI Model of Improvement to guide the test of a change to determine if the change is an improvement. The IHI provides tools that can be used in each step of this process in their Quality Improvement Essentials Toolkit (IHI, 2017), which can be found at https://www.ihi.org/resources/Pages/Tools/Quality-Improvement-Essentials-Toolkit.aspx. The DNP program curriculum includes courses in all elements of quality improvement and patient safety. Utilizing these widely accepted tools and processes can provide the DNP with the competencies they need to lead quality improvement initiatives in their organizations and practices.

IHI Patient Safety

The IHI has created a more effective way to identify events that do cause harm to patients and have created a selection of tools that can be used to enhance patient care safety. One important tool is Root Cause Analysis (RCA). This tool can be used by healthcare teams as they seek to understand and respond to the root causes of errors, in order to prevent future harm. A *root cause* is a latent vulnerability in a system that allows an incident to

TABLE 22.9 IHI Model for Improvement Foundational Questions

• What are we trying to accomplish?
o Action: Establishing Measurable Aims
• How will we know that a change is an improvement?
o Action: Establishing Measures
• What change can we make that will result in an improvement?
o Action: Selecting Change

occur (National Patient Safety Foundation, 2015). The key to solving a clinical problem in the long term is to truly understand the problem and the context in which it occurs. Otherwise, leaders are likely to focus on improvement efforts based on the symptom of the problem instead of real root causes.

The IHI provides healthcare organizations with the IHI Process: RCA^2: Improving Root Cause Analyses and Actions to Prevent Harm. This and its associated tools are available within the IHI Patient Safety Toolkit at the IHI website: https://www.ihi.org/resources/Pages/Tools/Patient-Safety-Essentials-Toolkit.aspx.

RCA development was led by the National Patient Safety Foundation (2015), which relabeled it as RCA^2 ("RCA squared") after panels of experts improved the RCA which now emphasizes consistency in the investigative process and focus on action plans that prevent future harm. The purpose of RCA^2 is to identify system vulnerabilities and implement strong actions that will eliminate or mitigate those vulnerabilities (National Patient Safety Foundation). Review teams strive to identify actions that prevent or minimize the chances of the event recurring and reduce the severity or consequences if it should recur. After a comprehensive investigation of root causes, including assessment of human factors and cognitive thinking, a tool such as the Action Hierarchy will assist teams in identifying which actions will have the strongest effect for successful and sustained system improvement. Table 22.10 describes the RCA^2 Process.

The IHI has created the Patient Safety Toolkit (IHI, 2019) to support the implementation of patient safety reviews including the RCA. These tools are described in the following section.

Cause-and-Effect Diagram

A cause-and-effect diagram is a tool used by organizations and teams to explore and identify the many causes that may contribute to an effect or outcome that is unwanted. This diagram also identifies the relationship between the cause and the effect and in doing so identifies areas for improvement. This tool is also known as the Ishikawa diagram for its creator. It is also known as the fishbone diagram. Specific categories of possible causes include materials, methods, equipment, environment, and people (IHI, 2019). Teams begin by identifying what outcome or effect they want to influence or change. They then generate lists of causes that contribute to these outcomes or effects for each category. They add these lists to the "fishbones" on the diagram. It is suggested that team members need to use the" 5 why's" approach until the needed level of detail is developed and the cause is defined enough to generate improvement strategies (IHI, 2019).

TABLE 22.10 RCA^2 Process

1. *Developing the RCA^2 team*
2. *Develop cause-and-effect diagram*
3. *Conduct "5 Why's" analysis*
4. *Create a flow diagram for the process involved in the error*
5. *Develop causal statements*
6. *Develop action plan, including strong and intermediate-strength action*
7. *Development measurement plan, including process and outcome measurements for action you have identified*

Source: National Patient Safety Foundation. (2015). *RCA2: Improving root cause analyses and actions to prevent harm.* https://www.ihi.org/resources/Pages/Tools/RCA2-Improving-Root-Cause-Analyses-and-Actions-to-Prevent-Harm.aspx

5 Why's to Finding the Root of the Problem

Taiichi Ohno, father of the Toyota Production System (IHI, 2019), which revolutionized automobile manufacturing with methods now known as *Lean*, developed this approach that assists teams to identify the root cause(s) of a problem by asking "Why?" and then to keep on asking it, at least five times (IHI, 2019). Ask "Why did this happen?" and then, don't stop at the answer to this first question. Ask "Why?" again and again, until you reach the root cause (IHI Patient Safety Toolkit).

Flowchart

Creating a flowchart is useful in a variety of patient safety activities, such as developing reliable processes and in the investigation of root cause development (IHI, 2019). Flowcharts are visual representations of steps in a process so therefore it is important to include team members who know the process well and can discuss how it works. This process not only allows all team members to learn more about the process but also helps them identify how changes can take place that lead to improvement. Brainstorming can be used by team members as they identify all of the steps in a process as it currently exists. Often one team member is responsible for creating the flowchart by using sticky notes to represent each step in the process. The flowchart tool provides symbols to indicate the start and end of the process, decision-making (yes/no question), activity or task, and the flow line (IHI Patient Safety Toolkit). The final flowchart should be reviewed for accuracy and updated as needed, as changes occur (IHI, 2019).

Developing Reliable Processes

This tool supports the development of reliable patient care processes that focus on reducing defects and increasing consistency, which will result in improved patient outcomes. This is achieved through the implementation of four steps: segmentation, visualization, standardization/simplification, and backup planning (IHI, 2019).

Segmentation is the first step and involves a segment of the population to begin testing the process. This allows teams to design processes for population segments and then move to another population and customize as needed (IHI, 2019). The second step, visualization, involves developing a representation of the sequence of steps, which most commonly involves a flow chart (IHI, 2019). This process helps identify each step of the process and identify points of vulnerability and potential errors. The third step of standardizing involves a review of the process steps to ensure they are based on roles and not dependent on specific staff, and are clearly defined. The fourth and last step involves the development of a backup plan to replace the new process being proposed if it is necessary to safeguard patients and staff. This process works best with processes that are not developed due to a significant error that could place patients in immediate jeopardy.

Failure Modes and Effects Analysis (FMEA)

FMEA is used when a new process is being developed that has the potential to cause harm to patients and/or staff. This tool provides a systematic analysis of this process and asks team members to participate in the following steps:

1. Failure Modes: What could go wrong?
2. Failure Causes: Why would the failure happen?
3. Failure Effects: What would be the consequences of each failure?

TABLE 22.11 Failure Modes and Effects Analysis Chart

Steps in the process	Failure Mode	Failure Cause	Failure Effect	Likelihood of Occurrence (1–10)	Likelihood of Detection (1–10)	Severity Severity (1–10)	Risk Profile Number	Actions to Reduce Occurrence of Failure
Step 1 Step 2								

Source: IHI Patient Safety Toolkit: https://www.ihi.org/resources/Pages/Tools/Patient-Safety-Essentials-Toolkit.aspx.

Team members contribute to the development of a flowchart that lists every mutually agreed-upon step in the process. They then create a table with a matrix of each step listed in the first column and each of the steps listed as the next three column headers (Table 22.11).

If the FMEA indicates a failure mode is likely to occur, team members should investigate the causes and eliminate those steps or components if possible. Consider the development of forcing functions, which is the addition of a physical constraint to the process that makes committing the error impossible. An example is the medical gas outlets that are designed to accept only gauges that match the medical gas. Verification, or a double-checking system, is also a possible action to reduce the cause of the failure.

Five Rules of Causation Statements

Through completion of the IHI tools of the Cause and Effect Diagram, 5 Why's, and the Flowchart, the RCA team will identify system and process vulnerabilities that are root causes of the sentinel event that has occurred. The *RCA²* process (National Patient Safety Foundation, 2015) describes the use of the *Five Rules of Causation* to communicate these findings. By applying the rules of causation, the result is a causal statement that will focus on correcting the system issues identified. The five rules of causation outlined in the *RCA²* are:

Rule 1: Clearly show the "cause and effect" relationship.
Example: A high volume of activity and noise in the emergency department led to (cause) the nurse being distracted when withdrawing the correct dose of a medication from a multidose vial.
INCORRECT: The ED is too loud.
CORRECT: The nurse had to withdraw medication from a multidose vial in an open area of the ED, increasing the likelihood that the dose would be incorrect.

Rule 2. Use specific and accurate descriptors for what occurred, rather than negative and vague words. Avoid negative descriptors such as: Poor; Inadequate; Wrong; Bad; Failed; Careless.
INCORRECT: The nurse was careless in her medication withdrawal technique.
CORRECT: The use of multidose vials for medications increases the opportunity for dosage errors.

Rule 3. Human errors must have a preceding cause.
INCORRECT: The nurse withdrew the wrong dose, which led to the patient being overdosed.
CORRECT: Medication administration for a medication supplied with a multidose vial requiring calculation of the correct dosage and withdrawal of the correct amount of

medication using a syringe necessitates a quiet environment for the nurse to perform a proper calculation and withdrawal of medication.

Rule 4. Violations of procedure are not root causes, but must have a preceding cause.

INCORRECT: The nurse did not follow the correct procedure for medication withdrawal from a multidose vial, which led to the patient receiving an overdose of the medication.

CORRECT: Noise and confusion in the ED medication prep area, coupled with the amount of time needed to calculate the correct dosage and withdraw the correct medication, increased the likelihood that the medication would not be the correct dose, resulting in the injection of an incorrect dose of a medication.

Rule 5. Failure to act is only causal when there is a preexisting duty to act.

INCORRECT: The nurse did not check the medication supplies at the start of her shift.

CORRECT: The presence of a multidose vial for a medication that is commonly provided in prefilled syringes was not known to the RN assigned to prepare the medication, which increased the likelihood that the medication dose would be incorrect, which led to an overdose of the medication to the patient.

The development of the RCA's *Causal Statement* is a critical step toward the correct identification of the root cause of the adverse event and the improvement of patient processes to reduce harm in the future. The final steps of the RCA include developing the action plan, including strong and intermediate-strength actions, and developing a measurement plan, including process and outcome measurements. These steps will assure the implementation of corrective action that will reduce repeated errors and create a safer patient care environment.

Preparation in this important process is critical to an organization's quality and patient safety programs. Hospital and other healthcare organizations have accrediting organizations that can assist them in maintaining safe and effective healthcare practices as well as safe environments of care. The Joint Commission is widely accepted as providing the most prominent and accepted quality and safety accreditation of healthcare organizations.

THE JOINT COMMISSION (TJC)

The Joint Commission (TJC), formerly known as the Joint Commission for Accreditation of Healthcare Organizations (JCAHO) was created in 1951 and is an independent, not-for-profit organization that accredits more than 20,000 U.S. healthcare programs and organizations (TJC, 2022a). TJC's mission is to ensure quality healthcare for patients, prevent harm, and improve patient advocacy (TJC). The Joint Commission standards emphasize the establishment of a consistent approach to clinical practice to reduce the risk of errors.

Currently, there are 250 accreditation standards, covering infection control medication safety, error prevention, and management, including reporting (TJC, 2022b). They also include staff credentialing, emergency management, patient rights, privacy, and education. Healthcare organizations are not required to be accredited by TJC, but if they do not have it or have lost it, they will lose their ability to bill federal payers, including Medicare and Medicaid. This would create a large financial burden for the organization. A hospital with no accreditation could still technically admit patients, as long as they have a state license, but there would be no way for them to collect payments for their largest third-party reimbursement source.

Patient safety is a major area of focus of TJC and they create annual National Patient Safety Goals for each of the nine healthcare organizations they accredit including:

- Ambulatory Health Care
- Assisted Living Communities
- Behavioral Health Care
- Critical Access Hospitals
- Home Care
- Hospital
- Laboratory
- Nursing Care Center
- Office-Based Surgery

The 2023 Hospital National Patient Safety Goals are described in Table 22.12 and include TJC standards that relate to that goal.

Sentinel Events (SE)

The Joint Commission created the formal Sentinel Event Policy for hospitals in 1996 that was designed to assist hospitals in the investigation of serious adverse events. The policy standardized the investigation and analysis of these patient safety events and assisted organizations in identifying needed system improvements that could reduce their occurrence.

TABLE 22.12 2023 Hospital National Patient Safety Goals

Patient Safety Goals	TJC Standard	Example
1. Identify Patients Correctly	NPSG.01.01.01	Use at least two ways to identify patients. For example, use the patient's name and date of birth. This is done to make sure that each patient gets the correct medicine and treatment.
2. Prevent Infections	NPSG.07.01.01	Use the hand-cleaning guidelines from the Centers for Disease Control and Prevention or the World Health Organization. Set goals for improving hand cleaning. Use the goals to improve hand cleaning.
3. Improve Staff Communication	NPSG.02.03.01	Get important test results to the right staff person on time.
4. Identify Patient Safety Risks	NPSG.15.01.01	Reduce the risk of suicide.
5. Prevent Mistakes in Surgery	UP.01.01.01	Make sure that the correct surgery is done on the correct patient and at the correct place on the patient's body.
	UP.01.02.01	Mark the correct place on the patient's body where the surgery is to be done.
	UP.01.03.01	Pause before the surgery to make sure that a mistake is not being made.

(continued)

TABLE 22.12 2023 Hospital National Patient Safety Goals (*continued*)

Patient Safety Goals	TJC Standard	Example
6. Use Medicines Safely	NPSG.03.04.01	Before a procedure, label medicines that are not labeled. For example, medicines in syringes, cups, and basins. Do this in the area where medicines and supplies are set up.
	NPSG.03.05.01	Take extra care with patients who take medicines to thin their blood.
	NPSG.03.06.01	Record and pass along correct information about a patient's medicines. Find out what medicines the patient is taking. Compare those medicines to new medicines given to the patient. Give the patient written information about the medicines they need to take. Tell the patient it is important to bring their up-to-date list of medicines every time they visit a doctor.
7. Use Alarms safely	NPSG.06.01.01	Make improvements to ensure that alarms on medical equipment are heard and responded to on time.

Source: The Joint Commission, https://www.jointcommission.org/standards/national-patient-safety-goals

The SE Policy defines a patient safety event as occurring outside of the natural course of the patient's illness or underlying condition and results in any *death, permanent harm, or severe temporary harm (TJC, 2022)*. Other events that are considered sentinel include the suicide of a patient in a facility staffed around the clock or within 72 hours of discharge, the unanticipated death of a full-term infant, the discharge of an infant to the wrong family, and abduction.

Accredited healthcare organizations are strongly encouraged, but not required, to report sentinel events to The Joint Commission. If the organization determines there is a sentinal event according to the SE policy, they are expected to notify the Office of Quality and Patient Safety (OQPS) of the type of SE that has occurred. Table 22.13 defines the steps an organization should take following a sentinel event.

TABLE 22.13 Sentinel Event Review Timeline

1. At the time of the patient safety event, notifies and mutually agrees with the Office of Quality and Patient Safety (OQPS) that a sentinel event has occurred.
2. Within 5 days of the sentinel event the organization notifies the Office of Quality and Patient Safety.
3. Prepare a thorough and credible comprehensive systematic analysis and corrective action plan within 45 business days of the event or of becoming aware of the event.
4. Submit its comprehensive systematic analysis and corrective action plan to The Joint Commission, or otherwise provide its response to the sentinel event using an approved methodology within 45 business days of the known occurrence of the event for Joint Commission evaluation.
5. Joint Commission OQPS staff will conduct a collaborative review with the organization's leadership or designee to determine whether the analysis and action plan is acceptable.

Source: The Joint Commission. (2022). Sentinel Event Policy.

The occurrence of an SE will not jeopardize an organization's accreditation status. But if the organization fails to respond to the SE appropriately the accreditation decision may be affected. The comprehensive systematic analysis is expected to identify the causal and contributory factors to any known sentinel event. A root cause analysis is one common type of comprehensive systematic analysis. The National Patient Safety Foundation has merged with IHI to provide guidance and support for the use of the RCA^2: Each organization can, however, determine its own internal process, tools, and methodologies to conduct the comprehensive analysis.

These methods must address the required questions presented in The Joint Commission's Framework for Root Cause Analysis and Corrective Actions form (TJC, 2022) that must be submitted within the 45 business days following the SE. This analysis should identify system vulnerabilities that can be eliminated or improved and not focus on identical healthcare workers' performance.

The Corrective Action Plan must include identifying corrective actions that will eliminate or reduce system hazards or vulnerabilities, as well as who is responsible for implementing these actions. Timelines and strategies for evaluating the effectiveness of the corrective actions are also included in the plan, as well as strategies to support and sustain the changes made.

The Joint Commission will review the submission of the comprehensive review and determine if the review was complete and if the corrective actions are acceptable. The OQPS will continue to monitor and support organizations in the completion of their corrective actions and their evaluations. The Joint Commission also collects and analyzes aggregate data from all SE reviews and action plans and maintains a database that is used to develop risk reduction strategies and advice for healthcare organizations. This information is disseminated through Sentinel Events Alerts and the Annual National Patient Safety Goals.

The goals of TJC are to ensure quality healthcare for patients, prevent harm and improve patient advocacy, and have created a system of standards that emphasize the consistent approaches to clinical practice and fair and equitable patient safety policies and processes as they support improved quality and reduction of errors.

CHAPTER SUMMARY

The nursing profession is assuming leadership in the transformation of healthcare delivery and quality improvement through the introduction of DNPs in both clinical and leadership roles. DNPs have been acknowledged by healthcare leaders for their respectability and reliability, particularly in the areas of QI and patient safety. Nursing organizations such as the AACN are leading the way in defining competencies for advanced, level nurses regarding leadership in quality improvement and patient safety. The NONPF has called for the adoption of the DNP as the terminal degree for nurse practitioners in 2025 in keeping with these expanded competencies and the national initiatives in QI and patient safety.

This chapter has sought to summarize the driving forces and significant events of the past 20 years that created the key national initiatives pertinent to the transformation of the U.S. healthcare system. Central to this healthcare transformation has been the development of health information technology, quality, and safety processes, and data-driven approaches related to monitoring and improving the quality of care provided in hospitals, primary care, and ambulatory services.

Underlying these efforts is the recognition that nursing, as well as all other healthcare professionals, must reduce the focus of discipline-specific strategies and approaches to quality and in its place recognize the interdisciplinary nature of healthcare delivery. With this recognition, the development of healthcare team strategies and approaches could realize the goals of healthcare reform through successful improvement of the quality of healthcare delivery, and create safe and effective systems of healthcare that meet the needs of patients and providers.

The DNP graduate is well-positioned to lead these efforts and add nursing's unique perspective to the transformation. Nurses at the level of the professional practice doctorate can and should be instrumental in the development of system-level changes that result in improved quality of care and increased patient safety in our increasingly complex healthcare system. It is clear that the collection and reporting of quality and safety measures are complicated and require oversight by someone with highly specialized expertise; a role that seems to describe a DNP. The range of competencies within the DNP's scope and expertise has expanded to included interpreting the data, discerning trends, understanding variation in the data and what it means, determining what and how to improve, and how to work with multidisciplinary teams to create integrated models of improvement that will yield improved patient outcomes. DNPs can create and implement innovative quality and safety programs that promote a culture of safety and quality. The next 20 years in healthcare quality and patient safety improvement will be defined by DNPs who have the knowledge and competency needed in healthcare practice and leadership.

CASE STUDY: MANAGEMENT OF A SENTINEL EVENT USING THE RCA^2 IN A HOSPITAL SETTING

(Disclaimer: This case has been adapted from the RaDonda Vaught case in Nashville, TN.)

Ronda Vaughn, RN, works for an understaffed hospital. On her current shift, she is a "float nurse" moving between units to provide care as needed. While in a surgical step-down unit, she gets a call to provide an anxious patient in radiology with a sedative medication prior to him getting an MRI. Ronda knows that the medication is not stocked on the radiology floor; she plans to withdraw the medication from the automatic dispensing cabinet (ADC) on her current floor and bring it to radiology, where the patient is waiting. At the same time, Ronda has been called to an overloaded ER to care for patients there. (Ronda later tells investigators that she was distracted and rushed by multiple duties at the time.) Because the order from the pharmacy had not yet been transferred to the ADC due to technological delays, Ronda had to select the medication manually. (Ronda later tells investigators that this was a common problem, and that many "workarounds" were needed to avoid technological delays and to keep units running smoothly.) Ronda quickly types the first two letters of the brand name of the medication into the ADC, forgetting that the ADC is programmed according to generic medication names. As a result, the incorrect medication appears on the screen—a paralytic agent—and Ronda fails to notice. She quickly clicks through four warnings, indicating that she is about to withdraw a paralytic drug, and withdraws it instead of the sedative. (Ronda later says to investigators that this was a case of "alarm fatigue," given the over-prevalence of warnings on the ADC.) She walks to the radiology floor and looks for the computer to scan the drug and patient's bracelet, per hospital policy, which would confirm the correct medication. Unable to locate a computer/scanner in the radiology department, she administers the drug, failing to look at the vial before doing so, on which both the drug name and "Warning: paralytic agent" are clearly printed. (Ronda later admits that she had become "complacent" and had simply assumed without checking that she had withdrawn the correct medication.) After administering the drug, Ronda immediately goes to the ER, leaving the patient alone. (Ronda later testifies that to her knowledge, the hospital had no policy to monitor patients receiving the sedative drug in question.) The patient suffers respiratory failure several minutes later, and after severe anoxic brain damage, is taken off life-support the next day.

As the chief quality officer, Dr. Julia Kale is notified of this patient's death. After gathering the details of these events, Dr. Kale notifies The Joint Commission's Office of Quality and Patient Safety (OQPS) and determines that this is considered a sentinel event. Dr. Kale discusses the TJC's Sentinel Event Policy and reviews the timeline for reporting with the OQPS manager. Dr. Kale notifies the hospital's leadership team and advises them of the steps and processes involved in completing the Comprehensive Systematic Analysis and Corrective Action Plan.

As a DNP, Dr. Kale is knowledgeable in the TJC's hospital's sentinel event protocols and the RCA² Process and tools. Dr. Kale initiates the following steps:

1. Convene the RCA² Team

Dr. Kale recognizes that event reviews should be initiated promptly and scheduled the RCA² team meeting within 48 hours of the event. The goal is to complete all RCA²-type activities within 30 days of the event. She will schedule three to four team meetings to complete the RCA² process. She schedules meetings 1.5 to 2 hours in length, with work time planned for individual members to complete interviews or locate and review publications and documents. She invites six team members that include herself as chief quality officer, the director of nursing, the patient representative, the charge nurse from the department involved, and two experienced frontline staff from the area involved (but not staff involved in the event). Dr. Kale informs the team members that their responsibilities will include attending meetings, conducting research and interviews, and identifying root cause contributing factors utilizing the IHI tools. They will also make the determination of the findings and recommendations that will be submitted to TJC.

2. Conduct the Comprehensive, Systematic Analysis
"5 WHY'S" ANALYSIS FINDINGS

Dr. Kale leads the team in creating a problem statement regarding the sentinel event (SE) and then as the question "Why?" until they feel the root cause or contributing factors have been identified

Problem Statement: A patient received the wrong medication, which was a high-risk paralytic drug, instead of the correct medication and was unattended when he went into respiratory failure several minutes later, suffered severe anoxic brain damage, and was taken off life-support the next day.

Why 1: Why did the patient receive the wrong medication?

Answer 1: Because the float nurse was not familiar with the environment (Radiology procedure room) that did not have a patient ID scanner. She ignored the ADC warnings for a paralytic medication and did not double-check the medication when she was unable to scan it. She did not double-check that it was the right medication and the right dose for the right patient and after giving the medication she left the patient alone

Why 2: Why did the nurse fail to double-check the medication when scanning was unavailable, and not monitor the patient after administering the medication?

Answer 2: Because the nurse was distracted and complacent due to being pulled to a new area of the hospital that did not have the appropriate equipment (ID scanner).

Why 3: Why was she distracted and complacent?

Answer 3: **Because the hospital was improperly staffed and the float nurse did not have the equipment she needed (ID scanner) and she admitted she had become complacent due to overwork and alarm fatigue.** She also was not aware of a policy of monitoring patients after giving them sedatives.

The team identified the root causes (in bold) that emerge even before five "why's" were asked—in this case, only three were necessary. This was the first step toward finding systemic solutions designed to prevent similar errors from occurring in the future.

3. Develop Cause-and-Effect Diagram

The team utilized the process of identifying contributing factors in this case by reviewing the materials, methods, equipment, environment, and people in a cause-and-effect diagram. Their findings were as follows:

Materials & Equipment: Lack of scanning equipment in the radiology department.

Methods: Lack of policies and procedures requiring monitoring of sedated patients and double-checking of unscanned medication.

Environment: Overworked and understaffed hospital, leading to distractions and undue time pressure.

People: Complacency on the part of the nurse in response to lack of appropriate materials/equipment, methods, and environmental factors involving "alarm fatigue."

These findings supported the findings of the 5 Why's process and did not warrant the development of a flow diagram.

4. Develop Causal Statements

The team determined there were four causal statements:

#1 There was no patient scanner in the radiology procedure room, which increased the likelihood that the patient's identification and drug order would not be available, and a drug error would occur.

#2 Distraction and alarm fatigue exist in nursing units when nurses are verifying new orders and accessing the ADC, which increases the likelihood that the nurse may override an ADC alert and select the wrong medication and dose.

#3 There was no policy or procedures requiring monitoring of sedated patients after sedation is given, which increased the likelihood that the patient who has a severe reaction would not receive timely emergency care.

#4 Nursing staffing practices that involve the use of float nurses and assigning nurses to unfamiliar environments and clinical procedures without orientation and supervision increase the likelihood that medication errors and inadequate patient supervision would occur.

The team held further discussions regarding the individual responsibility of nurses which they felt was compatible with both RCA (even if that's not its focus), and the underlying *just culture* on which it has an ethical foundation (Reason, 1997). The concept of just culture looks for systemic causes that avoid blaming individual nurses, unless the error was in some way intentional, as does the RCA^2 process. This is a valuable and important approach not only because systemic causes are *present* in adverse events and errors and are often the *primary* root cause (if not the only root cause), but because such a culture is vital for clinicians to feel free to report their own errors as well as those of their colleagues, due to its nonpunitive nature (Marx, 2001).

Further team meetings led to the completion of the comprehensive systematic analysis and action plan and review by stakeholders. The facility sent the report to TJC within 45 days after the SE.

CRITICAL THINKING QUESTIONS

1. What is the DNP's role with respect to quality and safety in nursing? Should DNP curricula have more of an emphasis on quality and safety?
2. Does the educational preparation of nurses have an impact on quality and safety? How should nurse leaders address educational preparation at their respective institutions?
3. How does the DNP-prepared chief nursing officer lead a continuous quality improvement organization with a focus on safety?
4. The DaRhonda Vaught case, on which the chapter case study is based, is a former Vanderbilt nurse who committed a fatal medication error, highlighted nurse accountability. Give an example of a policy or practice that promotes patient safety and reduces medical errors.
5. Are physicians and nurses treated equally with respect to consequences for medical errors?

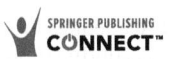

A robust set of instructor resources designed to supplement this text is located at http://connect.springerpub.com/content/book/978-0-8261-8137-4. Qualifying instructors may request access by emailing textbook@springerpub.com.

REFERENCES

Agency for Healthcare Research and Quality. (2014). *Quality indicators toolkit for hospitals*. http://www.ahrq.gov/professionals/systems/hospital/qitoolkit/index.html

Agency for Healthcare Research and Quality. (2022). *Offices, centers, and programs*. https://www.ahrq.gov/cpi/index.html

American Academy of Nurse Practitioners. (2022). *NP fact sheet*. https://www.aanp.org/about/all-about-nps/np-fact-sheet

American Association of Colleges of Nursing. (2015a). *Report from the task force on the implementation of the DNP*. http://www.aacn.nche.edu/news/articles/2015/dnp-white-paper

American Association of Colleges of Nursing. (2015b). *AACN QSEN modules*. https://www.aacnnursing.org/Faculty/Teaching-Resources/QSEN/QSEN-Learning-Module-Series

American Association of Colleges of Nursing. (2021). *The essentials: Core competencies for professional nursing education*. https://www.aacnnursing.org/Essentials

Auerbach, D. I., Martsolf, G. R., Pearson, M. L., Taylor, E. A., Zaydman, M, Muchow, A. N., Spetz, J., & Lee Y. (2015). The DNP by 2015: A study of the institutional, political, and professional issues that facilitate or impede establishing a post-baccalaureate doctor of nursing practice program. *Rand Health Q*, 5(1), 3.

Beeber, A. S., Palmer, C, Waldrop, J., Lynn, M. R., & Jones, C. B. (2019). The role of doctor of nursing practice-prepared nurses in practice settings. *Nursing Outlook*, 67(4), 354–364. https://doi.org/10.1016/j.outlook.2019.02.006

Carraccio, C., Englander, R., Gilhooly, J., Mink, R., Hofkosh, D., Barone, M. A., & Holmboe, E. S. (2017). Building a framework of entrustable professional activities, Supported by competencies and milestones, to bridge the educational continuum. *Academic Medicine*, 92(3), 324–330. https://doi.org/10.1097/ACM.0000000000001141

Center for Medicare & Medicaid Innovation. (2022). *Synthesis of evaluation across 21 Medicare models*. https://www.cms.gov/priorities/innovation/data-and-reports/2022/wp-eval-synthesis-21models-slides

Center for Medicaid and Medicare Services. (2022a). *Care-compare*. https://www.medicare.gov/care-compare
Center for Medicaid and Medicare Services. (2022b). *QualityNet*. https://qualitynet.cms.gov
Center for Medicaid and Medicare Services. (2022c) *Center of Innovation*. https://innovation.cms.gov
Deming, W. E. (2000). *The new economics for industry, government, and education*. The MIT Press.
Department of Health and Human Services. (2009). *HITECH final rule*. https://www.hhs.gov/hipaa/for-professionals/special-topics/hitech-act-enforcement-interim-final-rule/index.html
Department of Health and Human Services. (2010). *The Affordable Care Act, section by section*. http://www.hhs.gov/healthcare/rights/law/index.html
Englander, R., Cameron, T., Ballard, A., Dodge, J., Bull, J., & Aschenbrener, C. (2013). Toward a common taxonomy of competency domains for the health professions and competencies for physicians. *Academic Medicine*, *88*(8), 1088–1094. https://www.aacnnursing.org/Portals/42/Downloads/Essentials/Englander-2013.pdf
Gold, M., & McLaughlin, C. (2016). Assessing HITECH implementation and lessons: 5 years later. *Milbank Quarterly*, *94*(3), 654–687. https://doi.org/10.1111/1468-0009.12214
Institute for Healthcare Improvement. (2019). *Patient safety essentials toolkit*. https://www.ihi.org/resources/Pages/Tools/Patient-Safety-Essentials-Toolkit.aspx
Institute for Healthcare Improvement. (2022a). *About IHI*. https://my.ihi.org/portal/content/knowledge/openschool-courses.aspx
Institute for Healthcare Improvement. (2022b). *How to improve*. https://www.ihi.org/resources/Pages/HowtoImprove/default.aspx
Institute for Healthcare Improvement. (2022c). *Open school*. http://www.ihi.org/education/ihiopenschool/Pages/default.aspx
Institute of Medicine. (2001). *Crossing the quality chasm*. National Academies Press. https://pubmed.ncbi.nlm.nih.gov/25057539
Institute of Medicine. (2003). *Health professional education: A bridge to quality*. National Academies Press. https://pubmed.ncbi.nlm.nih.gov/25057657/#:~:text=Health%20Professions%20Education%3A%20A%20Bridge%20to%20Quality%20is%20the%20follow,competencies%20into%20health%20professions%20education.
Institute of Medicine. (2010). *The future of nursing: Leading change, advancing health*. National Academies Press. http://www.thefutureofnursing.org/sites/default/files/Future%20of%20Nursing%20Report_0.pdf
Langley, G. L., Moen, R., Nolan, K. M., Nolan, T. W., Norman, C. L., & Provost, L. P. (2009). *The improvement guide: A practical approach to enhancing organizational performance*, (2nd ed.). Jossey-Bass Publishers.
Marx, D. (2001). *Patient safety and the "just culture": A primer for healthcare executives*. Columbia University.
National Academies of Sciences, Engineering, and Medicine & National Academy of Medicine. (2021). *Committee on the future of nursing 2020–2030*. National Academies Press.
National Patient Safety Foundation. (2015). *RCA2: Improving root cause analyses and actions to prevent harm*. https://www.ihi.org/resources/Pages/Tools/RCA2-Improving-Root-Cause-Analyses-and-Actions-to-Prevent-Harm.aspx
Peden, C. (2013).The science and history of improvement. *Raising the standard: A compendium of audit recipes*, (3rd ed., pp 23–24). Royal College of Anaesthetists.
QSEN Institute. (2022). *Quality and safety education for nurses*. https://qsen.org
Reason, J. (1997). *Managing the risks of organizational accidents*. Routledge.
Sherwood G. (2021) Quality and safety education for nurses: Making progress in patient safety, learning from COVID-19. *International Journal of Nursing Sciences*. *8*(3), 249–251. https://doi.org/10.1016/j.ijnss.2021.05.009
The Joint Commission. (2022a). *Who are we?* https://www.jointcommission.org/who-we-are
The Joint Commission. (2022b). *Sentinel event policy and procedures* https://www.jointcommission.org/resources/sentinel-event/sentinel-event-policy-and-procedures
Wong, B., Baum, K., Headrick, E., Holmboe, S., Moss, F., Ogrinc, G., Shojania. K., Vaux, K., Warm, E., & Frank, J. (2020). Building the bridge to quality: An urgent call to integrate quality improvement and patient safety education with clinical care. *Academic Medicine*, *95*(1), 59–68. https://doi.org/10.1097/ACM.0000000000002937

CHAPTER TWENTY-TWO
Reflective Response

PAULA F. COE

This chapter on "The Role of the DNP in Quality Improvement and Patient Safety Initiatives," provides some great constructs of the role of the DNP in this particular sphere of nursing practice. As a practicing nurse with a DNP for over 8 years, it is my firm opinion that quality and safety are the most important spheres of my practice to influence not only entry-level nurses but also advanced-level nurses and nurse leaders on the importance of nursing practice initiatives and their relationship to outcomes in our respective institutions. To me it has always been the ability of the DNP to connect the dots for the bedside nurse as to the "why" they are doing certain procedures, tasks, and following best practices, and how they impact practice outcomes.

When nurses, quality improvement initiatives address patient outcomes in a positive way, real quality improvement takes place, and the outcomes are achieved. Many healthcare organizations are on the journey to nursing excellence seeking to achieve the prestigious American Nurses Credentialing Center Magnet® Designation. The empirical outcomes of nursing-sensitive indicators are a measure of performance that one needs to achieve in which to be successful in this endeavor. The role of the DNP-prepared nurse is pivotal to organizations receiving this recognition whether they are in the role of Magnet program direct or, director of nursing practice/education, or in other interprofessional roles in quality and safety. The DNP curriculum allows students to learn theories and practice that inform quality improvement structures and processes. Whether it be LEAN methodology, Six Sigma Training, Operational Excellence, or Plan, Do , Study, Act, having the knowledge, skills, and ability to teach and also guide nurses in these practices is critical in the role of the DNP-prepared nurse.

There is no doubt that the Radonda Vaught case and associated criminal charges had an impact across the healthcare continuum and especially on nurses regarding the impact of patient safety. Many hospitals and organizations took a critical look at compliance audits of their medication administration structures and processes, much like my organization did. Annual Culture of Safety Surveys inform nurse leaders of the opinion of the nursing staff regarding their perceptions of the punitive response to errors when they are made. Often there is a disparity between the leaders' perspective and response to errors versus bedside staff response. Using a model such as just culture (Marx, 2001) and having an algorithm to follow sets the expectation on all sides regarding how patient safety events and errors are responded to equitably and fairly. The role of the DNP-prepared nurse is paramount to the impact of quality and patient safety in the healthcare environment. Advanced practice providers educated at the doctoral level have an opportunity to shape the future of healthcare and specifically nursing practice across the continuum of care.

REFERENCES

Marx, D. (2001). *Patient safety and the "just culture": A primer for healthcare executives.* Columbia University

CHAPTER TWENTY-THREE

Stories of Successful Career Advancement Roles by DNP Graduates

TAMMY SLATER, VANESSA BATTISTA, JESSICA PETERS, LAURA O'ROURKE, AND VALERIE T. COTTER

CLINICAL PRACTICE/ADMINISTRATION ROLES

Vanessa Battista

I will be honest in saying that I was not "born to be a nurse." In fact, from an early age, I aspired to be a pediatrician. I always knew that I wanted to work in healthcare and with children and so I set my heart on becoming a medical doctor. It did not take long for me to realize in my freshman year at Boston College, however, that being a biology major and ultimately pursuing a career in medicine was not for me. I knew I still wanted to work with children in a healthcare setting but I was not sure exactly how and so I went to the career center on campus to explore my options. What ensued was a series of aptitude tests that all suggested a career in nursing, and I thought the tests were completely wrong as there was no way that I wanted to be a nurse; instead, I became a psychology major with the hopes of becoming a child psychologist. At the time, I erroneously was not aware that nursing offered more than wearing white, changing bed pans, and taking vital signs at the bedside.

Following my undergraduate education, I spent a year doing volunteer work as a case manager for abused children through the Jesuit Volunteer Corps (JVC) and part of my role was taking the children living in the shelter to their medical appointments. As such, I had my first experience working with a psychiatric nurse practitioner and was immediately enthralled by her ability to provide both therapeutic interventions and prescribe medications for children. Suddenly, a whole new vision of nursing was made clear to me, and I realized that maybe I did have a natural inclination to be a nurse. After completing my year as a Jesuit Volunteer, I knew that I wanted to return to graduate school, yet I was not entirely sure of the exact path I wanted to take. Pursuing my ongoing desire to work in a clinical setting, I landed my first job as a clinical research assistant working at the Eleanor and Lou Gehrig ALS Center at Columbia University where my immediate supervisor was a psychiatric and palliative care nurse practitioner. The rest, as they say, is history.

I thoroughly enjoyed my job as a clinical research assistant and went on to become a clinical research coordinator, serving to coordinate clinical trials for patients across multiple institutions. I found my work very gratifying and loved every minute of being with patients and was soon invited to lead the patient support group. It was during this time that I knew that I wanted to become a nurse and I remember writing my nursing school application describing how I wanted to hear people's stories to be a part of their illness journeys. With a supportive team behind me, I simultaneously switched to a position as a research coordinator in pediatrics and began nursing school at Columbia University with the goal to ultimately become a pediatric nurse practitioner (PNP). Three and a half years later, I proudly became the first person in my family to earn a master's degree and graduated as a PNP with a focus in behavioral health and palliative care, proving nearly a decade later that those aptitude tests actually were on to something.

While I was completing my master's studies I started to work as a research nurse in the pediatric neuromuscular center and then I assumed the role of PNP in the clinic when I finished my studies. I feel fortunate that my educational pursuits took place within an academic medical center and that I was steeped in an environment where clinical research was at the forefront and academic endeavors were highly valued. It was not uncommon for my days to include some combination of educational lectures, patient care, clinical trial visits, and stimulating conversations both with colleagues and with families. Pediatric palliative care (PPC) soon became my passion as there were not any treatments available for pediatric neuromuscular diseases and palliative care seemed like the natural way to support families as they made decisions about options for their children's care, yet my colleagues did not always consider it to be an acceptable service to offer to families. It was then that I learned that it was up to me to teach my team about PPC and how it was not synonymous with "giving up."

For me, PPC immediately felt like home as it brought together all my professional interests across the physical, emotional, social, psychological, and spiritual realms of care. I began to give informal presentations to our team to teach them how PPC was about making decisions and supporting families and not only about the end of life. I was invited to serve on the hospital's PPC committee and my desire to teach in a burgeoning field continued to grow stronger. PPC was a relatively new field at the time, and I remember one of my mentors telling me how exciting it was that I would get to be a part of moving the field forward. While I found this prospect thrilling, I also knew that it would soon be time for me to head back to school.

I did go back to school; in fact, I returned to Boston College, except this time I was a teacher and not yet a returning student. I was hired under a grant as a clinical faculty member to help build a PPC program in the School of Nursing and because patient care remained part of my passion and was at the root of clinical teaching, I also maintained a clinical practice. I quickly learned that I had a passion for teaching as I began to develop a curriculum and to teach in both the didactic and clinical settings, yet even as I began to teach, I still had a penchant for learning. I soon enrolled as a pastoral ministry student in the School of Theology and Ministry and began to audit doctoral nursing courses while continuing the ongoing debate of whether to enter a PhD or a DNP program. Although the question remained as to which degree I would pursue, I knew that, undoubtedly, I would earn a doctoral degree in nursing. Upon the conclusion of the teaching grant at Boston College, I continued to teach intermittently and returned to full-time clinical practice as a PPC nurse practitioner, as caring for patients was truly my passion. Ultimately, I knew that I wanted to be a leader, I wanted to teach nursing students, I wanted to implement clinical changes, and I wanted to remain an expert clinician and thus, it was clear that becoming a DNP was the right path for me.

A few years later, I excitedly enrolled in the Executive DNP and MBA program at Johns Hopkins University as part of the inaugural dual degree class. Given the nature of the Executive program, I fortunately was able to maintain a full-time clinical practice while pursuing my studies, although I soon learned that this was not for the faint of heart. The program was arduous and exhausting, yet I would not have traded this experience for anything. I thoroughly enjoyed every aspect of my DNP program, including learning from both faculty and my colleagues and embarking on my path as a leader. My DNP quality improvement project focused on advance care planning for adolescents and young adults living with neuromuscular disease, which allowed me to combine my passion for palliative care and neuromuscular diseases to make a clinical impact on this unique population. I took advantage of every opportunity that came my way and served on committees, engaged in projects and presentations, collaborated on publications, participated in experiential learning, and even conducted an independent study in storytelling. Given the nature of the dual degree program, I had the good fortune of remaining a clinician, while simultaneously seeing healthcare from a business lens and business from the lens of a healthcare provider, and I graduated as a confident leader feeling ready to conquer the world.

It seems that my career has come full circle as I ultimately did fulfill my childhood dream of becoming a doctor, in a way that I never could have imagined. Shortly after graduation I accepted a position as senior nursing director of palliative care at a large institution and having a doctoral degree was a requirement; immediately I experienced the benefits of having earned my DNP. My role as senior director requires that I use the leadership skills I learned in the DNP program regularly as I navigate the new position and serve as a member of both the palliative care leadership team and the institution's executive nursing committee. I use my critical thinking skills as I am part of decisions that affect my entire team as well as the institution, and I use my communication skills as I adapt to working with my leadership colleagues as well as the nurses and nurse practitioners on my team. I also serve as adjunct faculty at a school of nursing, which I would not be able to do without having a doctoral degree. Most importantly, I continue to use my clinical expertise as I maintain my practice as a PPC clinician, ultimately keeping patient care as the focus of my profession. I am immensely grateful for the professional opportunities available to me because of having earned my DNP and I look forward to all that lies ahead in the future.

CLINICAL PRACTICE/ACADEMIC ROLES

Jessica Peters

I began my nursing career as a bachelor's-prepared nurse in an urban teaching hospital within intermediate care. I was drawn to this practice environment initially because I was not sure about specialization at this point in my career, a concept that I still feel that I have challenges with to this day. I was hired with 10 other new graduates, oriented by travel nurses, and then, when their contracts ended, they were not renewed, thus within 6 months I was a resource nurse and shift manager. This concept and dynamic were present 20 years ago! While this was a challenging first 2 years, I learned very early on the value of nursing practice expertise. The majority of our patients were cared for by a practice group of acute care nurse practitioners who I depended on heavily to foster and support my nursing practice. I quickly realized they were experts in their patients and our health system, and viewed their patients as part of a system involving their support system and psychosocial components of their health. They were often the bridge between specialty consultation recommendations and the provider group that holistically and comprehensively cared for their patients. I knew very early in my career this was the nursing path I wanted.

After I completed my master's degree program to become an acute care nurse practitioner, I realized that advanced practice roles and responsibilities expanded beyond the immediate care of a specialty patient population group. Following my immediate nurse practitioner role assimilation, I was asked to participate on several institutional committees and serve on an interdisciplinary research group focusing on patient family experiences with prolonged critical care. I was afforded the opportunity to present our findings at several national conferences and participate as an author in the publication of some of the qualitative findings. I realized quickly that my master's education had not prepared me to present evidence-based practice initiatives or to participate on research teams as a clinical expert. I was drawn specifically to DNP education focusing on clinical scholarship and evidence-based practice.

Central to my DNP education was the relationship I had with the faculty, specifically my institutional mentors at Johns Hopkins Hospital and faculty mentors at Johns Hopkins University. Throughout my nursing career, I felt confident to navigate professional and educational opportunities because I always had role models and mentors who promoted my professional growth. I knew I wanted to "return" the mentorship I was so appreciative to receive. While I was in my DNP program, I completed a graduate certificate in nursing education and received grant support for my education. As part of this, I completed a teaching practicum as a teaching assistant in a critical care nursing practice course. I was also able to mentor and connect several students within the course to nursing opportunities in critical care.

When I was close to graduation, I was fortunate to have one of my practice mentors connect me with the director of the advanced practice specialty track at Johns Hopkins University. Once again, my ability to access and consistently engage with strong and passionate mentors facilitated my confidence and connection to transition to academic nursing practice. I have to admit I did not see myself transitioning to a full-time faculty position several years after completing my DNP program. I am continually reminded that I have the clinical practice expertise and am growing as a nurse educator because of mentors who have consistently connected me with professional growth opportunities. My hope is to continue to pass on the knowledge, mentorship, and expertise I am thankful to have obtained. Our profession is only as strong our ability to support and engage with our newest recruits, to provide them with examples of high-level dynamic and involved nursing practice, and professional opportunities to strengthen our profession and patient care.

CLINICAL PRACTICE/ADMINISTRATION ROLES

Laura O'Rourke

It is difficult for me to pinpoint the exact moment I knew I wanted to be a nurse. As far back as I can remember, it is all I have ever wanted to do, and I attribute this to a series of childhood events that set me down a path, ultimately leading me to where I am today. You could say I never really chose nursing; it chose me. Saturday mornings were spent watching medical docudramas, *Rescue 911* and *Trauma: Life in the ER*, while other children watched cartoons. I was devastated when I was not allowed to witness the birth of my younger sister at the ripe old age of five and eventually set up a make-shift emergency department (ED) on the sidewalk in front of our home, lemonade stand–style, after emptying out my parent's medicine cabinet. The most vivid memory propelling me down my path to nursing, the one I hold dearest, is rushing to the hospital in the middle of the night in my pajamas with my entire family to see my grandfather before he was whisked away to surgery for his long-awaited, life-saving heart transplant. I remember my inability to sleep, agonizing over my fears that he might not love me after receiving a donor's heart. My family spent what felt like an eternity at the hospital during his postoperative course, sleeping in the waiting room and eating out of the vending machines. With the fluorescent lights, constant alarms, and palpable hustle and bustle of the nursing staff, I just knew. I was not able to fully conceptualize it then, but I had found my calling. Or rather, it had found me.

Fast forward several years and I am enrolled in nursing school at the University of Texas at Austin. I completed my undergraduate degree and eagerly began my nursing career in acute care at a Level 1 trauma hospital. I focused on honing my nursing skills and clinical judgment and after several years of bedside care, returned to my alma mater to complete my master's program; I aimed to be a family nurse practitioner. I gravitated toward this patient population, colloquially referred to as "cradle to grave," because of the breadth, depth, and practice flexibility it provided. I unquestionably knew I wanted to work in the ED and had a detailed action plan on how to best prepare myself for this unique and clinically challenging role. Shortly after graduation, I uprooted my life and moved across the country to attend a rigorous 18-month postgraduate emergency medicine fellowship for nurse practitioners (NP) at Mayo Clinic in Rochester, Minnesota. The program was long and grueling but so incredibly worth my investment. Surrounded by the best and brightest in the world, I was prepared to practice autonomously, providing all aspects of emergency medical care, including but not limited to airway management, point-of-care ultrasound, and numerous advanced invasive procedures. The fellowship provided ample opportunities for quality improvement work and advanced leadership roles, most notably an education-focused chief fellow position, which I proudly accepted. After my successful completion of the program and subsequent national board certification as an emergency nurse practitioner (ENP), I began my advanced practice in a rural critical access ED while maintaining my involvement with the fellowship as an adjunct instructor.

My next move? Completion of my doctor of nursing practice (DNP) degree and post-master's certificate in nursing education at Johns Hopkins University School of Nursing (JHUSON). My interest in pursuing a terminal degree and specialized education certificate stemmed from my desire to lead patient care improvement initiatives while pursuing an academic leadership position. The course offerings within the executive track at JHUSON were perfect for my individual needs. Expertly mentored by world-renowned faculty and staff, I tailored my program deliverables based on my clinical experiences and interests in real-time in my current practice setting. I would be remiss if I failed to mention that I began coursework prior to the COVID-19 outbreak, blissfully unaware at that time of the monumental impact the pandemic would have on my life, both professionally and personally. Flexibility, resourcefulness, and an overtly dry sense of humor saw me through the evolution of my quality improvement project and final curriculum proposal.

The knowledge and expertise gained throughout my DNP journey have proven essential to my career advancement. Moreover, it has significantly shaped my view of the nursing profession and its impact on patient and learner outcomes. Specifically, my quality improvement project focused on improving nurse recognition of respiratory deterioration, utilizing in situ simulation to decrease preventable adverse medical events while simultaneously enhancing the training of redeployed nursing staff to the acute care setting from other hospital departments (i.e., float nursing staff) during the height of the pandemic. For my curriculum proposal, I developed an orientation handbook comprised of eight online modules geared at equipping graduate teaching assistants at JHUSON with varying educational training and backgrounds with a foundational understanding of pedagogy to help meet the ever-changing educational needs of nursing students.

Shortly after graduation, I passed the National League for Nursing Certified Nurse Educator examination and began my search for an academic leadership position. Had I not completed my doctorate, I am not certain I would be where I am today: the assistant program director for the emergency medicine fellowship at Mayo Clinic. Every step along my journey, from that late-night car ride in my pajamas up until now, has prepared me to be an effective nurse leader on an international stage and an expert in quality patient care and nursing education. I am eternally grateful to the nursing faculty and staff at each institution I have had the privilege of being a part of and earnestly look forward to continuing to positively impact patient and learner outcomes for many years to come.

CHAPTER TWENTY-THREE Reflective Response

TAMMY SLATER AND VALERIE T. COTTER

While each of these inspiring stories of successful career advancement roles by DNP graduates is unique, there are many common themes. First is their foundation in and passion for clinical practice, which has continued after completing their DNP. In contrast to recent studies, these nurse practitioners did not experience role ambiguity but successfully combined new or existing clinical practice roles with new academic and administration roles (Beeber et al., 2019; Dobrowolska et al., 2021). Being in major medical centers where there were opportunities to grow and mentors to help foster their professional development contributed to their success.

The mentoring process is a guiding relationship that occurs between an experienced professional and a novice who is transitioning into a new role or learning new responsibilities (Davis et al., 2023; Higgins & Newby, 2020). For each of these DNP leaders, interprofessional networking and interdisciplinary supportive teams helped create mentoring experiences that have encouraged professional growth and development while providing unlimited, open access to new and expanded opportunities resulting in innovative roles and responsibilities.

Since Benner's (1982) novice to expert model was first described over 40 years ago, it is well documented that clinically focused nurses engage in stages of increasing proficiency. Two of these DNP leaders recount their initial exposure to nursing by describing characteristics of nurses they encountered while performing other healthcare functions such as volunteering, working as a research assistant, leading patient support groups, and providing care to family members. These beginning attributes can closely be identified within the novice role (Benner, 1982). Each one also depicts how their novice nursing roles evolved from an advanced beginner into a proficient professional nurse with increasing competence (Benner, 1982). Compelling examples of these behaviors include how they learned to care for highly specialized patient populations, such as those in surgical critical care, pediatric palliative care, emergency, and trauma nursing, while they were new nurses in orientation. They pursued additional educational opportunities that enabled them to provide exemplary clinical care throughout their careers. Taking advantage of every available opportunity has allowed them to remain up to date with the latest treatments while participating in higher learning activities, which intuitively develops confidence. This confidence builds on itself and allows informal leadership roles to grow organically, and in turn facilitates the DNP graduate to transition into formal leadership positions.

Through their professional growth and development, they have benefited from many of the key components of an effective mentoring relationship, including (a) open communication and accessibility, (b) goals and challenges, (c) passion and inspiration, (d) caring personal relationship, (e) mutual respect and trust, (f) exchange of knowledge, (g) independence and collaboration, and (h) role modeling (Eller et al., 2014).

Dr. Battista portrays a perfect example of this by having been accessible for new experiences, identifying her passion in palliative care, pursuing the executive DNP and master of business administration (MBA) dual degree program, and obtaining the senior nursing director of palliative care position at a large institution. She maintains clinical expertise as a practicing nurse practitioner in pediatric palliative care. Additionally, Dr. Battista has become a professional role model through her adjunct clinical faculty position.

Dr. Peters was challenged as a new nurse learning how to provide exemplary care with limited resources; however, she embraced this opportunity and identified role models who were clinical experts in the field who fostered and supported her nursing practice. While studying to become an acute care nurse practitioner, she realized that advanced practice roles and responsibilities expanded beyond the immediate clinical care of a specialty patient population group. This realization led Dr. Peters to actively engage with and participate in several institutional committees in addition to serving on an interdisciplinary research group focusing on patient and family experiences relating to prolonged critical illness. This is an example of how through passion and collaboration, an exchange of knowledge occurs, and advanced practice leaders emerge. Knowing that clinical scholarship and evidence-based practice are crucial elements in professional practice, Dr. Peters pursued an executive DNP degree. Her accessibility to academic and clinically focused institutional mentors has empowered her to pursue a more formal leadership position in academia. She has developed a strong desire to be a role model and help mold future DNP nurse practitioner leaders.

Dr. O'Rourke took a similar path focusing on developing clinical skills within a specialized patient population. Her approach expanded her trauma nursing experience, and she was able to pursue an advanced practice degree and become a family nurse practitioner. She remained steadfast and determined as she wanted to practice clinically in the emergency department. Her dedication empowered her to apply and be accepted to an 18-month postgraduate emergency nurse practitioner fellowship. Additionally, the fellowship was structured to include advanced leadership roles such as an education-focused chief fellow position. Dr. O'Rourke accepted this position and has been able to collaborate and serve as an adjunct instructor. This is an excellent example of how she has been able to follow her passion while developing a strong knowledge base expanding her clinical acumen. These accomplishments enabled her to seek additional education within the executive DNP program and nurse educator certificate option.

One of the more important themes expressed by these DNP graduates is their thoughtful selection of which terminal degree in nursing (PhD vs. DNP) was best suited to their individual career goals. Each wanted to remain an expert clinician and implement clinical changes in healthcare organizations and have roles in academic nursing.

DNP-prepared nurses are well equipped to fully implement the science developed by nurse researchers prepared in PhD, DNS, and other research-focused nursing doctorates (AACN, 2022), but they also participate on research teams as clinical experts and as principal and co-investigators. In nursing, we currently characterize the DNP degree as a practice doctorate, similar to our colleagues in medicine, psychology, physical therapy, etc., with professional "clinical" doctorates.

What's unique to nursing is how our culture discourages DNP-educated nurses from pursuing research training and funding, and suggests that only the PhD prepares one for this career development. In contrast, physicians with an MD/DO degree in academic medical centers develop successful research careers through federal funding for research training and grant support despite not having a PhD.

Why have we established this cultural limitation in nursing? As we advance the requirement for the DNP as entry into advanced practice, we should support and encourage DNP-prepared nurses to develop their research careers as clinician-scientists. The DNP graduate is a valuable resource on an integrated research team where each team member brings specific expertise to address the research problem especially in pragmatic trials and implementation research. If we dare to generalize Benner's (1982) model to the professional growth of DNP-prepared nurses with experiential learning and formal research training, moving from novice to expert will include research opportunities.

REFERENCES

American Association of Colleges of Nursing [AACN]. (2022). *DNP education.* https://www.aacnnursing.org/Nursing-Education-Programs/DNP-Education

Beeber, A. S., Palmer, C., Waldrop, J., Lynn, M. R., & Jones, C. B. (2019). The role of doctor of nursing practice-prepared nurses in practice settings. *Nursing Outlook, 67*(4), 354–364. https://doi.org/10.1016/j.outlook.2019.02.006

Benner, P. (1982). From novice to expert. *American Journal of Nursing, 82*(3), 402–407.

Davis, L., Mullins, K., Fathman, A., & Donaworth, S. (2023). Mentoring novice NPs: Recommendations for navigating the transition to autonomous practice. *The Nurse Practitioner, 48*(2), 41–47.

Dobrowolska, B., Chrusciel, P., Markiewicz, R., & Palese, A. (2021). The role of doctoral-educated nurses in the clinical setting: Findings from a scoping review. *Journal of Clinical Nursing, 30*(19–20). 2808–2821. https://doi.org/10.1111/jocn.15810

Eller, L. S., Lev, E., & Feurer, A. (2014). Key components of an effective mentoring relationship: A qualitative study. *Nurse Education Today, 34*, 815–820.

Higgins, K., & Newby, O. (2020). DNP student mentorship: Empowering students and nurse practitioner organizations. *The Nurse Practitioner, 45*(5), 42–47. https://doi.org/10.1016/j.nedt.2013.07.020

CHAPTER TWENTY-FOUR

Analysis of the 2021 Essentials of Doctoral Education for Advanced Nursing Practice: Where Do We Go From Here?

JOAN ROSEN BLOCH, BRENDA DOUGLASS, AND AMANDA BROCK

INTRODUCTION

This chapter focuses on the American Association of Colleges of Nursing (AACN) 2021 The Essentials document that influences doctoral nursing education for advanced nursing practice. As noted throughout this book, the doctor of nursing practice (DNP) degree is widely recognized and accepted as one of two terminal doctoral degrees in the nursing discipline. Evidence is clear that many seek the DNP degree as preparation for the highest level of nursing practice (AACN, 2020; Dreher & Glasgow, 2017). What that means, of course, varies based on the advanced nursing practice role. Be that as it is, this chapter focuses on the AACN Essentials for advanced-level nursing education and its current and future implications for those seeking the DNP degree. Issues that pertain to real-world nursing practice also apply to academic nursing and the preparation of those seeking DNP degrees for professional advancement in nursing. Foremost for nursing education is the notion of curriculum and knowledge of the key AACN documents that influence nursing curriculum development. The bridge between academic nursing and clinical nursing practice is critical in preparing a competent nursing workforce that meets society's needs, across all levels of nursing academic degrees and nursing roles. It is our responsibility to continue to foster collaborations between academia and practice, and to ensure that these collaborations are meaningful and mutually beneficial.

The global coronavirus pandemic, also referred to as the COVID-19 pandemic, has had an extraordinary impact on how individuals think about their health and life. Nurses, as the largest professional group of the healthcare workforce, were greatly affected in nursing practice, nursing education, and nursing research (Bloch & Smith Glasgow, 2023; Boulton et al., 2022; Roush, 2022). Yet over the last decade even before the pandemic, there have been urgent calls to transform the American healthcare system (AACN, 2016; IOM, 2013). AACN, the key nursing organization that influences nursing education across the United States, responded to this call by disrupting the status quo and convening a task force to outline a new model to guide nursing education through the release of the 2021 Essentials: *Core Competencies for Professional Nursing Education* (AACN, 2021a). While the task force began their work before the global pandemic, its release during the pandemic created additional stress for many faculty who were already burdened by the effects of the pandemic on higher education (Boamah et al., 2022; Jeffries, 2020). Reimagining the transformation of nursing education with the new 2021 AACN Essentials seemed insurmountable in the context of shifting to the online teaching environment and escalating nursing faculty shortages (Bloch & Smith Glasgow, 2023; Jarosinski et al., 2022). Nonetheless, academic nursing faculty are embracing the disruption by placing significant emphasis on the alignment of undergraduate and graduate nursing program curricula with the new 2021 Essentials (Galura & Warshawsky, 2022; Welch & Smith, 2022). As we proceed, the environment of our times influences our professional nursing abilities to thrive and successfully meet the health and well-being needs of the people we serve. This important responsibility must not be taken lightly.

The 2021 AACN Essentials aims to transform nursing education curricula across undergraduate and graduate programs through a new Essentials model guided by a competency-based education (CBE) pedagogical approach for nursing education. Applied as intended, students should be better prepared upon graduation with the knowledge, skills, and attitudes needed for ethical and competent clinical reasoning and skills needed for nursing practice. These are indeed lofty goals. How leaders of the profession guide the curriculum necessary for real-world nursing practice is at stake. DNP students and graduates are germane to curricula discussions and tasked to ensure that their DNP education prepares them to take on the leadership needed in directing the vision and preparation for the future nursing workforce, across many roles and practice settings. As DNP students, we expect that you will read this chapter with your commitment as future doctoral-prepared nurses, accepting your professional responsibility of shepherding the nursing profession forward. This includes identification of your learning needs and finding the resources to meet those needs.

The DNP is widely recognized and accepted as one of two terminal doctoral degrees in the nursing discipline. Many nurses seek the DNP as preparation for the highest level of nursing practice. The achievement of the highest level of nursing practice varies depending on the level of clinical or administrative experience, professional identity, specialty practice, or absence of this in the case of BSN-DNP graduates. The DNP is an academic degree and is not synonymous with a particular nursing role. The variation in DNP graduate skill sets is attributed, in part, to the real-world nursing practice experience of the DNP student prior to entering the DNP program (AACN, 2022a).

Foremost to DNP education is the notion of curriculum and the influence of the AACN Essentials on curriculum development. Given the dire nursing faculty shortage (AACN, 2021b), which is not expected to lighten up any time soon, the Essentials are relevant to DNP students. With attainment of a DNP degree, nursing practice leaders are expected to have a prominent role in preparing the next generation of professional nurses. The evidence is clear that most DNP graduates have critical roles in academic nursing and are shaping the future of nursing education (AACN, 2022a). In Chapter 8, co-authored by Dr. Wittmann-Price, you learned that there are various academic roles you may have as either full-time or part-time faculty. While some may decide to transition into full-time faculty roles, others may focus on advanced nursing practice and be asked to share their practice expertise with future nursing students, across the wide array of academic programs and degrees. DNP education is designed to develop leaders in nursing to shepherd the nursing profession forward.

Tasked with the objective to provide an analysis of the 2021 AACN Essentials for DNP education and provide a vision for where we go from here, the authors of this chapter were strategically chosen. Each brings a slightly different perspective, but all are key stakeholders of DNP education, with great respect for clinical scholarship, research, and practice. Each author has extensive experience in real-world nursing practice, which garnered each, eventually, full-time academic faculty appointments. Two (JB and BD) are nurse practitioners and experienced DNP educators (one with a PhD degree and the other with a DNP degree). The third (AB), in the pipeline for a DNP degree, is a bioethicist and clinical research nurse with a medical school leadership appointment. In this role, this author (AB) leads research teams to ensure feasible and ethical implementation of complex interdisciplinary clinical research protocols. Together for this chapter, is a shared agenda to push forward the best DNP education for our discipline of nursing and our interdisciplinary stakeholders, including the patients and families we aim to serve. We bridge our perspectives, learning from each other, as we address what the 2021 AACN Essentials means for DNP education.

Reading the 2021 AACN Essentials as a standalone document is insufficient for students in doctoral nursing programs. What the 2021 Essentials mean for doctoral education for advanced nursing practice, and where we go from here, requires a broader and deeper understanding of the key AACN documents that have impacted and will impact the future of DNP education in nursing. Curriculum development, implementation, and evaluation is a dynamic process. It is important to note that educational standards among highly regulated and licensed healthcare professions (e.g., nurses, physicians, physical therapists) usually have an overseeing professional organization that recommends standards and guidelines for the profession's academic curricula. That is where the AACN comes in for nursing. Doctoral graduates practicing in advanced nursing practice roles have a responsibility to understand the broader implications of the 2021 Essentials for the nursing profession, as opposed to a narrow focus on the implications for their specific advanced nursing practice roles. Thus, this chapter begins by providing a thorough background of key AACN documents influencing DNP education and doctoral nursing education, in general. Then, because the 2021 Essentials are designed as a competency-based education model, the pedagogy and background of competency-based education are included in the discussion of the 2021 AACN Essentials. Throughout this chapter there are points to ponder, concluding with an assessment of the next steps from here.

■ BACKGROUND HISTORY OF THE AACN'S DNP ESSENTIALS AND OTHER KEY AACN DOCUMENTS INFLUENCING DOCTORAL NURSING EDUCATION

The history of the AACN Essentials for professional nursing education spans more than three decades. The AACN published the first Essentials in 1986, culminating in an educational framework with expectations for the preparation of nurses at 4-year colleges and universities (AACN, 2021a). As the DNP degree began to gain momentum as an important practice doctorate degree, the AACN took a strong position supporting the DNP degree. The AACN plays an integral role in supporting and guiding DNP education for advanced nursing practice. Figure 24.1 presents a timeline of key AACN documents influencing DNP education. Close to 20 years ago in October 2004, the AACN's endorsement of the practice doctorate in nursing through their *Position Statement on the Practice Doctorate in Nursing* calling for a transformational shift in the education of professional nurses (AACN, 2022a) was monumental. The adopted recommendations called for (it

512 ■ III: OPERATIONALIZING ROLE FUNCTIONS

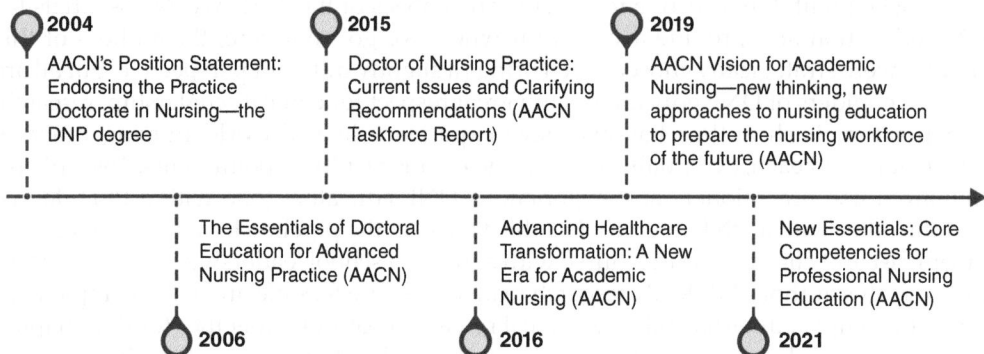

FIGURE 24.1 Timeline of Key American Association of Colleges of Nursing (AACN) Reports Influencing DNP Education

was never mandated) moving the level of academic preparation for advanced nursing practice from the master's degree to the doctorate level by 2015 (AACN, 2004). The practice doctorate in nursing, also referred to as a clinical doctorate prior to the 2004 AACN Position Statement, was not novel. However, this was an evolutionary movement for graduate nursing education recognizing the DNP as a terminal degree in nursing practice, thus preparing a graduate for the highest level of preparation in the profession. The 2004 AACN Position Statement informed the purpose of the professional practice doctorate and next steps in developing DNP educational standards, quality indicators for, and foundational curricular content, specifically core content areas and core competencies for practice-focused doctoral programs (AACN, 2004). Subsequently in 2006, two decades after the earliest AACN Essentials in 1986, the first curricular elements and core competencies required in programs conferring the DNP degree were published (AACN, 2006).

Nursing is the backbone of the U.S. healthcare system and a vital component of healthcare delivery. The DNP degree was developed to prepare advanced practice registered nurses (APRNs) beyond initial preparation in the discipline, including but not limited to, clinical nurse specialists, nurse anesthetists, nurse practitioners, and nurse-midwives for leadership in clinical practice (AACN, 2004). The timeline leading up to the emergence of the DNP degree began with two landmark Institute of Medicine (IOM) published reports. The first groundbreaking report in 1999, *To Err is Human: Building a Safer Health System*, brought transparency to alarming, preventable medical errors significantly impacting the quality of care and healthcare outcomes (IOM, 1999). The report also identified the high degree of fragmentation across a multitude of sectors in the U.S. healthcare system and made recommendations for a vision toward a safer and improved health system (IOM, 1999). The follow-up report, *Crossing the Quality Chasm: A New Health System for the 21st Century*, called for a sweeping overhaul of the healthcare system, thus closing the gaps by improving patient safety and quality of healthcare delivery (IOM, 2001). The report focused more broadly on restructuring a healthcare delivery system designed to innovate and improve care (IOM, 2001). In this second report, recommendations for the 21st century healthcare system established six aims in that healthcare should be safe, effective, client-centered, timely, efficient, and equitable care (IOM, 2001). The vision incorporated preparing a workforce with new skills and approaches together with leaders prepared to restructure the healthcare system. To narrow the quality chasm and redesign the U.S. healthcare system, a multifaceted approach far-reaching beyond healthcare, professionals and academia was necessary, involving payers, health plans, government officials, and regulatory and accrediting bodies.

The hallmark IOM reports (1999, 2001) were drivers in the 2004 AACN Position Statement with recommendations for advancing the level of academic nursing preparation to a terminal practice degree, the DNP. Nurses embody the largest profession of the healthcare workforce, and practice-focused doctoral nursing programs have a critical role in preparing leaders for nursing practice (AACN, 2022a). The DNP is an academic degree and is not specific to a particular clinical role. Accordingly, the critical need for nurses in advanced practice roles to design, evaluate, and continuously improve the context within which care is delivered was recognized in transforming healthcare and preparing DNP graduates (AACN, 2004). In alignment with the IOM (2001) recommendations, the AACN Position Statement (2004) endorsed DNP preparation, stating that: "Nurses prepared at the doctoral level with a blend of clinical, organizational, economic and leadership skills are most likely to be able to critique nursing and other clinical scientific findings and design programs of care delivery that are locally acceptable, economically feasible, and which significantly impact health care outcomes" (p. 3). With a practice doctorate it was anticipated that advanced practice clinical nursing roles would be enhanced so that DNP-prepared nurses would apply new knowledge and skills to improve health outcomes and healthcare systems.

A multitude of factors, which are still relevant today, influenced reenvisioning graduate nursing education for doctoral-level preparation including increasing patient care complexities; the rapid expansion of clinical scientific knowledge; national concerns about patient safety, quality, and outcomes; nursing personnel shortages; a higher level of preparation for nursing leaders who can design and assess care; shortages of doctoral-prepared nursing faculty; and increasing educational expectations for parity with other health professionals (AACN, 2004). In conjunction with the growing nursing practice demands and complexities within the healthcare environment, evidence established a clear relationship between higher levels of nursing education and improved patient outcomes (Aiken & Fagin, 1991; AACN, 2004). The expansion of scientific knowledge required for safe nursing practice and growing concerns regarding the quality of patient care delivery and outcomes were vital catalysts driving the impetus for the DNP, a practice doctorate degree (AACN, 2006). With the AACN endorsing DNP education, a rapid proliferation of DNP programs ensued, as illustrated in Figure 24.2 (AACN, 2022a, p. 10).

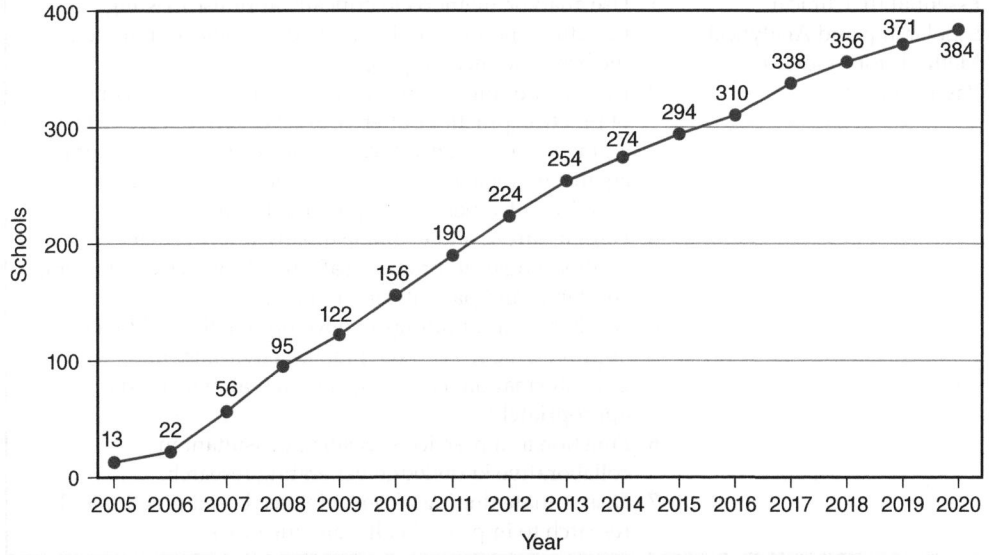

FIGURE 24.2 Number of Active DNP Programs 2005–2020

To better guide faculty, in 2006 the AACN released the first and only Essentials *of Doctoral Education for Advanced Nursing Practice,* also referred to as the DNP Essentials, as a foundation for curriculum development to prepare practice-focused DNP graduates. These DNP Essentials are comprised of eight foundational outcome competencies, each informed with comments regarding specialty competencies and content, for preparation of all DNPgraduates regardless of specialty (AACN, 2006). Table 24.1 provides an overview of the 2006 DNP Essentials. DNP students are highly encouraged to read the full document, which is available in the public domain on the AACN's website.

Table 24.1 An Overview of the 2006 AACN DNP Essentials

8 Key DNP Essentials	The DNP graduate is prepared to:
Essential I: Scientific Underpinnings for Practice	1. Integrate nursing science with knowledge from ethics, the biophysical, psychosocial, analytical, and organizational sciences as the basis for the highest level of nursing practice. 2. Use science-based theories and concepts to: -determine the nature and significance of health and healthcare delivery phenomena; -describe the actions and advanced strategies to enhance, alleviate, and ameliorate health and healthcare delivery phenomena as appropriate; and -evaluate outcomes. 3. Develop and evaluate new practice approaches based on nursing theories and theories from other disciplines.
Essential II: Organizational and Systems Leadership for Quality Improvement and Systems Thinking	1. Develop and evaluate care delivery approaches that meet current and future needs of patient populations based on scientific findings in nursing and other clinical sciences, as well as organizational, political, and economic sciences. 2. Ensure accountability for quality of healthcare and patient safety for populations with whom they work 3. Develop and/or evaluate effective strategies for managing the ethical dilemmas inherent in patient care, the healthcare organization, and research.
Essential III: Clinical Scholarship and Analytical Methods for Evidence-Based Practice	1. Use analytic methods to critically appraise existing literature and other evidence to determine and implement the best evidence for practice. 2. Design and implement processes to evaluate outcomes of practice, practice patterns, and systems of care within a practice setting, healthcare organization, or community against national benchmarks to determine variances in practice outcomes and population trends. 3. Design, direct, and evaluate quality improvement methodologies to promote safe, timely, effective, efficient, equitable, and patient-centered care. 4. Apply relevant findings to develop practice guidelines and improve practice and the practice environment. 5. Use information technology and research methods appropriately 6. Function as a practice specialist/consultant in collaborative knowledge-generating research. 7. Disseminate findings from evidence-based practice and research to improve healthcare outcomes

(continued)

Table 24.1 An Overview of the 2006 AACN DNP Essentials (*continued*)

8 Key DNP Essentials	The DNP graduate is prepared to:
Essential IV: Information Systems/Technology and Patient Care Technology for the Improvement and Transformation of HealthCare	1. Design, select, use, and evaluate programs that evaluate and monitor outcomes of care, care systems, and quality improvement including consumer use of healthcare information systems. 2. Analyze and communicate critical elements necessary to the selection, use and evaluation of healthcare information systems and patient care technology. 3. Demonstrate the conceptual ability and technical skills to develop and execute an evaluation plan involving data extraction from practice information systems and databases. 4. Provide leadership in the evaluation and resolution of ethical and legal issues within healthcare systems relating to the use of information, information technology, communication networks, and patient care technology. 5. Evaluate consumer health information sources for accuracy, timeliness, and appropriateness.
Essential V: HealthCare Policy for Advocacy in HealthCare	1. Critically analyze health policy proposals, health policies, and related issues from the perspective of consumers, nursing, other health professions, and other stakeholders in policy and public forums. 2. Demonstrate leadership in the development and implementation of institutional, local, state, federal, and/or international health policy. 3. Influence policy makers through active participation on committees, boards, or task forces at the institutional, local, state, regional, national, and/or international levels to improve healthcare delivery and outcomes. 4. Educate others, including policy makers at all levels, regarding nursing, health policy, and patient care outcomes. 5. Advocate for the nursing profession within the policy and healthcare communities. 6. Develop, evaluate, and provide leadership for healthcare policy that shapes healthcare financing, regulation, and delivery. 7. Advocate for social justice, equity, and ethical policies within all healthcare arenas.
Essential VI: Interprofessional Collaboration for Improving Patient and Population Health Outcomes	1. Employ effective communication and collaborative skills in the development and implementation of practice models, peer review, practice guidelines, health policy, standards of care, and/or other scholarly products. 2. Lead interprofessional teams in the analysis of complex practice and organizational issues. 3. Employ consultative and leadership skills with intra-professional and interprofessional teams to create change in healthcare and complex healthcare delivery systems.

(*continued*)

Table 24.1 An Overview of the 2006 AACN DNP Essentials (*continued*)

8 Key DNP Essentials	The DNP graduate is prepared to:
Essential VII: Clinical Prevention and Population Health for Improving the Nation's Health	1. Analyze epidemiological, biostatistical, environmental, and other appropriate scientific data related to individual, aggregate, and population health. 2. Synthesize concepts, including psychosocial dimensions and cultural diversity, related to clinical prevention and population health in developing, implementing, and evaluating interventions to address health promotion/disease prevention efforts, improve health status/access patterns, and/or address gaps in care of individuals, aggregates, or populations. 3. Evaluate care delivery models and/or strategies using concepts related to community, environmental and occupational health, and cultural and socioeconomic dimensions of health.
Essential VIII: Advanced Nursing Practice	1. Conduct a comprehensive and systematic assessment of health and illness parameters in complex situations, incorporating diverse and culturally sensitive approaches. 2. Design, implement, and evaluate therapeutic interventions based on nursing science and other sciences. 3. Develop and sustain therapeutic relationships and partnerships with patients (individual, family or group) and other professionals to facilitate optimal care and patient outcomes. 4. Demonstrate advanced levels of clinical judgment, systems thinking, and accountability in designing, delivering, and evaluating evidence-based care to improve patient outcomes. 5. Guide, mentor, and support other nurses to achieve excellence in nursing practice. 6. Educate and guide individuals and groups through complex health and situational transitions. 7. Use conceptual and analytical skills in evaluating the links among practice, organizational, population, fiscal, and policy issues.

Curricula for practice-focused doctorates in nursing are designed to prepare experts in a variety of nursing practice roles (AACN, 2006). While the DNP Essentials were intended to serve as core to all advanced nursing practice roles, the depth and focus of the competencies varied based on the specific advanced practice nursing role for which a student was preparing for (AACN, 2006). In the DNP Essentials, faculty of each DNP program was designated academic freedom to create innovative and integrated curricula to meet the competencies outlined in the Essentials document. Nonetheless, there has been some controversy over the years as to the level of consistency in addressing the DNP Essentials (Campbell-O'Dell & Dreher, 2017).

DNP programs continue to flourish. Nearly a decade after the 2006 Essentials and the 2004 AACN Position Statement were published, the DNP was widely recognized as one of two terminal degrees in nursing and the preferred pathway for the highest education level as a practice-focused degree in nursing (AACN, 2015). Findings from a national study commissioned by the AACN Board of Directors and conducted by the RAND corporation supported near-universal agreement among the nursing community on the value of DNP education in preparing nurses to meet future healthcare needs (Auerbach et al., 2015). The evolving healthcare landscape, higher education, and substantial growth in DNP programs presented a need for greater clarity and guidance concerning DNP curricular and practice expectations. This gave rise to the publication of the 2015 AACN report titled, *The Doctor of Nursing Practice: Current Issues and Clarifying Recommendations*. As a white paper, the report delineated clarifying characteristics of DNP graduate scholarship, the DNP project, resource efficacies, program length, curriculum considerations, practice experiences, and collaborative partnership guidelines (AACN, 2015). The white paper was an important resource in DNP education for faculty to prepare DNP graduates with the expanded knowledge, skills, and attitudes needed for future advanced nursing practice (AACN, 2015).

In 2016, *Advancing Healthcare Transformation: A New Era for Academic Nursing* (AACN, 2016) was a pivotal report in the evolution of DNP education. This report offered a strategic framework for engaging nursing and medical school deans, health system executives, and university presidents and chancellors in the collaborative work needed to spark clinical innovation, align critical resources, and fortify the public's health (AACN, 2016). Keenly aware of the central role of nursing in transforming healthcare, the report recognized the critical need for a coordinated response from academic and practice partners providing six actions for embracing a new vision for academic nursing (AACN, 2016). Achieving a new partnership necessitated that nursing faculty have a deeper involvement in clinical practice and greater opportunity to engage in the clinical innovation needed by evolving academic health systems. Preparing DNP graduates for their role in population health, health systems leadership, leadership, innovation, prevention and wellness programs, innovative models of care delivery, and continuity across transitions of care settings were fitting illustrations for DNP-prepared nurses.

Continuing to envision the future, the AACN's *Vision for Academic Nursing* (2019) report assessed trends and addressed overarching academic considerations and future goals related to meeting the needs of a dynamic, global society and a diverse patient population. Designed to address the fundamental aim of the AACN serving as a catalyst for excellence and innovation in nursing education, research, and practice, the report was intended to highlight the contemporary impact on academic nursing of evolving practice needs and nursing roles in the context of faculty resources, emerging learning and technologies, and learner profiles, in creating a competent, highly diverse, and adaptable nursing workforce (AACN, 2019). In the report, the importance of terminal degrees that were both research-focused and practice-oriented in academic nursing was highlighted, along with dual degrees (PhD and DNP) and increasing collaboration between education and practice. Overall, the recommendations was intended to inspire nursing education leaders to innovate and seek opportunities to advance the nursing profession within a changing environment (AACN, 2019).

2021 AACN's New *Essentials: Core Competencies for Professional Nursing Education*

In April 2021 a new educational framework, *The* Essentials: *Core Competencies for Professional Nursing Education* (also referred to as the Essentials), was approved and published by the AACN reflecting clearly defined expectations across the trajectory of nursing education and applied experience (AACN, 2021a). For AACN member schools, the Essentials represent new educational standards but also nursing education transformation in contemporary practice and adaptation to future changes within nursing education (AACN, 2021a; Giddens et al., 2022). The Essentials aim to transform how nurses are prepared in baccalaureate, master's, and DNP programs by transitioning to competency-based education (CBE) focusing on two levels of professional nursing education: entry-level and advanced-level nursing practice (AACN, 2021a). Level 1 subcompetencies focus on preparing students for entry into professional nursing practice, whereas level 2 subcompetencies prepare students for advanced nursing practice roles and specialties (Giddens et al., 2022). The Essentials assimilate 10 broad domains and eight core concepts threaded throughout that exemplify professional nursing practice (see Table 24.2). Each domain is informed by expectations for each level of nursing, interwoven concepts, competencies, and subcompetencies. A competency is defined as an observable ability of a health professional, integrating multiple components such as knowledge, skills, values, and attitudes that can be measured (AACN, 2021a). Because the 2021 Essentials is a paradigm shift guided by the CBE framework, there are many national conversations with excellent available resources by the AACN and nursing specialty organizations. The AACN's website is continually updated. Readers are encouraged to expand their knowledge around the Essentials domains (https://www.aacnnursing.org/Essentials/Domains) and concepts (https://www.aacnnursing.org/Essentials/Concepts).

COMPETENCY-BASED EDUCATION

As stated above, competency-based education comprises a major shift in the new Essentials and, although influenced by the AACN's *Vision for Academic Nursing* report (AACN, 2019), it constitutes a new direction for nursing (AACN, 2021a; Giddens et al., 2022). As defined by the AACN (2021a), CBE refers to a system of instruction, assessment, feedback, self-reflection, and academic reporting that is based on students demonstrating that they have learned the knowledge, attitudes, motivations, self-perceptions, and skills expected of them as they progress through their education (AACN, 2021a). In CBE, learning experiences are designed to be integrative, experiential, self-aware, reflective, active, interactive, developmental, and transferrable. Table 24.3 offers a quick overview of what CBE is and is not.

To fully appreciate and understand the implications of the new 2021 AACN Essentials for DNP education, a deeper dive into the pedagogical underpinnings of CBE is warranted. Pedagogy is an important construct when working in academia. Simply defined, pedagogy is the art and science of teaching. It includes the study of teaching materials, including the aims of education and how the goals of our education, across various disciplines, are to be achieved. Underpinning the broad array of pedagogies are

TABLE 24.2 2021 AACN Essentials: Domains and Concepts for Professional Nursing Practice

Domains for Nursing:	Concepts for Nursing Practice:
o **Domain 1:** Knowledge for Nursing Practice o **Domain 2:** Person-Centered Care o **Domain 3:** Population Health o **Domain 4:** Scholarship for Nursing Practice o **Domain 5:** Quality and Safety o **Domain 6:** Interprofessional Partnerships o **Domain 7:** Systems-Based Practice o **Domain 8:** Informatics and Healthcare Technologies o **Domain 9:** Professionalism o **Domain 10:** Personal, Professional, and Leadership Development	o Clinical Judgment o Communication o Compassionate Care o Diversity, Equity, and Inclusion o Ethics o Evidence-Based Practice o Health Policy o Social Determinants of Health

TABLE 24.3 Key Elements Explaining What Competency-Based Education Is and Is Not

Competency-Based Education	
What is it?	**What is it *not*?**
o A set of expectations which, when taken collectively, demonstrate what learners can do with what they know. o Demonstrated across all spheres of care and in multiple contexts. o Clear expectations made explicit to learners, employers, and public. o A result of determined (planned and repeated) practice. Visibly demonstrated and assessed over time.	o A checklist of tasks o A one and done experience or demonstration o Isolated in one sphere of care or context o Demonstrated solely on an objective test

Source: Adapted from Douglass, B., Scruggs-Corey, J., & Stanley, J. (August 11, 2021). *DNP Education and Practice: A Facilitated Conversation Embracing the Essentials.* Paper presented at the Fourteenth National Doctors of Nursing Practice National Conference.

various philosophies of education and learning theories, stemming primarily from the field of educational psychology (Chinn, 2008). Nursing pedagogies are built upon the unique ways of knowing for nursing as a discipline and practice profession (Billings & Halstead, 2005; Moyer & Wittmann-Price, 2008).

Excellent teaching does not just happen. It is a result of thoughtful reflection and action that occurs in a circular, ongoing process. Underlying ideas and values based on philosophies and theories of education are brought to the classroom, by either the teacher or the student (Chinn, 2008). A curriculum, in general, is the totality of the formal and informal content that imparts the knowledge, skills, attitudes, and values considered important in achieving the educational goals. Curriculum development is a process that takes much time and thought, requiring serious faculty attention, time, and effort (AAUP, 2015; Billings & Halstead, 2005; Moyer & Wittmann-Price, 2008). In and out of classroom and clinical placement experiences are designed to ensure learning occurs through an organized approach.

HISTORICAL BACKGROUND OF CBE IN NURSING EDUCATION

CBE is a leading pedagogical approach to clinical health education (Englander et al., 2013; Giddens et al., 2022). It is not new for nursing education. In 1978, legendary nurse-educator Dorothy J. de Bueno published an article on CBE based on the presentation she gave at the 1st National Nurse Education Conference (de Bueno, 1978). A year later, the National League of Nursing (NLN) published Report No. 23-1770 on competency-based curriculum and instruction (Peterson et al., 1979).

De Bueno (1978) explained that CBE can be conceptually interpreted in either a broad or narrow sense. Applied in a broad sense, CBE is used as the conceptual framework for curricula that allows the learner to be self-directed in the selection of their learning objectives and goals, learning experiences, and methods used to demonstrate achievement of their competencies (de Bueno, 1978). Applied in a narrow sense, desired competencies are identified. De Beuno explains that if acquisition of the competency cannot be demonstrated, the instructor establishes the learning activities to achieve it. However, the student is expected to negotiate with instructors to set priorities for their learning and to establish the sequence of learning activities.

Faculty across all nursing education programs are tasked with ensuring measurable outcomes aligned with the competencies in the 2021 Essentials. This is not an easy task, given that measurable outcomes may be more effective, not skill or knowledge oriented. We are reminded that even in 1978, de Bueno explicitly states that outcomes do not need to be only knowledge or psychomotor skills that are clearly observable to instructors, but CBE can include affective outcomes (1978), which are harder to articulate values and affective behaviors. CBE should be viewed as a philosophy of teaching as well as a framework for curriculum development. In 1979, the NLN advocated CBE as an educational approach that situates competencies based on real-world nursing practice with educational aims to ensure graduates are ready for nursing practice. The diagram that appeared in the 1979 NLN report (Peterson et al., 1979, p. 31) that compares a traditional nursing education approach with a CBE approach is as relevant today as it was four decades ago (see Table 24.4).

In CBE, both processes and outcomes of learning are important. The curriculum is designed to ensure students' readiness for practice, where clinical reasoning and skills are acquired. Learning processes shape knowledge, beliefs, and attitudes, which influences readiness for nursing practice. A careful review of the 2021 Essentials should clarify that the 2021 domains and concepts broaden students' understandings of the human condition, raising greater awareness of many factors contributing to multilevel influences of health and illness (determinants of health).

From its inception, there has been much discussion in the published literature about CBE and its value in clinical education (de Bueno, 1978; Englander et al., 2013; Giddens et al., 2022). Even in the 1970s, some hailed it as a revolutionary approach to clinical education, while others criticized it as a mechanistic approach that dehumanizes the student to a measurable product and outcome (de Bueno, 1978). De Bueno, a proponent of CBE for nursing, goes on to dispel some of the myths of CBE approaches. Her article is as relevant today as it was back then. If you can, read this seminal article. Think critically about the pedagogy that supports CBE and why nursing educators are urging CBE pedagogy in nursing education to better prepare new graduate nurses for

TABLE 24.4 The National League of Nursing's Comparison of the Traditional Model of Nursing Education Versus the New Competency-Based Educational Model*

TRADITIONAL MODEL	
General or theoretical idea of the field of practice	
Philosophy of program Terminal behavioral objectives Course behavioral objectives Unit behavioral objectives Instructional behavioral objectives Content/experiences (i.e., curriculum)	Tests of knowledge and skill objectives rather than competencies guarantees what?
NEW PERSPECTIVE	
Analysis of real world of practice	
Competencies validated by job analysis and practitioners Performance objectives (terminal and supporting or enabling objectives leading to demonstration of the competencies)	Evaluation of performance guarantees readiness for practice.
Blueprint of content reflecting necessary knowledge, skills, and attitudes to get to the specified competencies	

readiness to practice with the knowledge and skills needed for clinical reasoning at the pointofcare. While the 2021 Essentials may not address DNP education as explicitly as in prior AACN documents, the profession certainly depends on practiced-based leadership to steward the profession forward and ensure readiness for practice.

WHAT DO THE NEW 2021 ESSENTIALS MEAN FOR DNP STUDENTS AND GRADUATES?

Embarking on the recently published AACN Essentials (2021a), specifically with competency-based education (CBE), constitutes a substantial shift in preparing nurses for contemporary practice. In CBE, the most impactful change for the DNP student will be the approach of self-directed learning and self-assessments. For the DNP graduate, CBE can lead to learning that lasts well beyond their formal college education (Rauschenberger et al., 2021). For the sake of capturing a glimpse of what the new AACN Essentials (2021a) with the integrated CBE model means for DNP students and graduates, we discuss broad and narrow perspectives to consider.

In a broad context, as explained in the foregoing, CBE is used as the framework for curricula that puts emphasis on the student's responsibility for their learning. Competencies are observable, measurable, and the achievement of the competency must be validated through demonstrated performance (Giddens, 2020). As an illustration applying the new Essentials with a CBE approach, a student would be required to meet various subcompetencies and when one is met, the student could possibly progress to the next requirement. The subcompetencies over time would be designed to "paint a picture" of how the competency can be achieved (AACN, 2021). You may question, how can this benefit the DNP student and graduate?

Competencies are maturing progressively over time and become more sophisticated with ongoing practice and thus provide value to the DNP student and graduate. This is a challenge for provide adequate resources to a student with minimal or no nursing experience compared to a student who is a well-seasoned nurse. A post-master's DNP student may have stark differences in advanced-level preparation and experiences compared to the entry-level nurse in a bachelor of science (BSN) to DNP program. Variations exist in the different aspects of competency completion and the rate at which a student can progress to validate achievement of the next subcompetency. Challenges to the approach could also lead to the academic institution and/or program of study designing the curriculum and processes informing successive succession of competencies. Hence, hard stops could thwart the time frame for demonstrating achievement of subcompetencies occurring within a course.

Self-knowledge and the ability for a DNP student to assess their own performances critically and accurately has been identified as having value in CBE (Rauschenberger et al., 2021). A student who performs self-assessment can identify their strengths and weaknesses, therefore concentrating on mastery of competency in areas where opportunities for improvement exist. To illustrate, a DNP student who enters a program with extensive quality and safety practice experience meets subcompetencies quickly in Domain 5: Quality and Safety, while a newly minted BSN-to-DNP student needing additional knowledge development and skills requires broader development. Each of these student illustrations can successfully achieve mastery of the subcompetencies and therefore, competency; however, the time and resources to successfully achieve mastery could differ. CBE can bridge these gaps through teaching and learning strategies with performance expectations that are observable and measurable (Giddens et al., 2022). Nonetheless, in considering differences among student preparedness and the varied level of entry, questions arise. Should students perform their own self-assessment? Are students adequately prepared and ready to complete their own self-assessment of performance? Do students perceive benefit to completing their own self-assessments? What does evidence inform around self-assessments specifically as it relates to DNP students? In time the capacity to better answer these questions may be more transparent anecdotally and in the literature.

Through a self-directed learning approach, CBE is learner centered and can improve the quality of learning for the student (Rauschenberger et al., 2021). Over the more traditional academic concept of teaching what is to occur, CBE results in what learning is to occur (Curry & Docherty, 2017). To an experienced nurse's benefit, there may be a potential time and cost reduction when pursuing DNP preparation. In contrast this may not be applicable to the student without professional nursing experience who may require additional time for knowledge and skills development.

Preparation of DNP students and graduates for readiness for real-world nursing practice is another advantage of CBE. Let us look to the future and ask, what does the nursing workforce need to look like? How should nursing education programs prepare graduates to be "work ready"? What can graduates do with their education? While the domains and competencies are broad in scope and cross all levels and areas of nursing practice, the subcompetencies build from entry into advanced professional nursing practice (AACN, 2021a). A well-prepared DNP graduate has the knowledge, skills, and attitudes that are requirements for ethical and competent clinical reasoning and the skill sets needed for contemporary nursing practice. DNP graduates have a larger and more diverse skill set—particularly in the areas of leadership, evidence-based practice, critical thinking, and quality improvement—and greater knowledge of policy, economics, and the business side of nursing (AACN, 2022a). The new Essentials are informed by 10 domains, 45 competencies, and 204 Level 2 subcompetencies. Indeed, this would be a lofty goal if students were expected to meet all. However, curriculum design in preparing DNP students is intended to provide the learner sufficient and diverse opportunities to achieve and demonstrate the competencies (AACN, 2021a) and can be accomplished in various ways through different subcompetencies.

In what ways can achievement of the competencies and subcompetencies as a DNP student have utility for a new DNP? DNP students should have a contextual understanding of the value of the DNP as it aligns with the competencies. According to a recent report (AACN, 2022a), uncertainty remains concerning the skills and value of DNP graduates among some practice employers. Achievement of competencies and subcompetencies aligned to the Essentials (AACN, 2021a) could prove beneficial in providing a linkage to practice. Development of a portfolio using the Essentials as a framework for students to present to a potential or actual employer could be mutually beneficial. What can the DNP-prepared nurse *"bring to the table"*? It is helpful to have an understanding of how the Essentials (AACN, 2021a) and competencies may correspond with employers' expectations. Table 24.5 provides an example of some contextualizing of common competencies that employers are seeking in nurses and how this may be applied to the 2021 AACN Essentials for the DNPstudent and graduate.

Nursing graduates will need to be wellequipped with a wide range of competencies and skills presently and in the coming years (Giddens et al., 2022). The domains and competencies in the AACN Essentials "exemplify the uniqueness of nursing as a profession and reflect the diversity of practice settings yet share common language that is understandable across healthcare professions and by employers, learners, faculty, and the public" (AACN, 2021a, p. 1). An additional benefit of CBE is that DNP students and graduates may come away with a sense of responsibility for their own learning and the ability and desire to continue learning independently (Rauschenberger et al., 2021). This

TABLE 24.5 Example of Contextualizing Competencies with the 2021 AACN Essentials for the DNP Student and Graduate

Competencies	Concepts for Nursing Practice:
Able to work on a team	o **Domain 3:** Population Health
	o **Domain 6:** Interprofessional Partnerships
Clinical decision-making	o **Domain 1:** Knowledge for Nursing Practice
	o **Domain 2:** Person-Centered Care
Communication skills	o **All Domains**
Compassion & empathy	o **Domain 2:** Person-Centered Care
Diversity, equity, and inclusion	o **Domain 2:** Person-Centered Care
	o **Domain 7:** Systems-Based Practice
Evidence-based practice (knowledge and current)	o **Domain 1:** Knowledge for Nursing Practice
	o **Domain 4:** Scholarship for Nursing Practice
Flexibility and Endurance	o **Domain 10:** Personal, Professional, and Leadership Development
Leadership	o **Domain 4:** Scholarship for Nursing Practice
	o **Domain 9:** Professionalism
	o **Domain 10:** Personal, Professional, and Leadership Development
Organization and time management	o **Domain 5:** Quality and Safety
Problem-solving	o **Domain 1:** Knowledge for Nursing Practice
	o **Domain 5:** Quality and Safety

Source: Adapted from Rauschenberger et al.'s (2021) webinar, produced by the AACN.

could provide merit to embracing and pursuing lifelong learning, which is a critical component and expectation for nursing professionals (IOM, 2011).

The new Essentials (AACN, 2021a) and the CBE approach to learning pose more questions than answers at the present time. Additionally, they present quandaries in academia for programs and faculty who are diligently working to reenvision curricula with the new AACN Essentials (2021a) and shift to CBE learning structures. Nonetheless, it is an exciting time to embrace disruptions in the current health environment, ponder what the future can hold, and capture the opportunity for making positive change. In nursing education and as a DNP student, now is a time for choosing to look either back or forward. If time stands still in nursing education and no changes are adopted, but the healthcare landscape evolves and practice evolves over time, what would the DNP graduate look like? Would the DNP student be wellprepared and ready for contemporary practice? DNP students and graduates are expected to shepherd the profession forward and therefore, there is only one way—forge forward. In concluding this section, here are some points to ponder.

- As nursing education and practice transform, where do you see yourself as a DNP student and graduate?
- How can I intentionally enhance my knowledge of the new AACN Essentials (2021) and CBE?
- In examining the AACN Essentials (2021a), how do I foresee myself as a DNP student preparing for a practice-ready role as a DNP graduate?

In an era of increased acuity, workforce shortages, and complexities in healthcare, DNP students and graduates fervently should foster a pursuit of excellence. The new Essentials and CBE may be ambitious, but they reflect insight into what is touted as a well-prepared nursing graduate ready for the healthcare environment of the future.

AACN DOCUMENTS ADDRESSING PHD NURSING EDUCATION

With the successful acceptance of the practice doctorate, distinguishing curricular guidelines between DNP and PhD education has led to much debate and confusion (Cronenwett et al., 2011; McCauley et al., 2020; Smith et al., 2021). In parallel with the AACN's key documents for DNP education, the AACN has also published documents to guide PhD nursing education, first in 1986, then again in 2001, 2010, and 2022 (AACN, 2022b). It is important to note that PhD nursing programs offered by schools of nursing were novel in the 1990s. Before the 1990s, most of the PhD-prepared nursing faculty obtained their PhDs in non-nursing disciplines (e.g., sociology, psychology, epidemiology, education, health services research). While the AACN currently addresses DNP and PhD education, it is important to note the historical timeline of doctoral nursing education degrees, which is shown in Figure 24.3.

Although the AACN's 2010 document guiding nursing PhD education is not labeled "Essentials of Nursing PhD education," it is helpful to read this document and the subsequent document published in 2022 (AACN, 2010, 2022b). Differences in the presumed roles of DNP and PhD graduates drive the debates and discussions regarding expectations of each group and how to shepherd the profession forward.

Just because the AACN Essentials guideline exists, it doesn't necessarily mean it is the golden rule. It is a critical resource for faculty involved in designing curricula and courses taught at the doctoral level in schools of nursing. From the tables presented throughout this chapter, it should be evident that DNP and PhD curricula are fluid. There are overlapping themes and language in all the AACN documents. Table 24.6 provides a summary of the AACN's expectations for PhD graduates, published in 2010 (AACN, 2010). Table 24.7 is from the AACN's recent 2022 white paper on the research doctorate in nursing, summarizing the core curricular elements for PhD programs in nursing (AACN, 2022b). Comparing these tables to Table 24.2 and Table 24.3 illustrate the overlap in expectations of DNP and PhD graduates. You can begin to see that there is even a blurring of some curricular elements.

2021 ESSENTIALS FOR DOCTORAL EDUCATION FOR ADVANCED NURSING PRACTICE: WHERE TO GO FROM HERE?

It is hard to believe that three decades have passed since the DNP doctorate degree was developed and implemented. DNP graduates bring important nursing scholarship and leadership to the profession, with impressive roles in academia and healthcare practice, meeting many marketplace demands (Auerbach et al., 2015; Dreher & Glasgow, 2017; Rundio & Wilson, 2015). Since the inception of the DNP academic degree, debate has ensued about the right terminal academic degree for advanced nursing practice, including those credentialed as advanced practice registered nurses (APRNs) who first

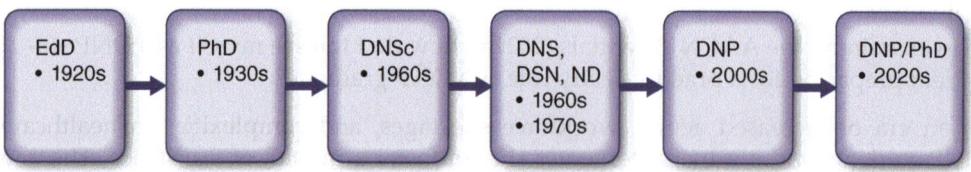

FIGURE 24.3 Doctoral Nursing Education Degrees: A Historical Timeline

TABLE 24.6 AACN's 2010 Document Guiding PhD Nursing Education: Expected Outcomes and Curricular Elements of PhD Programs in Nursing

Expected Roles of PhD Graduate	Outcomes Core	Curricular Elements
1. Develop the Science	• Master in-depth knowledge in a substantive area • Appreciate the history and philosophy of science • Understand the evolving nature of the nursing discipline • Critique and integrate different science perspectives in the conduct of research • Generate new ideas based on a critical evaluation of existing knowledge • Conduct original research • Utilize professional and research ethics and judgment in the conduct of research • Assume leadership in the conduct of culturally competent scholarship to improve nursing practice • Communicate research findings to lay and professional audiences and identify implications for policy, nursing practice, and the profession	• Sufficient formal and informal learning experiences to build scientific depth in an identified area of study • History and philosophies of science • Scientific methods, including team science • Advanced research design and statistical methods • Research ethics • Data, information and knowledge management, processing and analysis • Ways of knowing and habits of the mind • Concepts and components of scholarship • Mentored research experiences, including interdisciplinary mentors • Preparation of research grants and manuscripts for publication • Structured/guided clinical or practice experiences as needed to inform one's area of science and its application
2. Steward the Discipline	• Integrate the components of scholarship: research, teaching, mentoring, and service to the profession • Communicate scholarship including peer-refereed publications and presentations for professional interdisciplinary audiences • Understand the evolving roles and responsibilities of a nurse scholar • Lead in advancing the profession	• Theoretical/scientific underpinnings of nursing and other disciplines • Practice knowledge that informs nursing science and its application • Culture of nursing and practice environments • Strategies to influence health policy • Professional values • Scholarly writing • Leadership related to health policy and professional issues
3. Educate the Next Generation	• Conduct team science and participate and lead interdisciplinary research teams • Provide professional and research mentorship to others • Contribute to a global community of scholars • Contribute to the formal and informal education of future nurses through discovery, application, and integration	• Intra- and interdisciplinary communication skills • Leadership in intra- and interdisciplinary research teams • Mentoring • Leadership in culturally competent science • Art and science of teaching and learning • Mentored, integrative, applied experiences

Source: American Association of Colleges of Nursing [AACN]. (2010). *The research-focused doctoral program in nursing: Pathways to excellence.* https://www.aacnnursing.org/Portals/42/Publications/PhDPosition.pdf .Table 24.1.

TABLE 24.7 AACN's 2022 White Paper for Research Doctorate in Nursing: Summary of Core Curricular Elements that PhD Programs in Nursing Should Ensure Are expected Outcomes of Mastery and Skill Acquisition

PhD Nursing Core Curricular Items: Depth of knowledge and theoretical underpinnings are expected in the following substantive areas
• Philosophy, ethics, and the responsible conduct of research • Precision health • Effects of climate change on health • Determinants of health, health equity, and social justice (i.e., cultural humility, structural inequities in health, health disparities) • Health economics, patient-reported outcomes, health promotion and awareness, promotion of cultural safety, military, and LGBTI health • Global health and the conduct of global and rural health • Scientific methods, including team-based science • Advanced research design and statistical methods • Data methods, management, data analytics, and big data • Concepts and components of scholarship, design thinking, and innovation • Mentored research experiences, including interdisciplinary mentors and teams • Critical analysis of the extant literature • Grantsmanship and competencies in dissemination, both written and oral, to various audiences • Health policy engagement, implications of research on health policy and healthcare systems, and strategies to influence health policy and engage in advocacy • Skill-building in leadership through didactic and non-course elements to prepare the next generation of nurse leaders • Content on teaching and learning

Source: American Association of Colleges of Nursing [AACN]. (2022b). *The research-focused doctoral program in nursing: Pathways to excellence.* https://www.aacnnursing.org/Portals/42/News/Position-Statements/Pathways-Excellence-Position-Statement.pdf

obtained MSN degrees and built upon that with nursing practice–focused doctorate degrees (Dreher & Glasgow, 2017; McCauley et al., 2020). How will roles and competencies be different for APRNs who first obtain MSN degrees and build upon that with nursing practice–focused doctorate degrees? How will they differ? How will they differ from APRNs who obtain research-focused doctorate, PhD, degrees?

These questions still abound and the AACN has continually stepped in to provide clarity and guidance. Previous and current AACN position statements and Essentials documents will continue to influence where we go from here. Each doctoral-prepared nurse must ask themselves how their voice will be heard in the development of future AACN documents. Has the previous "graying" of nursing faculty turned the corner to a new voice shaping the future of nursing? We think so, as the great retirement and resignation of nursing was accelerated during COVID-19. Incentive packages for tenured faculty eligible for retirement packages and earning higher wages than their more junior counterparts has changed the academic nursing landscape. This should be viewed as a very exciting time for academic nursing—yielding the way to fresh perspectives from real-world nursing practice insights. Unprecedented numbers of nurses have sought doctoral education since the introduction of the practice doctorate in 2004 (AACN, 2020). It is exhilarating for students and professors, alike, to participate in the doctoral journeys of nurses passionate about learning more so they can better serve society's needs for caring and healing. Working together to build bridges and solutions to the *big* health problems that threaten all people is an important goal. Together, through nursing doctoral education, we have great opportunities to create important think tanks in which ideas for innovative solutions may be born.

The 2021 Essentials reinforce the notion that academia must be responsive to clinical healthcare practice needs. Nursing is not alone in adapting CBE approaches to disrupt our educational programs so our future workforce is better prepared for practice. Even our colleagues in medicine adapted CBE pedagogical approaches to better prepare their workforce to disrupt themselves by seeking innovative solutions (Englander et al., 2013; Englander & Carraccio, 2018; Holmboe et al., 2017). It took decades for some of the most disruptive innovations in nursing practice (e.g., nurse practitioner) and academic nursing (e.g., DNP) to take hold, despite tremendous initial push-back by mainstream academic nursing (Dunphy et al., 2009; McCauley et al., 2020). We have arrived at a critical junction. We *can* disrupt ourselves and put the profession of nursing first. It is a new day with tremendous opportunities for nurses with doctorate degrees—if only we all break down our guarded silos and genuinely collaborate across all roles and practice settings. It is critical that we all succeed, regardless of the differences in the alphabet soup of nursing degrees and credentials after our names. What is good for nursing is good for the people.

We must not accept the old saying, *nurses eat their young*, and look beyond incivility and microaggressions perpetuated by nurses to nurses in both academic and practice settings (Bloch & Smith Glasgow, 2023; Clark et al., 2021; McGee, 2021). As we go forward, trying to work together, remember the quote often attributed to Maya Angelou: *"people will forget what you said, people will forget what you did, but people will never forget how you made them feel"* (Angelou, 2021).

NURSES WITH DOCTORATE DEGREES: ETHICAL IMPERATIVE TO BREAK DOWN SILOS WHERE WE WORK TO ENHANCE COLLABORATIVE NURSING SCHOLARSHIP AND CLINICAL RESEARCH

It is clear from the 2021 Essentials that little attention is given to guiding doctoral nursing education, DNP or PhD. However, the DNP scholarly project is mentioned. Great debate and discussion over what a DNP scholarly project is or is not has ensued (Ketefian, 2013; Kirkpatrick & Weaver, 2013). Paramount to the discussion is the adamant refusal of DNP students to conduct research for their DNP scholarly project. The notion of what is research can be very contentious in nursing. What exactly is nursing research and nursing science is hotly debated in the literature as is also the question of who can do nursing science (Bloch & Smith Glasgow, 2023; Schnall, 2020). Must you be a nurse to conduct nursing research? The question of who is hired in schools of nursing to do research as tenured nursing faculty has raised many concerns as we witness PhD-prepared non-nurses given tenure-track positions, while PhD- and DNP-prepared nurses may be passed over and not offered tenure-track positions as they take on full-time academic nursing faculty positions (Algase et al., 2021; Bloch & Smith Glasgow, 2023; Schnall, 2020). We have no intention of answering these questions. We leave that to you to ponder and guide the next generation of doctoral students.

Nursing Research Is Clinical Research

With the explosion of DNP programs, much focus is on evidence-based practice (Melnyk & Finehout-Overholt, 2019), with many excellent DNP textbooks addressing DNP scholarship within the context of the DNP scholarly projects and evidence-based practice. Students who are deciding between a practice doctorate (DNP) or a research doctorate

(PhD) should decipher where they really would like to see themselves in either a role that is (a) entrenched in the real world of healthcare practice and clinical teaching or (b) behind the "ivy towers" entrenched in building and sustaining a program of research that advances nursing knowledge through competing for fiercely competitive research grants and living in a work environment where the old adage of "publish or perish" still prevails. Yet, these two worlds must intersect, for those with DNPs are demonstrating an important academic role educating future nurses. Therefore, such a dichotomy is unclear, and the nursing discipline should look at other disciplines (e.g., medicine, dentistry, law) where practitioners and researchers often move between both worlds. Merged communities of researchers and practitioners are essential for effective feedback loops of knowledge dissemination and translation necessary for evidence-based practice and practice-based evidence (Bloch, 2015; Bloch et al., 2016; Buchholz et al., 2015).

It is important not to lose sight of the importance of the patterns of knowing that underpin the nursing knowledge needed for nursing practice (Carper, 1978). Barbara Carper (1978) originally identified these patterns as empirical, aesthetic, personal, and ethical knowledge. All DNP students should read this original paper and reflect on how these patterns of knowing resonate with their expert nursing knowledge in their nursing practice roles. Empowered with the 2021 Essentials, guiding future curricula, think about these types of nursing knowledge described by Carper as we aim to promote the critical thinking and reasoning needed for various nursing practice roles in our complex healthcare system—for nursing roles in and out of hospital systems.

Translating clinical questions from nursing practice into research and then using relevant research findings to improve healthcare practice are aligned with the National Institutes of Health's (NIH's) clinical and translational science goals from the Center for Advancing Translational Sciences (NIH, 2022). Nursing scholarship concerning knowledge translation to practice for improving healthcare systems and health outcomes demands a thorough understanding of essential aspects of the clinical research process at the doctoral level (Buchholz et al., 2013). Preparing practice scholars with DNP credentials will require skills to interact with interdisciplinary colleagues about the evidence and clinical research. Clinical research designs, methods, and interpretation of data results using statistics are the same, no matter what discipline one is in. Nursing research is clinical research. According to the IOM (2002, p. 101):

> Clinical Research is a component of medical and health research intended to produce knowledge valuable for understanding human disease, preventing and treating illness, and promoting health. Clinical Research embraces a continuum of studies involving interactions with patients, diagnostic clinical materials or data, or populations in any of the following categories: (1) disease mechanisms (etiopathogenesis); (2) bi-directional integrative (translational) research; (3) clinical knowledge, detection, diagnosis and natural history of disease; (4) therapeutic interventions including development and clinical trials of drugs, biologics, devices, and instruments; (5) prevention (primary and secondary) and health promotion; (6) behavioral research; (7) health services research, including outcomes, and cost-effectiveness; (8) epidemiology; and (9) community-based and managed care-based trials.

Clearly the IOM's definition of clinical research is aligned to how nursing research is defined in our leading nursing textbooks. Yet, somehow, the concept of nursing research became siloed from the larger construct of clinical research. Nursing research textbooks either use the term research or nursing research, but rarely the term clinical research

(Gray et al., 2017; Melnyk & Fineout-Overholt, 2019; Polit & Beck, 2012). Conceptualizing nursing research within the broader construct of clinical research, as once was (IOM, 2002), may be illuminating and avoid barriers that prevent nurses involved in clinical research from collaborating, despite their roles either in practice or faculty roles. Perhaps we can use the 2021 Essentials to influence a paradigm shift, bringing more nurses with doctorate degrees together to push forward interdisciplinary and intradisciplinary clinical research. Relevant to the Essentials, the case study that follows highlights important lessons from clinical research conducted during the COVID-19 pandemic.

COVID-19 A Game Changer for Clinical Research and an Opportunity for the Nursing Profession

Clinical research priorities dramatically shifted to COVID-19 research in 2020. The world urgently depended on the scientific breakthroughs that occurred during the pandemic that brought life-saving therapeutic discoveries. The impact of the tremendous funding that was shifted to COVID through research enterprises that had the necessary clinical research infrastructure was a huge success. A plethora of scientific papers were published in a relatively short time. A recent PubMed search using COVID-19 as the keyword identified 312,876 articles published in less than 2 years, between January 2020 and November 15, 2022. Integral to the clinical and translational research enterprise are clinical research nurses (CRN). The CRN applies expert clinical research knowledge and skills to implement complex research protocols ensuring integrity and fidelity to the research protocol, while also protecting ethical and safe care to patients who are research participants (Showalter et al., 2022). Among academic nursing faculty and nursing practice, little is actually known about CRNs and their expertise in implementing clinical research protocols, not an easy task (Showalter et al., 2022). During COVID-19, the intersections between clinical care and clinical research just about collided.

Through the case study, we highlight key Essentials domains (or competencies) that can be applied to complex clinical research that occurs at academic health centers where opportunities for nursing scholarship, leadership, and research are abundant. The Essentials addresses the need for new specialties for transforming healthcare and emphasizes the importance of interprofessional partnerships (academia/practice) and across and within disciplines. Clinical research is a perfect vehicle to foster these types of critical relationships and expand opportunities for scholarship among DNP- and PhD- prepared nurse leaders.

The Essentials' Core Competencies for Professional Nursing Education, including interprofessional partnerships, systems-based practice, and professionalism, are always fundamental to the nursing profession, but especially in times of crisis. The AACN's New Era report (2016) identifies low levels of research collaboration between nursing schools with partner health systems, medical schools, and other professional schools. Transdisciplinary research programs should be supported to foster "university wide" research leadership and programs (p. 17). Of the more than 9,000 NIH-funded scientists in the healthcare workforce, only 3.7% were nurse scientists (AACN, 2016). Nurse scientists may be included in clinical research communities but are often lacking representation in the clinical research enterprise in many academic health centers. Many nurse scientists may not even be aware of such research infrastructures and the central role of clinical research nurses (CRN) in cutting-edge innovative research conducted at major biomedical research centers, not only in the United States, but globally. The case study reflects how the COVID-19 pandemic brought together nurse leaders who work full-time in research but were siloed and seemed like they were worlds apart. In the case study presented, will the 2021 Essentials and COVID-19 be a game changer?

CASE STUDY **Leadership and Ethical Dilemma for Two Doctoral-Prepared Nurses Implementing COVID-19 Research at an Academic Medical Center**

The two nurses, Drs. Smith and Quinn (names are fictitious), hold leadership positions that engage them full-time in research at a large hospital system associated with a leading academic medical center (AMC) renowned for its innovative, cutting-edge research. One reports to the health system's nursing department while the other reports to the school of medicine. Mary Smith, PhD, RN, CRNP, is the director of research and evidence based practice at this large AMC, and part of the nursing executive team. Dr. Smith oversees the implementation of nursing research and provides structured pathways for nurses to conduct nursing research within their practice environment. She has a formal academic partnership between the school of nursing and the AMC. In this role, Dr. Smith is responsible for maximizing the translation of evidence into nursing practice and providing resources and infrastructure for nurses to conduct nursing research. Dr. Smith and many of the other clinical nurses in the Department of Nursing give the impression to the clinical research nurses employed in the medical clinical research units that the clinical research conducted at the AMC is different from nursing research. The leadership team at the clinical research unit, through the school of medicine, seems to feel that there is an attitude that the AMC's interdisciplinary clinical research is less important than their nursing research department, which is under the Department of Nursing at the AMC.

Janet Quinn, DNP, RN, CRN-BC, is the director of the Center for Clinical Research at the same AMC. Dr. Quinn is not part of the nurse executive team in the department of nursing for her leadership position is in the school of medicine's clinical research unit, which is a National Institutes of Health–funded Clinical and Translational Science Award (CTSA) program hub. Dr. Quinn oversees a large staff of clinical research nurses (CRNs), technicians, bionutrition staff, and administrative staff. The CRN role is a direct care research position in AMCs and biomedical industries that have clinical research units, providing nursing care to complex patients who are also research participants.

At this AMC, the Center for Clinical Research implements hundreds of funded clinical research protocols and collaborates with a diverse group of clinical study teams. Dr. Quinn often feels disconnected from the rest of the institution because her nursing work is so specialized, and the significant contributions of her clinical research team often go unrecognized. Certainly, they are invisible heroes at the frontlines of clinical research where miraculous therapeutic discoveries occur. Yet, despite the research mission of the AMC, Drs. Smith and Quinn have never worked together and are unaware of the nuances of their individual research roles.

There is a long history of lack of integration of clinical care, clinical research, and nursing research. Yet, operations during COVID-19 changed that. During the COVID-19 pandemic Dr. Smith was the nursing representative tasked with implementation of COVID-19 protocols on the hospital nursing units, outside the Center for Clinical Research's clinical research unit. While Dr. Smith had vast experience in nursing research, she seemed to lack knowledge regarding the research enterprise infrastructure and support at the AMC's Clinical Research Center. It turns out that clinical research, except nursing research, is conducted through the well-funded and -staffed research infrastructure in the school of medicine.

(continued)

> Dr. Smith also was confronted with logistical research challenges due to the pandemic and needed more research support for the COVID-19 protocols that were taking place in the COVID units in the hospital. She reached out to Dr. Quinn seeking clinical research nursing. Dr. Smith was under the impression that the clinical research unit was vacant and that the CRNs needed assignments, which was incorrect. Unfortunately, Dr. Quinn was unable to assist Dr. Smith (and the department of nursing) due to several competing research priorities occurring on the clinical research unit, and a lack of training for the CRNs to be deployed to manage COVID-19 trials. Dr. Smith was left to implement COVID-19 protocols without the support of the Center for Clinical Research. Subsequently, Dr. Quinn tried to partner with Dr. Smith several months into the pandemic and initially was outright rejected by Dr. Smith. However, after several strategic meetings with other health system stakeholders, using the experience of the COVID-19 clinical research that was carried out on clinical units outside the clinical research unit, a relationship between the two nursing leaders has finally started to take hold. They are talking about finding ways to grow clinical research and nursing scholarship opportunities for all. While their first professional encounters were off-putting, they are slowly developing a professional relationship. Healthcare work environments can be stressful. When trust among *strangers* who are competing for institutional resources is not the culture of the work environment, it can be intimidating to forge productive professional relationships. It takes work and time. Hopefully, Drs. Smith and Quinn will eventually feel safe enough in their work environment and let their guard down so other nurses will flourish through their leadership.

What a shame for nursing when there are siloes between nurses, like these two nursing practice leaders who both lead research initiatives under the same umbrella organization. Applying the 2021 Essentials to this case study highlights how the case study can be framed in a constructive way for learning, which is outlined in Table 24.8. Consider how applying the 2021 Essentials to this case study gives insight into outcomes of collaborative professional relationships between Drs. Smith and Quinn that could benefit the organization, patients, and nursing staff.

Ethics is a core concept in the 2021 Essentials (AACN, 2021a). The ethical implications of the issues raised in this case study simulates many real-world nursing practice scenarios with changes only in the cast of characters and the clinical setting. The 2021 Essentials presents many ways for DNP students to translate what ethics means to them in advanced nursing practice. In this example, there is confusion about who does and what is clinical research and nursing research. Simple tweaks to the terminology used could foster improved understandings for better collaboration between these two nurse leaders. For example, the discipline of medicine often refers to the term translational science spectrum (NIH, https://ncats.nih.gov/translation/spectrum) while nursing often refers to evidence-based practice (Melnyk & Fineout-Overholt, 2019). Clinical research that occurs in hospital units when patients are also research participants require intentional collaboration between many stakeholders. Underpinning the case study are ethical issues that impacted the nursing staff in providing the best possible care to patients, which certainly was a challenge during the COVID-19 pandemic. Table 24.9 outlines some of the ethical implications within the case study.

TABLE 24.8 2021 Essentials Highlighted in the Case Study

2021 Essentials Domain of Knowledge	2021 Essentials Competency	Application to Case Study
Personal, Professional, and Leadership Development	Cognitive flexibility in managing change within complex environments	Although Drs. Smith and Quinn have different nursing backgrounds and nursing roles related to research, their combined knowledge would have a broader impact than their individual contributions. Self awareness and continuous reflection are important for leadership development. Neither Dr. Smith nor Dr. Quinn considered the impact of their inability to collaborate on the nursing profession and future opportunities to enrich scholarship among nurses through their university.
Interprofessional partnerships	Intentional collaboration Fostering positive team dynamics to strengthen desired outcomes	Drs. Smith and Quinn were not intentional. Rather than thinking of ways they could help each other, they came to an impasse. Were they just protecting their "own turfs" within the organization? Perhaps it could be better if they are reminded of core professional values of altruism, excellence, caring, ethics, respect, communication, and shared accountability.
Interprofessional partnerships	Foster an environment that supports the constructive sharing of multiple perspectives and enhances interprofessional learning	Clinical research professionals (e.g., project manager, research assistants) that conduct clinical research are integral members of the care team for participants on clinical research such as the research that occurred during COVID-19. They are often placed in clinical situations without the same expertise and training as clinicians. Drs. Smith and Quinn had an opportunity to combine efforts to foster bidirectional learning between the clinical staff and the research staff. There is always so much to learn when cutting-edge clinical research is conducted.
Systems-Based Practice	Participate in organizational strategic planning. Integrated healthcare systems are highly complex, and gaps or failures in service or delivery can cause ineffective, harmful outcomes. Cognitive shifting from focused to big picture is a crucial skill set.	Drs. Smith and Quinn were focused on their own roles and did appear to view collaboration as beneficial. Focused on their individual objectives, no system rewards existed for developing collaborative working relationships. The organization also did not prioritize the integration of clinical research prior to COVID-19. Having a voice at the table for strategic planning is imperative for nurses. Making explicit the implicit barriers for the workforce and their workflow is critical.

TABLE 24.9 Ethical Implications of the Case Study: Barriers to Collaboration During the COVID-19 Pandemic When Hospitalized Patients Are also Research Participants

Ethical Implication	Real-World Application
Inadequate nurse staffing	Nurses are "obligated to provide optimal patient care" according to provision 4 of the American Nurses Association Code of Ethics (ANA, 2015). When nurses find themselves in a situation where they have more patients than they can safely care for, it puts patients and staff at risk and causes moral distress. Staffing ratios during the pandemic were complicated due to isolation precautions, visitation restriction for caregivers, and staff illness. – Patients receiving investigational therapy require close oversight and additional monitoring necessitating lower nurse-to-patient ratios. – Additional personal protective equipment was not available early in the pandemic, and there was a shortage of N95 masks which limited the number of staff that could enter and exit the room of a patient with COVID. – Drs. Smith and Quinn could not think past some of the staffing issues associated with implementation of COVID-19 research protocols. Creative solutions were needed to implement clinical research during this pandemic. – Creation of a nursing-specific ethical framework and evidence-based logic for rationing and resource allocation of nursing resources during times of crisis is a missed opportunity for collaboration between Drs. Smith and Quinn. – "The need to balance multiple ethical values for various interventions and in different circumstances is likely to lead to differing judgments about how much weight to give each value in particular cases. This highlights the need for fair and consistent allocation procedures that include the affected parties: clinicians, patients, public officials, and others" (Emanuel, 2020).
Informed Consent	– The process of informed consent consists of (a) provision of complete and accurate information, (b) assessment of comprehension, and (c) safeguards to protect voluntary participation (American Nurses Association and International Association for Clinical Research Nursing, 2016). – Communication breakdowns between the research teams and the clinical teams can lead to a poor informed consent process. This was compounded by strict isolation precautions throughout the pandemic and an absent infrastructure. – Adherence to all three elements of informed consent is paramount in the conduct of clinical research. Interprofessional partnerships are critical to the safe care of participants on clinical trials. – Nurses administering investigational treatments without full knowledge of the protocol, and inability to answer questions in real time regarding the investigational treatment causes moral distress and burnout over time.

Appreciate Diverse Roles and Perspectives Among Nurses with Practice Doctorate Degrees: Seek Conceptual Clarity

Conceptual clarity is critical as there are key terms used in nursing, healthcare, and nursing education that are not uniformly defined. Language is critical and clear understanding of terms is mandatory. Given that communication is a core nursing concept in the 2021 Essentials, conceptual clarity is essential when communicating with others as we seek to transform nursing education guided by the 2021 Essentials. In our analysis of the 2021 Essentials, we found that definitions of key nursing terms are not necessarily consistent among the multiple AACN documents that we reviewed in this chapter. Respect for multiple realities and perspectives should be expected. Therefore, it is important to reach consensus within your working groups on explicit definitions of key terms. This will be salient when designing how to measure competencies for CBE curricula. Even the term competency for CBE curricula is vulnerable to misinterpretation (Englander et al., 2013). While the *2006 AACN* Essentials *for DNP Education* does not define competency, the 2015 AACN's *White Paper for DNP Education* defines competency (p. 11) in more depth than the 2021 Essentials (p. 56), and states that "nursing does not have its own universally agreed upon measurable competencies and tools to measure competencies" (p. 11). It is important to keep this in mind, especially for CBE curricula for DNP education. Become part of the virtual community on the AACN's Essentials website (https://www.aacnnursing.org/Essentials), which is continually updated with new resources and conversations.

With attention to language, the term *advanced nursing practice* presents confusion between the 2015 AACN's DNP white paper and the 2021 Essentials. The 2015 AACN document explicitly defines advanced nursing practice as separate from an advanced practice nurse (APN or APRN). However, the 2021 Essentials does not define APN. Since the 2015 AACN document remains an important document guiding DNP education, an analysis of the terms between both documents was conducted. Table 24.10 compares terms explicitly defined by the AACN's 2015 white paper with the 2021 Essentials. Of the 13 terms extracted from the 2015 DNP document, only 33.3% ($n = 4$) were defined the same in the 2021 Essentials.

TABLE 24.10 Comparing the AACN's Glossary Terms and Definitions that Are Relevant for DNP Education in the AACN 2015 White Paper with the 2021 Essentials

2015 Glossary Term and Its Definition	Does the Term Appear in the 2021 AACN Essentials' Glossary?	Is It Defined the Same?
Advanced nursing practice: Any form of nursing intervention that influences healthcare outcomes for individuals or populations, including the direct care of individual patients, management of care for individuals and populations, administration of nursing and healthcare organizations, and the development and implementation of health policy	No	n/a *(not in the glossary)*
Advanced practice registered nurse: The title given to a nurse who has met education and certification requirements and obtained a license to practice as an APRN in one of four APRN roles: certified registered nurse anesthetist (CRNA), certified nurse-midwife (CNM), clinical nurse specialist (CNS), and certified nurse practitioner)	Yes	No Not the same definition

(continued)

TABLE 24.10 Comparing AACN's Glossary Terms and definitions that are relevant for DNP Education in the AACN 2015 White paper with the 2021 Essentials (*continued*)

2015 Glossary Term and Its Definition	Does the Term Appear in the 2021 AACN Essentials' Glossary?	Is It Defined the Same?
Collaboration: When multiple health workers from different professional backgrounds work together with patients, families, caregivers, and communities to deliver the highest quality of care.	No	n/a *(not in the glossary)*
Competence: The array of abilities across multiple domains or aspects of performance in a certain context. Statements about competence require descriptive qualifiers to define relevant abilities, context, and stages of training. Competence is multidimensional and dynamic. It changes with time, experience, and setting.	Yes	Yes *(same source, but more concise)*
Healthcare outcomes: The end result of healthcare practices. There are many kinds of outcomes. How long people live following a healthcare treatment is one kind of outcome, known as survival. Other outcomes measure the effects a treatment has on people's lives, such as changes in their ability to function or changes in their quality of life. Outcomes also include undesirable events such as side effects of drugs. Another type of outcome is whether people needed to change to another kind of treatment.	No	n/a *(not in the glossary)*
Implementation science: The study of methods to promote the integration of research findings and evidence into healthcare policy and practice.	No	n/a *(not in the glossary)*
Informatics: Nursing informatics (NI) is a specialty that integrates nursing science, computer science, and information science to manage and communicate data, information, knowledge, and wisdom into nursing practice. NI supports consumers, patients, nurses, and other providers in their decision-making in all roles and settings. This support is accomplished through the use of information structures, information processes, and information technology.	Yes	No *(different, broader than just nursing informatics)*
Interprofessional collaborative practice: Working across healthcare professions to cooperate, collaborate, communicate, and integrate care in teams to ensure that care is continuous and reliable. The team consists of the patient, the nurse, and other healthcare providers as appropriate.	No	n/a *(not in the glossary)*
Interprofessional education: Involves shared learning experiences among health profession students across disciplines, with the goals of building strong clinical teams and improving health outcomes.	No	n/a *(not in the glossary)*
Population health: Inclusive of aggregates, community, and/or clinical populations that consider the environmental, occupational, and cultural, socioeconomic and other dimensions of health, and derives evidence from population-level data and statistics.	No	n/a *(not in the glossary)*

(*continued*)

TABLE 24.10 Comparing AACN's Glossary Terms and definitions that are relevant for DNP Education in the AACN 2015 White paper with the 2021 Essentials (*continued*)

2015 Glossary Term and Its Definition	Does the Term Appear in the 2021 AACN Essentials' Glossary?	Is It Defined the Same?
Public health: Public health is the science of protecting and improving the health of families and communities through promotion of healthy lifestyles, research for disease and injury prevention, and detection and control of infectious diseases.	No	n/a (*not in the glossary*)
Quality improvement: In healthcare quality improvement (QI) refers to routinely giving the right patients the right care at the right time and in the right place of service. Typically, QI efforts are strongly rooted in evidence-based procedures and rely extensively on data collected about processes, outcomes, and infrastructure.	Yes	No
Quality improvement in public health: The use of a defined improvement process, such as a four-step model Plan-Do-Check-Act, which is focused on activities that are responsive to community needs for carrying out change in public health practice and improving population health. It refers to a continuous and outgoing effort to achieve measurable improvements in the efficiency, effectiveness, performance, accountability, outcomes, and other indicators of quality in services or processes which achieve equity and improve the health of the community.	No	n/a

Source: This table was adapted from the glossary lists that appeared in the 2015 AACN's DNP white paper and the 2021 AACN Essentials. All definitions listed above are as they appeared in the 2015 AACN white paper.

CHAPTER SUMMARY AND CONCLUSIONS

Healthcare in the 21st century is experiencing a radical transformation exemplified by a cadre of trends contributing to what has been referred to as a healthcare revolution (AACN, 2019). Accordingly, nursing education has an obligation to be congruent in preparing DNP graduates for the current and future healthcare landscape (Giddens et al., 2022). Although the approach to align academic preparation to the practice arena is not novel, embarking on the recently published AACN Essentials (2021) specifically with competency-based education (CBE) constitutes a substantial shift preparing nurses for contemporary practice. Nursing graduates will need to be well equipped with a wide range of competencies and skills in order to elevate the profession and remain viable in evolving healthcare enterprises (Giddens et al., 2022).

In speaking to what CBE means for DNP students and graduates, we would be amiss not to recognize the impact the nursing workforce has on the nation's health and envisioning the future. Nursing comprises the largest healthcare profession, with about 4.2 million registered nurses nationwide (AACN, 2022a). For two decades nursing has been identified as the most trusted profession according to a Gallop poll (Gallop, 2022).

PhD and DNP programs provide complementary approaches to the highest level of nursing education (Cygan & Reed, 2019; Michael & Clochesy, 2016). While they may differ regarding goals and research competencies, they share important goals for shepherding the profession forward. The academic preparation leading to the PhD and the DNP are distinct yet share some common threads. As outlined above in this chapter, several concepts identified in the updated 2021 Essentials are germane to PhD and DNP educational preparation: ethics, health policy, and social determinants of health. The unique competencies of both groups of doctoral-prepared nurses must be combined and leveraged to ensure that the profession assumes a leadership role in the integration and translation of research into practice (Buchholtz et al., 2015; Michael & Clochesy, 2016).

During the unprecedented coronavirus pandemic, the crucial role of nursing was illuminated, and nurses are now commonly hailed as heroes. In looking forward, lessons learned and insights gained during the pandemic can be used as a springboard to prepare the next generation of nurses for the healthcare complexities, leadership, future disaster threats, and public health preparedness. Nurses will face many formidable challenges in the coming years (NASEM, 2021).

The AACN Essentials sets the stage for nurses seeking their terminal nursing practice doctoral degree. DNP faculty must be courageous to relinquish their traditional approach toward doctoral students, otherwise they may hinder potential innovation. The 2021 AACN Essentials will guide your curriculum and you then will guide the AACN and future AACN-guided curricula. You will be the driver of your role and success once you attain your DNP academic degree. Collectively, we must collaborate across all borders—across all doctoral degrees, clinical specialties, and nursing roles. Bridging nursing leaders together in nursing practice and academia creates infrastructure that will build a sound foundation for future generations of nurses. As stewards of the profession, reflect on the AACN Essentials (AACN, 2021a). Embrace curiosity as nursing scholars, and continue to ask and share our questions on how to push forward health and healthcare.

CRITICAL THINKING QUESTIONS

1. Explain how DNP program chairs should decide if PhD faculty will be involved in teaching DNP courses. Provide perspectives from the AACN 2021 Essentials that support this or do not support this position.
2. What gives you optimism or pessimism about the new 2021 AACN Essentials and the future of DNP education?
3. As nursing education undergoes revisions to align with the 2021 AACN Essentials, choose two of the Essentials that you would develop with your DNP classmates/faculty because either they are areas of interest or you bring expertise.
4. Think back to the best teachers you had in your nursing courses during your graduate nursing education. Reflect how and why their teaching strategies were effective. Could you align them into your CBE approaches when you serve as a DNP-prepared nursing educator as you share your clinical expertise with future students?
5. Reflecting on the previous question, try articulating your pedagogical approach in a three-sentence statement.
6. Given your expertise in nursing practice as a DNP student, assess your competencies among the 10 AACN CBE domains. Create a tailored plan for your DNP education in the domains where you seek additional competencies and explain why. Can you articulate how your plan will help you lead the profession forward when you graduate with your DNP degree.
7. Given the dire need for nursing faculty and the discordance in pay and sometimes respect in nursing academe and practice, explain how the Essentials core concepts

align with the concepts of intersectionality, microaggressions, and implicit bias in addressing incivility and bullying in nursing.
8. Explain why or why not the AACN should have more explicit DNP educational competencies in its efforts to transform nursing education to ensure DNP nurses are ready to lead nursing practice so new nurses are ready for practice equipped with clinical reasoning skills for nursing practice.
9. You are a tenured DNP faculty member who has a PhD in nursing, actively practice as a nurse practitioner, and engaged in community-based translational research. The newly appointed associate dean of nursing who has a DNP (nontenure track) in a college of health sciences decides that no PhD nursing faculty can teach in the DNP program. Why would you support or not support this new rule?

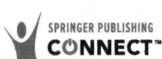

A robust set of instructor resources designed to supplement this text is located at http://connect.springerpub.com/content/book/978-0-8261-8137-4. Qualifying instructors may request access by emailing textbook@springerpub.com.

REFERENCES

Aiken, L., & Fagin, C. (1991). *Charting nursing's future*. J. B. Lippincott Company.

Algase, D., Stein, K., Arslanian-Engoren, C., Corte, C., Sommers, M. S., & Carey, M. G. (2021). An eye toward the future: Pressing questions for our discipline in today's academic and research climate. *Nursing Outlook, 69*(1), 57–64. https://doi.org/10.1016/j.outlook.2020.08.010.

American Association of Colleges of Nursing [AACN]. (2004). *Position statement on the practice doctorate in nursing*. https://www.aacnnursing.org/News-Information/Position-Statements-White-Papers/Practice-Doctorate

American Association of Colleges of Nursing [AACN]. (2006). *DNP Essentials*. https://www.aacnnursing.org/DNP/DNP-Essentials

American Association of Colleges of Nursing [AACN]. (2010). *The research-focused doctoral program in nursing: Pathways to excellence*. https://www.aacnnursing.org/Portals/42/Publications/PhDPosition.pdf

American Association of Colleges of Nursing [AACN]. (2015). *The Doctor of Nursing Practice: Current issues and clarifying recommendations*. https://www.aacnnursing.org/Portals/42/DNP/DNP-Implementation.pdf

American Association of Colleges of Nursing [AACN]. (2016). *Advancing healthcare transformation: A new Era for academic nursing*. https://www.aacnnursing.org/portals/42/publications/aacn-new-era-report.pdf

American Association of Colleges of Nursing [AACN]. (2019). *AACN's vision for academic nursing* https://www.aacnnursing.org/News-Information/Position-Statements-White-Papers/Vision-for-Nursing-Education

American Association of Colleges of Nursing [AACN]. (2020). *DNP fact sheet*. https://www.aacnnursing.org/News-Information/Fact-Sheets/DNP-Fact-Sheet

American Association of Colleges of Nursing [AACN]. (2021a). *The essentials: Core competencies for professional nursing education*. https://www.aacnnursing.org/Education-Resources/AACN-Essentials

American Association of Colleges of Nursing [AACN]. (2021b). *Data spotlight: Insights on the nursing faculty shortage*. https://www.aacnnursing.org/News-Information/News/View/ArticleId/25043/data-spotlight-august-2021-Nursing-Faculty-Shortage

American Association of Colleges of Nursing [AACN]. (2022a). *AACN position statement on the practice doctorate in nursing*. https://www.aacnnursing.org/DNP/Position-Statement

American Association of Colleges of Nursing [AACN]. (2022b). *The research-focused doctoral program in nursing: Pathways to excellence*. https://www.aacnnursing.org/Portals/42/News/Position-Statements/Pathways-Excellence-Position-Statement.pdf

American Association of University Professors [AAUP]. (2015). *AAUP (American Association of University Professors): Policy documents and reports*, (11th ed.). Johns Hopkins University Press.

Angelou, M. (2021, August 5). *Maya Angelou quotes: 31–44 of 44 quotes.* https://www.quotescosmos.com/people/Maya-Angelou-quotes-2.html#14

Auerbach, D. I., Martsolf, G. R., Pearson, M. L., Taylor, E. A., Zaydman, M., Muchow, A. N., Muchow, A. N., Spetz, J., & Lee, Y. (2015). The DNP by 2015: A study of the institutional, political, and professional issues that facilitate or impede establishing a post-baccalaureate doctor of nursing practice program. *Rand Health Q, 5*(1), 3.

Billings, D. M., & Halstead, J. A. (2005). *Teaching in nursing: A guide for faculty,* (2nd ed.). Elsevier Saunders.

Bloch, J. R. (2015). Will nursing faculty hinder or facilitate innovation in nurse executive DNP students? In A. Rundio & V. Wilson (Eds.), *The doctor of nursing practice and the nurse executive role.* Wolters Kluwer Health.

Bloch, J. R., Courtney, M. R., & Clark, M. L. (Eds.). (2016). *Practice-based clinical inquiry in nursing for DNP and PhD research: Looking beyond traditional methods.* Springer Publishing Company.

Bloch, J. R., & Smith Glasgow, M. (2023). Where are nurse-scientists? Academic nursing research at critical crossroads. *Nursing Outlook, 71*(2), 101894.

Boamah, S. A., Hamadi, H. Y., Havaei, F., Smith, H., & Webb, F. (2022). Striking a balance between work and play: The effects of work-life interference and burnout on faculty turnover intentions and career satisfaction. *International Journal of Environmental Research & Public Health, 19*(2), 809. https://doi.org/10.3390/ijerph19020809

Boulton, M., Garnett, A., & Webster, F. (2022). A Foucauldian discourse analysis of media reporting on the nurse-as-hero during COVID-19. *Nursing Inquiry, 29*(3), e12471. https://doi.org/10.1111/nin.12471

Buchholz, S. W., Budd, G. M., Courtney, M. R., Neiheisel, M. B., Hammersla, M., & Carlson, E. D. (2013). Preparing practice scholars: Teaching knowledge application in the Doctor of Nursing Practice curriculum. *Journal of the American Association of Nurse Practitioners, 25*(9), 473–480. https://doi.org/10.1002/2327-6924.12050

Buchholz, S. W., Yingling, C., Jones, K., & Tenfelde, S. (2015). DNP and PhD collaboration: Bringing together practice and research expertise as predegree and postdegree scholars. *Nurse Educator, 40*(4), 203–206. https://doi.org/10.1097/NNE.0000000000000141

Campbell-O'Dell, D. G., & Dreher, H. M. (2017). A critique of the 2006 Essentials of doctoral education for advanced nursing practice: Do they guide practice? In H. M. Dreher & M. E. S. Glasgow (Eds.), *DNP role development for Doctoral Advanced Nursing Practice* (pp. 527–549). Springer Publishing Company.

Carper, B. A. (1978). Fundamental patterns of knowling in nursing. *Advances in Nursing Science, 1*(1), 13–23. https://doi.org/10.1097/00012272-197810000-00004

Chinn, P. L. (2008). Philosophical foundations for excellence in teaching. In B. A. Moyer & R. A. Wittman-Price (Eds.), *Nursing Education: Foundations for practice excellence* (pp. 15–31). F. A. Davis Company.

Clark, C. M., Landis, T. T., & Barbosa-Leiker, C. (2021). National study on faculty and administrators' perceptions of civility and incivility in nursing education. *Nurse Educator, 46*(5), 276–283. https://doi.org/10.1097/nne.0000000000000948

Cronenwett, L., Dracup, K., Grey, M., McCauley, L., Meleis, A., & Salmon, M. (2011). The Doctor of Nursing Practice: A national workforce perspective. *Nursing Outlook, 59*(1), 9–17. https://doi.org/10.1016/j.outlook.2010.11.003

Curry, L., & Docherty, M. (2017). Implementing competency-based education. *Collected Essays on Learning and Teaching, 10,* 61–74. https://doi.org/10.22329/celt.v10i0.4716

Cygan, H. R., & Reed, M. (2019). DNP and PhD scholarship: Making the case for collaboration. *Journal of Professional Nursing, 35*(5), 353–357. https://doi.org/10.1016/j.profnurs.2019.03.002

de Bueno, D. J. (1978). Competency-based Education. *Nurse Educator, 3,* 11–14.

Douglass, B., Scruggs-Corey, J., & Stanley, J. (2021, August 11). *DNP education and practice: A facilitated conversation embracing the essentials.* Paper presented at the Fourteenth National Doctors of Nursing Practice National Conference.

Dreher, H. M., & Glasgow, M. E. S. (2017). *DNP role development for doctoral advanced nursing practice.* Springer Publishing.

Dunphy, L. M., Smith, N. K., & Youngkin, E. Q. (2009). Advanced nursing practice: Doing what has to be done-radicals, renegades, and rebels. In L. Joel (Ed.), *Advanced practice nursing* (2nd ed., pp. 2–22). F. A. Davis.

Englander, R., Cameron, T., Ballard, A. J., Dodge, J., Bull, J., & Aschenbrener, C. A. (2013). Toward a common taxonomy of competency domains for the health professions and competencies for physicians. *Academic Medicine, 88*(8), 1088–1094. https://doi.org/10.1097/ACM.0b013e31829a3b2b

Englander, R., & Carraccio, C. (2018). A lack of continuity in education, training, and practice violates the "Do No Harm" principle. *Academic Medicine, 93*(3S), S12–S16. https://doi.org/10.1097/acm.0000000000002071

Gallop, P. (2022). *Honesty/ethics in professions.* https://news.gallup.com/poll/1654/Honesty-Ethics-Professions.aspx

Galura, S., & Warshawsky, N. (2022). Initial evaluation of a Doctor of Nursing Practice - Executive track program: The development of a three-year process to implement the new AACN Essentials. *Journal of Professional Nursing, 42,* 276–280. https://doi.org/10.1016/j.profnurs.2022.07.014

Giddens, J., Douglas, J. P., & Conroy, S. (2022). The revised AACN essentials: Implications for nursing regulation. *Journal of Nursing Regulation, 12*(4), 16–22. https://doi.org/10.1016/S2155-8256(22)00009-6

Gray, J. R., Grove, S. K., & Sutherland, S. (2017). *Burns and Grove's the practice of nursing research: Appraisal, synthesis, and generation of evidence* (8th ed.). Elsevier.

Holmboe, E. S., Sherbino, J., Englander, R., Snell, L., & Frank, J. R. (2017). A call to action: The controversy of and rationale for competency-based medical education. *Medical Teacher, 39*(6), 574–581. https://doi.org/10.1080/0142159x.2017.1315067

Institute of Medicine [IOM]. (1999). *To err is human: Building a safer health system.* National Academies Press.

Institute of Medicine [IOM]. (2001). *Crossing the quality chasm: A new health system for the 21st century.* The National Academies Press.

Institute of Medicine [IOM]. (2002). Clinical research roundtable. In S. Tunis, A. Korn, A. Ommaya (Eds.), *The role of purchasers and payers in the clinical research enterprise: Workshop summary.* The National Academies Press.

Institute of Medicine [IOM]. (2013). *Health in international perspective: Shorter lives, poorer health.* http://www.iom.edu/Reports/2013/US-Health-in-International-Perspective-Shorter-Lives-Poorer-Health/Report-Brief010913.aspx

Jarosinski, J. M., Seldomridge, L., Reid, T. P., & Willey, J. (2022). Nurse faculty shortage: Voices of nursing program administrators. *Nurse Educator, 47*(3), 151–155. https://doi.org/10.1097/NNE.0000000000001139

Jeffries, P. R. (2020). Academic nursing dean's role during COVID-19: Lessons from the frontlines of higher education. *Nurse Educator, 45*(5), 229–230. https://doi.org/10.1097/NNE.0000000000000903

Ketefian, S. (2013). Is the DNP fulfilling its promise? *Dean's Notes, 35*(2), 1–2.

Kirkpatrick, J. M., & Weaver, T. (2013). The doctor of nursing practice capstone project: Consensus or confusion. *Journal of Nursing Education, 52*(8), 435–441. https://doi.org/10.3928/01484834-20130722-01

McCauley, L. A., Broome, M. E., Frazier, L., Hayes, R., Kurth, A., Musil, C. M., Norman, L. D., Rideout, K. H., & Villarruel, A. M. (2020). Doctor of Nursing Practice (DNP) degree in the United States: Reflecting, readjusting, and getting back on track. *Nursing Outlook, 68*(4), 494–503. https://doi.org/10.1016/j.outlook.2020.03.008

McGee, P. L. (2021). A descriptive study of faculty-to-faculty incivility in nursing programs in the United States. *Journal of Professional Nursing, 37*(1), 93–100. https://doi.org/10.1016/j.profnurs.2020.07.004

Melnyk, B. M., & Finehout-Overholt, E. (ed.). (2019). *Evidence-based practice in nursing and healthcare* (4th ed.). Wolters Kluwer.

Michael, M., & Clochesy, J. M. (2016). From scientific discovery to health outcomes: A synergistic model of doctoral nursing education. *Nurse Education Today, 40,* 84–86. https://doi.org/10.1016/j.nedt.2016.02.011. PMID: 27125154

Moyer, B. A., & Wittmann-Price, R. A. (Eds.). (2008). *Nursing education: Foundations for practice excellence.* F. A. Davis Company.

National Academies of Sciences, Engineering, and Medicine [NASEM]. (2021). *The future of nursing 2020–2030: Charting a path to achieve health equity.* The National Academies Press. https://doi.org/10.17226/25982

National Institutes of Health [NIH]. (2022). *Clinical and Translational Science Awards (CTSA) program.* National Center for Advancing Translational Scinces. https://ncats.nih.gov/ctsa

Peterson, C. J., Broderick, M. E., Demarest, L., & Holey, L. (1979). *Competency-based curriculum and instruction.* National League of Nursing [NLN] Report # 23-1770.

Polit, D. E., & Beck, C. T. (2012). *Nursing research: Generating, and assessing evidence for nursing practice* (9th ed.). Wolter Kluwer Health/Lippincott Williams & Williams.

Rauschenberger, Schulte, J., & Eerden, A.V. (2021). American Association of Colleges of Nursing [Producer]. *Introduction to competency-based education* [webinar]. https://www.aacnnursing.org/Essentials/Webinars-Programs

Roush, K. (2022). The Top News Stories of 2021: Nursing: A profession reshaped by COVID-19. *American Journal of Nursing, 122*(1), 13. https://doi.org/10.1097/01.NAJ.0000815384.08710.bb

Rundio, A., & Wilson, V. (2015). *The Doctor of Nursing Practice and the nurse executive role.* Wolters Kluwer Health.

Schnall, R. (2020). National Institute of Health (NIH) funding patterns in schools of nursing: Who is funding nursing science research and who is conducting research at schools of nursing? *Journal of Professional Nursing, 36*(1), 34–41. https://doi.org/10.1016/j.profnurs.2019.07.003

Showalter, B. L., Malecha, A., Cesario, S., & Clutter, P. (2022). Moral distress in clinical research nurses. *Nursing Ethics, 29*(7–8), 1697–1708. https://doi.org/10.1177/09697330221090613

Smith, G. L., Schultz, C. M., & Danforth, C. A. (2021). DNP or PhD? Dispelling misconceptions. *DNP or PhD? The Journal for Nurse Practitioners, 17*(9), 1122–1123. https://doi.org/10.1016/j.nurpra.2021.05.026

Welch, T. D., & Smith, T. B. (2022). AACN Essentials as the conceptual thread of nursing education. *Nursing Administration Quarterly, 46*(3), 234–244.

CHAPTER TWENTY-FOUR Reflective Response

MARY F. TERHAAR

The much-anticipated *New Essentials: Core Competencies for Professional Nursing Education* (AACN, 2021) is the result of intentional and inclusive deliberations that spanned some 5 years. Top-10 and small programs; rural and urban programs; full professors and clinical instructors; chief nursing executives; leaders from healthcare, industry, and public health; entrepreneurs; academics; scientists; clinicians; policymakers; informaticians; advocates; and consumers all worked their way through challenging conversations focused on moving the profession toward the goals set by the Robert Wood Johnson Foundation and the National Academy of Sciences. Their shared commitment was to lay a foundation for a future where nurses practice at the top of their license, advance the health of the nation, and have parity with other professionals in the health sector.

The chapter written by Bloch, Douglass, & Brock, academics from leading U.S. schools of nursing, guides the reader through a journey that brings nursing to an important inflection point. The authors describe the ontogeny of the Essentials in general and the Level 2 Essentials in particular, along with some of the growing pains that have attended progress, data that evidence uptake in education, impact on terminal degrees, and consequences both intended and unanticipated. They also foreshadow some speed bumps on the road ahead. There is much to celebrate here, and there is much that demands our curiosity and attention.

We can certainly celebrate that the number of terminal degree programs has mushroomed, that the number of graduates from these programs has moved the needle toward the goal to increase the number of nurses prepared with a terminal degree, that more young nurses are seeking to earn a doctorate, which promises more years of impact from their education and expertise, and that dissemination of the scholarly work of nurses is increasing in quality and quantity. These are accomplishments of which we can be proud.

An unflinching examination of progress demands attention.

First concern: The authors are unable to point to data that evidence improved outcomes on a scale that corresponds with the significant increase in the number of doctorally prepared nurses. The fault is not with the authors, but with the discipline and higher education that has yet failed to consistently support and demand advancement of the science and its application to practice in ways that deliver important and significant improvements.

Second concern: The number of DNPs in practice has not kept pace with the number of graduates because the majority of DNPs today are employed in nursing education. This is logical because expert clinicians can become expert educators who are so needed in our discipline. These DNPs inspire young nurses and can establish new paths for smooth entry into practice. This is fortunate for the students they prepare, and at the same time it is unfortunate for healthcare because the practice doctorate is so badly needed in the clinical arena.

Third concern: Situating entry to advanced practice at the doctoral level requires retooling of curricula for a different learner, a group characterized as bringing less practice and life experience to their program of study. Incremental change in curricula has not delivered on programs of study that prepare graduates for the practice environment they will enter. The reason the DNP was introduced was that science is expanding in scope and complexity, and education needs to keep pace. The curriculum needs to do a better job of keeping pace with today's healthcare delivery needs. Education needs to prepare lifelong learners who are masters in learning and applying all they learn in the service of their practice and the health of those they serve, regardless of the role. Today's learners and clinicians and educators must demonstrate their ability to sift through the morass of information available and select that which is trustworthy, accurate, and applicable to the challenges they and those they serve face. Residencies and internships proliferate to ease entry to practice. Our challenge is to ensure that our curricula in higher education are nimble and responsive to changes in market demands, deliver learning that builds competencies that matter, and prepare graduates who are knowledgeable, capable, confident, collaborative, safe, and embrace the need to be responsible for their own learning transition.

Fourth concern: There is good reason to lament that the growth in DNP programs has left PhD education behind in terms of the numbers of applicants and graduates. This is a reality that invites our unflinching gaze. The Robert Wood Johnson Foundation and the Bedford Falls Foundation have incentivized our discipline to find ways to accelerate the path to becoming a nurse scientist or nurse researcher.

CONCLUSIONS

I encourage us to:

- Fully release the MSN entry to advanced practice
- Fully embrace the post baccalaureate student aspiring to advanced practice and design for them
- Take a deep critical look at our programs
- Reimagine the graduates we prepare to assume the awesome responsibilities of managing increasingly complex health concerns, polypharmacy, mental health and other comorbidities, burgeoning diversity in society, aging, and the countless many other challenges graduates will encounter the day they enter their practice
- Push past the initial success we have achieved and press on to achieve the full potential of the DNP
- Remember the demands on our profession, the needs that informed the goals that led to the creation of the DNP, and make necessary course corrections so we can do better
- Reflect on the early critique of the DNP that anticipated some of the challenges we now face and recommit to mitigating those
- Embrace competency-based education described in the *New Essentials,* which forms the scaffold for brave and bold improvements in our curricula, operations, and practice
- Refresh the curriculum, pedagogy, simulation, and evaluation methods we employ to prepare nurses to practice at the top of their license

- Accept nothing less than practice-ready DNPs who have the demonstrated abilities to accomplish true transformation in healthcare and in health

In closing, I propose that if the past 10 years were the decade of the DNP and we now need to improve that curriculum and its outcomes, then the next 10 years can be the decade of the nursing PhD. This can be the decade in which we focus even more attention on those programs, those pedagogies, and the outcomes we achieve that form the foundation for all of our practice, education, and service.

CHAPTER TWENTY-FIVE

Today, Tomorrow, and the Future: What Are the Critical Issues Facing Doctoral Advanced Practice Nursing?

MARY ELLEN SMITH GLASGOW, DAVID CAMPBELL O'DELL, AND H. MICHAEL DREHER

INTRODUCTION: WHAT HAVE WE LEARNED SINCE THE DNP INCEPTION?

The DNP degree will confuse the public, patients, and other healthcare providers.
The DNP degree will just become an easy doctorate to earn.
The DNP degree really isn't a terminal nursing degree, the PhD is.
Where is the research that says the outcomes from master's-level advanced practice, indicates the need for doctoral-level advanced practice?

Many of these statements were made by seasoned academic nursing leaders in the early years of the evolution of the doctor of nursing degree (DNP), and some still persist. There was significant skepticism (and opposition) about the origins and need for the degree (Marecki, 2007; Meleis & Dracup, 2005). Some claimed the central argument for this new terminal degree would contribute to improving healthcare outcomes (Fain et al., 2008; Sperhac & Clinton, 2008). Others claimed the educational level of advanced practice nurses needed parity with other terminal healthcare practice professions (Partin, 2008; Upvall & Ptachcinski, 2007). The validity of these arguments were questioned and these questions remain; however, significant progress has been made and today the degree has become embedded in the educational preparation of nurses for advanced nursing practice and to advance the discipline, and in just less than 20 years.

The standardized model for the DNP was formally introduced in 2004 in a position statement by the American Association of Colleges of Nursing (AACN, 2004). Now, many years later, are we clear on the trajectory of those who have earned and are yet to earn the DNP degree? Is the academic preparation of the DNP truly yielding a return on investment not only for the individual earning the degree, but also for the nursing profession? Have the efforts of our DNP-prepared nursing colleagues produced the health outcomes and healthcare system improvements as expected? In the context of an always increasingly, complex healthcare system and declining health outcomes in the United

States where the average life expectancy in 2021 has dropped in the two previous consecutive years largely due to COVID-19 (Centers for Disease Control and Prevention, 2022), DNP graduates should be prepared to practice at the most advanced level of nursing by synthesizing, translating, and applying the most sophisticated evidence into clinical practice (Johansen, 2023; Root et al., 2018). Some suggest that once the number of DNP-prepared nurses reaches a certain threshold, nursing practice would shift much like a paradigm of thought and action. Have we encountered this shift as a result of the efforts of DNP colleagues? These and other concepts and challenges are explored in this chapter.

THE VISION FOR THE DNP DEGREE AND DNP-PREPARED NURSING COLLEAGUES

The basis of the DNP degree, as stated by the AACN in the early years of its development was to improve healthcare outcomes by applying research to practice (AACN, 2006). The translation of evidence into practice was the spirit and initial goal of this degree. This goal still remains but has shifted slightly depending on the DNP's academic preparation or employer's role and preferences. In a 2019 study, 59% of DNP-prepared nurses from key professional nursing organizations (American Academy of Nurse Practitioners, American Association of Nurse Executives, and American Association of Nurse Anesthetists) reported that the DNP was neither required or preferred by their current employers (Minnick et al., 2019). In a qualitative study conducted in 2019, 23 employers were unable to differentiate between the DNP and MSN-prepared advanced practice registered nurses' (APRNs') level of functioning, emphasizing the need for DNP-specific positions and job descriptions (Beeber et al., 2019). The DNP-prepared nurse today is expected to translate evidence into practice to improve healthcare outcomes. The degree model was prospectively developed, with additional competencies beyond the master's degree envisioned. In other words, all master's-prepared APRNs translate evidence in practice, but the DNP would expand this focus. This includes, but is not limited to changing practice process, improving quality processes, and collaborating to determine best practices for patients and healthcare service organizations. There is also a critical need for the DNP graduate to be grounded in innovation science and design-seeking methods to meet the challenges of the healthcare system (Holt et al., 2002; Root et al., 2018). Though these expectations are foundational, not all DNP academic programs ascribe to this goal as a requirement for graduation. Not all current DNP graduates see themselves in roles to improve healthcare outcomes, and employers hire DNP-prepared colleagues for reasons that may not be specific to improving health outcomes in practice settings. The DNP prepares nurses for clinical and nonclinical roles as they engage in professional activities ranging from direct patient care to clinical operations, systems operations and administration, informatics, and health policy. Given the relatively short history of the degree, many of these issues will continue to evolve. What we can acknowledge now is that DNP-prepared colleagues have a wide range of influence and are involved in all aspects of healthcare services, evidence-based practice, policy formation, technology growth and development, and contributions to academia.

CLINICAL DNP-PREPARED PRACTICE

In clinical realm of practice, the DNP is becoming the expected and preferred preparation for practice. Discussions that began in about 2010 around licensure, accreditation, certification, and education continue today. Recommendations on a deadline for the DNP to become the entry level for practice continue, and organizations continue to share perspectives and press for the urgency of DNP entry level. The initial goal set by the AACN in 2004 was for the DNP degree instead of the master's degree to be recognized as the entry level for advanced practice by 2015. This goal was missed. A summit organized by the National Organization of Nurse Practitioner Faculty (NONPF) in 2017 recommended the DNP degree as the entry level for advanced practice by 2025 (Idzik et al., 2021). The revised 2021 AACN Essentials framework includes competencies organized within 10 domains at two levels of nursing education: entry level and advanced level. An advantage of this approach is greater clarity and confirmation regarding the knowledge and skills of nursing school graduates (Giddens et al., 2022).

The Essentials: Core Competencies for Professional Nursing Education provides a framework for preparing individuals as members of the nursing discipline, reflecting expectations across the trajectory of nursing education and applied experience. *Competency-based education* is a process whereby students are held accountable for the mastery of competencies deemed critical for an area of study (AACN, 2021). *The Domains* constitute a descriptive framework for the practice of nursing. These Essentials include 10 domains that were tailored to reflect the discipline of nursing. The domains used in the Essentials are:

- Domain 1: Knowledge for Nursing Practice
- Domain 2: Person-Centered Care
- Domain 3: Population Health
- Domain 4: Scholarship for Nursing Discipline
- Domain 5: Quality and Safety
- Domain 6: Interprofessional Partnerships
- Domain 7: Systems-Based Practice
- Domain 8: Informatics and Healthcare Technologies
- Domain 9: Professionalism
- Domain 10: Personal, Professional, and Leadership Development

In addition to domains, there are featured *concepts* associated with professional nursing practice that are integrated within the Essentials. A concept is an organizing idea that represents important areas of knowledge. The concepts are Clinical Judgment; Communication; Compassionate Care; Diversity, Equity, and Inclusion; Ethics; Evidence-Based Practice; Health Policy; and Social Determinants of Health.

Competencies are organized within the domains, which are applicable across all areas of healthcare and across diverse patient populations. Concepts core to professional nursing practice are evident across the domains and competencies, reflecting broad application. Another key feature within the revised Essentials is a model that places all programs into one of two categories: entry-level and advanced-level nursing education. Level-1 entry-level programs will focus on preparing students for entry into professional nursing practice. Level-2 advanced-level programs will focus on the preparation of nurses for nursing practice in advanced nursing roles or advanced nursing specialties and thus includes requirements and competencies specific to the given specialty. These advanced-level subcompetencies complement and provide a foundation for the additional competencies required for achieving advanced role or advanced specialty practice. All DNP programs (postbaccalaureate and post-master's) demonstrate that graduates attain and integrate Level 2 subcompetencies and competencies for at least one advanced nursing practice specialty or advanced nursing practice role.

The Essentials celebrate the role of advanced practice nursing by stating that the DNP-prepared graduate is prepared to practice in a specialized role within the nursing discipline. This distinctive role is a hallmark of the DNP degree (AACN, 2021). However, some DNP programs enroll students without the education, training, or ability to practice in a designated advanced practice role. Though all roles are important, and every graduate has value in their abilities to contribute to the nursing discipline, not all DNP graduates are prepared for a clinical or executive or specialty role. For example, the DNP with an executive educational background will require progressive leadership experience before assuming a senior-level executive role. This creates confusion concerning what the DNP-prepared nurse can do and detracts from the expectations of what DNP graduates can contribute.

RESEARCH BY THE DNP-PREPARED PROFESSIONAL

The DNP graduate is expected to advance the discipline in a variety of scholarly ways. In preparation for the launch of the DNP degree there were attempts to rigidly distinguish the scholarship of the PhD (generate evidence) and DNP (translate evidence to practice; AACN, 2004). We and others say this artificial demarcation of the PhD and DNP student has actually limited the scientific development of our practice profession. As recently as 2021 at a national doctoral nursing education conference, there was still a robust debate on this issue. Some adamantly stated that DNP-prepared nurses do not perform research as that is the exclusive realm of PhD-prepared colleagues. It is still not uncommon for a DNP student in some academic programs to say, "We can't call it research." Others argued that research of discovery and translational research go hand-in-hand and that the DNP-prepared nursing professional has the education and position to build these research skills in the context of professional practice. Again, if the domain of DNP scholarship is applying or translating evidence into practice, according to Radzyminski (2023):

> This process has been termed translational science which has evolved into translational research. If, in fact, translational research is a recognized form of research methodology, and the DNP graduate is skilled in this form of research, then the DNP should be redefined as both a practice and research degree. (p. 1)

With declining enrollments in PhD in nursing programs since 2013 (AACN, 2022), and many of them not positioned with resources to generate clinical nursing science, we should consider a comparison with our physician colleagues who earn a parallel professional practice degree (MD or DO). The publication of their findings in respective medical journals is not diminished by not having a PhD degree. In this AACN report it is stated, "This downward trend [in PhD nursing program enrollment] over the last 8 years has created great concern among academic nursing leaders responsible for preparing future nurse scientists, educators, and leaders" (p. 1). While we agree not all DNP programs have the mission, institutional resources, and/or faculty available to mentor DNP students in advanced scholarly projects we do not see why the DNP degree, student, or graduate is not part of the discussion. This debate will no doubt continue, yet the shift to DNP-prepared nurses performing and participating in research of discovery and research of practice continues to grow in scope and sophistication.

LEADERSHIP AND HEALTHCARE MANAGEMENT BY THE DNP-PREPARED PROFESSIONAL

The original intent of the DNP degree was to enhance advanced practice preparation for clinical practice. Executive and leadership roles were later adopted with great success. The nurse executive is foundational to ensuring the voice and value of nursing are considered at an organizational level to create a culture of safety, quality, and equity, and to improve the health and well-being of those under their leadership. Despite time pressures and a myriad responsibilities, nurse executives are challenged at the same time to assess personal strengths and development opportunities to master the skills required to lead healthcare organizations into the future (Boston-Fleischhauer, 2020; Morse & Warshawsky, 2021). The number of DNP-prepared colleagues in leadership positions continues to grow to include DNP-prepared nurses in the C-suites of healthcare service organizations and systems. DNP-prepared colleagues serve on the boards of directors of various organizations. Leadership roles that impact organizations, systems, and municipalities are now realized.

DNP PROFESSIONALS IN ACADEMIA

One of the goals of developing more doctoral-prepared nurses is to favorably impact the number of nursing faculty, especially clinically relevant faculty. The number of DNP-prepared faculty in academia has grown over the past few years, with 60% of DNP graduates entering academia and an increase in DNP enrollments and decrease in PhD enrollments (AACN, 2020); however, one needs to ask if DNP-prepared faculty are meeting the original intent and vision of the DNP degree while engaged in teaching? One would argue that preparing the next generation of nurses and advanced practice nurses is integral to meeting the goals of the profession. The challenge of DNPs having the ability to achieve tenure is an ongoing discussion. For example, in a large academic health center that contains health-related schools such as nursing, medicine, pharmacy, and law, tenure tracks are generally not available to DNP-prepared faculty. Even though medicine, law, and pharmacy are professional degrees, only the DNP degree was omitted from serving in a tenure-track position and earning tenure. Issues of equity can be argued, yet the evolution of academia may impact the notion of tenure in the long-term. Clinical promotion tracks are also common in many academic institutions, an alternative path to tenure for clinical faculty. However, one needs to closely examine the academic rigor of DNP programs nationally and the scholarly output of DNP-prepared nurses. A primary concern has been the lack of rigor in both DNP education and scholarly projects (Dols et al., 2017; Terhaar et al., 2016). Are DNP-prepared nurses dissuaded from pursuing a tenure-track position because of deans' and senior faculties' lack of understanding of the DNP's scholarly focus on innovative value-based delivery models and health outcomes or lack of attention to academic rigor in scholarly projects and other scholarship? This debate is an area that requires further exploration. Are DNP-prepared faculty fully capable of teaching at the scope and depth of those PhD-prepared faculty with terminal degrees? The answer is a qualified yes; however, the courses taught by the DNP would be different and based on their academic preparation and clinical expertise. DNP-prepared faculty represent the practice of nursing and collectively offer knowledge and clinical expertise that non-advanced practice nurses do not possess. It is also important to note that the DNP and PhD designations have different strengths and are not interchangeable.

DNP EDUCATION: PREPARING DNP PROFESSIONALS FOR THE FUTURE?

DNP education under the guidance of the AACN, NONPF, and accrediting bodies are molding and shaping the future of education. However, are these entities successfully producing DNP-prepared professionals for practice, and what content may be deficient? With these considerations, are DNP-prepared graduates comparable in their knowledge and competencies irrespective of the academic program attended? Despite national accreditation standards, students from University A are many times not receiving the same content as those in University B. A troubling trend has been health systems selecting academic nursing programs from for-profit universities for nurses' education institution-wide (Buerhaus et al., 2014; Pittman et al., 2019). Research on nursing program outcomes showed a 14-fold increase in the number of graduates from for-profit programs between 2007 and 2016 (rising to 14.2% of total graduates in 2016), and yet, as an example, for-profit programs have the lowest pass rates on the NCLEX (68.1%, compared to 88.2% in public programs and 84.1% in nonprofit programs: Pittman et al., 2019). Data on national APRN certification exam pass rates were not available for for-profit universities. As we know, a strong foundation in research and associated fundamental course work is important for academic preparation for graduate school. Generally, graduates from for-profit universities are not exposed to scholarly or research-active faculty. As leaders, we should guide nurses to enroll in academic programs that prepare them to provide the best patient care and to generate or translate research, not the most cost-effective educational option (Smith Glasgow & Colbert, 2022). There is also a legitimate concern about the generation of knowledge from practice due to the wide variety in the quality and consistency of DNP programs across the United States. Growth has been rapid, with approximately 350 new DNP programs since 2005 (Root et al., 2018). The lack of consideration of academic rigor has a tacit impact on the abilities and reputation of DNP-prepared graduates.

Moreover, along with the inclusion of content, many DNP programs are not as academically rigorous as in the past in an effort to be competitive in recruitment efforts. When the DNP degree began, the average number of credit hours from MSN to DNP was over 70. Over time the number of overall credits dropped to under 50 credit hours, and later to close to 40 credit hours. BSN to DNP programs started at over 100 credit hours and now are closer to 70 hours—roughly the same as the amount of MSN to DNP credit hours in the early years of this degree. A DNP generalist degree is offered by some schools, whereas some programs offer only clinical tracks such as advanced practice roles. Diversity in educational offerings is appreciated, yet when exploring the future of DNP-prepared practice, are we able to identify the impact of DNP educational programs when there is significant variability of preparation for an advanced practice role?

As described above, the rigor of programs is variable in both hours and content. Accreditation has little impact on these programs as long as standards are met. What factors need to be considered when exploring academic rigor and content that influence the scope and depth of a DNP program? Before these ideas are explored, consider the quote attributed to Jim Jarmusch: "Fast, Cheap, and Good ... pick two. If it's fast and cheap it won't be good. If it's cheap and good it won't be fast. If it's fast and good it won't be cheap" (Waits, 2008). These words suggest the probable outcomes of DNP programs of different levels of content and number of hours. How does a DNP graduate of a program that requires no more than 24 credit hours for MSN to DNP that can be completed in less than 12 months compare to the skill set and capabilities of a graduate from a program that is 2 to 3 years (or more) in length requiring more than 55 credit hours? By all intents and purposes, these are two separate degrees that reflect the variability of

DNP education and practice that impacts practice and ultimately outcomes. McCauley and deans from top-ranked schools of nursing echoed the DNP's long history of inconsistency (McCauley et al., 2020).

As we explore the future of the DNP-prepared nurse and the impact this degree has on outcomes and practice, we must reflect more deeply on the preparation processes and attempt to identify systemic structural and external issues. A recent report from the AACN sheds light on the state of DNP education. Based on a 2-year study, the report contains data on national trends in DNP programs; insights from employers, graduates, and program administrators on the value and impact of DNP education; and recommendations for ongoing engagement with practice partners and certification organizations to support the DNP for entry into advanced practice nursing. Among its key findings: DNP graduates add unique value in areas such as evidence-based practice, organizational change, quality improvement, and leadership, but some employers are uncertain about their skill set and what roles they are prepared to assume (AACN, 2022). The diversity of academic rigor has been mentioned; yet, the cause of the inconsistent rigor may be more insidious and complex than expected. Consider this dichotomy: A state-run school or private not-for-profit academic institution typically has a geographic scope of influence. Though these schools may have an online presence, other school structures have maximized the delivery of curricula to offer services that may impact enrollment. For example, a listing of all available DNP programs is offered by Doctors of Nursing Practice, Inc. (2022). As of this writing there are 396 entries. There are 93 online only programs (23%). Hybrid curriculum delivery that includes both online and on-site modes are found in 141 programs (36%) as declared by the program leaders. On-site only programs are found in 13 programs (3%), again, as declared by the listing academic institutions.

Of the available programs listed in the University DNP Programs database housed on the Doctors of Nursing Practice, Inc. website, the number and percentages are displayed in the following table. It's important to note that the listing of this information is on a volunteer basis, at no charge to the institution, and is updated when the respective DNP program offers information for updates.

University DNP Program Characteristics from the Doctors of Nursing Practice, Inc. Database

Track Offered	Number	Percentage
Family Nurse Practitioner	154	39%
Adult/Geriatric Nurse Practitioner	77	19%
Pediatric &/or Neonatal Nurse Practitioner	45	11%
Acute Care &/or Emergency Nurse Practitioner	45	11%
Psychiatric Mental Health Nurse Practitioner	81	20%
Nurse Anesthetist (CRNA)	33	8%
Clinical Nurse Specialist	21	5%
Administration / Executive / Leadership	120	30%
Informatics	15	4%
Policy	10	3%

Source: Doctors of Nursing Practice (2022). American Association of Colleges of Nursing [AACN]. (2022b). *The research-focused doctoral program in nursing: Pathways to excellence.* https://www.aacnnursing.org/Portals/42/News/Position-Statements/Pathways-Excellence-Position-Statement.pdf

This database does not differentiate for-profit from not-for-profit academic institutions; however, the numbers of students per annual cohort tends to be higher in for-profits compared to non-profit schools, most likely due to decreased costs. For example, Chamberlain University declared about 180 students per annual cohort compared to a randomly selected program for comparison: Florida Atlantic University, with 50 students per annual cohort. Also, many healthcare organizations have agreements with for-profit in colleges and universities.

The above information suggests that enrollment in DNP programs is largest in Family Nurse Practitioner and Nursing Administration tracks, and that for-profit programs enroll and graduate larger numbers of students per annual cohort than nonprofit programs. Are programs that offer tracks outside of a specialty with fewer hours diluting the competence and reputation of DNP graduates?

DISGUISING THE FOCUS OF THE DNP DEGREE

As DNP programs develop, the focus on executive leadership and healthcare management has DNP graduates leading organizations more willing to promote change. Before continuing this discussion we must also acknowledge that there is a tremendous need for nurse educators, and there is a declared need for growing more nursing faculty. DNP-prepared faculty are clinically relevant and wellsuited to teach the next generation of nurses in a practice profession, thus improving health outcomes. The AACN does not endorse the nurse educator as an advanced practice specialty in contrast to the nurse executive. "The discipline of education encompasses an entirely separate body of knowledge and competence" (AACN, 2004, p. 13) and is not an area of advanced nursing practice. Rather, the AACN proposes a post-master's certificate in nursing education in addition to a program of study or additional electives in nursing education but this is not sufficient to adequately prepare nursing faculty for equally complex roles in the midst of a severe nursing faculty shortage. King et al. (2020) disagree with this approach, citing that 60% of 826 graduate nursing students surveyed reported concerns about the lack of curriculum and teaching-learning content in existing doctoral programs. The National League for Nursing (NLN) proposes a more inclusive collaborative approach for the DNP with respect to nursing faculty preparation (NLN, 2018). The AACN (2019) identified the importance of addressing potential faculty shortages as faculty age, noting in an earlier report that 31% of full-time nursing faculty were over 60 years of age (AACN, 2015). When we compare nursing executive leadership, informatics, health policy, and education roles and competencies, why is the nurse educator role excluded from the DNP as an accepted choice? To address this issue, some accredited academic programs have disguised the nurse educator DNP focus by using other terms such as DNP in educational leadership. This practice needs to be reevaluated.

A STEP BACK: REFLECTING ON THE SCIENTIFIC UNDERPINNINGS OF DNP EDUCATION

Scientific principles as described in the DNP Essentials, as originally described by the AACN in 2006, reflects the complexity of practice at the doctoral level in the context of a rich heritage of the conceptual foundation of nursing. An appreciation of nursing theory and a strong foundation in the natural and social sciences help to provide a foundation for the application of evidence to practice. The sciences provide a foundation for nursing practice that includes human biology, genomics, the science of therapeutics, psychosocial sciences, as well as the science of complex organizational structures. The description of the scientific underpinnings underscores the value of nursing conceptual frameworks in the paradigm of nursing with knowledge from ethics, biophysical, psychosocial, analytical, and organizational science as the basis for the highest level of nursing practice. The reader of this description will likely agree that the foundation of the scientific underpinnings draws from nursing science as a major underpinning for DNP education, which has decreased in emphasis (Yancey, 2015). This is likely the most significant threat to doctoral nursing education. As DNP-prepared practice may offer opportunities to impact systems and complex health dynamics, looking back at this first essential of doctoral education may reveal that we are not adequately preparing the DNP with the necessary foundation for practice. A few examples will help to illustrate this concern.

Consider a career progression for a DNP-prepared nurse practitioner in the field of stem cell therapies, or precision medicine. These foundations of practice are drawn from the sciences of biology, hematology, oncology, and genetics. Do DNP courses address the scientific underpinnings for advanced specialty practice? Another example to consider: An advanced practice nurse with a focus as a nurse executive has evolved into a role of a system-wide chief executive officer. Educational preparation may have included course content in organizational structure, behavior, and particular processes of human resource management and accounting, with scientific underpinnings that should be foundational to the DNP role evolution.

Questions are posed to challenge the scope and depth of DNP preparation. Are we (as a system of academic and practice leaders) adequately preparing our colleagues for contemporary scope and depth of practice? To better appreciate this approach, consider the work by Dr. Mark Risjord, a professor of philosophy at Emory University. His book, published in 2009, explored the philosophical foundations and evolution of nursing science and practice. The recommendations for the future of nursing practice from this thoughtful philosopher were surprising. Nursing has invested more than a century in the development of nursing science to differentiate and identify the uniqueness of the nursing profession. The recommendation of reintegration of nursing into other disciplines to strengthen our collective future is a paradigm that is not discussed or explored in most colleges of nursing (Risjord, 2009). Instead of identifying the unique qualities and contributions of nursing, perhaps it is time for nursing, and the DNP-prepared nurse, to demonstrate collective and collaborative efforts with medicine, pharmacology, sociology, psychology, biology, business management, organizational behavior, information technology, and political science to list a few.

Are the scientific underpinnings that we applaud and attempt to integrate into DNP curricula to assure the best graduate misaligned? Are there other scientific underpinnings that are valuable in building the foundation of DNP-prepared practice? These questions are raised to question the direction and future of the DNP-prepared nurse in practice. As the profession matures, and DNP-prepared colleagues need to rise to address the complexities of healthcare delivery, the foundations of practice need to be challenged and modified to meet future challenges.

HOW CAN DNP PREPARED NURSES BE MORE INFLUENTIAL?

The three main roles of DNP-prepared practice include practitioner, executive, and educator. Informatics specialist, policy developer, and researcher are elements that may be considered as subunits of practice, educator, and executive. Exploring these three areas of practice as we investigate ways to influence the nursing practice and the profession in the future is dependent not only on the DNP's capabilities but also on the state's scope of practice. In essence, to address fundamental changes needed in the U.S. healthcare delivery system, the DNP-prepared colleague must assume leadership. As an example to demonstrate two levels of influence, consider these two colleagues.

One DNP-prepared nurse practitioner takes on the role of chief nurse practitioner officer addressing the administrative needs of a large healthcare system, managing and promoting the utilization of nurse practitioners in that system. This role is equivalent to a medical director managing physicians. The difference speaks to the complementary, yet different role of nurse practitioner compared to a physician, yet the overlap shows that this role assures consistent communication, self-governance, and techniques to assure quality services are delivered and improved upon. Does this role afford the opportunity to increase influence? Most will agree that it does within that system and the collateral systems that influence the healthcare delivery of the practitioners under the leadership of the chief nurse practitioner officer.

Another example is a DNP nursing colleague with an interest and background in forensic nursing. She had a background in law enforcement and was an expert in her field. After graduation, she accepted a position in the U.S. Department of Justice to identify a growing number of sexual assaults occurring in a large metropolitan area on another continent. She used her DNP knowledge and competencies along with her forensic expertise to determine deficiencies in the law enforcement department in an urban area related to identifying and treating reported sexual assaults. Her contributions over time helped to significantly lower the rate of sexual assaults in the area while enhancing the skills and sensitivity of law enforcement agencies in this city. These DNP-prepared nurses offer a significant and sustainable impact on healthcare system outcomes.

Given the fundamental changes needed in the U.S. healthcare delivery system to improve quality care, how can DNPs in the three main nursing roles of practitioner, executive, and educator be more influential?

Nurse Practitioner Recommendations

For DNP-prepared nurse practitioners to substantively change the landscape of healthcare service delivery, full practice authority must be achieved. Working on a state-by-state level is not adequate in this effort as it leaves the scope of practice in a disparate situation where full practice authority cannot be realized unless condoned by a state board of nursing, leaving some but not all nurse practitioners without full practice authority. Additionally, as more nurse practitioners gain full practice authority, more will be able to be listed independently on insurance panels and provide comprehensive services according to the scope of education earned.

Nurse practitioners have a strong national voice in changing health policy and regulatory issues; yet, to make substantive and sustainable change, their voices must be more influential on public policy initiatives. The United States ranks 11 out of 11 comparable countries in access to care, administrative efficiency, equity, and healthcare outcomes (The Commonwealth Fund, 2022a). Clearly the current structures for healthcare delivery are not working adequately; yet, the United States has the most expensive healthcare system, with significant morbidities and a lower life expectancy. The United States has the highest suicide rates, highest chronic disease burden, and highest rate of obesity. To add to the challenge of policy initiatives, the United States has one of the lowest average number of physician visits per capita, and the lowest number of physicians per capita (The Commonwealth Fund, 2022b). Advanced practice nurses and those with doctoral preparation could impact many aspects of health policy. The opportunities are tremendous, and the challenges are equally immense.

One approach to addressing how nurse practitioners can impact the delivery of healthcare services in the United States is to emulate and enhance the current medical model that includes profit sharing in clinical practices. Though this may not be embraced by all, and this structure has not proven to impact improved health outcomes, it does achieve greater equity and influence practice, at the local and system levels.

One challenge for DNP-prepared nurses is that salaries for MSN-prepared nurse practitioners are not different than DNP-prepared practitioners. There is not a certification option to differentiate the for DNP-prepared versus MSN-prepared APRN. This salary discrepancy not only negatively impacts the perception of the caliber of services offered but negates the call to action to improve educational preparation for nurse practitioners. A DNP-prepared nurse practitioner has a wide scope of academic experiences that translate into service delivery in a more cost-effective and productive manner. A salary differential would underscore the value of the DNP-prepared nurse practitioner.

Finally, for the sake of this discussion, DNP-prepared nurse practitioners can influence the substance and sustainability of practice change when afforded time for scholarship. This is intrinsic to practice yet not always provided in many practices, or in larger healthcare systems. Time carved out on a weekly or monthly basis dedicated to practice scholarship will have a positive impact on healthcare services, outcomes, and long-range benefits for the healthcare system. Partnering with other doctoral-prepared nurses can demonstrate the connection between research of discovery and translational research of practice. Advocating for this opportunity rather than working in the industrial model of number of patients seen per hour (or per day) will support growth and innovation to improve practice.

Executive Recommendations

The doctoral-prepared nurse executive is poised to evaluate complex systems, determine strategic plans for change, and lead an organization into levels of sustainability and long-term success. Evaluating the depth and scope of a healthcare system and generating interventions that influence sustainable change can influence the culture of an organization consistent with its mission and vision. Organizations would be wise to refine job descriptions that reflect the expectations of DNP-prepared executive leadership. Job descriptions that address DNP competencies will assist in clarifying role confusion by employees and other stakeholders on the expectations of DNP-prepared nurse executives. Clarification of the role is essential to the newly hired DNP-prepared executive and stakeholders, including those in the C-suites and boards of directors/advisors of the organization. Universal buy-in will promote substantive change for the organization. Emphasizing the cost-effectiveness of the role of the DNP-prepared executive brings additional value to the organization.

Educator Recommendations

The DNP-prepared educator holds a unique position of translating evidence in clinical practice and serving as a role model to students. DNP preparation is intended to enhance healthcare outcomes. Many nursing faculty are divorced from clinical practice, which begs the question of their clinical skills and capabilities to educate the next generation of nurses. Nurses with current clinical skills are needed to adequately prepare nursing students for a complex clinical environment. One opportunity for DNP-prepared faculty to bridge education and practice are joint appointments. Nursing and medicine joint appointments are available in academic health centers promoting interdisciplinary practice. Joint appointments in nursing, psychology, physical therapy, social work, or pharmacy would also promote a culture of collaboration and collegiality that will positively impact students and graduates.

Employer Recommendations

To explore how DNP-prepared nurses may impact healthcare services in the future, the employer is a key stakeholder. In the United States, healthcare delivery has been shaped by the direction of employers who have determined mechanisms for payment and/or purchased employee health plans to address the healthcare needs of their employees and their families. As we compare healthcare outcomes and costs in the United States to other comparable countries, a large burden of financial responsibility, is addressed by the employer segment. The financial burden and the measurable lack of improved societal health outcomes is a call to action that change is needed.

Organizations like Kaiser Permanente, Cleveland Clinic, and the Uniformed Armed Services University, and others, have responded and implemented policies related to the integration of the DNP-prepared nurse into key roles and positions. In some states, the inclusion of an advanced practice nurse on an insurance panel is contingent on whether the advanced practice provider has a doctoral degree.

FINAL THOUGHTS

The essence of the DNP-prepared nurse is scholarship, expert practice, and leadership. Rigor and innovation are adjunctive and are required to transform healthcare delivery and improve outcomes. Academic programs preparing this generation of practice scholars must continuously examine the quality, rigor, and clinical relevance of the DNP academic program and scholarly projects. If we do not increase the consistency and academic quality of the DNP academic programs nationally, we have no one to blame except ourselves. The variability of academic quality needs to be evaluated and corrected if DNPs are to be universally respected. Nurse leaders in all settings (academia and practice settings) should bring attention to the need for DNP scholarly work dissemination (Root et al., 2018). Nurse executives and leaders will need to strongly advocate for scholarly time for DNPs in the practice setting to accomplish this goal. Healthcare is at a critical crossroads that requires DNP-prepared nurses to lead the transformation to advance healthcare quality and equity in a variety of practice settings and elevate the voices of nurses. Substantive changes need to be made. The cost to the student, university, and health systems need to be considered as we contemplate these changes. What will be the impact of increasing the length and cost of APRN educational preparation across the board in the United States? We are already seeing the impact of decreased available preceptors in APRN education post-COVID and requests for payment for preceptor services. Do we have the faculty and financial resources to implement this strategic goal during a severe nursing shortage or should we hit the pause button?

CRITICAL THINKING QUESTIONS

1. What core competencies differentiate the master's-prepared advanced practice nurse from the doctoral advanced practice nurse?
2. How will faculty implement a consistent, relevant DNP curriculum while meeting the needs of students with significant differences in clinical experience and proficiency?
3. How should DNP programs incorporate technology and knowledge management in their respective curricula?
4. Describe the role of the doctoral advanced nursing practice "clinical executive" of the future. What specific competencies does the doctoral advanced nursing practice clinical executive require?

5. How can a progressive doctoral-level nurse leader shape an institution through one's value system and passion for nursing?
6. Today, many nursing faculty are divorced from clinical practice. How can the doctoral advanced nursing practice "educator" change the current system and reconnect with the practice context of the nursing discipline?
7. What are the benefits and risks of the doctoral advanced nursing practice "educator" in academia? Please cite benefits and risks to the individual DNP educator and to the nursing profession as a whole.
8. Describe how the academy can develop the productive nurse scientist of the future with a decrease in PhD enrollment.
9. What effect will the transition to the entry-level doctorate for advanced practice and the dissolution of the master's degree have on the nursing profession? What is the impact of increasing the length and cost of APRN educational preparation?
10. What do you see as the role of the DNP-prepared nurse of the future?
11. Should doctoral nurse fellowships be instituted universally to address readiness to practice?

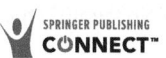

A robust set of instructor resources designed to supplement this text is located at http://connect.springerpub.com/content/book/978-0-8261-8137-4. Qualifying instructors may request access by emailing textbook@springerpub.com.

REFERENCES

American Association of Colleges of Nursing. (2004). *AACN position statement on the practice doctorate in nursing October 2004*. http://www.aacn.nche.edu/publications/position/DNPEssentials.pdf

American Association of Colleges of Nursing. (2006). *The essentials of doctoral education for advanced nursing practice*. http://www.aacn.nche.edu/DNP/pdf/Essentials.pdf

American Association of Colleges of Nursing. (2015). *The doctor of nursing practice: Current issues and clarifying recommendations*. Report from the Task Force on the Implementation of the DNP. https://www.aacnnursing.org/Portals/42/DNP/DNP-Implementation.pdf

American Association of Colleges of Nursing. (2019).*Vision for academic nursing white paper*. https://www.aacnnursing.org/Portals/42/News/White-Papers/Vision-Academic-Nursing.pdf

American Association of Colleges of Nursing. (2020). *The PhD pathway in nursing*. https://www.aacnnursing.org/Portals/42/news/surveys-data/PhD-Pathway.pdf

American Association of Colleges of Nursing. (2021). *The essentials: Core competencies for professional nursing education*. https://www.aacnnursing.org/Portals/42/AcademicNursing/pdf/Essentials-2021.pdf

AACN. (2022*). Nursing schools see enrollment increases in entry-level programs, signaling strong interest in nursing careers*. (aacnnursing.org)

Beeber, A. S., Palmer, C., Waldrop, J., & Lynn, M. R., & Jones, C. B. (2019). The role of doctor of nursing practice nurses in practice settings. *Nursing Outlook, 67*(4), 354–364. https://doi.org/10.1016/j.outlook.2019.02.006

Boston-Fleischhauer, C. (2020). Chief nurse executive readiness for the here and now. *JONA, 50*(6), 307–309. https://doi.org/10.1097/NNA.0000000000000889

Buerhaus, P. L., Auerbach, D. I., & Staiger, D. O. (2014). The rapid growth of graduates from associate, baccalaureate, and graduate programs in nursing. *Nursing Economics, 32*(6), 290–295. https://doi.org/10.1377/hlthaff.2019.00686

Doctors of Nursing Practice, Inc. (2022). *University DNP programs*. https://www.doctorsofnursingpractice.org/university-dnp-programs

Dols, J. D., Hernandez, C., & Miles, H. (2017). The DNP project: Quandaries for nursing scholars. *Nursing Outlook, 65*(1), 84–93. https://doi.org/10.1016/j.outlook.2016.07.009

Fain, J. A., Asselin, M., & McCurry, M. (2008). The DNP … Why now? *Nursing Management, 39*(7), 34–37.

Giddens, J., Douglas, J. P., & Conroy, S. (2022). The revised ASCN essentials: Implications for nursing regulation. *Journal of Nursing Regulation, 12*(4), 16–22. https://doi.org/10.1016/S2155-8256(22)00009-6

Holt, J. M., Talsma, A., Woehrle, L. M., Klingbeil, C., & Avdeev, I. (2022). Fostering innovation and design thinking graduate programs, *Nurse Education, 47*(6), 356–357. https://doi.org/10.1097/NNE.0000000000001206

Johansen, M. (2023). The value of a DNP degree. Nursing Management, *54*(1), 56. https://doi.org/10.1097/01.NUMA.0000905020.79954.e6

King, T. S., Melnyk, B. M., O'Brien, T., Bowles, W., Schubert, C., Fletcher, L., & Anderson, C. M. (2020). Doctoral degree preferences for nurse educators: Findings from a national study. *Nurse Educator, 44*(1), 144–149. https://doi.org/10.1097/NNE.0000000000000730

Idzik, S., Buchholz, S., Kelly-Weeder, S., Finnegan, L., & Bigley, M. B. (2021). Strategies to move entry-level nurse practitioner education to the doctor of nursing practice degree by 2025. *Nurse Educator, 46*(6), 336–341. https://doi.org/10.1097/NNE.0000000000001129

Marecki, M. (2007). Con: Is the Doctor of Nursing Practice (DNP) the appropriate doctoral degree for nurses? *American Journal of Maternal Child Nursing, 32*(3), 139. https://doi.org/0.1097/01.NMC.0000269560.89616.6b

McCauley, L., Broome, M. E., Frazier, L., Hayes, R., Kurth, A., Musil, C. M., Norman, L. Rideout, K. H., & Villarruel, A. (2020). Doctor of nursing practice (DNP) degree in the United States: Reflecting, readjusting, and getting back on track. *Nursing Outlook, 68*(4), 494–503. https://doi.org/10.1016/j.outlook.2020.03.008

Meleis, A., & Dracup, K. (2005). The case against the DNP: History, timing, substance, and marginalization. *Online Journal of Issues in Nursing, 10*(3), 3. www.nursingworld.org/MainMenuCategories/ANAMarketplace/ANAPeriodicals/OJIN/TableofContents/Volume102005/No3Sept05/tpc28_216026.aspx

Minnick, A.F., Kleinpell, R., & Allison, T. (2019). DNP labor participation, activities, and reports of degree contributions. *Nursing Outlook, 67*(1), 89–100. https://doi.org/10.1016/j.outlook.2018.10.008

Morse, V., & Warshawsky, N. E. (2021). Nurse leader competencies today and tomorrow. *Nursing Administration Quarterly, 45*(1), 65–70. https://doi.org/10.1097/NAQ.0000000000000453

National League for Nursing (2018). Headlines from the NLN: NLN releases a vision for doctoral faculty collaboration in nursing education. *Nursing Education Perspectives, 39*(5), 331–332. https://doi.org/10.1097/01.NEP.0000000000000392

Partin, B. (2008). Update on the DNP degree. *The Nurse Practitioner, 33*(3), 7. https://doi.org/10.1097/01.NPR.0000312992.70338.32

Pittman, P., Bass, E., Han, X., & Kurtzman, E. (2019). The growth and performance of nursing programs by ownership status. *Journal of Nursing Regulation, 9*(4), 5–21. https://doi.org/10.1016/S2155-8256(19)30011-0

Radzyminski, S. (2023). DNP: Research of not - That is the question. *Journal of Professional Nursing, 44*, 33–37. https://doi.org/10.1016/j.profnurs.2022.11.003

Risjord, M. (2009). *Nursing knowledge: Science, practice, and philosophy.* Wiley-Blackwell.

Root, L., Nunez, D.E., Velasquez, D., Malloch, K., & Porter-O'Grady, T. (2018). Advancing the rigor of DNP Projects for practice excellence, *Nurse Leader,* 261–265. https://doi.org/10.1016/j.mnl.2018.05.013

Smith Glasgow, M. E., & Colbert, A. M. (2022). Nursing's wicked problems – a path forward through transformative academic leadership and collaboration. *Nursing Administration Quarterly, 46*(4), 275–282.

Sperhac, A. M., & Clinton, P. (2008). Doctorate of nursing practice: Blueprint for excellence. *Journal of Pediatric Health Care, 22*(3), 146–151. https://doi.org/10.1016/j.pedhc.2007.12.015

Terhaar, M. F., & Sylvia, M. (2016). Scholarly work products of the doctor of nursing practice: One approach to evaluating scholarship, rigor, impact and quality. *Journal of Clinical Nursing, 25*(1–2), 163–174. https://doi.org/10.1111/jocn.13113

The Commonwealth Fund. (2022a). Mirror, Mirror 2021: Reflecting Poorly: Health Care in the U.S. Compared to Other High-Income Countries. https://www.commonwealthfund.org/publications/fund-reports/2021/aug/mirror-mirror-2021-reflecting-poorly

The Commonwealth Fund. (2022b). *U.S. health care from a global perspective, 2019: Higher spending, worse outcomes?* https://www.commonwealthfund.org/publications/fund-reports/2021/aug/mirror-mirror-2021-reflecting-poorly

Upvall, M. J., & Ptachcinski, R. J. (2007). The journey to the DNP program and beyond: What can we learn from pharmacy? *Journal of Professional Nursing, 23*(5), 316–321.

Waits, T. (2008, May 22). Tom Waits spills the beans to Tom Waits, Sound Effects Blog. *Boston Globe.* http://www.quotenik.com/tag/jim-jarmusch

Yancey, N. R. (2015). Teaching-learning processes: Why teach learning theory? *Nursing Science Quarterly, 28*(4), 274–278.

CHAPTER TWENTY-FIVE | Reflective Response 1

JANICE M. MILLER AND KATHY GRAY

RESEARCH BY THE DNP PREPARED PROFESSIONAL

Let's start at the beginning. Florence Nightingale was educated by her father, not in a formal university. Yet her inquisitive spirit led to data collection, changes in routines/processes, further data collection, and analysis (Nightingale, 1969). DNP education is not intended for a research-intense career. Yet any professional area of practice will have areas of shortcomings or inefficiencies where quality improvement is indicated. Such circumstances result in (and which we encourage) a spirit of inquiry that will fuel quality improvement.

Nurses select DNP programs of study intending to focus on practice-related concerns, rather than designing complicated research methodologies. A DNP does not prepare a professional for a rigorous research career yet prepares nurses to use some of the same tools to analyze effectiveness, efficiency, cost, beliefs, or experiences. An evaluation of 191 DNP projects (Turkson-Ocran et al., 2020) revealed six main themes: process improvement, clinician development, patient safety, patient outcome improvement, access to care, and workplace environment. Retrospective analyses, practice/process changes, and outcomes evaluation include many of the components of research. Does that mean it's not research?

Neal-Boylan (2020) discusses that nurses with PhDs conduct research, and that nurses with a DNP implement new treatment modalities and evaluate the outcome. Is implementing and evaluating outcomes research? Evaluating outcomes is pivotal to both research and quality improvement. Many lines are blurred, and most clinicians are less concerned with what type of degree a professional has than they are concerned with outcomes and the importance to healthcare. Have we experienced pushbacks when a PhD applies evidence to practice? Certainly not. It is welcome.

Academia is creating a problem where none exists. The nursing workforce shortage is a problem. The inability to afford life-saving medication is a problem. Whether or not a DNP's scope of work includes research is not a problem. Without oversimplifying or devaluing the important and rigorous training of PhDs, this is more of a discussion of turf and terminology. It's unfortunate that parties feel threatened, draw austere definitions, and waste energy. Florence Nightingale moved mountains as the earliest nurse researcher, and health and social advocate of our profession. And so can we.

HOW CAN DNP-PREPARED NURSES BE MORE INFLUENTIAL?

The authors describe practice, executive, and educator as the three main areas in which DNPS can be influential. They consider policy, research, and informatics as subunits of these. We disagree. If we continue in that mindset, we will never enlarge our footprint of influence. Everything stems from policy. Engagement in policy and informatics may have had their origins in practice, executive, and educator roles. Yet policy and Informatics can become main areas of influence themselves given the proper feeding and nurturing.

Influence involves systems thinking, identification of problems, stakeholders, their agendas, and the ripple effects of policy change. If these concepts are learned and nurtured in a doctoral program, they provide DNP-prepared clinicians and leaders with the confidence to establish connections, build coalitions, and leverage collective power.

Influence also results from DNP projects that focus on clinically based outcomes, evidence, and processes. Let's encourage scholarly projects in areas of policy and informatics, establishing our graduates as key opinion leaders. Everything stems from policy. Who better to influence health and social policy than the nurse? Who is better trusted than the nurse?

THE VISION FOR THE DNP DEGREE AND DNP-PREPARED NURSING COLLEAGUES

The statement that all master's-prepared APRNs translate evidence into practice and the DNP would expand this focus is true in part; however, it is much more than an expansion of the role of the master's-prepared nurse. APRNs at the master's level do not have a comprehensive toolbox required to effectively translate evidence into practice, they, they do not have mastery of the AACN DNP Essentials. (AACN, 2006). The focus of the master's degree is on developing the diagnostic, assessment, and planning skills required to practice in the different population foci, that is, the three Ps. APRNs at the master's level are typically not change agents who are able to evaluate and critique research, assess gaps, and develop process changes to improve patient outcomes. DNPs are systems thinkers who can translate the evidence, implement, and evaluate process changes on a micro and macro level to meet the Triple Aim of the Institute for Healthcare Improvement (IHI); to improve population outcomes, decrease cost, and improve patient outcomes. Systems thinking, change, population health, quality and safety, informatics, and health policy are crucial competencies required for the practice doctorate clinical scholar and executive leader.

In 2021, the AACN updated the Essentials in the publication: *The Essentials: Core Competencies for Professional Nursing*. In the report, 10 domains are listed, with expected competencies for entry-level nursing and advanced nursing levels. Competency-based education will provide consistency in graduate-level nursing education. The expectation of stakeholders will be that DNPs will have the knowledge and skills required to improve patient outcomes and meet the challenges of the 21st century in an already complex healthcare system. The competencies address diversity of practice settings and bridge the gap between education and practice. Our vision for advanced practice nursing is the DNP as the entry level to practice. The master's in nursing is no longer adequate to meet the challenges of the critical issues facing the healthcare system: artificial intelligence; data security; diversity, equity, and inclusion; post-COVID challenges; the healthcare consumer; population health; telehealth; and the shift from volume to value. "The world is now changing at a rate at which the basis systems, structures and cultures built over the past century cannot keep up with the demands being placed on them" (Kotter, 2014, p. 3).

LEADERSHIP AND HEALTHCARE MANAGEMENT BY THE DNP-PREPARED PROFESSIONAL

The doctorate-prepared nurse can provide direct or indirect patient care. Both roles are important in the healthcare system. Nursing leadership is needed more than ever since the pandemic has exposed the frailties of the healthcare system. Multiple changes, such as a shift from volume to value, telehealth, nursing shortages, diversity, equity, and inclusion, the aging population, increase in immigration, and artificial intelligence are imposing challenges on the healthcare system. Doctorate-prepared nurses in leadership roles are the catalysts to organizations' adoption of process improvements and an understanding of change theories such as those of Kotter and Lewin, the most applied theories according to a systematic review written by Harrison et al. (2021).

Innovation is the net result of systems thinking and the DNP in executive leadership, an indirect care role, has the tools to effect change based on sound research from randomized controlled trials and systematic reviews and all levels of research. We need strong nursing leaders prepared at the doctorate level who have the competencies and the tools to make organizational culture and process changes to meet these demands. The American Organization for Nursing Leadership (AONL) guides the development of nurse leaders. There are six leadership domains articulated by the AONL: communication and relationship building, leadership, knowledge of the healthcare environment, professionalism, business skills, and the leader within (Hughes et al., 2022). These leadership skills work in tandem with the domains and competencies of the AACN (2021) Essentials in preparing DNPs to transform healthcare in the 21st century.

DNP EDUCATION: PREPARING DNP PROFESSIONALS FOR THE FUTURE?

Smith et al. (2022) note that we should guide nurses to enroll in academic programs that are rigorous and not just the most cost-effective option. We agree with this statement and are concerned that there is no perceived consistency in the terminal nursing degree. We believe that all DNP programs should be accredited. Accreditation would ensure consistency and academic rigor. The 2021 AACN Essentials calls for a transition to competency-based education. In light of this transition, the number of credit hours do not need to be tightly regulated. The better question to pose is, Are DNP-prepared nurses meeting the competencies in clinical and executive roles that set them apart from the MSN-prepared nurse? If so, what are the competencies that set them apart and how can we articulate this to hospital administrators, legislators, and the public? Deans and other invested educators must educate the stakeholders regarding the value DNPs bring to the healthcare system. Where is the parity in salary and recognition with other professions prepared at the doctorate level? As a profession, we were remiss as educators and nursing leaders in our responsibility to the DNP-prepared nurse from the very onset of the practice doctorate endorsement by the AACN in 2006. Why are we still having this conversation in 2023, almost 20 years later? The goal of the revised Essentials is to provide consistency in preparing graduates from entry-level to advanced-level nursing practice. This consistency will provide stakeholders, hospital administrators, policymakers, and the public the assurance and confidence that DNPs are able to lead change and solve the complex problems facing society and the healthcare system of today.

NURSE PRACTITIONER RECOMMENDATIONS

The APRN in clinical practice should be included in the profit-sharing medical model. Physicians are paid based on relative value units (RVUs) from the yearly updated Centers for Medicare and Medicaid Services (CMS) fee schedule (2023). APRN services are billable and revenue producing. Too often their work is not recognized independently from their physician collaborator or assigned directly to the healthcare system. We believe there is an ethical issue to consider regarding this disparity. APRNs should meet with hospital administrators and legislators to voice these concerns. If the DNP were mandated as the entry to practice, APRNs would have parity with physicians and other healthcare providers who are prepared at the doctoral level. We believe that APRNs need to understand the current payment system and the revenue and value they bring into the organization. To date APRNs in 27 states plus the District of Columbia have full practice authority (AANP, 2022). When the DNP is required for practice entry, APRNs will have more influence and power to legislate for full practice authority in all states.

FINAL THOUGHTS: SHOULD WE HIT THE PAUSE BUTTON?

The authors conclude Chapter 25 by asking if we should hit the pause button concerning our goals to advance healthcare quality and equity and elevate the voice of the nurse. The answer is a resounding "NO."

There are several times when it may be reasonable to hit a pause button as one gathers information, strategizes, and builds partners. For example, the National Academy of Medicine (NAM) paused to release the *Future of Nursing 2020–2030* report. The release, intended to coincide with the Year of the Nurse was intentionally delayed as a result of COVID-19. Inequities that were long evident to those of us in healthcare were now at the forefront of discussions across the country. The NAM paused the release to leverage this opportunity of being in the public consciousness to refocus nursing's role (NAM, 2021).

But this is not such a time to push pause.

The authors recommend practices carve out time for DNP scholarly activity. Kesten et al. (2021) evaluated the activities in which DNPs engage routinely. They identified evaluating current evidence as the most frequently engaged in activity of DNPs. They further affirm the importance and value of ongoing practice scholarship. We agree. Momentum not capitalized upon devalues the DNP contribution to practice. Given the business- and metric-driven culture of practice, the DNP will need to make the case that such scholarly activity will benefit the practice or the revenue stream. DNP education prepares our students to create such discussion and buy-in. Persistently demonstrating relevance to the practice, service line, or organization will be crucial to carve out time. Procuring external financial support is another means to subsidize the DNP's salary to protect time for scholarly activity.

Nurses need doctoral education to develop skills to influence policy change and leadership, as well as the confidence to use these skills. Given the unprecedented, broad-based healthcare workforce shortage, the environment is ripe to look at policies and processes that can be updated and changed.

For example, full practice authority is expanding and under consideration after many states waived collaborative agreements during the pandemic. Physicians are retiring sooner than anticipated and we must take advantage of this time window.

Telehealth has tremendous advantages that improve access to care, and we wish it had been available when arranging and transporting a disabled parent to medical appointments. Patients now expect such convenience, and they expect payers to cover the visit. Further, we can't anticipate the next national or global events that will provide such opportunities. Thus, we must prepare DNP professionals, so they are equipped for rapid mobilization when the climate for change and progress emerges.

Each project in which DNP students engage improves a small slice of the healthcare pie. Each sector benefits from DNP project contribution to the knowledge base and the evidence. Who better knows the needs of the patient and the healthcare system than the nurse? What profession is more trusted than nursing?

Florence would agree with us: There is no time to pause.

REFERENCES

American Association of Colleges of Nursing. (2006). *The essentials of doctoral education for advanced nursing practice.* https://www.aacnnursing.org/essentials

American Association of Nurse Practitioners. (2022). *State practice environment.* https://www.aanp.org/advocacy/state/state-practice-environment

Centers for Medicare and Medicaid Services. (2022). Revisions to payment policies under the Medicare physician fee schedule quality payment program and other revisions to Part B for CY 2023. https://www.cms.gov/medicare/medicare-fee-service-payment/physicianfeesched/pfs-federal-regulation-notices/cms-1770-f

Harrison, R., Fischer, S., Walpola, R. L., Chauhan, A., Babalola, T., Mears, S., & Le-Dao, H. (2021). Where do models for change management, improvement and implementation meet? A systematic review of the applications of change management models in healthcare. *Journal of Healthcare Leadership, 13,* 85–108. https://doi.org/10.2147/JHL.S289176https://doi.org/10.2147/JHL.S289176

Hughes, R., Meadows, M. T., & Begley, R. (2022). AONL nurse leader competencies: Core competencies for nurse leadership. *Nurse Leader, 20*(5), 437–443. https://doi.org/10.1016/j.mnl.2022.08.005

Kesten, K., Moran, K., Beebe, S. L., Conrad, D., Burson, R., Corrigan, C., Manderscheid, A., & Pohl, E. (2021). Practice scholarship engagement as reported by nurses holding a doctor of nursing practice degree. *Journal of the American Association of Nurse Practitioners, 34*(2), 298–309. https://doi.org/10.1016/j.nurpra.2019.11.015

Kotter, J. (2014). *Accelerate: Building strategic agility for a faster-moving world.* Harvard Business Review Press.

National Academies of Science, Engineering and Medicine. (2021). *The future of nursing 2020–2030: Charting a path to achieve health equity.* The National Academies Press. https://doi.org/10.17226/25982

Neal-Boylan, L. (2020). PhD or DNP? That is the question. *Journal for Nurse Practitioners, 16*(2), A5–A6. https://doi.org/10.1016/j.nurpra.2019.11.015

Nightingale, F. (1969). *Notes on nursing.* Dover Publications.

Turkson-Ocran, R. N., Spaulding, E. M., Renda, S., Pandian, V., Rittler, H., Davidson, P. M., Nolan, M. T., & D'Aoust, R. (2020). A 10 year evaluation of projects in a doctor of nursing practice programme. *Journal of Clinical Nursing, 29*(21–22), 4090–4103. https://doi.org/10.1111/jocn.15435

CHAPTER TWENTY-FIVE Reflective Response 2

LORRAINE FRAZIER AND JUDY HONIG

TODAY, TOMORROW, AND THE FUTURE

While considerable progress has been made in embedding the doctor of nursing practice (DNP) degree in nursing education to advance nursing practice, variation in academic programs, faculty, and abilities of the graduates from varied degree programs causes confusion about the role among the public, patients, and other providers. Questions about the necessity of a doctorate when so many nurse practitioners (NPs) function effectively at the master's level still remain. The DNP, while not always a good return on investment for the individual nurse practitioner (who often makes the same pay as master's colleagues), is generally a good investment for the hiring institution, the patient population they care for, and the profession.

With poor health outcomes in the U.S. population a result of structural inefficiencies and inequities, DNPs should be in a position where they can oversee or influence healthcare service organizations at the institutional level. Until the DNP vision of effective application of translational science in patient care is evident by improved patient and healthcare outcomes, the DNP degree will not be preferred by the employer over the master's degree. As a result, DNP nurses will continue to function in positions where their education and experiential potential are not maximized, used, or valued. Although this may be due to inadequate job descriptions, the educational institution conferring the degree holds some accountability for preparing DNP graduates who function at the doctoral level. How many DNP programs prepare their graduates to design innovative models of delivering care or apply sophisticated and individualized use of evidence?

How can educators do a better job with this when faculty are not always experts in the area that they teach? One important strategy is to engage in faculty practice. DNP faculty must have a faculty practice and be expected to be clinical or practice scholars in the area of their teaching. Faculty who move between academia and practice convey a rich context to their students, so that DNP graduates are prepared for the realities of the complex healthcare roles and systems. In addition, engaging in practice is generative and seeds scholarship, innovation, uptake of evidence, and building evidence from practice data.

The variance in DNP programs, DNP nurses, and their jobs adds to the confusion regarding the degree, which has evolved from a clinical focus to emphasize nonclinical roles like leadership and health policy. The role of the DNP proficient in evidence-based care is fundamental to changing healthcare delivery in this country. Graduates who are not prepared to function at a DNP level not only lack the skills expected, they also lack the confidence to function at the doctoral level with their peers.

Perhaps there is a need to explore how many DNP graduates outside academia practice at a DNP level that reflects the vision of the degree.

The New Essentials will clarify the difference between entry-level and advanced-level nursing but does not distinguish between master's-level and DNP-level education. However, the New Essentials posit the expectation that all advanced-level competencies and subcompetencies are equally important and must be demonstrated—a one-size-fits-all model. No consideration is given to prioritizing, emphasizing, or weighing the importance of these capabilities depending upon the expected role of the graduate. While all the Essentials are important, some are clearly more critical than others for specific roles. (Examples are subcompetencies 1.2j Translate theories from nursing and other disciplines to practice and 4.3f Apply IRB guidelines throughout the scholarship process.) It is important that DNP graduates are competent to assume the role for which they are educated. Graduates prepared to assume clinical leadership may lack administrative experience and find it difficult to assume leadership at the executive level. This results in frustration on the part of the graduate, hiring institution, and colleagues who have experience.

Educational institutions vary in the inclusion of clinical or practice-based professionals for tenure. Most tenured professional degree holders at academic health science centers have programs of funded research. This may or may not include a practice role for the profession. The DNP must maintain a practice role to remain up to date in clinical practice. The DNP practitioner must be able to access and use evidence-based practice to provide appropriate care. An existing clinical practice helps ensure that the educator is teaching current practice guidelines and evidence. This practice focus of clinical faculty restricts them from engaging in the funded research necessary for achieving tenure.

Although DNP education does not prepare graduates for a funded research career that would provide a pathway to tenure in some institutions, scholarship for the DNP is critical for creating knowledge in clinical practice. DNP faculty have a responsibility to publish case studies and use of evidence-based research along with patient and population responses. They should also be able to apply the latest evidence when it is appropriate for their patients or population. Evidence-based practice is critical at the doctoral level and will ensure the confidence of the provider, patient, and institution.

Academia will need to revisit and broaden its perspective of nursing scholarship and give credibility to clinical scholarship. Boyer conceptualizes four overlapping and equally important areas of scholarship: discovery, integration, application, and teaching. Outcomes of clinical scholarship are derived from practice. Clinical scholars can contribute to knowledge in ways that fall outside traditional research methods and the academic status quo. The concept is not new and retains the rigor of scholarship: keen observation, analysis, interpretation, application, dissemination, and subject to peer review.

Clinical scholarship is a complex activity whose goal is the discovery, organization, analysis, synthesis, and transmission of knowledge resulting from client-oriented nursing practice. It is defined as that knowledge derived from the analysis and synthesis of observations of clients and families (Palmer, 1986).

Clinical scholarship is not the same as clinical research. While it starts with thoughtful patient observations, it leads to knowledge derived from a well-informed, perceptive, and clinically sound analysis (Diers, 1995).

Nursing scholarship is defined as those endeavors that methodically progress nursing education, research, and practice via in-depth investigation that is 1) noteworthy to the field, 2) innovative, 3) replicable, 4) expandable or replicable, and 5) amenable to diverse forms of peer review (AACN, 1999).

DNP EDUCATION: PREPARING DNP PROFESSIONALS FOR THE FUTURE

Perhaps the most important section of the chapter is the preparation of the future DNP. The New Essentials will drive programs toward a more intentional competency-based approach. The changing face of the DNP student also will impact the DNP degree and the influence of the graduates. The newly emerging DNP/NP candidate is a smart, BS-prepared nurse with limited and/or no nursing experience. The past reliance on service as a prerequisite is not realistic. The DNP curricula for this new generation of students will build on the RN competencies on a tabula rasa. In this new era, the student's education must be fully derived from their student experience in the DNP program. The post-BS DNP is the fastest growing DNP program and will be adding significant numbers of DNP NPs to the workforce.

Faculty who move seamlessly between the classroom and practice, exemplify the practice scholar, practice what they teach, and maintain a "practice lens" are crucial role models. Other fundamentals include creating a learning environment that fosters inclusion and interaction and maximizes knowledge and skill uptake; encourages reflective and evidence-based practice; offers an experiential immersion practicum where doctoral knowledge can be synthesized and applied; and considers a terminal project relevant to the role.

DISGUISING THE FOCUS OF THE DNP DEGREE

The DNP degree has evolved and as implemented is not a focused discipline-specific degree; programs vary greatly and often lack a distinct focus. A nurse with a DNP may be an advanced practice nurse, public health expert, nursing executive, or policymaker. This will continue to complicate DNP outcome studies. No metric can effectively capture the impact of nurses with DNP degrees across these broadly stated roles. In addition to multiple outcome roles, the rigor of DNP programs is unreliable and inconsistent, as mentioned, despite accreditation.

DNP programs need qualified doctorally prepared faculty who practice what they teach and who understand the principles of pedagogy specific to a practicing health professional. One strategy for DNPs opting to enter academia is to offer a series of elective courses for doctoral students who plan to combine their practice with teaching. Such targeted modules would establish a foundation for the DNP who pursues a faculty position. While education leadership may be a viable indirect nursing role, the content is distinct from principles of pedagogy. It is specious to rename education-focused DNP programs as DNPs in educational leadership for the purpose of accreditation.

HOW CAN DNP-PREPARED NURSES BE MORE INFLUENTIAL?

DNP graduates need to be pioneers and chart their course in practice by pushing boundaries and taking risks. Lifelong learning and scholarship must be an integrated thread in DNP programs. The newly minted DNP should be encouraged to think critically, problem solve- and disseminate (here is scholarship again). Because there is no overt distinction between an MS- or DNP-prepared NP, the DNP/NP should be encouraged to serve on committees that highlight their solid foundation in the context of care, including practice guidelines, evidence-based practice, and policy committees at the local, regional, national, and global levels.

REFERENCES

Diers, D. (1995). Clinical scholarship. *Journal of Professional Nursing*, *11*(1), 24–30. W. B. Saunders Company.

American Association of Colleges of Nursing. (1999). AACN position statement on defining scholarship in the discipline of nursing. *Journal of Professional Nursing*, *15*(6), 372–376. https://doi.org/10.1016/S8755-7223(99)80068-4

Palmer I. S. (1986). The emergence of clinical scholarship as a professional imperative. *Journal of Professional Nursing*, *2*(5), 318–325. https://doi.org/10.1016/s8755-7223(86)80032-1

Index

AACN. *See* American Association of Colleges of Nursing
abroad study program. *See also* Drexel DNP program's international study-abroad program; Duquesne University)
   international higher education, 434
   real-world experiences, 434
Academic Clinical Nurse Competencies, 216
academic coaching, 325
academic medical center (AMC), 202–203, 530–531
Academic Service Partnership Council (ASPC), 312
academic-service partnerships
   DNP essentials, 309
   DNP projects, 310
   education benefits, 310
   evidence-based practice (EBP), 318
   graduate nursing education (GNE) site, 311
   JH-JCN partnership, 317–319
   Minute Clinic practice sites, 311
   nurse-run clinics, 312
   practice experiences, 309
   practice partners, 310
   service benefits, 310
   university and rural hospitals, 311
   University of Pittsburgh Medical Center (UPMC), 312–314
Accreditation Commission on Education in Nursing (ACEN), 19, 179
Accreditation Commission for Midwifery Education (ACME), 110
ACEN, *See* Accreditation Commission on Education in Nursing
ACME. *See* Accreditation Commission for Midwifery Education
ACNM. *See* American College of Nurse-Midwives
"Acute Care Hospital at Home" waiver program, 421
administration roles
   Laura O'Rourke, 502–504
   Vanessa Battista, 499–501
administrative data, 275
advanced practice nursing roles
   clinical nurse specialists, 90–95
   DNP Essentials competencies, 389
   nurse anesthetist role, 85–87
   nurse-midwife role, 81–85
   nurse practitioner (NP), 87–90
advanced practice registered nurse (APRN), 534
   certified nurse midwife (CNM), 175–176
   certified registered nurse anesthetist, 178
   chronic illness management, 100
   clinical nurse specialist, 176–177
   communication styles, 97
   consensus model, 95–96, 413
   COVID-19 global pandemic, 184–186
   doctoral education value, 171–173
   education, 169–171
   evidence-based practice (*see* evidence-based practice)
   full practice authority, 414
   legislation, 173–174
   multistate licensure, 101
   nurse practitioner, 179–181
   opportunity for, 159
   practice outcomes, 97, 99
   prescription writing, 101
   regulation, 174
   role, 464
   services, 562
   uniqueness, 97
advancing research and clinical practice through close collaboration (ARCC) model, 148, 149
advocacy, 336
Affordable Care Act, 286, 292
Agency for Healthcare Research and Quality (AHRQ)
   Care Compare program, 480
   quality indicators (QI), 479–480
   quality indicators toolkit, 480–482

AHRQ. *See* Agency for Healthcare Research and Quality
alternate payment methods (APMs), 406–407
AMC. *See* academic medical center
AMCB. *See* American Midwifery Certification Board
American Association of Colleges of Nursing (AACN)
  AACN Position Statement, 512, 513
  2015 AACN report, 517
  active DNP programs, 513
  advanced practice registered nurses, 524, 526–527
  competency-based education, 478, 510
  coronavirus pandemic, 509–510
  DNP degree, 512
  DNP education, 510–511
  2006 DNP Essentials, 514–516
  domains, 474–475, 547
  history, 511–512
  PHD nursing education, 524–526
  Vision for Academic Nursing (2019), 517
2021 American Association of Colleges of Nursing (AACN) New essentials
  AACN 2015 White Paper, 534–536
  case study, 532–533
  competency-based education (CBE), 518–521
  conceptual clarity, 533–534
  concerns, 542–543
  contextualizing competencies, 522, 523
  domains and concepts, 518
American Association of Colleges of Nursing (AACN), 4, 170, 215
  advanced nursing practice, 189–190
  clinical executive, 187–188
  2004 position statement, 317
American Association of Critical-Care Nurses (AACCN), 408
American College of Nurse-Midwives (ACNM), 4, 83, 109
American Indian and Alaskan Native (AIAN) people, healthcare disparities, 425
American Medical Association (AMA), 5
American Midwifery Certification Board (AMCB), 110
American Nurses Association (ANA), 408
American Organization of Nurse Executives/Leaders (AONE/AONL), 561
  key questions, 191–192
  leadership competencies, 191
  MSN program reduction, 192
  Professional Practice Policy Committee, 191
anesthesia care team (ACT), 86
AONE/AONL. *See* American Organization of Nurse Executives/Leaders
applied statistician
  accuracy, 275–276

administrative data, 275
Bayes, 276
context, 274
data analysis, 270–273
data quality and bias, 274–275
data wrangling, 276–277
DNP Essentials, 282–283
employment of, 263
errors, 265–267
measurement, 267–269
p-value, 264–265
replication crisis, 273–274
research data, 275
risk, 276
sample size and accuracy, 269–270
validity, 269
APRN. *See* advanced practice registered nurse
ARCC model. *See* advancing research and clinical practice through close collaboration model
artificial intelligence (AI), 275
assessment, negotiation
  community, 368–369
  compensation possibilities, 369
  evaluation, 371
  implementation, 371
  language and attitude, 371
  negotiator, 369–370
  plan, 370
  practicing, 370
  self, 367–368
autonomy, 78

Bayesian analysis, 276
Bayesian theory of evidence, 125
BLS. *See* U.S. Bureau of Labor Statistics
Bologna process, 38
bundled payment, 407

Care Compare program, 480
carefronting, 326–327
CARES Act. *See* Coronavirus Aid, Recovery, and Economic Security Act
cause-and-effect diagram, 485, 494
CBE. *See* competency-based education
CCL. *See* Center for Creative Leadership
Center for Creative Leadership (CCL), 325
Center for Right Relationships (CRR) Global, 350, 351
Centers for Medicare and Medicaid (CMS) Innovation Center (CMMI), 471
Centers for Medicare and Medicaid Services (CMS), 406, 421
certified midwife (CM) credential, 109–110
certified nurse midwife (CNM)
  certification, 176
  credentials, 109–110

degree requirements, 175–176
midwifery programs, 175
specialty areas, 176
certified professional midwife (CPM), 85, 109–110
certified registered nurse anesthetist (CRNA), 5, 178
   anesthesia care team (ACT), 86
   certification, 86
   Mayo Clinic training program, 85
   military, 86
   practice guidelines, 86–87
   risk-adjusted mortality rates, 87
   salary benefits negotiation, 378
change theories, 157
chief nursing executives, 210–211
Children's Health Insurance Program (CHIP), 290
chronic disease management, 431
classical test theory (CTT), 267, 269
clinical DNP-prepared practice, 546–548
clinical inquiry process, 150
clinical nurse executive
   AACN report, 188
   Amanda Green, 200
   American Organization of Nurse Executives/Leaders, 190–192
   Barbara Wadsworth, 198–199
   Cecilia Page, 201
   COVID-19 pandemic, 187
   DNP program preparation, 192–193, 209–210
   DNP vs. other degree options, 195–197
   education, 210
   educational preparation, 197–198
   future aspects, 211
   healthcare settings, 188–189
   Kim Blanton, 200
   leadership case study, 202–206
   Lisa Thornsberry, 201
   Patty Hughes, 200
   practica experiences, 193–195
   responsibility, 188
   role of, 209
   Tukea Talbert, 199–200
clinical nurse specialist (CNS), 176–177, 375
   acute care, 375–376
   articulation, 376–377
   home health care, 375
clinical research, 527–529
clinical research nurses (CRN), 529
clinical scholar
   dissemination process, 234–237
   future aspects, 238–239
   inequity, 243
   PhD-prepared nurse research scholar, 242
clinical scholarship, 565
   action research oriented, 234
   components, 230–231
   definition, 229–230
   dissemination, 245
   elements, 230
   evidence-based practice, 231–234
   mentorship, 245
   new knowledge generation, 230
   translational practice knowledge, 245
CNM. *See* certified nurse-midwife
CNS. *See* clinical nurse specialist
COA. *See* Council on Accreditation
coaching approach
   business context, 323
   career transition, 326
   carefronting, 326–327
   conversation planning, 334–337
   data collection, 327–328
   emotional intelligence, 331
   executive, 325–326
   feedback, 328
   GROW framework, 327–328
   illustrative development plan, 329
   individual and organizational alignment, 332
   learning, 332
   political acumen, 332–334
   psychology and change management, 330
   sports linkage, 323–324
Columbia DrNP degree model, 21
Commission for Nursing Education Accreditation (CNEA), 218
communication
   collaboration, 394
   trust building strategy, 365–366
Community-Based Nurse Midwifery Program (CNEP), 84
community outreach, 432
competency, 518
competency-based education (CBE), 189, 297, 418, 547
   benefits, 522, 523
   broad sense, 519
   curriculum, 519
   elements, 518, 519
   historical background, 519–521
   narrow sense, 519
   pedagogical approach, 510
   pedagogy, 518–519
   self-assessment, 521–522
   self-directed learning approach, 522
   vs. Traditional Model of Nursing Education, 520
compromise, 350
confidentiality, 251
conflict resolution, 326
conservatism, 130
consultation, 325
contemporary nursing leadership, 67

content knowledge, negotiation, 356
contrary organizational dynamics, 350
conversation planning
  case study, 341
  cognitive biases, 335
  diversity, equity, and inclusion (DEI), 335–337
  ladder of Inference, 335, 336
  leadership presence, 337
  positioning, 334
  strategy sessions, 335
Copernicus's heliocentric model, 132
Coronavirus Aid, Recovery, and Economic Security (CARES) Act, 420
Corrective Action Plan, 491
Council on Accreditation (COA), 24
COVID-19 pandemic
  clinical practice changes, 419–420
  contingent labor, 423
  DNP nurse skills, 417–418, 431–432
  emergency preparedness, 426
  ethical triage, 427–428
  healthcare disparities, 425–426
  healthcare system initiatives, 418–419
  interventions, 423–424
  moral distress, 424
  moral injury, 425
  new care delivery models, 420–422
  postpandemic era, 426–427
  racial/ethnic health disparities, 389
  redeployment training, 423
  staffing, 422
CPMs. *See* certified professional midwife
credentialing group, 325–326
CRNA. *See* certified registered nurse anesthetist
CTT. *See* classical test theory
Culture of Health Initiative, 406
curriculum development, 519

data analysis
  Ascombe's quartet, 271–273
  chi-square results, 271
  convenience samples, 271
  design, 270
  effect sizes, 271
  frequency data error, 271
  homogeneity problems, 271
  overlapping distributions, 271, 272
  research question, 270
  residual analyses, 273
  sample size, 271
data wrangling, 276–277
DBA. *See* doctor of business administration
DEI. *See* diversity, equity, and inclusion
dental barriers, SDOH, 292–293
discrimination, 296
diversity, equity, and inclusion (DEI), 335–337
DNP. *See* Doctor of Nursing Practice

doctoral advanced practice nurse (DAPN), 52
doctoral nursing education
  doctoral-prepared nurse, 11–15
  history, 7–10
  nursing evolution, 10–11
  in United States, 10
doctorate of physical therapy (DPT), 4
doctor of business administration (DBA), 6
doctor of education (EdD), 6–7, 10
doctor of nursing (ND)
  Case Western Reserve University, 19–20
  post-master's model, 20
doctor of nursing practice (DNP) degree
  2004 AACN position statement, 22–23
  clinical doctorate, 21
  differentiation, 6–7
  Kentucky DNP model, 21–22
  positive outcomes, 32–34
  2022 program enrollment data, 24
  research issues, 25–31
  unresolved issues, 35–36
  U.S. Bureau of Labor Statistics (BLS), 23
  vision for, 546, 560
doctor of nursing practice (DNP)-prepared professional
  academia, 549
  accreditation, 550, 561
  forensic nursing, 554
  future DNP preparation, 566
  influencing factors, 559–560, 566
  leadership and healthcare management, 549, 561
  nurse practitioner, 554–556
  preparation processes, 551
  research by, 548, 559
  scientific underpinnings, 552–553
  University DNP Program Characteristics, 551
  vision for, 560
doctor of nursing practice (DNP) role
  AACN report, 53
  ANA's position statement, 53, 54
  BSN-prepared nurses, 54
  doctoral advanced practice nurse, 52
  global studies experiences (*see* Drexel DNP program's international study-abroad program; Duquesne University)
  minimum data set (MDS), 53
  practice-focused doctoral programs, 52
  profession, 55–66
  quality improvement (*see* quality improvement and patient safety)
doctor of occupational therapy (DOT), 27
doctor of philosophy (PhD)
  alternative nursing doctorate, 8
  health policy and advocacy, 401–402
  history, 7
doctor of psychology degree (PsyD), 8–9
doctor of social work (DSW), 4

doctoral advanced nursing practice
  applied statistician (*see* applied statistician)
  coaching approach (*see* coaching approach)
  decision making, law and ethics, 260–261. (*see also* law vs. morality)
  interdisciplinary/interprofessional collaboration, 390–399
  negotiation skills (see negotiation skills)
DOT. *See* doctor of occupational therapy
Drexel DNP-in-Dublin program
  case-based approach, 440
  doctoral student perspective, 441–442
  Irish women's history tour, 441
  medical walking tour, 440
  study experience, 440
  Trinity College School of Nursing and Midwifery, 440–441
Drexel DNP program's international study-abroad program, 443–444
  Drexel DNP-in-Dublin program, 438–442
  Drexel DNP-in-London Program, 438–439
  forward-thinking doctoral nursing faculty, 434
  funding, 436–438
  mandatory two-week intensive program, 435, 442
  short-term study-abroad program, 435
  undergraduate level, 435
Drexel DrNP program, 3, 25–26
Duquesne DNP-in-Italy global immersion opportunity
  activities and excursions, 446
  cultural activities, 446–447
  doctoral students' perspectives, 448–450
  global immersion experience, 446
  immersion activities, 447
  learning outcomes, 448
  prayer service, 447
Duquesne DNP-in-Singapore opportunity
  doctoral students' perspectives, 451–453
  International Council of Nurses (ICN) Congress, 450–451
  Transcultural Care and Global Health Perspectives, 451
Duquesne University, 194
  DNP Nurse Executive Curriculum, 194
  Duquesne DNP-in-Italy global immersion opportunity, 446–450
  Duquesne DNP-in-Singapore opportunity, 450–453
  global immersion experience, 453–454
  global-studies proposal, 445
  mission, 444
  Rome campus, 445
  school relationship, 444
  Transcultural and Global Health Perspectives, 445
dyad leadership model, 420

EBM. *See* evidence-based medicine
EBP. *See* evidence-based practice
EBQI. *See* evidence-based quality improvement
EC. *See* executive coaching
economic instability, 305
economic stability, 288–291
education models, 308
electronic health records (EHR), 470
electronic medical record (EMR), 407
emergency preparedness, 426
emotional intelligence (EQ), 331
empathy, 304–305
employer-based commercial health plans, 404
enterostomal therapist (ET), 374–375
entrustable professional activities (EPAs), 474
Essentials of Doctoral Education for Advanced Nursing Practice, 393
ethics, 260, 531
evidence
  classic theories, 121–125
  fingerprint, 125
  good evidence, 130–132
  inductive reasoning, 127–130
  knowledge, 125–127
  levels, 35
  logic of, 127
  quality, 139–141
  types, 35
  VAERS system, 133
evidence-based interventions, 476
evidence-based medicine (EBM)
  criticisms, 135
  evidence hierarchy, 135
  proponents, 135
  terminology, 133–134
evidence-based practice, 34
evidence-based practice (EBP), 391
  benefits, 144–146
  clinical scholarship, 231–234
  competencies, 158
  culture, 154–159
  definition, 153
  dissemination, 235–237
  DNP students and clinician's preparation, 166
  vs. evidence-based medicine, 133–135
  evolution, 151–154
  funding, 148
  healthcare system performance rankings, 144
  implementation science, 153
  language, 153–154
  models, 148
  organizational readiness, 155
  research and quality improvement, 151–152
  shared mental model, 155–156
  spirit of inquiry, 165
evidence-based quality improvement (EBQI), 145, 146, 149–150

executive coaching (EC), 325–326
    influencing without authority, 340
    leadership athleticism, 346–347
    leadership team, 338–340
    nonverbal communication, 337
    nursing or healthcare experience, 338–339
    readiness, 338
external coach, 326

faculty, 308
faculty development, 472
failure modes and effects analysis (FMEA), 486–487
fair play argument, 254
family nurse practitioner (FNP), 413
    Courtney Hicks, 379–381
    informal mentorship, 387
    leadership opportunities, 387
    Mary Grace Renfrow, 381–383
    Mary Marasa Radcliff, 383–386
    student education, 388
Federal Trade Commission (FTC), 90
financial health, 288–291
Fisher-based analyses, 276
flowcharts, 486
FMEA. *See* failure modes and effects analysis
forensic nursing, 554
forward-thinking communities, 288
"Four Horsemen of the Apocalypse" Behaviors, 359
free rider, 254
full practice authority (FPA), 414
funded programmatic studies, 140

gender differences, negotiation strategies, 352–354
geocentric theory, 132
geocentrism, 132
global study programs
    Drexel University (*see* Drexel DNP program's international study-abroad program)
    Duquesne University (*see* Duquesne University)
    international programs, 459–460
good theory of evidence, 121–122

healthcare costs, 405
healthcare disparities, 425–426
health-care improvement, 469
health education and promotion, 431
health equity issues
    DNP education and preparation, 296–297
    domains, 297–298
    empathy, 304–305
    social determinants of health (*see* social determinants of health)
    social justice, 304–305
    social processes and values, 305
health information technology, 476
Health Information Technology for Economic and Clinical Health Act of 2009, 470
health insurance, 404
Health Insurance Portability and Accountability Act (HIPAA) of 1996, 252
health literacy, 288
health policy and advocacy
    competence, 407–409
    credentialing process, 414
    DNP degree, 403–404
    healthcare costs, 405
    health insurance access, 404–405
    local/institutional level, 414
    organization, 409
    population health, 405–406
    practice doctorates evolution, 401–403
    quality of care, 406–407
    state level, 414
Healthy People 2030, 295
Healthy People initiative, 285–286
Hill-Burton Act, 68
2023 Hospital National Patient Safety Goals, 488–490, 489–490
HRO principles, 395–396
hybrid degree, 27–28
hypothetico-deductivism, 124

IHI. *See* Institute of Healthcare Improvement
implementation science, 153
inadequate insurance coverage, health-care, 292
Indiana University Nursing History, 8
inductive inferential techniques, 122–123
inductive reasoning
    color of swans, 128
    counterinstance, 130
    empirical evidence, 128–130
    falsificationism, 129
    generalization, 127
    logical positivists, 128
    probabilistic inferences, 129
    scientific hypothesis, 129
information, negotiation, 357
informed consent, 533
inquiry, 336
Institute of Healthcare Improvement (IHI), 480
    cause-and-effect diagram, 485
    failure modes and effects analysis, 486–487
    flowcharts, 486
    Model for Improvement, 483
    Open School, 483
    patient safety, 484–485
    profound knowledge, 483
    quality improvement, 483–484
    reliable patient care process, 486
    rules of causation statements, 487–488

5 Why's, 486
institutionalized medicine, 11
interdisciplinary/interprofessional collaboration
   academia, 392–394
   clinical practice, 394–395
   COVID-19 pandemic, 399
   DNP education, 390–391
   DNP graduates, 390
   leadership, 395–397
   partnerships for care, 399
   scholarship, 391–392
internal coach, 326
international nurse recruitment
   academic medical center (AMC), 202–203
   challenges, 203
   questions to consider, 203–204
   strategies, 204
   understaffing, 202
interprofessional collaborative practice, 535
Irish Healthcare System, 440
IRT. *See* item response theory
item response theory (IRT), 269

Jefferson Health-Jefferson College of Nursing (JH-JCN) partnership, 317–319
John Wooden's Pyramid of Success, 324
Joint Commission for Accreditation of Healthcare Organizations (JCAHO), 488
justice, 260

Kentucky DNP model, 21–22

ladder of inference, 335, 336
law vs. morality
   confidentiality, 251
   enforcement, 252
   internal moral states, 252
   lawbreakers, 254–255
   mens rea principle, 252
   Mill's harm principle, 250
   moral obligation, 256
   moral principles, 253
   normative dominance, 255–256
   objective morality, 257
   procedural nature, 253
   professional ethics, 251
   public and private sphere, 251
   social ethics, 251
   theories, 253–254
   violation, 260
leadership
   competencies, 322
   interdisciplinary/interprofessional collaboration, 395–397
   interventions, coaching, 326
"Lean In" movement, 353
listening technique, trust building strategy, 366

master of science in nursing (MSN), 403
Master's Family Nurse Practitioner (FNP) program, 13
Master's of social work (MSW), 4
MEAC. *See* Midwifery Education Accreditation Council
measurement error, 267
Medical Executive Committee, 414
medical-legal partnerships (MLP), 305
Medicare, 292
mens rea principle, 252
mentoring, 325
mentors
   mentorship, 466, 467
   types, 462
mentorship, 325
   clinical scholarship, 245
   nurse educator shortage, 224–225
Merit-Based Incentive Payment System (MIPS), 90
metamemory, 138
miasma theory, 132
midwifery, 372–373
Midwifery Education Accreditation Council (MEAC), 109
midwifery education program accreditation, 109
moral distress, 424
moral injury, 425
MSN-prepared nursing faculty, 17
MSW. *See* master's of social work
Myers-Briggs Type Indicator (MBTI), 328

NACNEP. *See* National Advisory Council on Nurse Education and Practice
National Advisory Council on Nurse Education and Practice (NACNEP), 13
National Association of Clinical Nurse Specialists (NACNS), 24–25
National Council of State Boards of Nursing (NCSBN), 89, 352, 217
National Institute of Nursing Research (NINR), 14
National League for Nursing (NLN), 216–217, 552
National Organization of Nurse Practitioner Faculty (NONPF), 13, 214–215, 297, 473, 547
National Organization of Public Health Nurses (NOPHN), 64
natural law theory, 253–254, 260
NCSBN. *See* National Council of State Boards of Nursing
negotiation skills
   assessment, 367–371
   barriers, 358–360
   collaborative relations, 349
   conflicts, 349–350
   definition, 350

negotiation skills (*cont.*)
  DNP role in, 350–352
  elements for, 357–358
  executive leadership position, 339–340
  gender differences, 350, 352–354
  human resources, 352
  midwifery, 372–373
  negotiators mistakes, 360
  organizational culture, 350
  political and symbolic frames, 352
  rank and privilege, 354–355
  steps in, 358
  strategic view, 350–351
  systems theory, 351–352
  tactical view, 355–358
  traits, 356–357
  trust building strategy, 365–366
neighborhood and built environment, 294–295
Nightingale nursing model, 62–63
NINR. *See* National Institute of Nursing Research
NLN. *See* National League of Nursing
non-normal distribution, 266
NONPF. *See* National Organization of Nurse Practitioner Faculties
nonverbal communication, 337
NOPHN. *See* National Organization of Public Health Nurses
Novice Academic Nurse Educator Competencies, 217
NP. *See* nurse practitioner
nurse educator
  diversity, 225–226
  qualifications, 217–218
  resiliency and self-care, 226
  undergraduate students, 221–222
nurse educator shortage
  baccalaureate colleges/universities, 213–214
  COVID-19 pandemic, 223
  data, 213
  mentorship model, 224–225
  nursing faculty, 224–225
  qualified nursing faculty needs, 214
  regulatory agencies, 214–217
nurse-midwife, 109
  educational programs, 83–84
  formal educational program, 81
  maternal-child needs assessment, 82
  natural childbirth methods, 83
  West African tribal folklore, 81
Nurse Practice Development Unit, 460
nurse practitioner (NP)
  accreditation, 179
  certifications, 180–181
  consensus model for APRN regulation, 89–90
  COVID-19 pandemic, 179
  degree requirements, 180
  disciplinary underpinnings, 97, 98
  educator recommendations, 555
  employer recommendations, 556
  executive recommendations, 555
  federal funding, 88–89
  formal practice, 88
  healthcare services, 88
  health-care service delivery, 554
  pediatric care providers, 88
  regulatory changes, medical education, 89
  role and population, 179
  salary discrepancy, 555
Nurse-Scientist Graduate Training Grants Program, 9
Nurse Training Act (NTA), 68
nursing informatics (NI), 535
nursing scholarship, 565

objective morality, 257
occupational therapy (OT) service, 293
Office of Quality and Patient Safety (OQPS), 490
organizational culture, 350

paraphrasing, trust building strategy, 366
patient confidentiality, 249
Patient Protection and Affordable Care Act (ACA), 100, 151, 404
Patient Safety and Accountable Care Act (ACA), 470–471
PCC. *See* positive psychology coaching
pedagogy, 518–519
pediatric palliative care (PPC), 500
pediatric psych/mental health practitioner (PMHPNP), 146
personal integrity, negotiation, 356
pharmacy doctorate (PharmD), 4
PhD. *See* doctor of philosophy (PhD)
physical therapy (PT) service, 293
PICO(T) question, 154, 166
Plan-Do-Study-Act (PDSA) cycle, 484
PMHPNP. *See* pediatric psych/mental health practitioner
policy development, 432
population distribution, 265
population health, 405–406, 535
positive psychology coaching (PCC), 326
positivism, 254, 260
poverty and economic instability, 289
power, 334, 356–357
PPC. *See* pediatric palliative care
practice doctorate, 9
practice-focused doctoral programs, 277
practice knowledge, 29
practice knowledge generation, 31
practice mentor, 462
practice/research-oriented doctorate, 27
preceptee expectations, 463
preceptors
  case exemplar, 461–462

clinical, 464
    expectations, 463
preceptorship, 462, 467
Professional classification for nurse, 66–69
professional ethics, 251, 252
professional identity, 322
    COVID-19 pandemic, 322
    domains, 321
    health professions' literature, 322
    leadership development programs, 322–323
    professional practice, 322
professionalizers, 5
professional nurse roles
    early classical professions, 56
    emergence, 61–63
    Melosh's definition, 56
    new DNP graduates, 57
    public health nurses, 63–66
    recognized professionalism of nursing, 66–69
    sociological schools of thought, 58–61
profound knowledge, 483
psychiatric-mental health nursing, 9
public health nurse, 66
    generalist role, 66
    knowledge and skills, 63
    post–World War II advancements, 68–69
    privately funded voluntary agencies, 65
    public health initiatives, 64
    social activism, 64
p-value, 264–265, 282

Quality and Safety Education for Nurses (QSEN) project, 479
quality improvement and patient safety, 149, 477
    Agency for Healthcare Research and Quality (AHRQ), 479–482
    Annual Culture of Safety Surveys, 497
    DNP Program Progress, 473
    DNP role competencies, 475–476
    educational strategies and tools, 476, 478
    health-care improvement, 469
    health professional education, 470
    Institute of Healthcare Improvement (IHI), 483–488
    The Joint Commission (TJC), 488–491
    nursing's leadership role, 471–472
    project, 391–392
    Quality and Safety Education for Nurses project, 479
    21st century DNP education, 472–473
quality indicators (QI), 479–480
QualityNet, 480
quality of care, 406–407

RCA. *See* root cause analysis
reflection, 336
regulatory practice boards, 322

relative value units (RvUs)-based compensation, 369
reliable patient care process, 486
research, 147–148
research data, 275
research-focused nursing doctorate, 27
resiliency, nurse educator, 226
responsible practitioner, 249
Re-visioning PhD Education Project, 401–402
Robert Wood Johnson Foundation (RWJF), 402
role-taking, 61
root cause analysis (RCA), 484–485

sampling error, 267
scholarship, 277. *See also* clinical scholarship
scientific evidence, 138–139
scientific inquiry model, 29, 30
scientific rigor, 139
SDOH. *See* social determinants of health
Sentinel Event (SE) policy
    comprehensive systematic analysis, 491
    Corrective Action Plan, 491
    definition, 490
    The Joint Commission, 491
    review timeline, 490
    root cause analysis process and tools, 493–495
SE policy. *See* Sentinel Event policy
settlement house movement, 64
social activism, 64
social cohesion, 296
social determinants of health (SDOH)
    Affordable Care Act, 286
    determinants, 285–286
    economic stability, 288–291
    education, 287–288
    Future of Nursing 2030 report, 286
    health and healthcare barriers, 291–294
    Healthy People 2030, 285–286
    inequities, 286
    issues, 287
    neighborhood and built environment, 294–295
    screening tools, 287
    social and community context, 295–296
social ethics, 251
social interactions, professional roles
    DNP role themes, 59–60
    doctorally prepared advanced practice nurse, 59
    functionalist view, 58
    role-taking, 61
    symbolic interactionist view, 59
social justice, 304–305
sociological schools of thought, 58–61
structural-functional theory, 58
successful career advancement roles
    academic role, Jessica Peters, 501–502, 506

successful career advancement roles (*cont.*)
  administration roles, Laura O'Rourke, 502–504, 506
  administration roles, Vanessa Battista, 499–501, 506
  Benner's model, 505, 507
systems thinking approach, 390
system-wide organizational EBP models, 156–157

technology-enabled care delivery, 420–422
telehealth, 407, 421, 432
The Joint Commission (TJC)
  accreditation standards, 488
  mission, 488
  patient safety, 489
  Sentinel Events (SE), 489–491
time needs, negotiation, 357
TJC. *See* The Joint Commission
traditionalists, 5
Transcultural Care and Global Health Perspectives, 451
transdisciplinary research programs, 529
translational research, 37–38
transportation barrier, SDOH, 293
Tri-Council for Nursing, 408

University of Pittsburgh Medical Center (UPMC), 308
  Academic Service Partnership Council (ASPC), 312
  standardization, 313
  student feedback surveys, 314
UPMC. *See* University of Pittsburgh Medical Center
U.S. Bureau of Labor Statistics (BLS), 23, 176
USPHS. *See* U.S. Public Health Service
U.S. Public Health Service (USPHS), 64

Vaccine Adverse Event Reporting System (VAERS), 133
VAERS. *See* Vaccine Adverse Event Reporting System
validity, 269
verbal ability, negotiation, 356
Veterans Administration (VA) medical centers, 407
virtual care models, 432
vision care, 292

Well-Being Initiative, 424
Work Progress Administration (WPA), 67
WPA. *See* Work Progress Administration